Analgesia and Anesthesia for the Ill or Injured Dog and Cat

Analgesia and Anesthesia for the Ill or Injured Dog and Cat

Karol A. Mathews
Guelph
ON, CA

Melissa Sinclair
Guelph
ON, CA

Andrea M. Steele
Guelph
ON, CA

Tamara Grubb
Uniontown
WA, USA

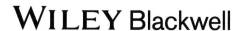

The right of Karol A. Mathews, Melissa Sinclair, Andrea M. Steele and Tamara Grubb to be identified as the authors
of this work has been asserted in accordance with law.

Registered Office
John Wiley & Sons, Inc., 111 River Street, Hoboken, NJ 07030, USA

Editorial Office
111 River Street, Hoboken, NJ 07030, USA

For details of our global editorial offices, customer services, and more information about Wiley products visit us at
www.wiley.com.

Wiley also publishes its books in a variety of electronic formats and by print-on-demand. Some content that appears
in standard print versions of this book may not be available in other formats.

Library of Congress Cataloging-in-Publication Data

Names: Mathews, Karol A., editor. | Sinclair, Melissa, editor. | Steele, Andrea M., editor. |
    Grubb, Tamara, editor.
Title: Analgesia and anesthesia for the ill or injured dog and cat / Karol A. Mathews, Melissa Sinclair,
    Andrea M. Steele, Tamara Grubb.
Description: Hoboken, NJ: Wiley, [2018] | Includes bibliographical references and index. |
Identifiers: LCCN 2017033962 (print) | LCCN 2017036345 (ebook) | ISBN 9781119036517 (pdf) |
    ISBN 9781119036456 (epub) | ISBN 9781119036562 (pbk.)
Subjects: LCSH: Veterinary anesthesia. | Analgesia. | Pain–Treatment. | Dogs–Diseases. |
    Cats–Diseases. | MESH: Analgesia–veterinary | Anesthesia–veterinary | Pain Management–veterinary |
    Dogs–injuries | Cats–injuries
Classification: LCC SF914 (ebook) | LCC SF914 .A49 2018 (print) | NLM SF 914 | DDC 636.089/796–dc23
LC record available at https://lccn.loc.gov/2017033962

Cover Design: Wiley
Cover Image: Photo credit – Karol A. Mathews

Set in 10/12pt Warnock by SPi Global, Pondicherry, India

10   9   8   7   6   5   4   3   2   1

Contents

List of Contributors   *viii*
Preface   *ix*
Acknowledgements   *x*

1   General Considerations for Pain Management upon Initial Presentation and during Hospital Stay   *1*
Karol Mathews

2   Physiology and Pathophysiology of Pain   *8*
Tamara Grubb

3   Physiologic and Pharmacologic Applications to Manage Neuropathic Pain   *17*
Karol Mathews

4   Physiology and Pharmacology: Clinical Application to Abdominal and Pelvic Visceral Pain   *51*
Karol Mathews

5   Physiology and Management of Cancer Pain   *64*
Karol Mathews and Michelle Oblak

6   Movement-Evoked and Breakthrough Pain   *68*
Karol Mathews

7   Pain: Understanding It   *70*
Karol Mathews

8   Recognition, Assessment and Treatment of Pain in Dogs and Cat   *81*
Karol Mathews

9   Pharmacologic and Clinical Application of Sedatives   *112*
Melissa Sinclair

10 Pharmacologic and Clinical Application of Opioid Analgesics   *119*
Melissa Sinclair

11 Pharmacologic and Clinical Application of Non-Steroidal Anti-Inflammatory Analgesics   *134*
Karol Mathews

12 **Pharmacologic and Clinical Principles of Adjunct Analgesia** *144*
Karol Mathews and Tamara Grubb

13 **Pharmacologic and Clinical Application of General Anesthetics** *165*
Melissa Sinclair

14 **Local Anesthetic Techniques** *171*
Alexander Valverde

15 **Integrative Techniques for Pain Management** *204*
Cornelia Mosley and Shauna Cantwell

16 **The Veterinary Technician/Nurse's Role in Pain Management** *217*
Andrea Steele

17 **Optimal Nursing Care for the Management of Pain** *219*
Andrea Steele

18 **Preparation and Delivery of Analgesics** *230*
Andrea Steele

19 **Cardiovascular Disease as a Co-Morbidity for Anesthesia and Analgesia
of Non-Related Emergencies** *244*
Tamara Grubb

20 **Kidney Disease as a Co-Morbidity for Anesthesia and Analgesia of Non-Related
Emergencies** *255*
Melissa Sinclair

21 **Liver Disease as a Co-Morbidity for Anesthesia and Analgesia of Non-Related
Emergencies** *263*
Melissa Sinclair

22 **Managing the Aggressive Patient** *270*
Andrea Steele and Tamara Grubb

23 **Analgesia and Anesthesia for Pregnant Cats and Dogs** *279*
Karol Mathews and Melissa Sinclair

24 **Analgesia and Anesthesia for Nursing Cats and Dogs** *294*
Karol Mathews, Tamara Grubb, Melissa Sinclair and Andrea Steele

25 **Physiologic and Pharmacologic Application of Analgesia and Anesthesia
for the Pediatric Patient** *308*
Karol Mathews, Tamara Grubb and Andrea Steele

26 **Analgesia and Anesthesia for the Geriatric Patient** *328*
Karol Mathews, Melissa Sinclair, Andrea Steele and Tamara Grubb

27   **Analgesia and Anesthesia for Head and Neck Injuries or Illness**   *336*
Karol Mathews, Melissa Sinclair, Andrea Steele and Tamara Grubb

28   **Torso, Thorax and Thoracic Cavity: Illness and Injury**   *356*
Karol Mathews, Tamara Grubb and Andrea Steele

29   **Torso and Abdomen: Illness and Injuries**   *375*
Karol Mathews, Tamara Grubb and Andrea Steele

30   **Pelvic Cavity/Abdomen, Perineum and Torso: Illness and Injuries Urogenital System and Perineum**   *391*
Karol Mathews, Tamara Grubb and Andrea Steele

31   **Musculoskeletal Injuries and Illness**   *409*
Karol Mathews, Melissa Sinclair, Andrea Steele and Tamara Grubb

32   **Vertebral Column (Vertebrae and Spinal Cord)**   *423*
Karol Mathews, Tamara Grubb and Andrea Steele

33   **Integument Injuries and Illness**   *439*
Karol Mathews, Tamara Grubb and Andrea Steele

34   **Environmental Injuries**   *454*
Karol Mathews, Tamara Grubb and Andrea Steele

     Index   *465*

List of Contributors

Shauna Cantwell, DVM, MVSc, Dipl.ACVAA, CVA, CVSMT/CAVCA, CTN
Medicine Wheel Veterinary Services, Inc.
Ocala, FL, USA

Tamara Grubb, DVM, PhD, DACVAA
Associate Clinical Professor, Anesthesia & Analgesia
College of Veterinary Medicine
Washington State University
Pullman, Washington, USA

Karol A. Mathews, DVM, DVSc, DACVECC
Professor Emerita, Department of Clinical Studies
Emergency & Critical Care, Health Sciences Centre
Ontario Veterinary College, University of Guelph
Guelph, Ontario, Canada

Cornelia Mosley, Dr.med.vet., Dipl.ACVAA, CVA
Anesthesia and Integrative Pain Management
VCA Canada, 404 Veterinary Emergency and Referral Hospital
Newmarket, Ontario, Canada

Michelle Oblak, DVM, DVSc, DACVS, ACVS
Fellow of Surgical Oncology
Assistant Professor, Department of Clinical Studies
Institute for Comparative Cancer Investigation
Ontario Veterinary College, University of Guelph
Guelph, Ontario, Canada

Melissa Sinclair, DVM, DVSc, DACVAA
Associate Professor, Department of Clinical Studies
Anethesiology, Health Sciences Centre,
Ontario Veterinary College, University of Guelph
Guelph, Ontario, Canada

Andrea M. Steele, MSc, RVT, VTS(ECC)
ICU Technician
Emergency & Critical Care, Health Sciences Centre
Ontario Veterinary College, University of Guelph
Guelph, Ontario, Canada

Alexander Valverde, DVM, DVSc, DACVAA
Associate Professor, Department of Clinical Studies
Anesthesiology, Health Sciences Centre,
Ontario Veterinary College, University of Guelph
Guelph, Ontario, Canada

Preface

All injured, and many ill, patients are in pain, but deciding on how painful the patient is, and the best pain management strategy for many, can be challenging. General considerations for pain management upon presentation are detailed and, as many patients will require anesthesia to manage their problem or to facilitate further diagnostics, basic information gathering is also outlined. Selecting an appropriate, safe analgesic and anesthetic regimen can be difficult, compounded by the anatomical location involved and associated co-morbidities. This book addresses these concerns, detailing pharmacologic and physiologic mechanisms applicable to groups (pregnant, nursing, pediatric, geriatric) and etiologies of pain. In addition to a step-by-step approach through various scenarios based on anatomical location of illness or injury, the veterinary technician/nurse's role in managing these patients, and the methods of analgesic delivery, are detailed.

Acknowledgements

While the authors have years of experience managing ill or injured cats and dogs, specific details of a colleague's practice, or publications, were sought and shared. For their contribution, we would like to thank: Drs. Alexa Bersenas, Alice Defarges, Robin Downing, Mark Epstein, Steve Escobar, Bernard Hansen, Fiona James, Mark Papich, Bruno Pypendop, Marc Raffe, Margie Scherk, Kelly St. Denis, Bob Stein and Bonnie Wright.

As a target audience test, we would like to thank Dr. Felicia Uriarte, McLean House Call Veterinary Services, Barrie, Ontario, Canada for reviewing the approach to the scenarios.

We would like to thank Dr. Kathrine Lamey, Metro Animal Emergency Clinic, Dartmouth, Nova Scotia, Canada, for contributing photographs of patients presenting to her clinic. These are included in many scenarios to illustrate some of the injuries our patients' experience, and to highlight the degree of pain experienced.

For pharmaceutical assistance and researching details of usage, global availability, approval of veterinary analgesics and government controls, we would like to thank Heather Kidston, RPh, FSVHP, Pharmacy Manager, Ontario Veterinary College Health Sciences Centre, University of Guelph, Guelph, Ontario, Canada. We would also like to thank Greg Soon BSc(Pharm), Pharmacist – ICU, Peterborough Civic Hospital, Ontario, Canada for his assistance in contributing publications and specific details on human-only-approved analgesics used in various scenarios in this book.

Where specific information is not available in the veterinary literature, we would like to thank Lorne Porayko MD, FRCP(C), CIM Consultant in Critical Care Medicine & Anaesthesiology, Victoria, BC, Canada, for sharing the information available for humans, and his experiences with some aspects, which are incorporated for human comparison into the various topics.

1

General Considerations for Pain Management upon Initial Presentation and during Hospital Stay

Karol Mathews

The quest for relief from pain is pursued in human medicine because its existence is known since the patient can verbalize their pain: what it feels like, where it is and the relief they feel when treatment is appropriate. As we all have experienced pain of various degree and duration, it is an excellent topic for comparison and understanding with our veterinary patients. As veterinary patients cannot tell us how painful they are, we as veterinarians and veterinary technicians/nurses have to understand what can cause pain and how pain manifests itself, which is discussed throughout this book, and how best to treat it.

Upon presentation immediate and appropriate treatment for the presenting problem should begin. Managing these problems frequently relieves some of the pain experienced (e.g. cooling a burn). The analgesic procedures are included in the scenarios; however, for definitive management of the presenting problem, the reader is referred elsewhere. Initial management is also based on inclusion/exclusion of pre-existing problems, medications and when the patient was last fed. An additional factor is the aggressive nature of the patient and how to deal with that (Chapter 22). Frequently, patients require diagnostic imaging and some may require surgical management. Specific analgesic/anesthetic protocols will be required for each circumstance. Preparation for intubation and assisted ventilation is essential. As cardiac arrhythmias may occur within 12–24 h (if not already present) following trauma, continuous ECG monitoring must be included in the ongoing patient assessment.

While management procedures contribute to a reduction in the pain experienced, analgesics are an essential component of case care in the urgent and emergent trauma, and for many critically ill, patients. Some degree of inflammation is present in these patients and is associated with great energy expenditure, the demands for which frequently cannot be met. The addition of pain, a great utilizer of energy, can contribute to associated morbidity, especially in the more seriously affected patients. In addition to the pain experienced by the primary problem, there is an additive effect of pain due to placement/presence of IV, urinary, thoracic, abdominal catheters and drains. Many undergo frequent manipulations and procedures that contribute to the overall pain experienced. Prior to analgesic and anesthetic selection, the pharmacologic aspects and contraindications for the various agents must be considered due to the fragile organ function of many of our ill or injured patients. Refer to the pharmacology and clinical application of sedatives (Chapter 9), opioids (Chapter 10), non-steroidal anti-inflammatory analgesics (Chapter 11), adjunct analgesia (Chapter 12) and anesthetics (Chapter 13). As pain is an individual experience associated with specific situations, general dosing of analgesics may not be appropriate. Refer to Chapter 8 for analgesic dosing suggestions for various levels of pain and the individual scenario chapters.

Analgesia and Anesthesia for the Ill or Injured Dog and Cat, First Edition. Karol A. Mathews, Melissa Sinclair, Andrea M. Steele and Tamara Grubb.
© 2018 John Wiley & Sons, Inc. Published 2018 by John Wiley & Sons, Inc.

A common misconception is that analgesics mask physiological indicators of patient deterioration (e.g. tachycardia in response to hypotension) and are, therefore, withheld. Evidence to support that analgesics *do not* mask signs of patient deterioration is reported in both the human and veterinary literature [1]. In fact, improved outcomes of well-managed pain in trauma patients is reported [2]. Our clinical observations show that when opioids are administered as a slow push or as a continuous rate infusion to treat pain an appropriate heart rate in response to hypotension, hypoxia, hypovolemia or hypercarbia still occurs. As tachycardia frequently occurs in the painful patient, treating the pain and eliminating this component as a cause for tachycardia, the persistence or recurrence of increased heart rate alerts the clinician to potential patient deterioration. If appropriate analgesia is not administered, tachycardia may be assumed to be pain and not patient deterioration. It is essential to obtain intravenous (IV) access, collect blood for laboratory evaluation and commence fluids while initiating opioid analgesia. Where hemorrhage or other hypovolemic states may exist, the severity of intravascular volume loss may be masked by the pain-induced "artificial" blood pressure (BP) reading. With administration of an analgesic, the pain-induced sympathetic response is reduced, allowing the BP reading to reflect the true intravascular volume. Heart rate will still reflect volume loss. Studies confirm that opioids do not result in a deterioration in hemodynamics when administered to dogs with 30% blood loss. Should BP drop below normal during opioid administration, this reflects that hypovolemia and fluid administration should be increased to that required for the patient. Where blood loss is identified, continuous monitoring of BP and laboratory evaluation is essential to identify the patient requiring a blood transfusion. The biochemistry results will identify organ dysfunction and will assist with selection of an analgesic protocol—and an anesthetic protocol should this be required.

Another concern expressed by many veterinarians is the potential for adverse reactions associated with analgesic drug administration, especially so for cats. However, current evidence, based on many studies investigating the efficacy and tolerability of analgesics of several drug classes, indicates that adverse effects are minimal when used appropriately [3]. This applies to both cats and dogs [4]. Adverse effects, primarily those associated with opioid use, such as respiratory depression, are extrapolated from humans and are over-emphasized in dogs and cats. In thirty years of practice in the critical care setting, this author has witnessed only two such incidences, both associated with fentanyl patch application in very small dogs. With respect to ventilation, opioid administration after a traumatic incident frequently improves ventilation rather than impairs it. This has been confirmed by arterial blood gas assessment by the author. Based on the physiologic abnormalities present in the ill or injured cat and dog, selection, dosing and method of administration of analgesics require careful consideration to ensure efficacy without the potential for adverse effects. As an example, non-steroidal anti-inflammatory analgesics (NSAIAs) should never be administered to any ill or injured patient upon presentation (Chapter 11). The administration of NSAIAs in the emergent patient should be withheld until the volume, cardiovascular, liver and kidney status of the patient is determined to be within normal limits and there is no potential for deterioration, such as ongoing or occult hemorrhage. Human patients with severe or poorly controlled asthma, or other moderate to severe pulmonary disease, may deteriorate with **cyclooxygenase 1 (COX-1) selective NSAIA** administration [5]. It is not known whether this may occur in cats and dogs; however, as bronchodilator physiology is similar across species, this may still be a concern. As asthmatic patients receive glucocorticoid therapy, NSAIA would be contraindicated. COX-1 selective NSAIAs are not recommended for any patient scenario included in this book.

Concerns for opioid immunosuppressive effects, and subsequent infection, have been reported in the human literature. Based on the author's experience working with critically ill patients all receiving opioids, infections potentially associated with opioid use were not identified. However, as the immunosuppressive potential of some opioids, especially morphine, was raised [6], a two-month prospective study was carried out at the author's institution, including all patients (ICU and surgical ward) with a variety of problems receiving opioids. Fentanyl, hydromorphone and buprenorphine were opioids used predominantly, in addition to NSAIAs, which demonstrated a 6/140 (4.3%) new infection rate. Survival rate was 98% with 2% euthanasia due to poor prognosis (e.g. neoplasia, severe head trauma). As with other reported studies, the tibial plateau levelling osteotomy (TPLO) procedure was the major orthopedic procedure represented in the infection rate (two of the six patients acquiring infections). Interestingly, critically ill patients rarely acquired infection, whereas the TPLO procedure is performed in healthy dogs. An earlier study investigating surgical site infections (SSIs) in dogs at the same institution receiving opioids during hospitalization included 846 dogs over a 45-week period and identified 26 (3%) SSIs [7]. A recent study in healthy dogs reported that morphine and buprenorphine did not alter leukocyte production, early apoptosis or neutrophil phagocytic function [8]. It is important to add that pain, and associated stress, is immunosuppressive and the withholding of analgesics based on a potential problem may increase morbidity rather than prevent it. In addition, the effect of hospitalization alone on the stress response in cats [9] and dogs [10, 11] has been described and this stress could have profound effects on the immune system [12], especially when associated with trauma [13]. Pain will compound this stress, illustrating the importance of appropriate analgesia [14].

Many ill or injured animals will require diagnostic and emergency procedures where analgesia, to facilitate restraint, is essential. As each animal will present with varying levels of injury or illness and experience different levels of pain, one cannot apply a standard regimen for all patients. An opioid is the analgesic of choice for initial management; however, dose and method of administration is patient- and situation-dependent and is described in the individual scenarios in this book. In the immediate post-traumatic event, the stress response may reduce the pain experienced below that expected for the associated injury. Therefore, bolus administration of analgesics is not advised due to the potential for adverse effects (panting, nausea, vomiting, dysphoria) when the amount administered is excessive for the degree of pain experienced. "A single dose does not fit all"; therefore, titration to effect is essential. The opioid requirement can be increased as the "stress analgesic response" diminishes. Other important considerations are all drug interactions within the patient and drug compatibilities within the infusions. Refer to Chapter 9 for more detail on sedatives, Chapter 10 (opioids), Chapter 11 (NSAIAs), Chapter 12 (adjunct analgesia), Chapter 13 (anesthetics) and Chapter 18 (preparation and delivery of analgesics).

The aggressive patient will require a different approach and this is patient- and situation-dependent. Patients may be aggressive upon presentation from pain and fear, or may be aggressive in a strange environment. Animals may appear to be stable when acting aggressively upon admission; however, endorphin and epinephrine release can mask the seriousness of the patient's clinical condition. Chemical restraint rather than force is the humane and often safer way to deal with these animals. Assess the patient from afar and, where time permits, obtain a thorough history, including potential current drug therapy, before selecting a method of restraint. Once the reason for the aggression has been identified, frequently associated with significant pain and fear in traumatized animals, a more direct approach to management can follow. Details and drugs/dosages are given in Chapter 22. Respiratory distress may appear as a combination of panic and aggression; therefore, provide "flow by" oxygen initially as this will relieve some stress. If possible, use an open mask (without the diaphragm) to concentrate oxygen towards the nose of the cat or dog, but without touching the face. As soon as possible following sedation, place two or three drops of ophthalmic local anesthetic drops (e.g. proparacaine) into the entry of the nasal passages, then five minutes later place nasal cannulae (prongs, Figure 1.1) or nasal catheter in the dog. For smaller dogs, use an oxygen cage, if available, immediately following sedation. Cats may be better oxygenated in an induction

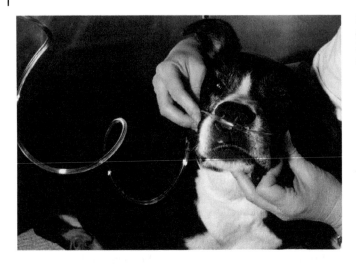

Figure 1.1 Placement of nasal cannulae following placement of 2–3 drops of ophthalmic local anesthetic.

chamber, an oxygen hood or a cage; administer an analgesic intramuscular prior to placing in the oxygen rich environment if possible. Refer to Chapter 28 for details.

Of utmost importance to consider is that a continual painful experience is detrimental to the overall well-being and healing process of humans and animals, resulting in prolonged hospital stay, which increases the potential for secondary problems such as hospital-associated infections. Another potential outcome in veterinary patients is euthanasia due to increasing costs. Also of importance is the association between inadequately treated acute pain and the development of chronic pain. This has been reported in human patients occurring after traumatic, surgical and painful medical conditions [2]. While considering all the negative physiological effects associated with the experience of pain, above all, inadequate analgesia resulting in ongoing pain is inhumane.

It is important to question the owner about pre-existing co-morbidities as cardiovascular, hepatic and renal problems will influence the pain and anesthetic management protocol. It is also important to enquire as to pre-existing orthopedic problems (e.g. osteoarthritis of various joints) as careful handling or manipulation of these areas in general, and whilst under general anesthesia for diagnostic purposes, is essential to avoid increasing the degree of pain.

General anesthetics (inhalant, propofol, barbiturates) may be required for surgical or diagnostic procedures for any ill or injured patient and the approach to prevention of pain applies to all. Special considerations for the individual patient are required (refer to Chapter 13 for details and the scenarios in this book for guidance). It is important to note that general anesthetics only block conscious perception of pain for the duration of anesthesia; however, nociceptive input still occurs and will be experienced by the patient upon recovery. Ketamine, however, has anti-hyperalgesic and analgesic properties. The practice of "preventive" analgesia is to reduce the impact of the total peripheral nociceptive barrage associated with noxious pre-, intra- and post-operative or traumatic stimuli [11]. The term "preemptive analgesia" is restricted to analgesic administration prior to the onset of pain, such as in the pre-operative setting with the intention of reducing nociceptive input and potential peri-operative pain. However, this single event of analgesic administration is inadequate to manage post-operative, and frequently intraoperative, pain. Where moderate to severe pain is to be expected, and is frequently associated with injured and some ill patients, one or more classes of analgesics (based on pain severity) with a demonstrated preventive effect should be administered in addition to an opioid. These analgesics (NSAIAs, local anesthetics, N-methyl-D-aspartate (NMDA) antagonists (e.g. ketamine)) not only reduce the inhalant requirement (MAC reduction) and severity of acute post-surgical pain but may in some cases also reduce the incidence of chronic (persistent) post-operative pain. The efficacy of a multi-modal regimen, combining drugs with pharmacologic action at different sites in the pain pathway, provides optimal analgesia to treating pain, while reducing the dosage of each drug and, therefore, reducing the potential for adverse effects of any single drug that would otherwise require high dosing. Of utmost importance is the utilization of neuraxial analgesia and local blocks wherever possible, both intraoperatively and post-operatively (refer to Chapter 14 for details on the application of all potential techniques for the individual patient). As pain transmission is complex, all nociceptive pathways must be blocked to effect optimal analgesia [15] (refer to Chapter 2). Refer to the pharmacology and clinical application of sedatives (Chapter 9), opioids (Chapter 10) and adjunct analgesia (Chapter 12) for further details.

Illness or injury results in an inflammatory response either local to the area involved or systemically. The presence of inflammation increases the degree of pain experienced following a surgical procedure when compared to that of a routine procedure. As an example, ovariohysterectomy in patients with metritis or pyometra will require higher dosing of analgesics during and after ovariohysterectomy and for longer duration when compared to that of a routine elective procedure. Also, in addition to the potential establishment of chronic pain due to inadequate pain management, inadequately treated pain associated with abdominal or thoracic incisions prevents normal ventilation/oxygenation. Controlled walking and other rehabilitation exercises are essential for post-operative orthopedic repair to ensure appropriate "stress" for bone healing, enhance periosteal blood flow and to maintain muscle mass to support the limb. Without adequate analgesic administration, frequently requiring at least two classes of analgesics, movement will be too painful, resulting in non-use bone and muscle atrophy. Above all, "facilitating pain" to control movement following surgery is unethical. When in hospital, controlled leash walking and integrative techniques (refer to Chapter 15) should be included in the post-operative management protocol, neither of which can be tolerated when in pain. Similar discharge home instructions, with analgesia, must be given.

When considering analgesic selection, the adverse effects must be minimal due to the fragile organ function of these patients. Other important considerations are drug interactions within the patient. Drug metabolism and clearance is primarily via the liver and kidney; where a patient is identified with organ dysfunction, an NSAIA is contraindicated. However, opioid analgesics can still be administered. Initial dosing to effect is required to reach therapeutic levels; however, the dosing intervals may be extended and the hourly infusion rates may be reduced based on patient assessment as the metabolism and excretion may be reduced. The ongoing dosing with adjustments will be dependent on the individual patient. To optimize efficacy and safety, evaluation of cardiovascular, hepatic respiratory and renal systems is essential to guide ongoing pain management. Refer to the appropriate chapters (Chapter 19, cardiovascular; Chapter 20, kidney; and Chapter 21, liver) for information on drug metabolism and excretion, and adjustments in the delivery regimen, for patients with significant organ dysfunction (refer to Chapter 18).

Pregnant (Chapter 23), nursing (Chapter 24) and pediatric (Chapter 25) patients may present with an injury or illness associated with various degree of pain, which must be managed to prevent the consequences noted above. Of importance, is that the newborn and infant animals feel pain and, in fact, have increased sensation when compared to a similar stimulus in an adult. It is extremely important to prevent/treat pain in these patients as permanent hyperalgesia/allodynia may manifest due to the extreme plasticity of the central nervous system in these young animals.

Sedation must not be interpreted as analgesia; therefore, midazolam or dexmedetomidine should only be used as adjuncts in addition to analgesics for stable patients requiring more "restraint" or sedation than the analgesic alone can provide. Refer to Chapter 9 for details.

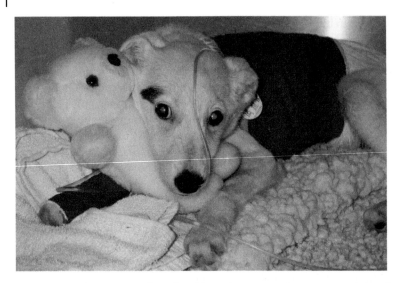

Figure 1.2 A clean, warm and comfortable environment reduces stress and, therefore, pain.

Of great importance is that analgesia should be withdrawn slowly to avoid an abrupt return to a hyperalgesic state should pain still be present. Where the recurrence of pain is identified, return to the previous dose for several more hours and attempt withdrawal very slowly when appropriate.

Analgesia and sleep is the goal; therefore, it is essential that optimal patient care be provided to avoid further pain (Figure 1.2) and stress. Based on the anxiety and stress our patients experience whilst in the hospital and the detrimental effect this has on their well-being and recovery, it is essential that the nursing care described in Chapter 17, and in all the scenarios presented, is implemented. The requirement for ongoing analgesia is the dual responsibility of the veterinary technician/nurse and the veterinarian and is outlined in Chapter 16. The analgesic/sedative and anesthetic regimen must be tailored to the individual patient according to the problem at hand. See suggestions and recommendations for individual case scenarios throughout this book and review other chapters to optimize analgesic and anesthetic management.

To complete the picture of managing pain in all conditions in small animal practice, consult references [4] and [16].

References

1 Brock, N. (1995) Treating moderate and severe pain in small animals. *Can Vet J*, 36: 658–660.

2 Randall, J., Malchow, M. D., Black, I. H. (2008) The evolution of pain management in the critically ill trauma patient: Emerging concepts from the global war on terrorism. *Crit Care Med*, 36: S346–S357.

3 Robertson, S. A. (2008) Managing pain in feline patients. *Vet Clin North Am Small Anim Pract*, 38: 1267–1290.

4 Mathews, K. A., Kronen, P. W., Lascelles, D. X., *et al.* (2014) WSAVA: Global Pain Council Guidelines for Recognition. *Assessment and Treatment of Pain in Small Animals*, 55(6): E10–E68.

5 Jenkins, C. (2000) Recommending analgesics for people with asthma. *Am J Ther*, 7(2): 55–61.

6 Odunayo, A., Dodam, J. R. and Kerl, M. E. (2010) Immunomodulatory effects of opioids *J Vet Emerg Crit Care*, 20(4): 376–385.

7 Turk, R., Singh, A. and Weese, J. S. (2015) Prospective surgical site infection surveillance. *Dogs Veterinary Surgery*, 44: 2–8.

8 Monibi, F. A., Dodam, J. R., Axiak-Bechtel, S. M., *et al.* (2015) Morphine and buprenorphine do not alter leukocyte cytokine production capacity, early apoptosis, or neutrophil phagocytic function in healthy dogs. *Res in Vet Sci*, 99: 70–76.

9 Quimby, J. M., Smith, M. L. and Lunn, K. F. (2011) Evaluation of the effects of hospital visit stress on physiologic parameters in the cat. *J Feline Med Surg*, 13: 733–737.

10 Bragg, R. F., Bennett, J. S., Cummings, A. and Quimby, J. E. (2015) Evaluation of the effects of hospital visit stress on physiologic variables in dogs. *J Am Vet Med Assoc*, 246: 212–215.

11 Hekman, J. P., Karas, A. Z. and Dreschel, N. A. (2012) Salivary cortisol concentrations and behaviour in a population of healthy dogs hospitalized for elective procedures. *Applied Animal Behavior Science*, 141: 149–157.

12 Calcagni, E. and Elenkov, I. (2006) Stress system activity, innate and T helper cytokines, and susceptibility to immune-related diseases. *Annals of the New York Academy of Sciences*, 1069, 62–76.

13 Molina, P. E. (2005) Neurobiology of the stress response: Contribution of the sympathetic nervous system to the neuroimmune axis in traumatic injury. *Shock*, 24(1): 3–10.

14 Dahl, J. B. and Kehlet, H. (2011) Preventive analgesia. *Curr Opin Anaethesiol*, 24, 331–338.

15 Woolf, C. (2004) Pain: Moving from symptom control toward mechanism-specific pharmacologic management. *Annals of Internal Medicine*, 140: 441–451.

16 Epstein, M. E., Rodan, I. and Griffenhagen, G. (2015) AAHA/AAFP pain management guidelines for dogs and cats. *J Feline Med Surg.*, 17: 251–272.

Further Reading

Attard, A. R., Corlett, M. J., Kidner, N. J., *et al.* (1992) Safety of early pain relief for acute abdominal pain. *Br Med J*, 305: 554–556.

Mathews, K. A. (ed.) (2017) *Veterinary Emergency & Critical Care Manual*, 3rd edn. LifeLearn, Guelph, Ontario, Canada.

2

Physiology and Pathophysiology of Pain

Tamara Grubb

Pain is defined by the International Association for the Study of Pain (IASP) as "an unpleasant sensory and emotional experience associated with actual or potential tissue damage, or described in terms of such damage" [1]. This is useful in that it describes the utility of pain to protect the individual from injury – an appendage placed on something excessively hot causes activation of the pain pathway, the appendage is reflexively withdrawn and tissue damage is prevented, or at least reduced from what it would have been had withdrawal of the appendage not occurred. Although the definition may seem to impart a simple process, the initiation, propagation and subsequent sensation of pain is not at all simple. Pain is a very dynamic and complex phenomenon that involves integration of a variety of receptors, neurotransmitters, neural fibres, neural pathways and both discrete and diffuse anatomic locations. As described, pain can be a normal physiologic response to tissue damage causing withdrawal from a painful stimulus, and as such is called "physiologic" or "protective" pain. Pain can also be an abnormal response causing a situation of intense and/or prolonged pain that is not protective from tissue damage, and as such is called "pathologic" or "maladaptive" pain, among other names (including "clinical pain"). A basic understanding of the pain pathway is important for the appropriate and effective treatment of pain. This understanding will facilitate (1) selection of the most effective analgesic drugs based on the origin of the pain and (2) integration of techniques like multi-modal and preventive (or "preemptive") analgesia to create balanced analgesic protocols.

I. Pain versus Nociception

An understanding of "nociception", versus "pain", is important. *Nociception* describes the physiologic/pathologic process that occurs in mammals, birds, reptiles, amphibians, etc. and likely many other species, in response to a noxious stimulus. The prefix "noci", which means "harm" or "injury", is part of many of the terms describing the process (nociceptive, nociceptor, etc.). *Pain* is defined as a cognitive or emotional response to nociception that occurs in the higher centres of the central nervous system (CNS), such as the cerebral cortex. There are those that believe animals experience only nociception and not pain because they feel that animals do not have the cognitive, and certainly not the emotional, response. However, most animal pain experts, and those of us working with animals, completely disagree with this, especially since animals learn to anticipate and avoid painful situations, which can be indicative of a cognitive response. And as we manage our patients on a daily basis, we certainly recognize the emotional response which is demonstrated in their behaviour (refer to Chapter 8). Pain

Analgesia and Anesthesia for the Ill or Injured Dog and Cat, First Edition. Karol A. Mathews, Melissa Sinclair, Andrea M. Steele and Tamara Grubb.

technically doesn't occur in anesthetized patients since the cognitive or emotional response would be prevented by the anesthetic. However, response to noxious stimuli that occurs under anesthesia is often still described as pain because the noxious surgical stimulus activates the pain pathway and causes the pain-mediated changes described in this chapter. Although the pain centres in the brain don't recognize the pain during anesthesia, it is waiting there for the brain to perceive in recovery.

II. The Pain Pathway in Physiologic Pain

The pain pathway is composed of a series of integrated anatomical structures and physiologic processes that are dynamic and may change their structure or process according to pain source, intensity and/or duration. These changes can be a part of the normal pain response but can also lead to pathologic pain, as discussed in Section III. The processes involved in the pain pathway (Figure 2.1) include transduction, transmission, modulation and perception. Some authors

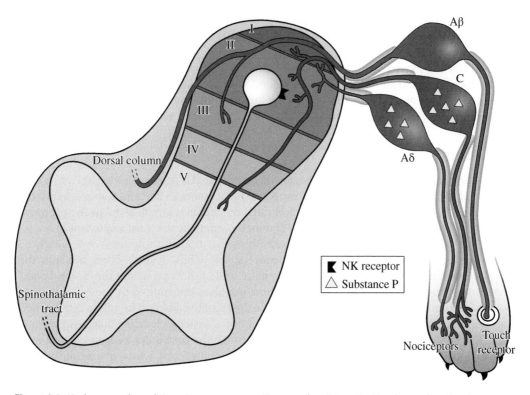

Figure 2.1 Under normal conditions, innocuous sensations or a low-intensity stimulus, such as touch or vibration, is transmitted from the periphery to laminae III and IV of the dorsal horn by means of A-beta fibres; the signal is then relayed to the brain by way of the dorsal column somatosensory pathway. Noxious thermal or mechanical input (transduction), the protective nociceptive "first pain" experience, activates the A-delta fibres, which have small receptive fields, and functions as a warning and is protective to the animal. With increased intensity of the stimulus, C-fibres also conduct impulses along with A-delta fibres. C fibres have a larger receptive field compared with A-delta fibres and are responsible for the "second pain" experience. The A-delta and C fibres enter the dorsal horn of the spinal cord, wherein A-delta fibres almost solely and C fibres predominantly terminate in laminae I and II. The A-delta and C-fibre ganglions express Substance-P (S-P), and the neurokinin-1 (NK1 (S-P)) receptors are expressed in the neurons of lamina II. The signal is then relayed to the brain by way of the spinothalamic tract. *Source:* [9]. Reproduced with permission of Elsevier.

include projection (between modulation and perception) as a separate process. There is also an endogenous analgesic, or "anti-nociceptive", pathway with both ascending and descending components.

A. Transduction

Pain starts when a specialized, high-threshold peripheral sensory receptor, or "nociceptor", is depolarized by a noxious, or "nociceptive", stimulus. The nociceptors are actually not receptors in the traditional sense of the word but are the free nerve endings of A-delta and C nerve fibre dendrites from primary afferent neurons [2]. Most of the nociceptors, especially those from C fibres, are polymodal, meaning that they can be depolarized by a variety of noxious stimuli, including mechanical, thermal and chemical stimuli. For the most part, the nociceptors have no spontaneous depolarization and are high threshold, meaning they respond only to noxious stimuli and not non-noxious stimuli like touch [2]. Depolarization of the nociceptors *transduces* the mechanical information from these stimuli into an electrical impulse. Various ion channels are associated with transduction. These include purinergic, sodium, calcium and potassium channels along with a variety of transient receptor potential (TRP) ion channels. The latter include the transient receptor potential vanilloid (TRPV) receptors that are a major component of pain sensation (especially TRPV1) from heat, cold and chemical stimuli.

The density and exact distribution of nociceptors are species-dependent and often impacted by other factors such as age and disease. In general, they are highly represented in the skin and located throughout most structures in the body including the muscles, tendons, bone, viscera, peritoneum, pleura, periosteum, meninges, joint capsules, blood vessels, etc.

B. Transmission

Once the nociceptor has been depolarized, an action potential is *transmitted* to the CNS by the A-delta and C fibre dendrites from their respective nociceptors as described above. Primarily sodium (Na_v 1.1–1.9), but also potassium and calcium, channels are involved in the propagation of the action potential. The Na_v 1.7–1.9 channels seem to be the most important in nociception [3]. A-delta fibres are small myelinated fibres that transmit impulses very rapidly. C fibres are small, unmyelinated and transmit more slowly. Thus, A-delta fibres transmit the "first pain", which is the initial sharp, protective pain, while C fibres transmit the "second pain", which is described as "dull, achy" pain. In addition, impulses transmitted by the A-delta fibres have small receptive fields in the spinal cord, while the receptive fields of impulses carried by C fibres are more diffuse, making pain from A-delta fibres easier to localize than pain from C fibres. The pain impulse passes from both fibres through the first-order neuron in the dorsal root ganglion (DRG) and then to the dorsal horn of the spinal cord, where neurotransmitters (primarily glutamate and S-P) are released.

C. Modulation

The A-delta and C fibres terminate in various lamina in the dorsal horn of the spinal cord (A-delta primarily in lamina I with some in V; C primarily in II), where a variety of scenarios may occur. There is not a direct 1:1 relationship between the number of impulses that enter and those that leave the dorsal horn. The impulses may be sent directly to the brain without change or may be *modulated* (amplified or inhibited) by interneurons or descending projections. They can bifurcate, sending branches that ascend or descend several spinal cord segments (Lissauer's tracts) before synapsing. In the simplest process, the signal from the first-order neuron causes a release of an excitatory amino acid (primarily glutamate but also aspartate) and/or a neuro-peptide (S-P or neurokinin) which crosses the neuronal synapse to activate the second-order neuron in the dorsal horn, which is most likely to be an alpha-amino-3-hydroxy-5-methyl-4-isoxazolepropionic acid (AMPA) or a kainate (KAI) receptor.

Once the second-order, or "projection", neuron, is activated, the signal travels to the con-tralateral side of the dorsal horn and is transmitted (or "projected") up an ascending (or "projecting") tract. The ascending tracts are species-specific (and not well described in all species) as to their presence, location and importance. The tracts primarily include the spinothalamic (STT), spinocervicothalamic (SCT), spinoreticular (SRT) and spinomesence-phalic tracts (SMT), with the STT and SCT likely playing the most prominent roles in most mammals [4].

D. Perception

There is no specific pain centre in the brain, and nociceptive impulses from the ascending tracts may arrive primarily at the thalamus, hypothalamus and structures of the midbrain. At these locations, the second-order neurons synapse and the impulses are transmitted to vari-ous cortical and subcortical regions, including the somatosensory cortex, periaqueductal gray (PAG) region, reticular formation and the limbic system. This diverse pattern of distri-bution results in a variety of outcomes, which include pain perception, but also initiation of descending facilitatory (which increase pain) and inhibitory (which decrease pain) processes, wakefulness, behavioural reactions, emotional changes (at least in humans), etc. A third-order neuron transmits the impulse from the thalamus to the somatosensory cortex where the pain signal is "perceived" and identified by location, type and intensity. For intensity, depolarization of neurons is either "all" or "none" so varied pain intensity does not result from different stimulus strength but rather from the number of stimuli. Perception and interpretation of the impulse in the somatosensory cortex initiates a behavioural response, which can manifest itself in a number of ways, including withdrawal from, or aggression towards, the source of the pain. Impulses at the reticular system activate autonomic and motor responses, and impulses at the limbic system are responsible for emotional responses (at least in humans).

E. Endogenous Analgesic Pathways

1. Descending Inhibitory Pathway

Descending inhibition of ascending afferent pain impulses can be activated in various sites, including the cortex, thalamus, midbrain, brainstem and dorsal horn of the spinal cord. The inhibitory process is primarily controlled by the PAG, which appears to be a "coordinating centre" for the endogenous analgesic system. The main effective site of the descending pathway is the dorsal horn of the spinal cord, where a descending projection neuron from the PAG will synapse in the gap between the axon of the sensory first-order neuron and the second-order neuron, releasing neurotransmitters, including endogenous opioids (endorphins, enkephalins, dynorphins), serotonin (5-HT), norepinephrine, gamma-aminobutyric acid (GABA) and gly-cine. This alleviates propagation of the pain impulse at the synapse by release of inhibitory neurotransmitters that bind to both presynaptic and postsynaptic sites. Presynaptic binding causes decreased release of excitatory neurotransmitters into the synapse, and postsynaptic binding causes decreased propagation of the pain stimulus on the second-order neuron. The endogenous system is likely most effective in alleviating mild pain and can provide a brief period of relief for moderate to severe acute pain during high-stress states (like survival situations).

2. Ascending Analgesic Pathway

A-beta receptors and fibres, which travel with the A-delta and C nociceptors and fibres, are myelinated and have a rapid conduction velocity. These generally conduct non-noxious (non-nociceptive) stimuli such as touch and movement and can also recruit inhibitory neurons in the dorsal horn of the spinal cord (gate control). This appears to be part of the explanation for why rubbing a painful site may actually decrease the level of pain. Wide dynamic range (WDR) receptors or neurons may also initiate inhibitor responses to pain in the dorsal horn of the spinal cord. These neurons receive input from A-beta, A-delta and C fibres and respond to all forms of input, from light touch to noxious stimuli, in a graded fashion depending on stimulus intensity. The WDR output from normal A-beta activation is likely inhibitory.

III. The Pain Pathway in Pathologic Pain

With tissue injury, pain does not end with recognition of pain in the cortex and removal of the body part from the noxious stimuli. Ongoing mild to moderate pain from tissue that is currently injured is not necessarily "pathologic" – it can still be "protective" – but pain that is more intense than necessary for protection, and pain that continues after the injury has healed, is indeed pathologic pain. If pain is not necessary for protection, it serves no biologic purpose and results in needless decreased quality of life for the patient. Pathologic changes that occur in the pain pathway include peripheral sensitization, recruitment of fibres that normally don't carry noxious stimuli (A-beta fibres), central sensitization and dysfunction of the descending inhibitory pathway. These changes can cause more significant conditions, including hyperalgesia and/or allodynia. Hyperalgesia is an exaggerated pain sensation to a normally low-level pain stimulus and allodynia is a pain sensation from a normally non-painful stimulus, such as light touch. These changes may become permanent, or at least long-lasting, causing chronic pain states, which are often difficult to treat with standard analgesic therapy. An even more sinister type of pain, neuropathic pain, can be caused or enhanced by these changes.

To prevent or reduce pathologic pain, early administration of appropriate analgesics and careful surgical technique and tissue handling are essential. In addition, **multi-modal analgesia**, meaning utilization of more than one drug class and/or analgesic technique [5], is more likely to prevent the development of pathologic pain and is almost always required to treat pathologic pain once it has occurred because of the complexity of the pain pathway and the variety of changes that occur with the onset and progression of pathologic pain. There is no single therapy that can treat the myriad pathway alterations. The discussion below includes a description of pain pathway changes induced by pathologic pain and a list of drugs or compounds that affect the pain pathway at each step. The lists are by no means exhaustive.

A. Transduction

With tissue injury, damaged structural cells and damaged, and recruited, inflammatory cells (e.g. neutrophils, mast cells, macrophages and lymphocytes) release a variety of intracellular compounds that accumulate in the area of the injury which expands as cells on the periphery of the original injury site are also damaged, enlarging the painful area. Such a very large variety of compounds can be involved (e.g. H+, K+, prostaglandins, interleukins, tumour necrosis factor, bradykinin and S-P) that this group of compounds is often called the "sensitizing soup". The result is continued tissue damage as the "soup" expands and causes injury to adjacent cells, creating an ever-widening area of damage, recruitment of more A-delta and C nociceptors, and activation of the arachidonic acid pathway and inflammation. In addition, the "soup" causes a reduced depolarization threshold of nociceptors, which decreases the level of stimulus needed to activate A-delta and C nociceptors; induces changes in A-beta nociceptors, which makes them responsive to noxious stimuli (these normally only transduce touch and other non-noxious stimuli); and causes activation of "silent nociceptors" (likely C nociceptors) that were not participating in the pain transduced from the original injury. These processes create *peripheral sensitization*, which is a major component of hyperalgesia and also contributes to allodynia.

Example drugs or compounds effective at this site: non-steroidal anti-inflammatory drugs (NSAIDs), local anesthetics, capsaicin.

B. Transmission

With the recruitment of additional A-delta and C fibres and transformation of A-beta fibres to transmit noxious stimuli, the number and frequency of nociceptive impulses transmitted to the dorsal horn of the spinal cord are increased, thus amplifying the pain signal. Na + channels (especially Na_v 1.8) can become hyperexcitable and exhibit spontaneous electrical activity or pathological electrical activity [3].

Example drugs or compounds effective at this site: local anesthetics, opioids, $alpha_2$ agonists, tetrodotoxin.

C. Modulation

The processes that occur at the spinal cord in pathologic pain are numerous and complex. These processes can contribute to allodynia and central sensitization, and include (but are not limited to):

- The increased frequency and intensity of pain impulses reaching the dorsal horn (i.e. increased "afferent traffic") activate not only the AMPA and KAI receptors but also the N-methyl-D-aspartate (NMDA) receptors, which are normally dormant. Activation of the NMDA receptors, which is integral to the process of central sensitization, occurs secondary to "flooding" of the second-order synapse with excitatory neurotransmitters from the increased afferent input and from additional input from WDRs.
- As stated, the WDR neurons receive input from A-beta, A-delta and C fibres and respond to all forms of input (from light touch to noxious stimuli) in a graded fashion depending on stimulus intensity. Repetitive firing of A-beta and C fibres causes a noxious stimulus at the WDR.
- Central activation of the arachidonic acid pathway occurs with repetitive noxious stimuli, which may also influence NMDA-receptor activation and activity along with contributing to centrally mediated hyperalgesia.
- Non-neuronal cell types, such as astrocytes and microglia, that normally do not play a role in pain transmission can be activated or altered and can enhance pain transmission with repetitive stimuli [6].
- A-beta fibres can sprout into lamina 1 of the spinal cord and activate neurokinin (NK)-1 receptors.
- Nerve injury may also disrupt the A-beta-fibre-mediated inhibition and the GABA-mediated inhibition of pain transmission neurons in the dorsal horn [7–9]. The loss of this activity may be within interneurons, which ultimately releases the "brake" on central sensitization of dorsal horn neurons. The loss of this inhibitory process may contribute to spontaneous pain, hyperalgesia or allodynia following nerve injury [7–9].

Example drugs or compounds effective at this site: opioids, NMDA-receptor antagonists (ketamine, amantadine), $alpha_2$ agonists, local anesthetics, gabapentin, NE and 5-HT uptake inhibitors, tricyclic antidepressants, NSAIDs.

D. Perception

Previous pain experiences, agitation, fear, sensory triggers (smells, sounds, etc.), sensory distractors (smells, music, presence of a loved one, etc.), culture, social status, sleep deprivation and myriad other things can alter the perception of pain – at least in humans. It would appear that, at the very least, previous pain experiences may impact perception in animals because they do develop avoidance responses to repetitive noxious stimuli, which could be interpreted as a cognitive learned response. A curious phenomenon that occurs in humans, but is not yet reported in animals, is loss of cerebral gray matter in chronic pain states [10]. Whether this is caused by the pain itself or is an attempt to reduce the magnitude of the perception of pain is unknown.

Example drugs or compounds effective at this site: opioids, alpha$_2$ agonists, some general anesthetic drugs, NMDA-receptor antagonists, tricyclic antidepressants, NE and 5-HT uptake inhibitors.

E. Descending Inhibitory Pathway

Decreased efficacy of the descending inhibitory limb of the pain pathway may play a large role in the initiation, maintenance and degree of pathologic pain [11]. Reduced opioid receptor function with subsequent reduced response to IV or intrathecal opioids, altered or reduced levels of endogenous norepinephrine and serotonin activity at the spinal and supraspinal levels, and disruption of A-beta-mediated inhibition all contribute to the abnormal response of the descending inhibitory limb [9]. The loss of this inhibitory process, which serves as the "brake" in the pain pathway, may contribute to spontaneous pain, hyperalgesia and/or allodynia [7–9].

Example drugs or compounds effective at this site: Endogenous opioids, serotonin and norepinephrine reuptake inhibitors affect this portion of the pathway, as do drugs that increase the inhibitory neurotransmitter GABA and cannabinoids.

IV. Specific Types of Pain

A. Neonatal/Pediatric Pain

In both humans and animals, neonates and pediatric patients do feel pain. Untreated pain in neonates can cause amplified pain sensation as the patient ages and may lead to chronic pain in adulthood (refer to Chapter 25).

B. Neuropathic Pain

Various studies have identified the decreased efficacy of the descending inhibitory pathways in animals with neuropathic lesions and have demonstrated reduced opioid receptor function [13, 14]. Because descending inhibition normally acts as a spinal "gate" for sensory information, reduced inhibition increases the likelihood that the dorsal horn neuron will fire spontaneously or more energetically to primary afferent input [15]. While opioid receptors are less responsive in neuropathic pain, it appears that descending noradrenergic inhibition, and increased sensitivity of spinal neurons to alpha$_2$ agonists, may occur with peripheral inflammation and nerve injury [15]. Refer to Chapter 3 for a detailed discussion.

C. Visceral Pain

The physiology/pathophysiology of visceral pain is very complex and comprises afferent and efferent innervations, autonomic nervous system modulation, and central processing.

Peripheral and central sensitization may occur [16, 17]. Refer to Chapter 4 for details, as the understanding of these processes is important in managing the specific visceral pain experienced within the thorax, abdomen and pelvis.

D. Breakthrough Pain

Breakthrough pain (BTP) is described as an abrupt, short-lived and intense pain that "breaks through" the around-the-clock analgesia that controls persistent pain [18, 19]. This may occur in the post-operative setting or intermittently at home in animals on chronic pain medication for cancer or neuropathic pain. If a single analgesic agent is being used, consider the addition of other analgesics of a different class (refer to Chapter 6 and information contained in scenarios throughout this book). When BTP occurs at home, a careful history is required to obtain clues about the cause and pattern of BTP. It may be difficult to administer oral medication when animals exhibit excruciating pain. If this cannot be controlled, parenteral or transdermal administration has to be considered in addition to oral medication. The dose and/or dosing frequency of the around-the-clock analgesic should be adjusted for patients with end-of-dose BTP. In addition to pharmacologic therapy, non-pharmacologic strategies are often helpful in alleviating pain and anxiety. (refer to Chapter 15).

E. Stimulus-Evoked/Movement-Evoked Pain

As the name suggests, stimulus-evoked/movement-evoked pain does not occur when the patient is resting quietly with no movement or touch. While managing pain in situations other than when the patient is at rest can be challenging, this pain should not be ignored by preventing movement, as movement is essential for a normal recovery. Consider analgesic protocols and procedures specifically prepared for the individual patient and their associated pain stimulus (refer to Chapter 6). An example of stimulus-evoked pain is pressing around the surgical wound to assess the presence/degree of mechanical hyperalgesia. The response and extent of the anatomical area eliciting pain will indicate the degree of pain and solicit a review of the analgesic protocol.

References

1 Merskey, H. and Bogduk, N. (1994) *Classification of Chronic Pain: Descriptions of chronic pain syndromes and definitions of pain terms.* IASP Press, Seattle.

2 Woolf, C. J. and Ma, Q. (2007) Nociceptors: Noxious stimulus detectors. *Neuron*, 55(3): 353–364.

3 Levinson, S. R., Luo, S. and Henry, M. A. (2012) The role of sodium channels in chronic pain. *Muscle Nerve*, 46(2): 155–165.

4 Kajander, K. C. and Giesler, G. J., Jr (1987) Effects of repeated noxious thermal stimuli on the responses of neurons in the lateral cervical nucleus of cats: Evidence for an input from A-nociceptors to the spinocervicothalamic pathway. *Brain Res*, 436(2): 390–395.

5 Lamont, L. A. (2008) Multimodal pain management in veterinary medicine: The physiologic basis of pharmacologic therapies. *Vet Clin North Am Small Anim Pract*, 38(6): 1173–1186.

6 D'Mello, R. and Dickenson, A. H. (2008) Spinal cord mechanisms of pain. *Br J Anaesth*, 101(1): 8–16.

7 Taylor, B. K. (2001) Pathophysiologic mechanisms of neuropathic pain. *Curr Pain Headache Rep*, 5: 151–161.

8 Woolf, C. J. (2004) Dissecting out mechanisms responsible for peripheral neuropathic pain: Implications for diagnosis and therapy. *Life Sciences*, 74: 2605–2610.

9 Mathews, K. A. (2008) Neuropathic pain in dogs and cats: If only they could tell us if they hurt. *Vet Clin North Am Small Anim Pract*, 38(6): 1365–1414.

10 Apkarian, A. V., Sosa, Y., Sonty, S., *et al.* (2004) Chronic back pain is associated with decreased prefrontal and thalamic gray matter density. *J Neurosci*, 24(46): 10410–10415.

11 Ren, J. and Ruda, R. (2002) Descending modulation in persistent pain: An update. *Pain*, 100(1–2): 1–6.

12 Cui, M., Honore, P., Zhong, C., *et al.* (2006) TRPV1 receptors in the CNS play a key role in broad-spectrum analgesia of TRPV1 antagonists. *J Neurosci*, 26(37): 9385–9393.

13 Zimmerman, M. (2001) Pathobiology of neuropathic pain. *Eur J Pharmacol*, 429: 23–37.

14 Mayer, D. J., Mao, J. and Price, D. D. (1995) The development of morphine tolerance and dependence is associated with translocation of protein kinase C. *Pain*, 61: 365–374.

15 Tanabe, M., Takasu, K., Kasuya, N., *et al.* (2005) Role of descending noradrenergic system and spinal alpha$_2$-adrenergic receptors in the effects of gabapentin on thermal and mechanical nociception after partial nerve injury in the mouse. *Br J Pharmacol*, 144: 703–714.

16 Joshi, S. K. and Gebhart, G. F. (2000) Visceral pain. *Current Review of Pain*, 4(6): 499–506.

17 Knowles, C. H. and Aziz, Q. (2009) Basic and clinical aspects of gastrointestinal pain review. *Pain*, 141: 191–209.

18 Payne, R. (2007) Recognition and diagnosis of breakthrough pain. *Pain Med*, 8(suppl. 1): S3–S7.

19 McCarberg, B. H. (2007) The treatment of breakthrough pain. *Pain Med*, 8(suppl. 1): S8–S3.

Further Reading

Shilo, Y. and Pascoe, P. J. (2014) Anatomy, physiology and pathophysiology of pain. In: Egger, C. M., Love, L. and Doherty, T. (eds), *Pain Management in Veterinary Practice*. Wiley-Blackwell, Oxford: 9–29.

3

Physiologic and Pharmacologic Applications to Manage Neuropathic Pain

Karol Mathews

Neuropathic pain is re-defined by the International Association for the Study of Pain (IASP) as pain caused by a lesion or disease of the somatosensory nervous system and may be generated by either the peripheral or central nervous system, or both [1]. A very broad term is "neurogenic pain". There follows a plethora of changes in the peripheral nervous system (PNS), spinal cord, brainstem and brain as damaged nerves fire spontaneously and develop hyper-responsivity to both inflammatory and normally innocuous stimuli [1]. Refer to Chapter 2 for details on the anatomy and physiology of pain transmission in general.

Neuropathic pain is frequently associated with chronic pain. However, it also occurs in the acute setting either pre-operatively, when associated with trauma, or a neoplastic or inflammatory condition encroaching on neural tissue, or post-operatively, where transient or persistent iatrogenic injury has occurred. Patients noted to be at risk of progression to persistent pain include those with severe pain and those with injury to any part of the peripheral or central nervous system (CNS). The importance of being aware of the animals "at risk" of development of chronic neuropathic pain in the acute setting is to ensure that appropriate intervention is instituted pre-, intra- and post-operatively, and practising meticulous surgical technique to prevent such a debilitating situation, which may be difficult to diagnose once established at a later date.

In the chronic setting, the clinical signs have been insidious and present for weeks to several months with an obvious lesion being difficult to find. As pain in general can be difficult to recognize and isolate in many veterinary patients, neuropathic pain can be extremely difficult to identify unless we appreciate the occult nature of many of the predisposing causes. Frequently, neuropathic pain induces a response which may be interpreted as a primary behavioural problem and may, therefore, go untreated. Two major events occur in the development of chronic neuropathic pain: (1) abnormal peripheral input and (2) abnormal central processing. The situations where pain may be a cause for behavioural changes are:

- in the acute pain setting (at home or in the hospital);
- at a later period following a traumatic or surgical; experience
- due to a chronic primary lesion affecting the:
  - ○ somatosensory and visceral peripheral nerve(s),
  - ○ the meninges, vertebral column, spinal cord and its nerve roots, or
  - ○ a lesion in the brain.

Analgesia and Anesthesia for the Ill or Injured Dog and Cat, First Edition. Karol A. Mathews, Melissa Sinclair, Andrea M. Steele and Tamara Grubb.

I.   Physiology of Neuropathic Pain

The origin of neuropathic pain may be difficult to diagnose unless an obvious predisposing lesion or injury to the nervous system is easily identified, or a genetic predisposition exists. Understanding the physiology and events that occur in the nervous system, originating from poorly managed acute pain, chronic pain or from primary lesions within the nervous system is important, as individual mechanisms causing pain are targets for therapeutic consideration. Some lesions may be amenable to surgical therapy, whereas others will require specific pharmacological intervention.

A.   The Patient's Experience

Enhanced sensation at a certain level of tactile stimulus in areas normally hypoesthetic at rest [2, 3], for example:

- paresthesias (tingling, prickling, burning);
- hyperesthesias (heightened sensation to a nociceptive stimulus); and
- dysesthesias (unpleasant or painful sensation).

With these experiences the spontaneous actions of a dog or cat, in response to these sensations, can easily be interpreted as behavioural by the owner.

B.   The Quality and Pattern of Altered Sensitivity

The quality and pattern of altered sensitivity in neuropathic pain differs from transient or inflammatory pain. As examples:

A cold stimulus or warm stimulus, such as applying a cold or warm pack to an acutely injured joint or muscle to reduce the inflammatory pain in the "normal" or "naive" painful individual, would result in an excruciating painful experience in a patient with neuropathic pain [2]. This difference in "experience" is due to a reorganization of sensory transmissions within the nervous system which occur following nerve injury. These comprise alterations in expression of neurotransmitters, neuromodulators, receptors, ion-channels, especially the tetrodotoxin-resistant (TTR-X) sodium channels [4], and structural proteins. Some of these changes are involved in the reparative process but others contribute to neuropathic pain. Examples of neural response to injury include:

1. The A-beta (touch) fibres may sprout into the laminae II region of the dorsal horn, the same area as central terminals of C fibres (nociception), where Substance-P (S-P) and its receptors (neurokinin-1(NK_1)) are expressed [2] (Figure 3.1).
2. Due to nerve injury, the disruption of the glial ensheathment allows the adjacent denuded axons of A-beta fibres and C fibres to make contact facilitating both electrical (aphaptic) and chemical (via diffusible substances) cross-excitation [5]. A cross-after-discharge can also occur whereby normal A-beta fibres can activate C fibres [2, 5]. This occurs when light, innocuous stimuli are applied to the area subserved by the nerve-injured area, and the stimuli transmitted by the A-beta fibres are processed in the dorsal horn as C fibre sensory afferent stimuli with subsequent pain transmission [2] (see Figure 3.1).
3. During the healing process, there may also be a connection between the A-beta fibres and the C fibres. Therefore, the transmission of a normal innocuous "touch" stimulus elicited during transduction of the A-beta fibres is coupled to the axon of the C fibre. Subsequent transmission is then via the C fibre, where it is interpreted centrally as a noxious stimulus (allodynia) [2] (see Figure 3.1).

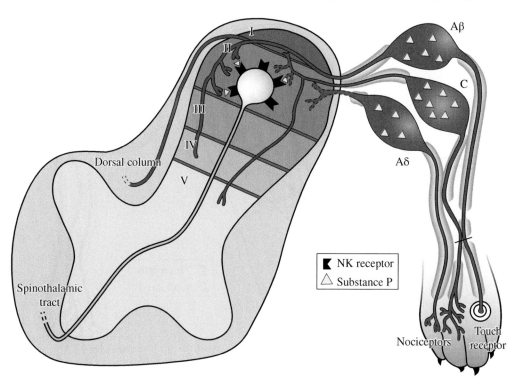

Figure 3.1 Nerve-injury-induced structural and neurochemical reorganization. *Source:* [9]. Reproduced with permission of Elsevier.

4. With (1), (2) or (3), dorsal root ganglion neurons in A-beta fibres now express SP and neurons in lamina II express a greater number of NK_1 receptors for pain transmission.

5. Normal touch and nociception are depicted in Figure 3.2 for comparison to nerve-injury-induced structural and neurochemical reorganization (see Figure 3.1).

C. Immune Response Mechanisms in Neuropathic Pain

1. Peripheral Nervous System Response

Injury to nerves results in an inflammatory response at the site of nerve injury, which is similar to that occurring following damage to non-neural tissue. Infiltration of inflammatory cells, as well as activation of resident immune cells in response to nervous system damage, leads to subsequent production and secretion of various inflammatory mediators. These mediators promote neuroimmune activation and sensitize primary afferent neurons contributing to pain hypersensitivity. Also, the activated macrophages at the site of nerve injury produce pro-inflammatory substances such as tumour necrosis factor (TNFα) and interleukin-1 β (IL-1β), which are known to produce pain in experimental animals when given subcutaneously or applied directly to the nerve [6].

2. Central Nervous System Response [7]

The pathway for sensory transmission from the periphery through the spinal cord to, and in, the cortex plays an important role in chronic pain, including inflammatory and neuropathic pain. Spinal microglia are activated after peripheral nerve injury and may release many bioactive

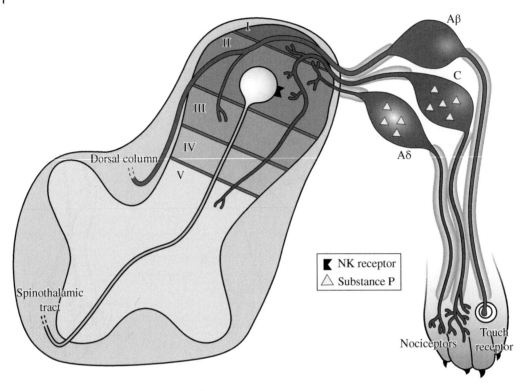

Figure 3.2 Normal transduction and transmission of touch (A-beta fibre) and nociception (A-delta and C fibres) to the dorsal horn. *Source:* [9]. Reproduced with permission of Elsevier. Refer to Chapter 2 for details.

molecules such as cytokines, chemikines and neurotrophic factors. An increased density of microglia has been reported in the ipsilateral dorsal horn laminae I to III following peroneal nerve ligation in mice. Anatomically, these areas are where primary sensory afferents innervating mechanoreceptors and nociceptors project. Also, biochemical changes along the neuronal sensory pathway may be an additional cause of microglia activation.

D. Endogenous Descending Facilitatory Systems [8]

Endogenous descending facilitatory systems, or facilitatory influences from the brainstem or forebrain, have been characterized. Descending facilitation reduces the neuronal threshold to nociceptive stimulation. One physiological function of descending facilitation is to enhance an animal's ability to detect potential danger signals in the environment. Descending facilitation is activated after injury, contributing to secondary hyperalgesia.The rostral ventromedial medulla (RVM) neurons undergo plastic changes during and after tissue injury and inflammation (**neuronal plasticity**).

E. Descending Inhibitory Pathway [9]

1. Opioid Receptor Function

In animals with neuropathic lesions, the activity of the inhibitory pathway is approximately 50% lower when compared to normal controls, with reduced opioid receptor function and efficacy of both intrathecal or intravenous (IV) administered morphine. Because descending inhibition normally acts as a spinal "gate" for sensory information, reduced inhibition increases the likelihood that the dorsal horn neuron will fire spontaneously or more energetically to primary afferent input. Of note, the decreased responsiveness to morphine could be prevented by pre-treatment of the animals with an N-methyl-D-aspartate (NMDA) receptor antagonist. These findings are explained by uncoupling of the m-opioid-receptor from a G-protein and/or changing opioid receptor-gated ion channel activity, both of which are processes that require phosphorylation at various intracellular sites including an NMDA-receptor.

2. Alpha₂ Adrenergic Receptor Function

In neuropathic pain, the descending noradrenergic inhibition, and increased sensitivity of spinal neurons to alpha₂ agonists, may occur with peripheral inflammation and nerve injury [2]. Norepinephrine is released in the spinal dorsal horn by descending noradrenergic axons, which mainly originate from the locus ceruleus (LC) and adjacent nuclei in the brainstem, and produces analgesia by stimulating alpha₂ adrenergic receptors [10]. Norepinephrine and, to a lesser extent, serotonin (5-HT) are major components of the endogenous descending pain inhibitory system [9, 10]. Chronic neuropathic pain may, in part, result from altered or reduced levels of endogenous norepinephrine and serotonin activity at both the spinal and the supraspinal levels [10].

3. The A-beta Fibre Mediated Inhibition and the GABA-Mediated Inhibition

The A-beta fibre mediated inhibition and the gamma-aminobutyric acid (GABA) mediated inhibition of pain transmission in the dorsal horn may also be disrupted [2, 11]. The loss of this activity may be within interneurons which ultimately release the "brake" on central sensitization of dorsal horn neurons. The loss of this inhibitory process may contribute to spontaneous pain, hyperalgesia or allodynia following nerve injury [5, 11].

F. To Summarize Neuropathic Pain

Neuropathic pain is a clinical syndrome of pain due to abnormal somatosensory processing in the peripheral or central nervous system and may include spontaneous pain, paresthesia, dysthesia, allodynia or hyperpathia. Neuropathic pain serves no beneficial purpose to the animal and can be regarded as a disease in itself. The pathophysiology of neuropathic pain is complex and incompletely understood. There are three pivotal phenomena intrinsic to the development of neuropathic pain:

- **Central sensitization**, i.e. the process of "windup" and the resulting transcriptional changes in dorsal horn neurons leading to altered synaptic neurotransmitter levels and number of receptors.
- **Central disinhibition**, i.e. an imbalance between the excitatory and inhibitory side of the nervous system.
- **Phenotypic change of mechanoreceptive A-beta fibres** (light touching) to produce SP so that input from them is perceived as pain.

II. Clinical Relevance of Physiology to Pharmacology

Refer to Chapters 9, 10 and 12 for discussion, dosing and warnings, for the following.

A. Opioids/Opiates

Opioids/opiates bind to opioid receptors both peripherally and centrally. Peripherally, they prevent neurotransmitter release and nociceptor sensitization, especially in inflammatory tissue. Centrally, opioids modulate afferent input into the substantia gelatinosa of the dorsal horn where the C fibres terminate, as well as in cortical areas which blunt the perception of pain [12]. As opioids have a specific effect on C fibre input and not A-beta fibres, where tactile allodynia (A-beta stimulus) is a component of the pain syndrome, opioids may not be beneficial. Therefore, the effectiveness of the opioids is dependent on the underlying mechanism causing the pain. In addition, opioid receptor function and efficacy is decreased in the central inhibitory pathway in neuropathic pain. Based on this, methadone is probably the preferred opioid to manage neuropathic pain in the acute setting because, in addition to the opioid analgesic properties, it is also an NMDA receptor antagonist, uncoupling the opioid receptor blocking effect, and a serotonin re-uptake inhibitor [13]. Oral methadone is not effective in dogs.

B. Tricyclic Antidepressant Analgesic (TCA) Effects

TCA effects are through multiple mechanisms: NMDA antagonism, voltage-gated sodium channel blockade, enhance the activity of adenosine and GABA receptors, anti-inflammatory effects and inhibition of serotonin and norepinephrine reuptake enhancing adrenergic transmission resulting in sustained activation of the descending pain inhibitory pathway [11]. Based on the safety profile of amitriptyline reported in the human literature, and the TCA most consistently reported to produce analgesic effects in humans with neuropathic pain, it is also recommended for some veterinary patients [14]. (Refer to Chapter 12 for further details on the TCAs to avoid toxicity with dug combinations.)

C. Gabapentin

Gabapentin activates the descending noradrenergic system as measured by increasing cerebrospinal fluid (CSF) norepinephrine levels [15, 16]. The analgesic effect is due to gabapentin's ability to bind with the high affinity alpha$_2$ delta subunits of voltage-dependent calcium channels, blocking calcium currents both at the spinal and supraspinal level and blocking maintenance of spinal cord central sensitization [15, 16].These findings indicate the responsiveness of the noradrenergic inhibitory system in neuropathic and chronic pain; however, this effect does not appear to be present where chronic pain is not established [17]. However, gabapentin has been shown to be effective in certain acute pain situations.

D. NMDA Receptor Antagonists

The NMDA receptor is located on post-synaptic neurons in the dorsal horn. It has various binding sites that regulate its activity, which include glutamate, magnesium, glycine and polyamine binding sites. Nerve injury causes an increase in spinal glutamate, which opens the NMDA ionophore channel causing an influx of calcium resulting in a cascade effect leading to spinal windup. The channel may be blocked by NMDA receptor antagonists, such as ketamine [13] and amantadine. In animal models of neuropathic pain, both the allodynic and hyperalgesic state were sensitive to NMDA receptor antagonists.

1. Ketamine
Ketamine is a non-competitive NMDA antagonist. This property may minimize neuronal cell death caused by trauma, hypoxia or ischemia. Where inflammation is a major component of ongoing pain, ketamine's anti-pro-inflammatory effects, preventing exacerbation of inflammation and modulating inflammation when already initiated, can be an added benefit.

2. Amantadine

Amantadine is an NMDA antagonist through stabilizing the NMDA channels in the closed state, as opposed to ketamine's action, which blocks the channels, thus conferring its safety profile [18]. Amantadine may not be an effective analgesic when used alone, but it confers a synergistic effect when administered in combination with an opioid, nonsteroidal anti-inflammatory drug (NSAIA) or gabapentin/pregabalin. It can be incorporated into a chronic pain management regimen [19] or, where acute or chronic neuropathic pain exists/is suspected, can be introduced during weaning of ketamine in the acute setting in preparation for discharge home with other analgesics, such as an NSAIA and/or gabapentin.

E. Local Anesthetics

Sodium channels are responsible for the voltage-dependent sodium flux that serves to depolarize the excitable membrane. In a neuroma formed after nerve injury, there is an upregulation of distinct types of tetrodotoxin-insensitive (or tetrodotoxin-resistant (TTX-R)) sodium channels, including C-afferent neurons and small diameter dorsal root ganglion neurons, which may serve as ectopic generator sites. This channel is blocked by local anesthetic agents at plasma concentrations that do not produce an afferent conduction block [20]. The TTX-sensitive (TTX-S) sodium channels are preferentially expressed in large and medium dorsal root ganglion neurons and are reported to be four times more sensitive than TTX-R sodium channels to lidocaine therapy. Systemically administered lidocaine has been shown to be effective in the treatment of several neuropathic pain disorders. When administered systemically, at doses that do not produce anesthesia or slow cardiac conduction, lidocaine provides analgesia separate from the direct local anesthetic properties by blocking the ectopic afferent neural activity at the NMDA receptor within the dorsal horn [13]. Several veterinary studies have shown the benefit of lidocaine infusions during anesthesia in dogs [21]. No veterinary studies have evaluated lidocaine's analgesic efficacy when used alone in neuropathic pain states; however, when added to a multi-modal regimen, the author has noted patient improvement. Infusions of lidocaine have led to a significant improvement in human patients experiencing chronic neuropathic pain [22]. Based on the different sensitivity of lidocaine on the TTX-R and TTX-S sodium channels, the response to lidocaine therapy varies depending on the neural lesion and sodium channel involvement [20]. In human medicine, patients report that the pain associated with spontaneous ectopic discharges seems to be responsive to lidocaine therapy in most instances; however, this type of pain may also be mediated by alpha-adrenergic receptor sensitization, which may not respond to lidocaine [22]. Also, not all neuropathic pain symptoms in humans include ectopic discharges; therefore, this type of pain may respond differently to lidocaine therapy [22]. The clinical importance of this is that, when neuropathic pain is suspected in dogs and cats, lack of lidocaine responsiveness should not be interpreted as the non-existence of neuropathic pain but that the underlying mechanism is not primarily involving the TTX-S sodium channel. Lidocaine infusions have been evaluated in cats with no apparent benefit when used alone [23]. However, a multi-modal assessment has not been reported. Caution is advised as, depending on dosage, they can be associated with adverse effects in this species [23]. (Refer to Chapter 12 for details.)

F. Alpha$_2$ Adrenergic (Alpha$_2$) Agonists

Alpha$_2$ agonists, medetomidine and dexmedetomidine, function in the inhibitory pathway by binding receptors in the LC which receives efferent noradrenergic axons from the periaqueductal gray matter (PAG); the noradrenergic axons then extend to the spinal cord. Activation in the LC appears to indirectly contribute to analgesia at the level of the dorsal horn through these descending projections [24]. The alpha$_2$ receptor is coupled through G-proteins to hyperpolarize spinal projection neurons and to inhibit transmitter release from small primary afferents. Spinally administered alpha$_2$ agonists have been shown to reverse the dysesthetic and allodynic components of pain states observed after peripheral nerve injury in rats and humans. Medetomidine and dexmedetomidine have been used as a continuous rate infusion (CRI) in dogs [25].

G. Nonsteroidal Anti-Inflammatory Analgesics (NSAIAs)

NSAIAs act peripherally at sites of inflammation but also have a direct spinal cord action by blocking hyperalgesia induced by the activation of spinal glutamate and SP receptors [26]. Spinal prostanoids are thus critical for the augmentation of pain processing at the spinal cord level [26]. The proposed mechanism is that the CNS injury increases COX-2 expression. Prolonged elevation of COX-2 contributes to inflammation, programmed cell death, free radical-mediated tissue damage and alterations in cellular metabolism. The action of COX-2 inhibitors decreases synthesis of prostanoids and free radicals. However, because of this dominant metabolic reaction, COX-2 inhibition results in shunting arachidonic acid away from the cyclooxygenase pathway down alternative enzymatic pathways (e.g. cytochrome P450 epoxygenases), resulting in the synthesis of potentially neuroprotective eicosanoids [27]. The author of this study proposes that COX-2 inhibition blocks delayed cell death and neuroinflammation. Of interest, inhibition of cyclooxygenase -2 (COX-2) has been shown to benefit recovery after injury to the brain or spinal cord in laboratory animals [27]. Inhibition of COX-1 may also be of benefit as COX-1 also plays an important role in spinal cord pain processing and sensitization after surgery and inflammation.

H. Acupuncture

There is a sound physiological mechanism for the analgesic effects of acupuncture [28]. Acupuncture is the stimulation of specific anatomic points in the body to produce therapeutic or analgesic effects. Placement of fine-gauge needles may decrease muscle spasms when inserted into trigger points. Placement of needles at specific acupuncture points can induce the release of a variety of neurotransmitters, which can affect the processing of sensory input, including blockade of C fibre input and amplification of the inhibitory system, as previously discussed (Gate Control theory of pain). Proper needle placement, with administration of various frequencies of electrical stimulation, releases endorphins, serotonin and norepinephrine. Another benefit of acupuncture therapy is, when performed in an aseptic manner, that there are no associated adverse effects such as those which may occur with any pharmaceutical agent. (Refer to Chapter 15.)

III. Diagnosing Neuropathic Pain

Commonly in veterinary medicine a major focus for assessing neurologic injury following surgery or trauma, or where a medical problem exists, is loss of motor and sensory function, or in certain illnesses, primarily a loss in motor function. In this setting, damage or disease of axons (axotomy) and/or myelin disrupts the ability to conduct nerve impulses, causing hypoesthesia and numbness (as described by humans), and potentially loss of motor function. However, testing for hyperalgesia and allodynia (see Box 3.1) should also be undertaken to identify the presence of this pathologic state (neuropathy) [29, 30]. As nerves are protoplasmic extensions of live cells, the neurons respond actively to injury – surgery, trauma and inflammatory states. The developing

---

Box 3.1 Simple tests for the assessment of stimulus-evoked neuropathic pain

---

The tests are performed on normal (uninjured) skin. The description of the sensation is included to give the reader an impression of what a cat and dog may also experience when tested. Tests using temperature or stroking stimuli would require a shaved area which could be performed once an area of involvement was identified using the pinprick or pressure tests.

Allodynia

- Manual light pressure of the skin
  - Normally non-painful but elicits a dull, burning pain in the affected area when compared to an unaffected area.
- Light manual pinprick with a sharpened wooden stick or stiff von Frey hair
  - Sharp superficial pain elicited in the affected area but not in the unaffected area.
- Stroking skin with a brush, gauze or cotton applicator
  - Sharp, burning, superficial pain in affected area but not in the unaffected area.
- Manual light pressure at the joints
  - Deep pain is elicited at the joints of the affected area but not in the unaffected area.
- Thermal cold
  - Contact of the skin with objects at 20 °C is painful, often burning, temperature sensation in affected area but not the unaffected area.
- Thermal warm
  - Contact of the skin with objects at 40 °C is a painful, burning temperature sensation in the affected area but not the unaffected area.

Hyperalgesia

- Manual pinprick of the skin with a safety pin
  - Sharp superficial pain normally painful but the stimulus produces a more exaggerated response in the affected area compared to the unaffected area.
- Thermal cold
  - Contact of the skin with coolants such as acetone or cold metal is normally painful, often a burning, temperature sensation, which produces a more exaggerated response on the affected area when compared to the unaffected area.
- Thermal heat
  - Contact the skin with objects at 46 °C.
  - Painful burning temperature sensation.
- Algometer
  - A-delta and C fibre activity arising from nociceptors and A-beta fibre activity arising from mechanoreceptors.
- The response is a lower threshold and tolerance, or suprathreshold, response to stimuli.

Source: Data adapted from [83] with permission of Wolters Kluwer Health.

---

pain is due to injury or disease that damages the axon or soma of sensory neurons or disrupts the myelin sheath that surrounds many axons (dysmyelination and demyelination); as a result, ectopic firing of these nerves tends to occur [30].

Based on the various branches from the sensory pathways to subcortical areas in the brain, the "emotional" aspects of pain, in addition to the sensation of pain, are experienced, which alters the animal's "personality". In addition to obvious signs of pain, a change in behaviour, such as "dullness" or occasional aggression, may also be noted by the owner. A comparison will be made to the human clinical and research setting as a potential resource for recognizing, diagnosing and treating neuropathic pain in veterinary patients. In the human setting, the diagnosis of neuropathic pain may be based solely on history and examination findings as judged by an experienced clinician. This requires five of eight features suggestive of neuropathic pain [29, 30]:

1. History consistent with nerve injury.
2. Pain within but not necessarily confined to an area of sensory deficit:
   - Detected on neurologic examination of the cat or dog where light touch is not perceived but hyperalgesia is produced with increasing, normally non-painful, test.
3. Pain in the absence of ongoing tissue damage
   - An area of pain or lameness localized on neurologic examination.
4. Character of pain: burning, pulsing, shooting, stabbing
   Identified in cats and dogs based on behaviour described by the owner:
   - Jumping from rest or walk.
   - Targeting/looking at a specific area but may not bite it, consistently the same area.
5. Paroxysmal or spontaneous pain
   Identified in cats and dogs based on behaviour described by the owner:
   - Spontaneously chewing the area affected.
6. Associated dysesthesias
   Identified in cats and dogs based on behaviour described by the owner and is frequently constant:
   - Chewing, biting at a specific area.
7. Allodynia, secondary hyperalgesia, hyperpathia.
   Based on behaviour described by the owner,
   - Vocalization, as severe pain frequently exists.
8. Associated autonomic features in dogs and cats are panting and increased heart rate.

Obviously, it is difficult to apply all these features to veterinary patients but a selected few can be applied. In addition, cats also manifest pain by progressive behavioural changes of hiding, inappropriate urination in addition to exhibiting specific behaviours of pain. The authors of one study believe that (1) clinical vigilance, with regard to history taking, where an "unexpected" level of pain is still present after the time course post-surgery or post-trauma, and (2) the sensory examination (Box 3.1) remain the key factors in the diagnosis of neuropathic pain in the acute setting [29, 30]. In addition to trauma-induced neuropathic pain, examples of human post-surgical neuropathic pain include gynecological surgery, inguinal hernia repair, laparotomy or thoracotomy and those with ischemic limbs following vascular surgery. Other examples include post-intercostal catheter insertion, compartment syndrome secondary to coagulopathy, acute cancer pain, spinal abscess, vasculitis and others with no precipitating cause identified [29]. From the patient population identified with acute neuropathic pain in this study, we can definitely make the assumption that there is the potential for this to occur in veterinary patients. Case examples can be found in Chapter 8 (Figure 8.9) and Chapter 32 (Figure 32.2).

Neuropathic pain scales are published in human medicine. The Neuropathic Pain Scale and the LANSS Pain Scale are utilized in human medicine in attempts to gain greater precision in the description and diagnosis of neuropathic pain. Where chronic neuropathic pain is experienced, these scales are valuable in localizing the lesion based on history of illness or injury and descriptions of pain experienced. As the descriptions (dull, aching, burning vs sharp, lancinating, etc.) are used to diagnose the type of neuropathic pain in humans, these scales are of no value in veterinary patients. However, client observation of behaviour may identify the sharp, lancinating, ectopic firing pain; however, this may also coexist with constant dull, burning and aching pain.

In veterinary medicine, pain severity and precise localization can be difficult to assess [31]. However, with recent history, physical examination with attention to detail and experience, pain assessment can be made in the majority of cases. Chronic neuropathic pain, however, may be difficult to suspect because the presenting signs may be subtle and client observations may be vague. Therefore, in the acute setting, there is the possibility of an acute-on-chronic problem. A veterinary study investigating the prevalence and characteristics of pain among dogs and cats examined as outpatients at a veterinary teaching hospital identified a slightly higher prevalence of neuropathic pain (dogs, 8%; cats, 7%) than occurs in humans [32]. In this study a total of 1153 dogs and 652 cats were examined as outpatients at the Ohio State University Teaching Hospital during 2002. Of these, 231 (20%) dogs and 92 (14%) cats had evidence of pain. The characteristics of pain were recorded from the examination of these patients. The categories of pain were:

- **Inflammatory pain** considered to be initiated by chemical inflammatory mediators released by tissue damage).
- **Neuropathic pain** defined as pain caused, or initiated, by a primary lesion or dysfunction in the peripheral or central nervous system. Pain was then further categorized as:
  1. **Primary hyperalgesia** (peripheral sensitization) was considered to exist when the animal responded adversely to light touch directly on the area of the body from which the pain originated (i.e. the area of primary hyperalgesia).
  2. **Secondary hyperalgesia** (central sensitization) was considered to exist when the animal responded adversely to a light touch to an uninjured area surrounding the area of primary hyperalgesia.
  3. **Allodynia** (pain elicited from non-injured tissues by non-noxious stimuli) was considered to exist when the animal responded adversely to a light touch applied to normal (non-injured) tissues distant from the area of primary hyperalgesia.
  4. **Hyposensitivity** (an apparently reduced pain response when pain would have been expected to be present because of a tissue or nerve injury) was considered to exist when a dog or cat with obvious tissue or nerve damage demonstrated reduced or no signs of pain during physical examination.

Some conditions are well known to cause neuropathic pain in cats and dogs (see Section IV), but the major challenge is the recognition of the not-so-well-known, or previously unreported, conditions that cause neuropathic pain. In addition to history taking and neurologic examination, electrodiagnostic methods are available for veterinary patients

IV.   Neuropathic Pain Associated Conditions

A.   Neuropathic Pain Associated with Trauma: Accidental and Surgical

1.   Intraoperative Considerations for the Prevention of Neuropathic Pain
Specific details are described for surgical procedures on peripheral nerves in veterinary surgical texts. Neural tissue at the surgical site should be identified and handled with care; however, there often is not the same emphasis for many surgical procedures where neural tissue may be inadvertently incorporated in the surgical procedure. As nerve ligation is a model for the study of neuropathic pain, it may be prudent to identify neural tissue and ensure that this is not incorporated in ligatures at any surgical site to prevent the potential for development of neuropathic pain that may be difficult to identify and treat at a later date. Should transection or excessive manipulation or traction of neural tissue be necessary, application of lidocaine 2% to neural tissue at least five minutes prior to handling (then dissect away from neural tissue) is recommended to reduce the painful experience upon recovery. Lidocaine confers its effect earlier than bupivacaine;

however, where time permits, bupivacaine 0.5% may be preferred due to its having a longer duration of effect. Overall, gentle handling of tissue to reduce the inflammatory response is essential.

2. Inguinal Hernia Repair

Inguinal hernia repair is a relatively common procedure in veterinary medicine. The potential for nerve injury during the repair may be similar to that for human patients. Three distinct chronic pains were identified in a human male study. The most common and most severe pain was somatic, localized to the common ligamentous insertion to the pubic tubercle. The second and third were visceral and ejaculatory pain. Some patients had post-operative numbness at 2 years, which was most common in the distribution of cutaneous branches of the ilioinguinal and iliohypogastric nerves [33]. Again, an association of numbness and pain may occur in veterinary patients, and such assessment would be beneficial during follow-up examination.

3. Pelvic Fractures

A high incidence of chronic pain was present in a follow-up study of human patients at a median of 5.6 years after pelvic fracture repair [34]. Most of these patients had a combination of somatic nociceptive, visceral nociceptive and neuropathic pain. While assessing complications associated with motor function in veterinary patients, it is recommended to perform a sensory examination (see Box 3.1) or electrodiagnostics to identify the potential of established neuropathic pain to be a cause of, or be coexistent with, motor deficits. Pelvic fractures and repair may result in:

- injury to the femoral nerve with notable lameness;
- injury to the cauda equina within the lumbosacral canal and is composed of the:
  o seventh lumbar (L7) nerve,
  o the sacral nerve roots,
  o coccygeal nerve roots.

Injury of these roots causes deficits of sciatic, pudendal, pelvic, perineal and caudal rectal nerve function.

Motor dysfunction is readily recognized in these injuries in veterinary patients.

Sensory dysfunction, such as subtle hypoesthesia (which may reflect hyperalgesia depending on the stimulus) or hyperesthesia, must consistently be evaluated. Careful observation of the specific area being "attacked" by the patient is essential as this may suggest the presence of either persistent or intermittent neuropathic pain.

4. Pudendal Nerve Entrapment

Pudendal nerve entrapment is a potential problem following perineal hernia repair or pelvic/sacral trauma. The injury may happen during trauma/surgical procedure, or at some later point should the nerve become entrapped in a post-surgical/traumatic fibrous scar. Pudendal nerve entrapment in humans is a cause for chronic, disabling perineal pain (ano-rectal, urogenital, especially when sitting), urinary hesitancy, frequency, urgency, constipation/painful bowel movements and sexual dysfunction in both sexes [35]. The diagnosis of pudendal nerve entrapment was based on clinical factors, neurophysiologic studies and response to pudendal nerve infiltrations. Human patients, refractory to conservative management, underwent surgical decompression with 60% responding measured by a > 50% reduction in visual analogue score (VAS), a > 50% improvement in global assessment of pain or a > 50% improvement in function and quality of life [35]. Pudendal nerve entrapment may be suspected in dogs and cats:

- where there is a historical event compatible with an entrapment;
- where the owner describes similar findings to those occurring in humans;
- if constant licking occurs at a site subserved by the pudendal nerve;
- if pain can be elicited on rectal or vaginal examination, lifting of the tail or when forced to sit.

Also:

- Pain on rectal examination can commonly be elicited in dogs with cauda equina syndrome (see Section IV.A.3 and IV.B).
- Electrodiagnostic testing would be a valuable tool to confirm clinical suspicion.

5. Limb Nerve Entrapment

Iatrogenic nerve entrapment is a complication of surgical limb procedures, but notably during limb fracture repair. A case report describing neuropathic pain in a cat after sciatic nerve entrapment during femoral fracture repair [36] is discussed to demonstrate the importance of lesion localization and underscores the importance of vigilance and awareness required to recognize this complication. The day after fracture repair, deep pain was absent in this cat, but severe pain was present on manipulation of the coxofemoral joint. Corticosteroid therapy was instituted for 48 h with no improvement. Hind limb amputation was performed because of lack of function. At 38 days after amputation, the cat was presented again because of continually progressive behavioural changes of hiding, inappropriate urination and shaking of the stump. This was treated as a primary urinary tract problem; in addition, amitriptyline was prescribed. The urinary clinical signs did improve; however, shaking of the stump and difficulty in walking and standing gradually worsened. On repeat presentation at 60 days after amputation, pain could not be elicited at the hip joint or stump of this cat; however, neuropathic pain was suspected. Treatment with morphine, lidocaine and ketamine was instituted until the signs of pain resolved. The duration of treatment was 37 h: ramping up to effect over 18 h, with a gradual reduction during the remaining 19 h (details given in the section on treatment using ketamine). After this, the cat seemed to be pain-free and was discharged home on amitriptyline at a dosage of 10 mg every 12 h for 21 days. At 10 months, the cat appeared to be free of pain [36]. This case illustrates the presence of neuropathic pain even when hypoesthesia was present and when there was evidence for central pain. Frequently, amputation is performed because of motor nerve injury; however, it is important to identify the exact level of the lesion to ensure that the nerve injury is relieved so as to prevent ongoing or potential future development of neuropathic pain. Another potential cause for nerve entrapment is that due to heterotopic calcification, otherwise known as "heterotopic osteochondrofibrosis", associated with hematoma formation at a site of trauma. Similar ossification due to injury, hematoma and unstable fractures may entrap a peripheral nerve potentially resulting in delayed neuropathic pain.

6. Amputation

Phantom limb pain is a known syndrome in human patients, but also may occur in veterinary patients. The cause may be due to peripheral sensitization as a result of spontaneous activity from sprouting regenerating nerve endings or neuroma formation (Figure 3.3) which gives rise to secondary changes in otherwise silenced small dorsal root ganglia cells, central sensitization or cortical reorganization [37]. There has been an association of severity of pre-amputation pain to post-amputation phantom pain. Prevention of phantom pain by pre-operative epidural analgesia and post-operative local anesthesia, however, resulted in variable responses. There appears to be no consistent, effective treatment. Many therapies – including surgical exploration, tricyclic antidepressants, sodium channel blockers, topical capsaicin and gabapentin, all used with efficacy in other neuropathic states – may be ineffective or unproven in controlled studies of phantom limb pain. Interestingly, neuropathic pain occurs in 60% of humans following limb amputation but usually not until one year post surgery. This highlights the ongoing changes occurring in the peripheral and central nervous systems established by a precipitating event prior to experiencing neuropathic pain in some patients and conditions. Phantom limb pain is rarely reported in veterinary medicine [36]. Potential clinical signs, other than those

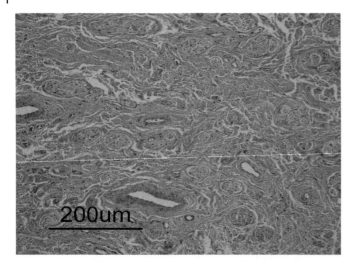

Figure 3.3 Neuroma at tail amputation site resulting in persistent abnormal behaviour which resolved with revision of the amputation site and removal of tail dock amputation site (Figure 3.4).

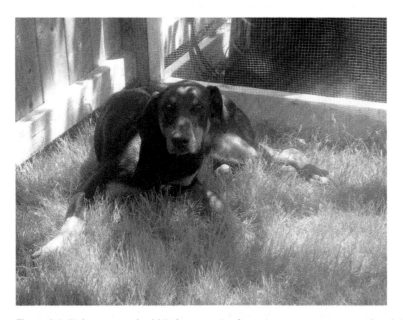

Figure 3.4 Eighteen-month-old Doberman pinscher prior to neuroma removal and after surrender to Humane Society. New owners noted a great difference following tail dock revision.

occurring in nerve entrapment noted above, may be chewing at the stump, intermittent unprovoked crying or "jumping up or away", indicating lancinating pain due to ectopic firing. This has been interpreted as a dog's "bad behaviour" resulting in surrender (Figure 3.4) or euthanasia. Following revision of the tail dock and removal of a neuroma (see Figure 3.3), the dog is now pain-free (Figure 3.5). Cosmetic surgery should be abolished in North America, as it is in the rest of the world, due to the lifetime suffering of many animals, and this injury induced by veterinarians is contrary to the Veterinarian's Oath.

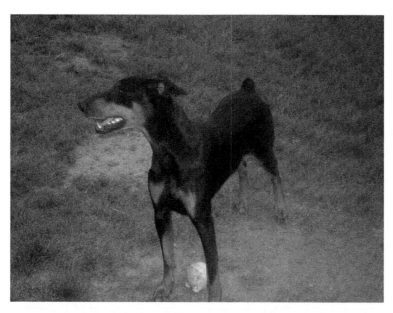

Figure 3.5 Doberman following revision of tail-dock site and removal of a neuroma.

B. Lumbosacral Lesions

A common cause for neuropathic pain in dogs is degenerative lumbosacral stenosis or cauda equina syndrome. Many other terms have been used to describe this syndrome, which is due to soft tissue and bony changes, possibly in conjunction with abnormal motion of the lumbosacral joint, impinging on the nerve roots or vasculature of the cauda equina [38]. There are many causes for lumbosacral lesions (degenerative lumbosacral stenosis, the most common disease of the cauda equina in large-breed dogs, idiopathic stenosis, discospondylitis, trauma, neoplasia, inflammatory disease, vascular compromise and congenital abnormalities) and are discussed in detail elsewhere [38]. A full description of the physical examination to identify subtle abnormalities is well described and beyond the scope of this chapter [38]. However, inclusion of a rectal examination and palpation of the lumbosacral joint with manipulation of the tail is one of many manoeuvres to include in the neurologic examination [38]. A thorough focused neurologic examination in dogs exhibiting signs of pain as described for humans with pudendal entrapment, dysesthesias or motor dysfunction secondary to sciatic or caudal rectal nerve compression is important as results of diagnostic imaging may be misleading. A study evaluating the severity of clinical signs (lumbosacral pain, paresis, lameness, urinary and fecal incontinence and dysesthesias) to severity of cauda equina compression using diagnostic imaging, revealed a lack of correlation [39]. While correlation of clinical signs and diagnostic imaging was poor, the authors recommend pursuing MRI as MRI is invaluable in accurately identifying the underlying disease process as well as giving the surgeon in-depth pre-operative knowledge of both site and extent of the lesion. In dogs with minimal MRI changes, the authors commented that cauda equina neuritis may be the cause of pain. Cauda equina neuritis has been described in dogs where marked interstitial and perivascular infiltration with mononuclear cells, axonal degeneration and demyelination were present [40].

C. Spinal Cord Injury

Spinal cord injury may be due to trauma, ischemia, hemorrhage or extradural compression (e.g. intervertebral disc extrusion; see C.1 below) resulting in persistent or intermittent somatic or visceral neuropathic pain. Several problem-based conditions discussed may also apply to lesions associated with spinal cord injury.

1. Intervertebral Disc Herniation/Extrusion

A common cause of neuropathic pain is intervertebral disc herniation/extrusion (IVDH/E). Dogs and cats are almost always painful upon presentation (or exhibit pain during the neurologic examination), some excruciatingly so. The occurrence of acute cervical disc extrusions occur at C2–C3, C3–C4 and C4–C5 in chondrodystrophic breeds, where C5–C6 and C6–C7 are the most common sites in large breed dogs. Signs of pain are low head and neck carriage, neck guarding, stilted and cautious gait, and spasms of cervical spinal muscles. Pain can also be identified if the animal is lame. Radicular pain (root signature or referred pain) is observed with impingement of nerve roots C5–C8. Pain may also be elicited during neurologic examination with manipulation of the affected limb. Surgical treatment is recommended as conservative management using corticosteroids, muscle relaxants and cage rest has a high recurrence rate [41]. The reason given for this is the presence of a large amount of disc material present in the spinal canal and difficulty with total immobilization of the cervical region. Based on the pathophysiology of neuropathic pain, and the experience of this for the individual, it would be inhumane not to adequately treat the patient with severe to excruciating pain. Surgical treatment is recommended in this situation to prevent further compromising neurologic function. However, the pain may not be relieved in some cases where extruded disc material is still present and impinging on nerve roots. Occasionally, re-exploration is required when the pain is excruciating and non-responsive to multi-modal analgesic therapy. Thoracolumbar IVH/E also results in pain and neurologic dysfunction of varying degree in both cats and dogs. Spinal hyperesthesia, kyphosis and reluctance to walk are obvious signs of pain and may occur without neurologic deficits in a percentage of cases. Despite the lack of motor neurologic dysfunction, these dogs can have substantial spinal cord compression, as seen on diagnostic imaging. Where surgery is not an option, for the most profoundly neurologic dogs, dexamethasone at 0.1 mg/kg IV then prednisone starting at 1 mg/kg, tapering the dose over 10–14 days. This treatment is based on an anti-inflammatory effect aiming to reduce vasogenic edema. The use of corticosteroids is not considered routine; however, the individual situation may indicate this therapy. A COX-2 preferential or selective NSAIA for the less neurologic and more stable dogs is recommended where corticosteroids have not been administered. If recurrence of clinical signs occurs following surgical treatment, it may be related to a second disc extrusion, cicatrix formation at the previous surgery site or hyperesthesia resulting from surgical manipulation, residual hemorrhage or disc material. As with cervical disc disease, pain management is extremely important to avoid continuing acute pain and establishment of chronic neuropathic pain. The reader is referred to Coates [41] for a review of conservative versus surgical treatment and recurrence rates of thoracolumbar IVDD. Electroacupuncture, reported by Joaquim [42], and anecdotal reports, is another modality to consider as this can be as effective as decompressive surgery for recovery of ambulation and improvement in neurologic deficits in dogs with long-standing severe deficits attributable to thoracolumbar IVDD. Thoracolumbar IVDD in cats does occur but at a much lower rate than dogs and is reported in both older and younger (<5 years of age) cats. Similar diagnostic and surgical techniques are recommended in cats as in dogs. (Refer to Chapter 15 for non-pharmacologic techniques and suggested readings.)

2. Fibrocartilaginous Embolic Myelopathy (FCEM)

FCEM is noted to be painful upon acute disc extrusion as the owners note a yelp followed by the neurologic deficits. Pain may also be elicited upon presentation, but pain abruptly subsides in most dogs. The reader is referred to da Costa [43] for further information on this topic. Rarely, dogs with FCEM remain extremely painful for several days requiring constant analgesic administration titrated to effect (personal observation). This may be due to secondary hemorrhage or release of vasoactive substances at the site of ischemia.

3. Discospondylitis and Vertebral Osteomyelitis

Discospondylitis and vertebral osteomyelitis are most commonly reported in medium- to large-breed dogs, but may occur in any dog or cat. The most common presenting sign is mild to severe spinal pain. This may or may not be associated with neurologic deficits or fever [44]. As any bacterial, or fungal, organism may be the etiologic agent, a definitive diagnosis should be attempted with culture and sensitivity performed on both aspirates from the affected area and blood cultures. As the diagnostic yield from blood cultures in veterinary medicine in general is low, aspirates from the lesion are recommended. Cytological examination of the aspirate should be performed immediately as an aid in selection of empirical therapy prior to receiving the antibiogram, which may take several days. Suggested antimicrobial drugs can be found in Thomas (p. 180) [44].

4. Vascular Innervation as a Cause of Spinal Pain

Myelinated fibres of spinal cord blood vessels in dogs and cats may function in sensory innervation. It may be that the innervation of blood vessels shares pathways with nerves supplying other structures in the bony vertebral canal and also contribute to pain development in this area [45].

D. Potential Sources of Neck and Back Pain in Cats and Dogs

The above are examples of the more common clinical conditions causing neuropathic neck and back pain in cats and dogs. However, there are several others that should be considered. The reader is referred to Webb for a review on this topic [46].

V. Primary Lesions of the Peripheral or central Nervous System

A. Peripheral Nervous System

1. Polyradiculoneuritis

Polyradiculoneuritis is most commonly associated with motor nerve and ventral nerve root, and ventral horn motor dysfunction, although a milder but significant dorsal nerve root and dorsal root ganglial inflammation can result in hyperesthesia with touch and manipulation. This is made worse by the fact that the animal cannot withdraw from the stimulus. Electrophysiologic studies in dogs with acute polyradiculoneuritis did reveal a sensory dysfunction in some affected dogs [47]. Physiotherapy, a recommended management for these dogs, can be extremely uncomfortable. It is important for the caregiver to be cognizant of this when treating these patients and to consider adding some form of pain management based on severity of pain (based on Section II), especially in the first several days of the incident. Do not administer corticosteroids.

2. Malignant Peripheral Nerve Sheath Tumours (MPNSTs)

MPNSTs, previously called schwannomas or neurofibromas, are a primary cause of chronic neurogenic lameness in dogs and cats [48]. A fairly common, yet sometimes difficult, lesion to identify initially is a tumour involving the PNS. Where a source for limb pain and lameness cannot be identified in either the thoracic or the pelvic limbs, an MPNST should be considered. Ultrasonographic examination and fine-needle aspirate (US-FNA) of an identifiable mass are frequently diagnostic and complementary to CT and MRI, which allow evaluation of proximal nerve structures and the spinal cord. Where limb dysfunction occurs, potentially due to both motor and sensory dysfunction (hyperesthesia or hypoesthesia), and amputation is the suggested treatment, it is essential that the primary lesion also be removed. This may require a hemilaminectomy should the tumour extend into, or beyond, the proximal nerve roots. Leaving the tumour will continue to cause chronic pain, and result in an extremely poor quality of life. Masses within subcutaneous tissue and within muscle with local invasion of neural tissue can present similarly to nerve sheath tumours. There are many other neurologic conditions causing lameness in dogs and cats, a discussion of which is beyond the scope of this chapter; however, the reader is referred to a review on the topic in McDonnell *et al.* [48].

3. Diabetic Neuropathy

Diabetes mellitus is a well-recognized cause of neuropathic pain in humans. Both dogs and cats also can develop a neuropathy associated with this endocrinopathy, although cats have a much more dramatic clinical presentation when compared to dogs, whose neuropathy is often sub-clinical. Despite the subclinical nature of canine diabetic neuropathy, peripheral sensory nerve conduction slowing has been identified. The small number of early reports of diabetic-associated neuropathy in cats concentrated on the clinically obvious motor dysfunction, consisting of a palmigrade and plantigrade stance and gait and a generalized weakness, with no mention of peripheral sensory abnormalities. However, an extensive electrophysiologic, biochemical and histological study performed on feline diabetic neuropathy definitively demonstrated equal involvement of both sensory and motor nerves in these cats, with the sensory dysfunction involving both the most proximal dorsal (sensory) nerve roots as well as the entire length of the peripheral sensory nerves in both the thoracic and pelvic limbs [49]. It is the presence of this sensory neuropathy and radiculopathy that may explain the observation that many cats with diabetes resent having their paws touched, reminiscent of people suffering from the "diabetic hand and foot" with diabetes [49]. Where these behaviours are observed in dogs or cats, a trial of amitriptyline is suggested to see whether behavioural patterns improve.

B. Central Pain Syndrome

The examples of central pain presented here highlight the importance of history taking with respect to either obvious or subtle changes in behaviour. Questions must be asked relating to potential behaviour elicited by the cat or dog, extrapolated from the human experience (crawling insects, itchiness, etc.), such as "scratching motion without touching the skin", continually biting or attacking an area on the body, frequently turning (looking) at the same area or yelping for no reason (lancinating pain). The physical and neurologic examination as well as the diagnostic modalities presented here can be considered for all patients with suspect central pain syndrome.

1. Tumours of the Central Nervous System

In humans, tumours involving pathways subserving somatic sensibilities of pain and temperature – such as the dorsal horn, spinothalamic, spinoreticular and spinomesencephalic tracts, and the cerebral cortex – can result in pain. The area of pain experienced is that which is subserved by the location and the pathway involving the neoplastic process. This is referred to as "central pain". In humans, the highest incidence of these tumours is within the spinal cord, lower brainstem and ventroposterior thalamus. Hemi-hyperesthesia and hyper-responsiveness resembling the central pain syndrome in humans has been reported in a dog with a forebrain oligodendroglioma [50]. This 4-year-old Boxer dog presented with alterations in behaviour, mentation and circling, but the most notable clinical finding was right-sided hemi-hyperesthesia and hyper-responsiveness. Exaggerated responses, such as flinching, jumping away from the stimulus and biting, were elicited by non-noxious stimuli, such as a light pinprick and pinching of the skin, applied to various areas on the right side of the body. The clinical impression was that the dog was experiencing a significant amount of pain during the examination. Similar stimuli applied to the left side did not elicit a response. While the lesion in this case was highly suspicious for a brain tumour due to the altered mentation and circling, the recognition of hyperesthesia required a careful and methodical examination. Spinal cord lesions causing central pain may be more subtle, non-specific and more difficult to diagnose unless a similar examination is performed. Primary vertebral neoplasia, or primary or metastatic neoplasia involving vertebrae, cause neck/back pain, which may be moderate to severe.

2. Congenital/Developmental Lesions

Chiari-like malformation with syringomyelia (also known as syringohydromyelia) is a cause for central pain syndrome associated with moderate to severe neuropathic pain in humans and dogs [51]. This appears to be a genetic disorder in Cavalier King Charles spaniels and is characterized by a mismatch between the caudal fossa volume and its contents (the cerebellum and caudal brainstem) [51]. Due to obstruction of normal cerebrospinal fluid movement through the foramen magnum via the normal outflow pathways, syringomyelia, a fluid-filled cavitation and dilation of the central canal within the spinal cord, results. The behaviour exhibited by affected dogs is suggestive of neuropathic pain, since it has the characteristics of allodynia, or dysesthesia. For example, dogs appear to dislike touch to certain areas of skin and may be unable to tolerate grooming or a neck collar. Signs may be unilateral, such as scratching on one side only, at rest and whilst walking, and often without making skin contact [51]. For details on diagnostic findings and therapeutic suggestions, the reader is referred to Rusbridge [51], Plessas [52] and Ortinau [53] for treatment outcomes. Another congenital lesion affecting the nervous system resulting in pain is cervical spondylomyelopathy (CSM), or wobbler syndrome, commonly seen in large- and giant-breed dogs; however, may also occur in chondrodystrophic breeds. CSM is characterized by compression of the spinal cord and/or nerve roots, which leads to neurologic signs and/or severe neck pain.

3. Meningitis, Arteritis and Vasculitis

Vasculitis associated with the meninges and spinal cord can be a cause for central pain. The recommended diagnostic tests, however, differ from the above due to the inflammatory nature of these diseases. Vasculitis has been identified as a cause of neuropathic pain in Beagle dogs, and has been termed "Beagle pain syndrome". This pain syndrome associated with a generalized vasculitis, perivasculitis and vascular thrombosis. The small- to medium-sized muscular arteries in many organs, including the cervical meninges, are consistently involved. The clinical signs, laboratory abnormalities and vascular lesions suggest that the condition is immune-mediated. There are many diseases that produce inflammation of the meninges, especially involving the cervical region, resulting in a varying severity of cervical pain. These include granulomatous meningoencephalomyelitis (GME), aseptic meningitis and breed-associated aseptic meningitis seen in such breeds as the Bernese mountain dog.

VI. Neuropathic Pain and Management of Visceral Origin

This is discussed in Chapters 29 and 30.

VII. Treatment

Neuropathic pain cannot be adequately managed with a single pharmacologic class unless tapering from a multi-modal regimen. Severe pain requires several classes of medications and procedures. A report on pain management in the trauma patient reported that with aggressive pain management the military has decreased acute and chronic pain conditions [13]. The individual medications discussed here are intended to be administered in conjunction with those from a different class to block the various mechanisms involved in sensory transmission. Prior to, and often during, any surgical procedure, various different analgesics and analgesic modalities can be used to reduce the inciting nociceptive afferent impulse. Many of these can be continued post-operatively to reduce both peripheral and central sensitization (see Section II, and Chapter 12, 14 and 15).

Pain management must be based on the complexity of neuropathic pain, and considered throughout the hospital stay. An individual plan should be formulated based on severity of injury, invasiveness of the surgical procedure (controlled injury), the anatomical area of surgery (assumed descending order of discomfort: oral cavity, rectum/vagina/testicles/penis, thorax, abdomen, limbs) the definite, or potential, involvement of neural tissue and pain experienced pre-operatively.

A. Acute Pain Management

1. Opioids/Opiates

As previously mentioned, opioid receptors in the descending pathway may be reduced or inactivated in neuropathic pain; therefore, opioid efficacy is inadequate when used alone but will contribute to some degree of analgesia in a multi-modal regimen. Of interest, the closer the nervous system lesion is to the CNS, the less effective the opiates are [54]. For example, peripheral nerve injuries tend to respond better to opioid therapy than nerve root injuries, which respond better than spinal cord injuries [54]. Because neuropathic pain is not as responsive as non-neuropathic conditions to opioids, titration of the dose to effect, while avoiding side effects, is suggested. Notable side effects in dogs and cats are dysphoria, panting, inappropriate antidiuretic hormone secretion with oliguria and edema, urinary retention, nausea and vomiting, inability to ambulate, ileus and respiratory depression, as a very infrequent finding. Should pain appear to worsen with increasing doses of an opioid, opioid-induced hyperalgesia (OIH) should be considered [55]. Ketamine administration will reverse OIH but requires titration to effect as high dosages may be required.

i. *Fentanyl, morphine, methadone and hydromorphone*

Frequently used systemic opioids are fentanyl, morphine, methadone and hydromorphone. It has been recommended that should side effects occur, switching to another opioid is recommended, as higher dosages may be better tolerated in any individual given a different opioid [54]. Fentanyl and methadone appear to have fewer side effects than morphine and hydromorphone at higher dosages, especially in cats. Methadone also has SRI activity and NMDA receptor antagonism, which is beneficial in neuropathic pain. The shorter half-life of fentanyl also makes it the best choice in patients with CNS pain, as withdrawal for assessment is more easily planned.

With the understanding that opioids may be ineffectual in some neuropathic pain states, it may be unwise to increase the dose to that which results in noticeable side effects. With the understanding that opioids may be ineffectual in some neuropathic pain states, it is unwise to increase the dose to that which results in noticeable side effects, such as nausea and vomiting, which will raise intracranial pressure (ICP) and therefore, be of concern in head-injured patients. Cortical depression may mask signs associated with increasing ICP and delay treating for this. Also, peripheral neurologic signs may appear to be worse as bladder emptying, and limb motion beyond the area of spinal injury, is significantly decreased with opioid use. As an example, the author has noted continual lack of voluntary bladder emptying in cats with sacrococcygeal injuries while receiving an opioid. With a 1 mL/min titration of diluted naloxone (0.1 mL (0.4 mg/mL naloxone) diluted in 5 mL saline) to ensure that analgesia is not totally reversed, while gently palpating the urinary bladder to initiate voluntary micturition, it is possible to reverse the inhibitory effects of the opioid on detrusor function should this be a factor. While urinary catheter placement is frequently required in these patients, testing bladder function is required for prognostication. Therefore, reversal of opioid effects is essential prior to informing the client of a potential bad prognosis that may result in euthanasia. Detrusor dysfunction may occur following systemic or epidural use of opioids, regardless of cause of pain, but usually in the post-operative setting where high dosages may have been used intraoperatively. The author uses the naloxone titration technique to reverse side effects of opioids, especially if the patient is dysphoric or vomiting. Where detrusor dysfunction is suspected, gentle compression of the bladder during naloxone titration, as above, until voiding occurs, avoids an excessive dose of naloxone where analgesia is still required. The above mixture of naloxone is used for small dogs and for larger dogs a mixture of 0.25 mL naloxone (0.4 mg/mL) diluted in 10 mL saline is used for titration. Once the side effects are reversed, and a "pleasant" state of rest is achieved, or the patient is aware and can respond during the neurologic assessment, titration is halted. A frustrating situation for both criticalists and neurologists is the requirement for withdrawal from analgesics prior to neurologic examination. It is suggested that an appointment be made, which is strictly adhered to, for the neurologic assessment so withdrawal of the analgesics can be planned and, therefore, long periods of time where the patient is without analgesic therapy can be avoided.

Opioids alone are not recommended for neuropathic pain, but if prescribed, and should pain appear to worsen with increasing doses, OIH should be considered [55]. This has rarely been observed by the author and managed by titration of ketamine to effect, which resulted in analgesia and sleep. Evidence suggests a role for COX-2 inhibitors in the modulation of OIH in humans; however, while OIH is modulated by COX-2 activity, it probably has a less important role than the NMDA receptor system [55]. Evidence in human patients suggests that opioid tolerance and OIH does occur acutely and within one month of continuing opioid use. This is a point to consider in veterinary patients as there may be the potential for opioid tolerance to occur and, therefore, it should not necessarily be interpreted as a worsening of the underlying condition. A recent review identified OIH to occur in rats, mice and humans, following acute or chronic opioid administration [55].

ii. Tramadol

There are no reports in the veterinary literature assessing the efficacy of tramadol in neuropathic pain. Based on lack of efficacy for managing severe pain, which neuropathic pain is, tramadol should not be prescribed (collective anecdotal reports). Also with long-term use, where efficacy may be established for mild to moderate pain, the efficacy has been reported to decrease and also confirmed with pharmacokinetic studies [56]. In addition to lack of efficacy, common side effects associated with tramadol administration include sedation and dysphoria, especially in cats [56]. (Refer to Chapter 10.) It is also reported to decrease the seizure threshold in certain human patients. Due to its inhibitory effect on serotonin re-uptake, there may be some minor effect on pain; however, tramadol should not be used in patients that may have received monoamine oxidase inhibitors such as selegiline (Anipryl®) or in combination with other SRIs. (Refer to Chapter 12.) Tramadol has been reported to enhance NSAIA toxicity resulting in duodenal perforation in dogs when combined with an NSAIA [57].

2. N-Methyl-D-Aspartate (NMDA) Receptor Antagonists

i. *Ketamine*

In one study assessing the efficacy of ketamine (0.5 mg/kg IV as a bolus before surgery, 10 µg/kg/min during surgery, and 2 µg/kg/min for 18 h after surgery) for amputation pain, where neuropathic pain is certainly a concern, an improvement in post-operative pain scores was noted over a three-day duration when compared to an opioid-alone regimen [58]. It is the experience of the author that low doses of ketamine (<0.5 mg/kg IV loading dose and < 1.0 mg/kg/h CRI), even in combination with opiates, ±lidocaine, ±NSAIAs, are frequently inadequate to manage severe/excruciating pain in dogs and cats with multiple and massive bite wounds, severe pancreatitis, multiple orthopedic injuries/post-operative, and post-operative cauda equina syndrome or cervical disc herniation, as examples. Most of these cases have a component of neuropathic and inflammatory pain. As an example of a rare potential requirement, a dog with severe refractory cauda equina pain existing prior to surgical correction, which was worse immediately following surgery and with titration of morphine, required a titrated dose of ketamine to 4 mg/kg to manage the violent post-operative behaviour associated with neuropathic pain and potential OIH, where morphine was titrated to a high dose in an attempt to manage the severe neuropathic pain. This was followed by 4 mg/kg CRI (in combination with low-dose morphine) for several hours to maintain "sleep" overnight. The ketamine CRI was slowly reduced over 16 h in order to assess analgesic requirements and avoid the hyperalgesic state. Following this, the dog appeared comfortable and demonstrated normal behaviour and appetite on a reducing dose of morphine. Addition of an NSAIA would be recommended; however, it wasn't in this case because of a previous administration of corticosteroids.

Case Example

The 6 kg cat with neuropathic pain associated with hind limb amputation reported above [36], received medetomidine 100 µg, morphine 1.5 mg and ketamine 2 mg given intramuscularly. A CRI of Lactated Ringer's solution containing morphine (0.06 mg/mL), lidocaine (0.24 mg/mL) and ketamine (0.06 mg/mL) of solution was established. The initial infusion was started at 5 p.m. at 5 mL/h. This was increased to 11 mL/h the following morning at 8 a.m., increased to 18 mL/h at 9 a.m., increased further to 24 mL/h at 10 a.m. and then decreased at 11 a.m. to 11 mL/h, when the cat began to show signs of excessive sedation. The infusion was continued for a further 19 h for a total of 36 h. No adverse effects of lidocaine were noted; however, refer to Chapter 12 for cardiac and dosing cautions. Amitriptyline 10 mg PO q12h was continued for 21 days. This treatment led to resolution of the neuropathic pain the cat had experienced for 60 days post amputation [36]. Similar acute treatment strategies are reported in human patients with reflex sympathetic dystrophy.

When considering analgesic therapy, it is prudent to also be aware of potential adverse effects, especially in critically ill or traumatized patients. Reports in the literature have documented concerns for increased ICP with ketamine administration; however, this was documented in subjects where the PCO_2 was not controlled. Where PCO_2 was held constant within the normal range, an increased ICP did not occur during ketamine administration [59]. This highlights the importance of avoiding hypoventilation during pain management in patients with head trauma. It has also been shown that ketamine does not directly dilate cerebral vessels accompanied by an increased blood flow that may potentially increase ICP [59]. In fact, when combined with a benzodiazepine, ketamine attenuated the increasing ICP in patients with an already increased ICP. Ketamine demonstrated no adverse effects on cerebral hemodynamics in head trauma patients, and in fact reduced the ICP [60]. Neuroprotection is another potential benefit of ketamine administration as it is safe and, as a non-competitive inhibitor of the NMDA receptor, may protect against further ischemic and glutamate-induced injury while managing pain in a head-injured patient. This may minimize neuronal cell death caused by trauma, hypoxia or ischemia. As pain in head-injured dogs and cats can be difficult to manage, especially when there are other neurologic and orthopedic injuries, the addition of low-dose ketamine may be of benefit in a multi-modal analgesic regimen. However, beginning with a low dose initially with frequent assessment is required. While ketamine was found to be neuroprotective in animal models, it is also an inhibitor of the GABA receptor and may increase cerebral oxygen consumption at high-end ketamine dosages (>5 mg/kg), doses higher than recommended for analgesia. Co-administration of a GABA agonist (e.g. propofol) may decrease these effects if higher dosages of ketamine are required. Compared with analgesia/sedation with opioids, a greater cerebral perfusion pressure is maintained with ketamine sedation and the need for vasopressors is reduced.

Dosing

Ketamine 0.2–1.0 mg/kg, ideal body weight in the overweight/obese patient, titrated to effect, followed by the effective dose as an hourly CRI. Where severe pain/hyperalgesia is present, higher dosages will be required; therefore, titration to effect is necessary to deliver the appropriate dose. From experience, the hourly infusion based on the effective dose maintains an "effective" dose during the painful period. Slowly reduce the hourly rate when appropriate.

Ketamine has a relatively short elimination half-life (1–1.6 h); therefore, the analgesic effect of a single low dose will be short-lived requiring a CRI to maintain analgesia.

ii. Amantadine

Amantadine is an oral NMDA receptor antagonist with similar activity to that of ketamine and is not suitable for acute pain but mentioned here to be considered in patients receiving ketamine and the requirement for an NMDA receptor antagonist following discharge. In this setting, amantadine should be administered during ketamine weaning in preparation for discharge home. It can be incorporated into a chronic pain management regimen with an NSAIA and/or gabapentin. A human study reported amantadine accelerated the pace of functional recovery during active treatment in patients with post-traumatic disorders of consciousness; however, the rate of improvement decreased when treatment was discontinued at four weeks, indicating the need for slow weaning and potential long-term requirement [61].

Dosing

Based on pharmacokinetic studies 3–5 mg/kg, ideal body weight in the overweight/obese patient, q12h is recommended.

3. Sodium Channel Blockers

i. Lidocaine

Systemically administered low-dose lidocaine has been shown to be effective in the treatment of several neuropathic pain disorders including improvement in humans experiencing chronic neuropathic pain [62, 63]. Based on the different sensitivity of lidocaine on the TTX-R and TTX-S sodium channels, response to lidocaine therapy will vary depending on the neural lesion and sodium channel involvement [63]. In human medicine, patients report that the pain associated with spontaneous ectopic discharges appears to be responsive to lidocaine therapy in most instances; however, this type of pain may also be mediated by alpha-adrenergic receptor sensitization, which may not respond to lidocaine [63]. Also, not all neuropathic pain symptoms in humans are due to ectopic discharges; therefore, this type of pain may respond differently to lidocaine therapy [63]. The clinical importance of this is where neuropathic pain may be suspected in dogs and cats, lack of lidocaine responsiveness should not be interpreted as the non-existence of neuropathic pain but rather the underlying mechanism is not primarily involving the TTX-S sodium channel. Lidocaine infusions have been evaluated in healthy laboratory cats with no apparent benefit when used alone [64], and may be associated with adverse effects in this species when used at an anesthetic MAC reduction dose, which is much higher than an analgesic dose. (Refer to Chapter 12 for further guidance.)

Lidocaine may be useful in managing the head trauma patient during periods of increasing ICP, such as occurs during vomiting or "gagging". Lidocaine has been reported to lower ICP during endotracheal intubation. The author has used lidocaine 1 mg/kg bolus, to treat impending tentorial herniation and suggests a 1–2 mg/kg/h CRI, in some cases, to reduce the opioid requirement in this acute setting for the ensuing 24 h only.

Lidocaine has been shown to be **neuroprotective** following a cerebral ischemic event in laboratory animals by limiting the expansion of infarction. At doses recommended below, lidocaine attenuated neuronal apoptotic cell death in the penumbra and may potentially be a useful intervention for the prevention and treatment of ischemic cerebral injury which may occur during a particular intracranial surgical procedure or following traumatic brain injury (TBI) and cerebrovascular accident [65].

- Dogs – Awake: 1–2 mg/kg, IV (give over 2–5 min) followed by 1–2 mg/kg/h, ideal body weight in overweight/obese patients. The infusion dose should be reduced after 6–8 h for cases requiring prolonged infusions for pain control to avoid CNS side effects, nausea and vomiting, and the potential signs noted above in humans.
- Cats – awake: 0.25–0.5 mg/kg IV (give over 10 min) followed by CRI 0.25–0.5 mg/kg/h, ideal body weight in overweight/obese patients. Dosages up to 1 mg/kg/h may be considered where required. As there are no reports on this suggestion in cats, continuous ECG monitoring and assessment for nausea are required. Until multi-modal regimen studies including lidocaine produce demonstrable benefits, follow the ventricular tachycardia protocol for cats [66]. Discontinue after 6–8 h or sooner should adverse signs or no improvement be noted. (Refer to Chapter 12 for further guidance.)

ii. Lidocaine Dermal Patches

Lidocaine 5% dermal patches (Lidoderm™ patch, Endo pharmaceuticals) are frequently used in humans with neuropathic pain due to a variety of causes. The low systemic concentrations achieved by transdermal lidocaine application suggest that efficacy is achieved via block of peripheral rather than CNS sodium channels [67]. Successful results with application of this patch have been obtained in children suffering from intractable and disabling neuropathic pain which originated at, and around, the site of previous surgical procedures. These sites were identified at a nephrectomy scar, laminectomy scar, inguinal area scar from a cardiac catheterization procedure and laparotomy scar where surgical involvement of a nerve was suspected [67]. Worthy of note, is that these procedures, and many others where nerve entrapment may occur, are performed in cats and dogs. Pharmacokinetic studies of the lidocaine patch in dogs found that lidocaine peak levels occurred at 9.5–12 h after patch application, reached steady-state concentrations between 24 and 48 h and levels decreased dramatically at 60 h post application. Low plasma lidocaine concentrations remained for 6 h after patch removal [67]. No analgesic efficacy studies have been reported in dogs or cats.

iii. Tocainide, Mexiletine and Flecainide

These agents are analogues of lidocaine and have also been shown to relieve neuropathic pain in some human patients. Again, there are no veterinary reports on analgesic efficacy in dogs or cats with neuropathic pain; however, mexiletine is used chronically in dogs with cardiac arrhythmias.

4. Alpha$_2$ Receptor Agonists

Dexmedetomidine is the alpha$_2$ agonist currently used in small animal veterinary patients (refer to Chapter 9). Dexmedetomidine may be administered via several routes including the epidural, perineural, parenteral, alone or in combination with several other medications. As an example of its use in neuropathic pain in the dog, this author has administered medetomidine 1–3 µg/kg/h, in addition to low-dose fentanyl (3–4 µg/kg/h) and corticosteroids, for management of the severe pain associated with meningitis. Intra- and post-operative pain management for intervertebral disc herniation is another example for alpha$_2$ agonist administration to otherwise healthy dogs. The sedative effect outlasts the analgesic effect so patients may be painful while sedated, requiring frequent assessment. Muscle relaxation is also apparent with clinical doses. It should be noted that the MAP may increase by 10–20% and heart rate may decrease slightly with the CRI. A slight increase in arterial blood pressures may be preferred to hypotension in these cases. Human guidelines for TBI patients indicate that raising arterial pressure to maintain MAP above 80 mmHg is of benefit. Also, in human TBI and neurosurgical patients, dexmedetomidine did not raise ICP; in fact, it may offer cerebral protection by attenuation of global or focal ischemia [68]. Other important considerations are that it produced "cooperative sedation" allowing neurologic examination and was compatible with neurophysiological monitoring [69]. The alpha$_2$ agonists induce hyperglycemia at higher dosages; however, at the CRI doses given below this doesn't occur, or only minimally, in dogs and may be similar in cats. Human medicine guidelines for TBI propose to maintain blood glucose levels between 7.8 and 10 mmol/l (140–180 mg/dl) in the subgroup of patients vulnerable for brain injury [69]. Regardless of species, monitoring is important to ensure excessive hyperglycemia does not occur with or without alpha$_2$ agonist administration. The decision to use dexmedetomidine is at the discretion of the clinician. Always use the lowest effective dose.

- As an adjunct, dexmedetomidine 0.5–1 µg/kg, ideal body weight in overweight/obese patients is administered as a 15 min loading dose IV followed by 0.5–1 µg/kg/h CRI, conferring good analgesia with minimal cardiovascular effects at these doses and rates in stabilized patients.
- For difficult to physically manage stable painful animals, following the above loading dose, a CRI: 1–3 µg/kg/h combined with an opioid may be required.

5. Regional Analgesia

There are significant benefits to the use of regional analgesia, epidural analgesia or continuous peripheral nerve blocks (CPNB). Regional analgesia improved pain control, improved outcomes and produced greater satisfaction over systemic analgesia in human patients [13]. As an example, placement of a wound diffusion catheter into the surgical wound following amputation is highly recommended. For all regional analgesia/anesthesia techniques, refer to Chapter 14 for placement, dosing instructions and management to avoid potential adverse effects. While the benefits of local analgesia far outweigh the potential risks, these risk factors must also be considered. In human medicine the major risks for this technique are local anesthetic toxicity and nerve injury; however, phrenic nerve blockade, inadvertent epidural or subarachnoid spread, infection and hematoma have also been reported to occur infrequently [13].

6. Non-Steroidal Anti-Inflammatory Analgesics (NSAIAs)

The NSAIAs have been shown to be very effective analgesics for moderate to severe pain in both cats and dogs. However, no veterinary studies specifically assessing the efficacy of managing neuropathic pain have been reported. Where neuropathic pain is assumed to be present, such as with limb amputation and crushing injuries, the addition of a parenterally administered NSAIA to an opioid improves analgesia and pain scores compared to an opioid alone (unpublished data). It has been shown that NSAIAs are of benefit in CNS injury in laboratory animals. COX inhibitors also attenuate development of opioid tolerance in animals; however, the OIH modulation appears to have a less important role than that of the NMDA receptor system [55]. Prior to NSAIA therapy, the individual patient must be identified for potential adverse effects, and the absolute contraindication for co-administration with corticosteroids (refer to Chapter 11).

7. Gabapentin

Gabapentin has been recommended for acute post-operative pain in human patients where the most benefit appears to be where chronic pain is present [70, 71]. However, these studies indicate that perioperative administration of gabapentin to animals with nerve injury may reduce the potential establishment of, or ongoing, neuropathic pain. It is the author's observation that gabapentin has reduced the pain in dogs and cats suffering from refractory neuropathic pain secondary to cervical or thoracolumbar IVDD or pelvic trauma. Initially, gabapentin is administered in combination with an opioid and an NSAIA, but gradually these analgesics may be tapered and gabapentin remain as the sole method of analgesia. There is an extremely wide dose range for gabapentin and it should be given to effect. The dose-limiting side effect is usually sedation, which may be beneficial in the acute setting. See Section VII.B.2 for ongoing administration. Anecdotal evidence appears to indicate its value in managing acute, chronic and neuropathic pain in dogs and cats in a multi-modal regimen and continued as a sole analgesic. Follow-up assessment is essential to ensure it is effective and to manage the dose to avoid adverse effects. Conditions where gabapentin is indicated:

- In dogs and cats suffering from neuropathic pain secondary to cervical or thoracolumbar IVDD or pelvic trauma/surgery.
- The chronic neuropathic pain associated with feline onychectomy appears to be responsive to high dosages of gabapentin (Dr K. St. Denis, personal communication).
- A case report suggested that gabapentin produced desirable effects in managing traumatic and orthopedic pain in cats [72].
- Perioperative in addition to an opioid, ± an NSAIA, where neural tissue is involved or chronic pain/hyperalgesia is established prior to surgery.
- Following recovery from cardiopulmonary arrest, or seizures for animals that are extremely restless, disoriented, vocalizing and/or manic, the author has found gabapentin useful in treating these patients. Dosing to effect and resolution of these signs is the goal. Sedation in this instance is appropriate! Careful lowering of the drug is recommended.

Comments

As pain is an individual experience, as is the underlying cause, it is expected that pain experienced from direct involvement of neural tissue is extremely painful requiring a higher dosage of gabapentin initially than recommended for non-neural involvement. Clinical usage and experience with various scenarios, and pharmacokinetic studies, are assisting with recommendations for prescribing. As examples, a study of post limb amputation in dogs showed no benefit with a dose of gabapentin 5 mg/kg q12h for three days [73]. Another canine study examining efficacy of gabapentin 10 mg/kg q12h added to an opioid post-intervertebral disc surgery reported no detectable reduction in pain behaviour compared to the control group receiving opioid analgesia alone, although a trend to lower pain levels was present. With more information from pharmacokinetic studies, the dosing and frequency must be increased for the neuropathic pain associated with these conditions. However, a case series reported significant improvement with gabapentin 6.5 mg/kg q12h for long-term management of musculoskeletal pain, or following head trauma, in three cats [72]. These reports highlight the need for individual dosing based on the underlying cause of pain.

8. Acupuncture

As neuropathic pain is difficult to manage with pharmaceutical agents, there is a growing interest in the use of acupuncture as an adjunct to a multi-modal pharmaceutical regimen. For the past 12 years at least, the National Institute of Health has listed pain management as an indication for acupuncture therapy. Based on sound physiological evidence for the benefit of acupuncture in both acute and chronic pain states, acupuncture is highly recommended in the management of neuropathic pain. Acupuncture has more recently become a widely accepted treatment for pain in veterinary medicine. The relief of pain by acupuncture can be explained neurophysiologically and has a role in treatment for neuropathic pain (refer to Chapter 15).

B.   Chronic Neuropathic Pain Management

Any chronic pain condition can subsequently develop a neuropathic component due to the continual nociceptive barrage and subsequent maladaptive changes in the functioning of the nervous system. A common cause for this maladaptive pain condition is osteoarthritis, but any acute painful condition not appropriately managed, and not necessarily directly as a consequence of neural pathology, may establish as chronic neuropathic pain.

1. Amantadine

The only study reporting the chronic use of amantadine in the veterinary literature showed improved activity and lameness scores in refractory canine osteoarthritic pain when used in combination with meloxicam 0.2 mg/kg orally loading dose followed by 0.1 mg/kg orally q24h thereafter, compared to meloxicam (Metacam®, Boehringer-Ingelheim) alone [19]. The dose of amantadine used in this randomized, blinded, placebo-controlled study was 3–5 mg/kg orally q24h; however, based on recent pharmacokinetic studies, 3–5 mg/kg, ideal body weight in overweight/obese patients, orally q12h is suggested (refer to Chapter 12 for further details). This study gives hope to the potential benefit of amantadine in managing chronic neuropathic pain similar to that of ketamine in the acute pain setting.

2. Gabapentin

Frequently, some animals need several weeks to months for resolution of their pain, potentially requiring a lifetime of medication. Gabapentin as an adjunct, or as sole analgesic, is recommended where acute or chronic neuropathic pain exists. Frequently, two or more classes of analgesics are required, an NSAIA and gabapentin for example. When the pain is well managed for a period of time, introduce a slow reduction in the NSAIA with subsequent withdrawal where there is no regression. If gabapentin alone maintains the analgesic state, careful lowering of the drug dosage is recommended to assess ongoing dosing requirement. Where the q8h treatment is difficult for the owner, initially reducing, then eliminating, the middle dose is suggested to assess ongoing requirement. Otherwise, a small reduction in each dose is suggested.

As dosing to effect is the method by which the appropriate dose is selected, once this effect is reached, twice daily rather than three times daily treatment may suffice. Gabapentin is primarily eliminated unchanged by the kidneys in the cat with ~40% hepatic metabolism in dogs [56]. Dogs and cats with renal, or hepatic (dogs), insufficiency may require less frequent dosing due to slower elimination. Tapering of the dose is important, as stopping the drug abruptly will lead to rebound pain, which may be severe, should analgesia still be required.

Dosing

The author's method of dosing is to start with 10 mg/kg, ideal body weight in overweight/ obese patients, PO q8h in dogs, or higher in cats, then increase or decrease to effect (dose range 5–25 mg/kg). Dosages up to 30 mg/kg q8h are given to some cats with severe pain (e.g. post-onychectomy neuropathy). Gabapentin is also used in human patients for management of neuropathic pain associated with diabetes, cancer and primary nerve compression [54]. The combined number needed to treat (NNT) for gabapentin, at a set dose, to be effective for one patient to experience pain reduction in the management of painful polyneuropathy and postherpetic neuralgia, were 6.4 and 4.3, respectively, indicating that not all patients may benefit from gabapentin; however, dosing to effect is required in the individual veterinary patient, some requiring high dosages.

3. Pregabalin

Pregabalin has a similar pharmacologic profile as gabapentin and is used to manage neuropathic pain in humans [70, 71]. It is reported in humans that pregabalin appears to have less mental confusion and sedative side effects than those reported with gabapentin. Based on pharmacokinetic studies in dogs, a dose of 4 mg/kg PO q12h is suggested; however, analgesic efficacy has not been established for veterinary patients.

4. Non-Steroidal Anti-Inflammatory Analgesics

Where there are no contraindications, an NSAIA is recommended in a multi-modal regimen for chronic neuropathic pain. See Section VII.A.6 and Chapter 11 for further details.

5. Tricyclic Antidepressants

Imipramine and amitriptyline are two commonly recommended tricyclic antidepressants (TCAs) for veterinary patients. Based on the greater adverse effects of imipramine reported in human medicine, amitriptyline is recommended. The TCAs are effective analgesics for managing neuropathic pain conditions in humans, and the analgesic effects of these drugs appear to occur at lower than antidepressant doses [54]. In veterinary medicine, the TCAs may be effective adjunctive analgesics for a range of neuropathic conditions, or for sole use in inflammatory bowel disease and selective cases of idiopathic cystitis in cats, aka feline interstitial cystitis [14] which, with long duration, acquires a neuropathic component due to central sensitization. Refer to Chapter 4 for details. It has been reported that it can take 2–4 weeks for these drugs to achieve maximal effectiveness; however, clinical improvement may appear earlier, especially when combined with other analgesics, or when used in combination with corticosteroids for feline inflammatory bowel disease. When other traditional analgesics have failed to achieve complete analgesia, the addition of amitriptyline may prove successful in managing the refractory, chronic pain.

Dosing

The recommended dose, based on ideal body weight in overweight/obese patients for amitriptyline for dogs is 1–2 mg/kg orally q12–24h, and for cats 2.5–12.5 mg/cat orally q24 h. These products may be distasteful requiring some creative method of administration.

VIII. Future Therapeutic Modalities

A. Vanilloid Receptor 1 Antagonists

The identification and cloning of the vanilloid receptor 1 (TRPV1) represented a significant step in the understanding of the molecular mechanisms underlying the transduction of noxious chemical and thermal stimuli by peripheral nociceptors [74, 75]. The TRPV1 receptor is also expressed in the CNS and appears to play an important role in pain mediated by central sensitization. Refer to Chapter 2. The TRPV1 antagonists currently being investigated effectively reduce thermal hyperalgesia and mechanical allodynia associated with inflammatory and osteoarthritic pain in research models. With identification of both a peripheral and central role of the TRPV1 receptor, the future potential of TRPV1 antagonists as analgesics for neuropathic pain may be a consideration.

B. Serotonin and Norepinephrine Re-Uptake Inhibitor Mixed Compound

As the descending inhibitory system appears to be dysfunctional in neuropathic pain states, serotonin re-uptake inhibitor (SRI) and norepinephrine re-uptake inhibitor (NRI) mixed compounds are being investigated for analgesic efficacy.

Duloxetine, a mixed SRI and NRI (SNRI) with potency at both transporters, was the first re-uptake inhibitor approved for the treatment of diabetic neuropathy [76, 77]. In dogs, bioavailability is poor and clinical efficacy is lacking [56].

Venlafaxine is also an SNRI. It is also a TCA and has very similar effects to amitriptyline and has been shown to be effective in at least one-third of human patients with neuropathic pain [78]. Venlafaxine plus gabapentin in the management of painful diabetic neuropathy showed significant pain relief relative to placebo plus gabapentin. Oral administration of 2 mg/kg resulted in an elimination half-life of approximately 3 h, indicating a q8–12 h administration. As for other adjunctive analgesics, there is no knowledge of plasma concentrations that are effective for analgesia in dogs or cats. The predominant metabolite, O-desmethylvenlafaxine (ODV), is not detected in dogs; therefore, any pharmacologic effects are produced by the parent drug [79]. The pharmacokinetics of venlafaxine have not been reported in cats. There are no clinical studies reported in cats and dogs receiving venlafaxine; however, it has been used at 2.5 mg/kg/day for juvenile canine narcolepsy and cataplexy. Toxicity is reported at 10 mg/kg. There is potential for GI hemorrhage when combined with tramadol in humans.

Based on the unfavourable profile of duloxetine, future studies in dogs and cats favour venlafaxine [56].

Cannabinoids are third in line for treatment of diabetic neuropathy and postherpetic neuralgia where gabapentin and TCAs fail in human patients. Interestingly, opioids (methadone also has NMDA antagonism) are fourth in line. As medical cannabinoids become available/legal for veterinary patients, these may be considered in a treatment plan for the management of spinal cord injury pain.

IX. Conclusion

Cats and dogs share a similar nervous system to humans. They also encounter similar surgical, traumatic, inflammatory and metabolic conditions. As humans experience neuropathic pain associated with these, and other pathologic situations, it would seem reasonable to assume that cats and dogs also share this experience. Neuropathic pain is difficult to diagnose in veterinary patients as they are unable to verbalize their pain. By assuming neuropathic pain may exist based on the history of events each patient has experienced, a focused client history and neurologic examination may identify a lesion resulting in persistent or spontaneous pain. Should neuropathic pain be diagnosed, it is important to identify the particular cause responsible for generating a particular pain because this represents the first anatomic target for treatment. While it is impossible to discriminate burning from prickling and lancinating from stabbing in veterinary patients, behavioural patterns described by owners may assist with lesion localization. Once neuropathic pain is diagnosed, a trial multi-modal analgesic plan and/or acupuncture session(s) should be prescribed with instructions for owners to observe behaviour. Dosing of the analgesic can be titrated to the patient's needs while avoiding adverse effects. Where a particular analgesic may be ineffectual, an alternate class should be tried. This approach was used in a case series of three dogs with poor response to conventional analgesic therapy [80]. A trial of amitriptyline 1.1 mg/kg q12h successfully managed the pain in one dog but not another; however, the second dog responded to gabapentin 14.3 mg/kg q12h. A third dog was administered gabapentin 12.5 mg/kg q12h but with no improvement; improvement was noted with amitriptyline 1.3 mg/kg q12h. The trial period for these dogs ranged from two to four weeks, but where the response was positive, this occurred quite rapidly [80].

The revised consensus statement from the Canadian Pain Society for pharmacological management of chronic neuropathic pain states that gabapentinoids, TCAs and SNRIs represent first-line treatments for chronic neuropathic pain either individually or in combination [81]. When these agents fail, conventional opioid analgesics provide important avenues of treatment, bearing in mind their associated risks and adverse effect profiles. Cannabinoids are now considered to be third-line agents based on recent evidence of efficacy, but they also require judicious prescribing practices [79].

These recommendations are also made based on a more recent systematic review and meta-analysis of pharmacotherapy for neuropathic pain in humans [82]. The findings concluded that (1) strong recommendation for use and proposal as first-line treatment in neuropathic pain for tricyclic antidepressants, serotonin-noradrenaline reuptake inhibitors, pregabalin and gabapentin, (2) a weak recommendation for use and proposal as second line for lidocaine patches, capsaicin high-concentration patches and tramadol (ineffective in dogs) and (3) a weak recommendation for use and proposal as third line for strong opioids and botulinum toxin A. Topical agents and botulinum toxin A are recommended for peripheral neuropathic pain only [82].

As research into the neurobiological mechanisms of neuropathic pain continue, specific therapies for its management will eventually appear in the human clinical setting and subsequently investigated for veterinary clinical use.

References

1 Niv, D. and Devor, M. (2006) Refractory neuropathic pain: The nature and extent of the problem. *Pain Practice*, 6(1): 3–9.

2 Taylor, B. K. (2001) Pathophysiologic mechanisms of neuropathic pain. *Current Pain and Headache Reports*, 5: 151–161.

3 Woolf, C. J. (1992) Excitability changes in central neurons following peripheral damage: Role of central sensitization in the pathogenesis of pain. In: Willis, W. D., Jr (ed.), *Hyperalgesia and Allodynia*. New York: Raven Press, 221–243.

4 Novakvic, S. D., Tzoumaka, E., McGivern, J. G., *et al.* (1998) Distribution of the tetrodotoxin-resistant sodium channel PN3 in rat sensory neurons in normal and neuropathic conditions. *J Neurosci*, 18: 2174–2187.

 5 Amir, R. and Devor, M. (2000) Functional cross-excitation between afferent A- and C-neurons in dorsal root ganglia. *Neuroscience*, 95: 189–195.

 6 Ellis, A. and Bennett, D. L. H. (2013) Neuroinflammation and the generation of neuropathic pain. *British Journal of Anaesthesia*, 111 (1): 26–37.

 7 Zhang, F., Vadakkan, K. I. and Kim, S. S. (2008) Selective activation of microglia in spinal cord but not higher cortical regions following nerve injury in adult mouse. *Mol Pain*, 4: 15–31.

 8 Zhuo, M. (2005) Cellular and Synaptic Insights into Physiological and Pathological Pain. *Can. J. Neurol Sci*, 32: 27–36.

 9 Zimmermann, M. (2001) Pathobiology of neuropathic pain. *Review European Journal of Pharmacology*, 429: 23–37.

10 Dickenson, A. (2013) The neurobiology of chronic pain states. *Anaesthesia and Intensive Care Med*, 14: 11484–487.

11 Woolf, C. J. (2004) Dissecting out mechanisms responsible for peripheral neuropathic pain: Implications for diagnosis and therapy. *Life Sciences*, 74, 2605–2610.

12 Sacerdote, P., Limiroli, E. and Gaspani, L. (2003) Experimental evidence for immunomodulatory effects of opioids. *Adv Exp Med Biol*, 521: 106–116.

13 Malchow, R. J. and Black, I. H. (2008) The evolution of pain management in the critically ill trauma patient: Emerging concepts f rom global war on terrorism. *Crit Care Med*, 36[Supp]: S345–S357.

14 Chew, D. J., Buffington, C. A. and Kendell, M. S. (1998) *et al.* Amitriptyline treatment for severe recurrent idiopathic cystitis in cats. *J Am Vet Med Assoc*, 213: 1282–1286.

15 Kukkar, A., Bali, A., Singh, N., *et al.* (2013) Implications and mechanism of action of gabapentin in neuropathic pain. *Arch. Pharm. Res*, 36: 237–251.

16 Hayashida, K., DeGoes, S., Curry, R., *et al.* (2007) Gabapentin Activates Spinal Noradrenergic Activity in Rats and Humans and Reduces Hypersensitivity after Surgery. *Anesthesiology*, 106: 557–62.

17 Seib, R. K. and Paul, J. E. (2006) Preoperative gabapentin for postoperative analgesia: A meta-analysis. *Can J Anaesth*, 53: 461–469.

18 Blanpied, T. A., Clarke, R. J. and Johnson, J. W. (2005) Amantadine inhibits NMDA receptors by accelerating channel closure during channel block. *J Neurosci.*, 25: 3312–3322.

19 Lascelles, B. D. X., Gaynor, J., Smith, E. S., *et al.* (2008) Evaluation of amantadine in a multimodal analgesic regimen for the alleviation of refractory canine osteoarthritis pain. *J Vet Intern Med.*, 22(1): 53–59.

20 Challapalli, V., Tremont-Lukats, I. W., McNicol, E. D., *et al.* (2005) Systemic administration of local anesthetic agents to relieve neuropathic pain. *Cochrane Database of Systematic Reviews*, 19(4) (Art. No.: CD003345).

21 Smith, L. J., Bentley, E., Shih, A., *et al.* (2004) Systemic lidocaine infusion as an analgesic for intraocular surgery in dogs: A pilot study. *Vet Anaesth Analg*, 31: 53–63.

22 Mao, J. and Chen, L. L. (2000) Systemic lidocaine for neuropathic pain relief. *Pain*, 87: 7–17.

23 Pypendop, B. H., Ilkiw, J. E. and Robertson, S. A. (2006) Effects of intravenous administration of lidocaine on the thermal threshold in cats. *Am J Vet Res*, 67: 16–20.

24 Yaksh, T. L., Pogrel, J. W., Lee, Y. W., *et al.* (1995) Reversal of nerve-ligation induced allodynia by spinal alpha 2 adrenoreceptor agonists. *J Pharmacol Exp Ther*, 272: 207–214.

25 Valtolina, C., Robben, J. H., Uilenreef, J. *et al.* (2009) Clinical evaluation of the efficacy and safety of a constant rate infusion of dexmedetomidine for postoperative pain management in dogs. *Veterinary Anaesthesia and Analgesia*, 36: 369–383.

26 Malmberg, A. B. and Yaksh, T. L. (1992) Hyperalgsia mediated by spinal glutamate or substance P receptor blocked by spinal cyclo-oxygenase inhibition. *Science*, 257: 1276–1279.

27 Strauss, K. I. (2008) Antiinflammatory and neuroprotective actions of COX-2 inhibitors in injured brain. *Brain, Behaviour, and Immunity*, 22: 285–298.

28 Karavis, M. (1997) The neurophysiology of acupuncture: A viewpoint. *Acupuncture in Medicine*, 15(1): 33–42.

29 Hayes, C., Browne, S., Lantry, G. and Burstal, R. (2002) Neuropathic pain in the acute pain service: A prospective survey. *Acute Pain*, 4: 45–48.

30 Baron, R., Binder, A. and Wasner, G. (2010) Neuropathic pain: Diagnosis, pathophysiological mechanisms, and treatment. *Lancet Neurol*, 9: 807–19. (Excellent Review. Also lidocaine patch and detailed discussion.).

31 Anil, S. S., Anil, L. and Deen, J. (2002) Challenges of pain assessment in domestic animals. *J Am Vet Med Assoc*, 220(3): 313–319.

32 Muir, III, W. W., Wiese, A. J. and Wittum, T. E. (2004) Prevalence and characteristics of pain in dogs and cats examined as outpatients at a veterinary teaching hospital. *J Am Vet Med Assoc*, 224: 1459–1463.

33 Cunningham, J., Temple, W. J., Mitchell, P. *et al.* (1996) Cooperative hernia study. Pain in the postrepair patient. *Ann Surg*, 224(5): 598–602.

34 Meyhoff, C. S., Thomsen, C. H., Rasmussen, L. S., *et al.* (2006) High Incidence of Chronic Pain Following Surgery for Pelvic Fracture. *Clin J Pain*, 22: 167–172.

35 Popeney, C., Ansell, A. and Renney, K. (2007) Pudendal entrapment as an etiology of chronic perineal pain: Diagnosis and treatment. *Neurol Urodyn*, 26(6): 820–827.

36 O'Hagan, B. J. (2006) Neuropathic pain in a cat post-amputation *Aust Vet J*, 84: 83–860.

37 Woolf, C. J., Shortland, P. and Coggeshell, R. E. (1992) Peripheral nerve injury triggers central sprouting of myelinated afferents. *Nature*, 355: 75–77.

38 De Risio, L., Thomas, W. B. and Sharp, N. J. H. (2000) Degenerative sacral stenosis. *Vet Clin North Am Small Anim Pract*, 301: 111–132.

39 Mayhew, P. D., Kapatakinn, A. S., Wortman, J. A., *et al.* (2002) Association of cauda equine compression on magnetic resonance images an clinical signs in dogs with degenerative lumbosacral stenosis. *J AM Anim Hosp Assoc*, 38: 555–562.

40 Griffiths, I. R. (1983) Polyradiculoneuritis in two dogs presenting as neuritis of the cauda equina. *Vet Rec*, 112: 360–361.

41 Coates, J. R. (2000) Intervertebral disk disease. *Vet Clin North Am Sm Anim Pract*, 30(1): 77–110.

42 Joaquim, J. G. F., Luna, S. P. L., Brondani, J. T., *et al.* (2010) Comparison of decompressive surgery, electroacupuncture, and decompressive surgery followed by electroacupuncture for the treatment of dogs with intervertebral disk disease with long-standing severe neurologic deficits. *J Am Vet Med Assoc*, 236(11): 1225–1229.

43 da Costa, R. C. and Moore, S. A. (2010) Differential Diagnosis of Spinal Diseases. *Vet Clin North Am Small Anim Pract*, 40(5): 755–763.

44 Thomas, W. B. (2000) Diskospondylitis and other vertebral infections. *Vet Clin North Am Small Anim Pract*, 30(1): 169–182.

45 Heavner, J. E., Coates, P. W. and Racz, G. (2000) Myelinated fibres of spinal cord blood vessels – sensory innervation? *Current Review of Pain*, 4(5): 353–355.

46 Webb, A. A. (2003) Potential sources of neck and back pain in clinical conditions in cats and dogs. *The Veterinary Journal*, 165: 193–213.

47 Cuddon, P. A. (1998) Electrophysiologic assessment of acute polyradiculoneuropathy in dogs: Comparison with Guillain-Barre syndrome in people. *J Vet Int Med*, 12: 294–303.

48 McDonnell, J. J., Platt, S. R. and Clayton, L. A. (2001) Neurologic conditions causing lameness in companion animals. *Vet Clin North Am Small Anim Pract*, 31: 17–38.

49 Mizisin, A. P., Shelton, G. D., Burgess, M. L., *et al.* (2002) Neurological complications associated with spontaneously occurring feline diabetes mellitus. *J Neuropathol Exp Neurol*, 61(10): 872–874.

50 Holland, C. T., Charles, J. A., Smith, S. H. and Cortaville, P. E. (2000) Hemihyperesthesia and hyper-responsiveness resembling central pain syndrome in a dog with a forebrain oligodendroglioma. *Aust Vet J*, 78(10): 676–680.

51 Rusbridge, C. and Jeffery, N. D. (2008) Pathophysiology and treatment of neuropathic pain associated with syringomyelia. *The Veterinary Journal*, 175: 164–172.

52 Plessas, I. N., Rusbridge, C., Driver, C. J., *et al.* (2012) Long-term outcome of Cavalier King Charles spaniel dogs with clinical signs associated with Chiari-like malformation and syringomyelia. *Vet Rec*, 171: 501, doi: 10.1136/vr.100449.

53 Ortinau, N., Vitale, S., Akin, E. Y., *et al.* (2015) Foramen magnum decompression surgery in 23 Chiari-like malformation patients 2007–2010: Outcomes and owner survey results. *Can Vet J*, 56: 288–91.

54 Wallace, M. S. (2001) Pharmacologic treatment of neuropathic pain. *Current Pain and Headache Reports* 5: 138–150.

55 Lee, M., Silverman, S. and Hansen, H. (2011) A Comprehensive Review of Opioid-Induced Hyperalgesia. *Pain Physician*, 14: 145–161.

56 Kukanich, B. (2013) Outpatient oral analgesics in dogs and cats beyond nonsteroidal antiinflammatory drugs: An evidence-based approach. *Vet Clin North Am Small Anim Pract*, 43: 1109–25, doi: 10.1016/j.cvsm. (2013).04.007.

57 Case, J. B., Fick, J. L. and Rooney, M. B. (2010) Proximal duodenal perforation in three dogs following deracoxib administration. *J Am Anim Hosp Assoc*, 46: 255–8.

58 Wagner, A. E., Walton, J. A., Hellyer, P. W., *et al.* (2002) Use of low doses of ketamine administered by constant rate infusion as an adjunct for postoperative analgesia in dogs. *J Am Vet Med Assoc*, 221: 72–75.

59 Schwedler, M., Miletich, D. J. and Albrecht, R. F. (1982) Cerebral blood flow and metabolism following ketamine administration. *Can Anaesth Soc J*, 29: 222–226.

60 Botero, C. A., Smith, C. E., Holbrook, C., *et al.* (2000) Total intravenous anesthesia with a propofol-ketamine combination during coronary artery surgery. *J Cardiothorac Vasc Anesth*, 14: 409–415.

61 Giacino, J. T., Whyte, J., Bagiella, E., *et al.* (2012) Placebo-Controlled Trial of Amantadine for Severe Traumatic Brain Injury. *N Engl J Med*, 366: 819–826.

62 Challapalli, V., Tremont-Lukats, I. W., McNicol, E. D., *et al.* (2005) Systemic administration of local anesthetic agents to relieve neuropathic pain. *Cochrane Database of Systematic Reviews*, 19(4) (Art. No.: CD003345).

63 Mao, J. and Chen, L L. (2000) Systemic lidocaine for neuropathic pain relief. *Pain*, 87: 7–17.

64 Pypendop, B. H., Ilkiw, J. E. and Robertson, S A. (2006) Effects of intravenous administration of lidocaine on the thermal threshold in cats. *Am J Vet Res*, 67: 16–20.

65 Lei, B., Popp, S., Capuano-Waters, C., *et al.* (2004) Lidocaine attenuates apoptosis in the ischemic penumbra an reduces infarct size after transient focal cerebral ischemia in rats. *Neuroscience*, 125 691–701.

66 Mathews, K. A. and O'Sullivan, L. (2017) Ventricular arrhythmias: Acute therapy. In: Mathews K. A. (ed.), *Veterinary Emergency & Critical Care Manual*, 3rd edn. LifeLearn, Guelph, Ontario, Canada.

67 Weil, A. B. and Ko, J. (2007) The use of lidocaine patches compendium. *Compend Contin Educ Vet*, 29: 208–216.

68 Kamtikar, S. and Nair, A. S. (2015) Advantages of dexmedetomidine in traumatic brain injury: A review. *Anaesth Pain & Intensive Care*, 19(1)87–91.

69 Tang, J. F., Chen, P., Tang, E. J., *et al.* (2011) Dexmedetomidine Controls Agitation and Facilitates Reliable, Serial Neurological Examinations in a Non-Intubated Patient with Traumatic Brain Injury. *Neurocritical Care*, 15(1): 175–181.

70 Hurley, R. W., Cohen, S. P., Williams, K. A., *et al.* (2006) The Analgesic Effects of Perioperative Gabapentin on Postoperative Pain: A Meta-Analysis. *Reg Anesth Pain Med*, 31: 237–247.

71 Clarke, H., Bonin, R. P., Orser, B. A., *et al.* (2012) The Prevention of Chronic Postsurgical Pain Using Gabapentin and Pregabalin: A Combined Systematic Review and Meta-Analysis. *Anesth Analg*, 115: 428–42.

72 Lorenz, N. D., Comerford, E. J. and Iff, I. (2012) Long-term use of gabapentin for musculoskeletal disease and trauma in three cats *Journal of Feline Medicine and Surgery*, 15: 507–512.

73 Wagner, A. E., Mich, P. and Uhrig, S. R. (2010) Clinical evaluation of perioperative administration of gabapentin as an adjunct for postoperative analgesia in dogs undergoing amputation of a forelimb. *Am Vet Med Assoc*, 236: 751–756.

74 Kuner, R. (2010) Central mechanisms of pathological pain: Review. *Nature Medicine*, 1258–1266.

75 Cui, M., Honore, P., Zhong, C., *et al.* (2006) TRPV1 receptors in the CNS play a key role in broad-spectrum analgesia of TRPV1 antagonists. *J Neurosci*, 26(37): 9385–9393.

76 Jones, C. K., Peters, S. C. and Shannon, H. E. (2005) Efficacy of duloxetine, a potent and balanced serotonergic and noradrenergic reuptake inhibitor, in inflammatory and acute pain models in rodents. *J Pharmacol Exp Ther*, 312: 726–732.

77 Patel, D. S., Deshpande, S. S., Patel, C. G., *et al.* (2011) A dual action anti-depressant. *Indo Global J Pharm Sci*, 1: 69.

78 Saarto, T. and Wiffen, P. J. (2007) Antidepressants for neuropathic pain. *Cochrane Database of Systematic Reviews*, 4 (Art. No.: CD005454).

79 Howell, S. R., Hicks, D. R., Scatina, J. A., *et al.* (1994) Pharmacokinetics of venlafaxine and O-desmethylvenlafaxine in laboratory animals. *Xenobiotica*, 24: 315–27.

80 Cashmore, R. G., Harcourt-Brown, T. R., Freeman, P. M., *et al.* (2009) Clinical diagnosis and treatment of suspected neuropathic pain in three dogs. *Aust Vet J*, 87: 45–50.

81 Moulin, D.E., Clark, A. J., Gilron, I., *et al.* (2007) Pharmacological management of chronic neuropathic pain – Consensus statement and guidelines from the Canadian Pain Society. *Pain Res Manage*, 12(1): 13–21.

82 Finnerup, N. B., Attal, N., Haroutounian, S., *et al.* (2015) Pharmacotherapy for neuropathic pain in adults: A systematic review and meta-analysis. *Lancet Neurol*, 14(2): 162–173.

83 Harden, R. N. (2005) Chronic neuropathic pain: Mechanisms, diagnosis, and treatment. *Neurologist*, 11(2): 111–122.

Further Reading

Hayashi, A. M., Matera, J. M. and Fonseca Pinto, A. C. (2007) Evaluation of electroacupuncture treatment for thoracolumbar intervertebral disk disease in dogs. *J Am Vet Med Assoc*, 15(6): 913–918.

Moore, S. A. (2016) Managing neuropathic pain in dogs: Review. *Front. Vet. Sci*, 3: 12, doi: 10.3389/fvets.2016.00012.

4

Physiology and Pharmacology: Clinical Application to Abdominal and Pelvic Visceral Pain

Karol Mathews

The pathophysiology of visceral pain, involving both the abdominal and pelvic structures, is extremely complex and occurs in both the acute and chronic states associated with several etiologies. There is also a component of neuropathic pain associated with many of these scenarios. In addition to the pain associated with the underlying pathology, the emotional state has important modulatory influences on visceral pain.

I.   Neurophysiology Reviews [1–3]

A brief description of gastrointestinal (GI) and pelvic neurophysiology is presented as it relates to pain mechanisms and approach to treatment. The majority of thoracic and abdominal visceral organs, except the pancreas, are dually innervated by parasympathetic (craniosacral) and sympathetic (thoracolumbar) outflows. The lower abdominal viscera, including the small and large intestine and the urogenital organs, are innervated by thoracolumbar (lumbar splanchnic nerve and hypogastric nerve) and sacral (pelvic nerve) outflows. Spinal afferents are classified as mucosal, muscle or tension-sensitive, muscle/mucosal (also known as "tension/mucosal"), serosal and mesenteric afferents. The majority of these afferents are mechanosensitive, having characteristics of response to a mechanical stimulus.

A.   Afferent and Efferent Innervations

1. **The vagus (the tenth cranial nerve, or CN X)**, a mixed nerve, comprises 75% of the afferent limb and 25% of the efferent of the thoracic viscera and upper abdominal viscera.
2. **The pelvic nerve** innervates the lower GI tract and pelvic viscera.
3. **The serosal layer** of the GI tract and its adjacent mesentery, are innervated by C and A- delta afferents. These afferents are commonly found in both the lumbar splanchnic nerve and the pelvic nerve. It is purported that the excitation of the serosal afferents during ischemia is partly due to the release of prostanoids.

B.   Autonomic Nervous System [4]

Innervation of the GI tract and pelvic viscera comprises an extrinsic and intrinsic system, referred to as the "autonomic nervous system".

Analgesia and Anesthesia for the Ill or Injured Dog and Cat, First Edition. Karol A. Mathews, Melissa Sinclair, Andrea M. Steele and Tamara Grubb.
© 2018 John Wiley & Sons, Inc. Published 2018 by John Wiley & Sons, Inc.

1. The **extrinsic component** consists of both parasympathetic and sympathetic branches.
2. The **intrinsic component** consists of the nervous system residing within the submucosal and myenteric plexuses. All systems communicate extensively.
3. **Parasympathetic neurons** – (craniosacral) have:
   a. **Pre-ganglionic** fibres that synapse in or on ganglia near, or on, the target organ.
   b. **Post-ganglionic** fibres that release neuropeptides including Substance-P (S-P). Innervation of mechanoreceptors and chemoreceptors within the GI mucosa transmit sensory information, via the afferent limb of the vagus, to the central nervous system (CNS). The CNS response back to the GI tract is via the efferent limb of the vagus nerve to smooth muscle, secretory and endocrine cells.
4. **Sympathetic innervations:**
   a. The thoracic, abdominal and pelvic viscera are supplied by the T1 to L3 segments of the thoracolumbar spinal cord.
   b. Sympathetic neurons synapse at the celiac, superior and inferior mesenteric and hypogastric ganglia outside of the GI tract.
   c. Post-ganglionic neurons are adrenergic, releasing norepinephrine as the neurotransmitter.
   d. The sympathetic nerve fibres consist of approximately 50% afferent sensory fibres from the GI tract to the CNS and 50% efferent motor fibres to the GI tract.

C. Central Processing [2]

Within the anterolateral quadrant of the spinal cord:

1. The **spinoreticular**, **spinomesencephalic** and **spinohypothalamic tracts** mainly activate largely unconscious and/or automatic responses to visceral sensory input, including alterations in emotion and behaviour.
2. The **spinothalamic tract** transmits conscious sensation by its projection via sensory nuclei of the thalamus to the somatosensory cortex (SI/II **lateral pain system**), anterior cingulate cortex (**medial pain system**) and the **insula**. This widespread distribution of afferent pathways to areas beyond those required for localization alone may account for the strong emotional component of visceral pain and differences between patients with chronic visceral pain and acute visceral pain in the degree of activation of these pain areas.
   The main function of the **lateral pain system** is to provide intensity and localization of the stimulus; the **medial system** modulates affective pain behaviour with stimulation of important autonomic and descending inhibitory pathways.
3. **Insula** and the **orbital prefrontal cortex** have important roles in sensory integration and in the higher control of autonomic visceromotor and behavioural responses.
4. In the **dorsal columns**, another visceral pain pathway exists which passes via ipsilateral dorsal column nuclei to the contralateral ventroposterolateral nucleus of the thalamus similar to that from somatic afferents.

D. Peripheral Sensitization

Peripheral sensitization of primary afferent neuron terminals within the gut results [2, 3]:

1. **in a decrease** in the intensity and/or amplitude of the stimulus required to initiate their depolarization; and
2. **in an increase** in the number and/or amplitude of neuronal discharges in response to a given chemical or mechanical stimulus;
3. **from the release** of pro-inflammatory substances such as bradykinin, tachykinins, prostaglandins, interleukins, serotonin, adenosine triphosphate, tumour necrosis factor and

protons, at the site of injury or illness. These mediators are algogenic and act directly on receptors located at sensory nerve terminals, where they depolarize these neurons and initiate nociceptive inputs to the spinal cord. These substances also activate local immunocytes and/or mast cells or sympathetic varicosities, further releasing algogenic substances (e.g. norepinephrine) on sensory nerve endings. Growth factors, such as nerve growth factor, are present both in gut tissues and in mast cells and are released during mast cell degranulation. These factors are involved in neuronal plasticity but may also change the distribution of receptors to algogenic mediators, and the threshold of sensitivity to mechanical and chemical stimuli, resulting in hyperalgesia.

4. **in an increased** expression of sodium channels, which may contribute to the hypersensitivity of peripheral neurons that result from illness or injury.

Neurokinin (NK)-1 receptor and its agonist S-P are present in pain pathways in both the CNS and PNS. NK-1 receptors are also present in visceral tissues such as the bladder, esophagus and colon.

E. Central Sensitization (Inflammation-Induced)

Central sensitization develops, and is maintained by, S-P and N-methyl-D-aspartate (NMDA) mediated events. NMDA receptors are also involved in the processing of acute nociceptive inputs from non-inflamed abdominal and pelvic viscera.

II. Clinical Relevance of Physiology to Pharmacology

Refer to Chapter 12 for more in-depth details of individual drugs.

A. Dorsal Horn Targets for Analgesics [3]

1. **Presynaptic receptors:** opioid (μ, δ, κ), alpha$_2$ adrenergic, GABA$_A$, 5-HT$_3$, CCK.
2. **Post-synaptic receptors:** opioid (μ, δ, κ), alpha$_2$ adrenergic, NMDA, GABA$_A$, 5-HT$_{1 \text{ and } 3}$, NK$_{1, 2 \text{ and } 3}$.
3. **Blockade of NMDA receptors by**, for example, **ketamine** has been shown to have clear analgesic benefits in GI pain in animal models [2] and in a model of human esophageal sensitivity [2]. In addition, dogs receiving dosages of ketamine 3 to < 30 mg/kg/h had no effect on GI motility [4]. Ureter nociceptive response in rats was significantly inhibited by ketamine [5]. **Lidocaine** is also an NMDA antagonist.
4. **Blockade of alpha$_2$ delta subunit** of calcium channels at central nociceptor terminals by **ketamine, gabapentin and pregabalin** have proven efficacy in managing neuropathic pain [2]. Gabapentin and pregabalin reduce the visceral hyperalgesia in human patients with inflammatory bowel syndrome, and in rats with visceral pain induced by septic shock, inflammation, colonic glycerol and stress [3]. A case report presents the efficacy of ketamine in alleviating visceral inflammatory pain associated with fulminating ulcerative colitis in a pediatric patient [6].
5. **Serotonin re-uptake inhibitors** have also demonstrated a reduction in visceral sensitivity experienced in inflammatory bowel syndrome in humans [3].
6. **Tetrodotoxin-sensitive** (TTX-S) and **tetrodotoxin-resistant (TTX-R) sodium channels of visceral sensory afferents** are blocked by **kappa opioid receptor** (KOR) agonists (e.g. butorphanol) attenuating mechanotransduction of visceral afferents during noxious colon distension [5]. However, in the author's experience butorphanol is only effective for

mild to moderate visceral pain, not associated with a surgical procedure, and has not been effective in moderate to severe pain associated with visceral pathology. KOR agonists have no effect when injected spinally [5]. Where butorphanol is not totally effective, added lidocaine may be effective. The TTX-S sodium channels are preferentially expressed in large and medium dorsal root ganglion (DRG) neurons and are reported to be four times more sensitive than TTX-R sodium channels to **lidocaine** therapy. See point 7 below.

7. **Central C fibre activity** is **selectively blocked** by **lidocaine** when administered intravenously. When lidocaine is applied to nerves, voltage-gated sodium channels present in nociceptive fibres (**A-delta and C nociceptive**) are blocked. In addition to the analgesic properties:

   a. **Systemic lidocaine** treatment in human surgical patients experience less pain, and more rapid return of bowel function than those in a control group [7]. Post-operative ileus is caused, in part, by the activation of several nerve reflexes. Lidocaine has been hypothesized to alter sympathetic tone to the smooth muscle by suppressing transmission through afferent sensory pathways [8].

   b. **Local application of a local anesthetic.** Inhibitory reflexes are activated as soon as the parietal peritoneum is entered. A spinal reflex originating in the gut and a peripheral reflex transmitted through the prevertebral ganglia are also affected. This sympathetic action can be blocked by local anesthetics, which may be the result of a blockade of inhibitory reflexes originating from the myenteric plexus [3].

   c. **Epidural anesthesia and analgesia** used in conjunction with general anesthesia have the potential to attenuate post-operative ileus by blocking the spinal reflexes and the sympathetic innervation of bowel. This shifts the autonomic balance in favour of parasympathetics with direct excitatory effect on intestinal smooth muscle and increased motility [3].

   d. **Lidocaine 1.5 mg/kg relieved the pain of renal colic** in human patients more effectively than 0.1 mg/kg morphine. Changing the smooth muscle tone and reducing the transmission of afferent sensory pathways, lidocaine causes a significant reduction in pain [8].

8. **Neurokinin 1 (NK-1) receptor** antagonism by **maropitant** contributes to analgesia, especially in patients with GI pain. Maropitant decreased the anesthetic requirements during visceral stimulation of the ovary and ovarian ligament in dogs suggesting the potential role for NK-1 receptor antagonists to manage ovarian and visceral pain [9].

B. Peripheral Sensitization Targets for Analgesics

Anti-prostaglandins, opioids μ- and k-opioid agonists lessen the nociceptive response to either peritoneal administration of irritants or intestinal distension. K-agonists act peripherally to prevent visceral pain and are more active in inflammatory conditions. Studies demonstrate the efficacy of using specific partial opioid agonists/antagonists to counteract analgesic-related constipation [2].

C. Reduction/Modulation of the Transmission of Nociceptive Information

Reduction/modulation of the transmission of nociceptive information from visceral spinal afferents can occur with "**gating**" **influences** from "converging" viscerosomatic nociceptive and non-nociceptive neurons, resulting in transient inhibition of transmission [2]. An example in humans is the reduction in abdominal pain with application of a hot-water bottle on the abdominal wall. Some neurons in the dorsal horn of the spinal cord are also strongly inhibited when a nociceptive stimulus is applied to any part of the body distinct from their excitatory receptive fields. As an example, counter-irritation, such as rubbing, which we instinctively do for minor injuries, provides temporary relief. Pain thresholds in the viscera are increased by viscerosomatic inputs (e.g. hard prodding of the abdomen in the presence of visceral pathology/pain), which is a reason to apply gentle pressure, producing less pain than a hard prod (and so reducing the chance of an attack on the examiner!), when assessing for pain. Viscerosomatic inputs also account for "referred" pain (e.g. pain elicited upon abdominal palpation originating from thoracic inflammation; author's observation).

D. Epidural Site for Analgesic Administration

This is highly recommended where appropriate. Refer to Chapter 14.

III. Sources of Abdominal Pain

Acute abdominal pain may be caused by several mechanisms arising secondary to:

- visceral stretching as occurs with obstruction, torsion;
- capsule stretching as a result of solid organ (liver, spleen, pancreas) swelling due to inflammation, hemorrhage or neoplasia;
- inflammation as occurs in peritonitis and inflammatory bowel disease and cholecystitis/cholelithiasis;
- invasion/compression of nerves by tumours.

While acute pain such as surgery or trauma can be severe, where an acute incident occurs on established chronic abdominal pain, one can expect this to be more painful than a naive painful event based on the hyperalgesic state established by the chronic pain.

Abdominal rigidity elicited upon abdominal palpation is a sign of visceral/peritoneal abdominal pain. However, another reported cause of elicited abdominal rigidity, erroneously interpreted as pain, is poor abdominal palpation technique in that a hard, forceful, rather than a soft and gentle, increase in abdominal depth for examination technique is used. Bradycardia or normal heart rate may be present due to the vagal component, masking the sympathetic response normally elicited with pain. Therefore, the heart rate obtained must be interpreted based on the degree of potential vagal involvement. This is key in monitoring response to analgesics, as opioids also contribute to the vagal response where lowering of the heart rate may not be associated with adequate analgesia. Pain assessment should be based not only on heart rate response but also on behaviour and examination (refer to Chapter 8). Opioid analgesics should not be withheld due to concerns for metabolism in hepatic illness as a minimal amount of functional tissue is required to metabolize the opioid. The key is titration to effect, as with any case, followed by careful monitoring to assess duration of effect, which may be quite a bit longer than a patient with normal liver function. Avoid a continuous rate infusion (CRI) until the duration can be established and a lower dose for CRI planned. Where peritonitis is present, somatic innervations from the parietal peritoneum will also influence heart rate; therefore, both visceral and somatic pain are a feature.

A. Gastrointestinal System

Common, extremely painful, visceral conditions seen in dogs and cats, but not limited to:

1. Gastroesophageal
Esophageal lesions, reflux esophagitis, gastric ulceration/perforation, gastric dilation/volvulus and neoplasia.

2. Intestinal
Inflammatory bowel – see Section III.A.7, foreign body, torsion, ulceration/perforation, neoplasia.

3. Colonic
Inflammatory, constipation, foreign body, torsion, ulceration/perforation and neoplasia.

4. Liver and Gallbladder
Inflammation, biliary obstruction, cholelithiasis, neoplasia and abscess.

5. Pancreas
See Section III.A.8.

6. Spleen
Splenic torsion, hematoma, abscess and neoplasia.

With prolonged inflammation in some of these conditions, and direct involvement of neural tissue (pancreatitis), continual visceral afferent stimulation results in central sensitization, which frequently contributes to a secondary pain hypersensitivity in the GI tract resembling secondary hyperalgesia in the skin [10]. Because of the involvement of the neural pathways, these conditions are considered to result in neuropathic pain.

The following are illnesses that cause neuropathic pain in humans and are assumed to produce the same pain syndromes in cats and dogs.

7. Inflammatory Bowel Disease
Inflammatory bowel disease occurs in dogs and cats. From a neuropathic perspective, inflammatory bowel disease is similar to other conditions of persistent afferent barrage to the dorsal horn. True "nociceptors" may be "disguised" within the mechanoreceptors that have either a low or high threshold for response that encode for the intensity of the stimulus in the GI tract [5]. Both classes of mechanoreceptors are capable of processing and transmitting sensory input in the noxious range. Also, both low- and high-threshold mechanoreceptors are capable of becoming sensitized in the presence of inflammation [4]. The presence of silent fibres and their recruitment during inflammatory conditions has also been documented [1, 11]. Therefore, visceral afferent fibres innervating the GI tract are capable of changing their behaviour during organ inflammation to increase the peripheral barrage into the spinal cord giving rise to visceral pain and hyperalgesia [1, 11].

Visceral pain can influence the sensitivity of somatic structures, including the skin and muscle (i.e. viscerosomatic hypersensitivity). Human patients with irritable bowel syndrome often experience somatic and cutaneous hyperalgesia, which is thought to be the result of central sensitization. These clinical observations have been confirmed in a study of experimental cystitis, where mice exhibited cutaneous thermal hyperalgesia. Similar to viscerovisceral hypersensitivity, chronic somatic pain can also influence the sensitivity of the visceral organs [11].

8. Pancreatitis/Pancreatic Pain
Abdominal pain is a key feature of both acute and chronic pancreatitis in dogs and humans, but not consistently so in cats. In chronic pancreatitis and pancreatic cancer, damage to intrapancreatic nerves, and invasion by immune cells, supports the maintenance and exacerbation of neuropathic pain and the abdominal pain syndrome in humans [12]. Similarly, pancreatic cancer cells infiltrate the perineurium of local extrapancreatic nerves, which may in part explain the severe pain experienced by our patients. In recent years, the involvement of a variety of neurotrophins and neuropeptides in the pathogenesis of acute and chronic pancreatic pain was discovered [12].

In a human study, electrical stimulation of the GI tract with concurrent recordings using the electroencephalogram showed that pain in chronic pancreatitis leads to changes in cortical projections of the nociceptive system [13]. Similar findings have also been described in somatic pain disorders, among them neuropathic pain [13]. Potentially, these mechanisms exist in both cats and dogs explaining the apparent severe to excruciating pain experienced in some animals with repeated episodes of pancreatitis.

9. Analgesia

Analgesia for GI illness or injury is dependent on the underlying problem, whether surgery is performed, whether an acute or chronic, acute-on-chronic presentation and which of mild, moderate or severe pain is experienced. For details on managing specific cases, refer to case scenarios of the abdomen, pelvis and perineum in Chapter 29 and Chapter 30. Treatment from these cases can be extrapolated to other conditions of the abdomen, in combination with the physiology and clinical relevance of specific analgesic information presented here, and in Chapter 12. Where neuropathic pain is a potential painful experience due to chronicity, refer to Chapter 3.

Lumbosacral placement of analgesics may extend to T10 conferring abdominal analgesia. Refer to Chapter 14.

B. Urogenital System

1. Urologic System

Physiologic information derived from laboratory animals unless otherwise noted [5].

i. Kidney

As with other abdominal organs, capsular stretch is a cause of severe kidney pain. Causes for this are kidney parenchymal inflammation, toxicity, acute injury, nephroliths, hydronephrosis and neoplasia. The renal nerves involved in nociception, both myelinated and unmyelinated fibres, are derived from sympathetic and parasympathetic (vagus) nerves [5].

ii. Ureter

Pain is the only conscious sensation arising from the ureter. Afferents from the ureter are mostly found in the L2–L3 and S1–S2 DRGs in laboratory animals. Retrograde injection of a dye in one ureter revealed a large number of labelled small-diameter neurons containing S-P and calcitonin gene-related peptide (CGRP) in the DRGs of the contralateral side, suggesting that pain originating from one ureter can spread bilaterally to a wide referral site. Recordings from the thoracolumbar (T12–L1) spinal dorsal horn neurons have documented that all excitatory neurons respond to distending pressures > 20 mmHg, thus suggesting that ureter afferents are largely involved in signalling a painful stimulus [5]. Ureteral calculi are a common medical problem where pain is generated by local inflammation and smooth muscle contraction. The **pain of renal colic** in human patients was relieved more effectively with lidocaine 1.5 mg/kg than morphine [8]. The NMDA receptor processing of acute nociceptive inputs from non-inflamed viscera has also been identified in the ureter [3], and ketamine has been shown to inhibit nociceptive reflexes evoked from the normal ureter. Ketamine resolved the pain of renal colic in humans where morphine did not.

iii. Bladder

- **A-delta and C fibre mechanosensitive afferents**, with significant recruitment of "silent" afferents, are activated by inflammation of the bladder. The silent afferents are mechanically insensitive afferent neurons that develop mechano-sensitivity during inflammatory states. These sensations are transmitted to the CNS via sympathetic (lumbar splanchnic and hypogastric nerves) and parasympathetic (pelvic nerve) afferents [5].

- The **pelvic nerve** afferents project via S1–S4 dorsal roots. The pelvic nerve is the major pathway for sensation from the lower urinary tract. The pelvic nerve afferents are more abundant in the muscle than in the suburothelium and are widely distributed throughout the bladder, including the dome, body and trigone. Distension of the bladder can induce sensations in the perineal area, including the perineum and penis. Perineal sensations are thought to be mediated via the pelvic nerve afferents, which enter the sacral spinal segments having a dermatomal distribution in the perineal area [5].
- **Lumbar splanchnic nerve** terminals innervate the dorsal trigone and neck regions of the bladder and are predominantly found in the suburothelium. The lumbar splanchnic nerve afferents project via L2–L5 dorsal roots. The midline suprapubic sensation associated with bladder over-distension is mediated via lumbar splanchnic nerve afferents entering the thoracolumbar spinal cord; these segments of the spinal cord are known to innervate the suprapubic dermatomes and myotomes [5].

iv. Common, Painful, Urologic Conditions Seen in Dogs and Cats

- Bacterial cystitis, cystic calculi and interstitial cystitis (IC) are common problems in cats and dogs. Where the underlying problem is not treated, the afferent fibre barrage generated from the inflamed bladder results in a slowly developing, and maintained, increase in the excitability of spinal cord dorsal horn neurons producing central sensitization [10].
- **Idiopathic cystitis in domestic cats/feline interstitial cystitis (FIC)** is a well-recognized problem in cats and is an example of visceral inflammation resulting in neurogenic pain [14, 15]. Human patients with IC suffer bladder pain and urinary urgency. Studies in cats with IC have demonstrated abnormalities in the bladder, sensory neurons, CNS and sympathetic efferent neurons. These cats have decreased excretion of glycosaminoglycan (GAG), increased bladder permeability and neurogenic inflammation. The reduced protection of bladder uroepithelium by lowered GAG levels may facilitate increased contact of urine with the primary afferent nerve terminals innervating the bladder resulting in a local release of neurotransmitters, and neurogenic inflammation. High affinity S-P receptors have also been identified in the bladders of cats with FIC with associated increase in S-P [11]. Stress has been identified as a component of FIC in cats (see Section VI). Multi-modal therapy is frequently required based on the neurogenic inflammation, afferent, efferent and CNS stress component (refer to scenarios in Chapter 29 and Chapter 30).

2. Female Reproductive System: Review
i. Physiologic Information from Studies Performed in Rats and Mice [4]
Neuroanatomical information from the dog. Nociceptive transmission is via:

- **Projections from the uterine horn** run through the L1–L2 roots. The sympathetic and visceral afferent fibres via the hypogastric nerve (HGN) and parasympathetic and visceral afferents via the pelvic nerve (PN). The PN afferents are more sensitive to mechanical stimulation compared with HGN afferents, which mostly respond to discrete probing of the surface of the uterine horn and respond only to a high intensity of uterine distension. The uterine PN afferents are also sensitive to chemical stimulation, indicating sensitivity to inflammation, more so than the HGN.
- **Afferents from the vaginal canal** predominantly enter the spinal cord via the L6–S1 with HGN afferents responding best to vaginal and cervical distension, and probing of the internal surface of the cervix. Sensory afferents are via the pudendal nerve.
- **Projections from the mid-portion of the uterine cervix** are equally distributed in L6–S1 and L1–L2 roots. The majority of afferents also respond to chemical stimuli.

The intensity of pain sensation is primarily influenced by estrogen; both the PN and HGN afferents are more sensitive, including an expanded receptive field, in the proestrous stage compared with diestrous/metestrous stages. As with other visceral pathology, somatic and cutaneous hyperalgesia may also be experienced due to potential for central sensitization.

ii. Analgesia

In veterinary medicine, the preferred method of treatment for patients with **ovarian/uterine pathology** is ovariohysterectomy as endometrial hyperplasia, endometritis may persist or recur, and pyometra if left untreated can be fatal. Refer to [16] management.

Vaginal hyperplasia and prolapse is painful and may result in urethral obstruction at the papilla. As a rare occurrence, unrelenting pain may occur due to tearing of the vagina during copulation or artificial insemination, or human abuse. Careful examination of the vagina under anesthesia is essential to identify a potential lesion which may also result in sperm peritonitis [17].

Epidural anesthesia/analgesia is highly recommended (refer to Chapter 14). Refer to abdomen, pelvis perineum case scenarios in Chapter 29 and Chapter 30 for recommended perioperative analgesia and anesthesia. Lumbosacral epidural block of dogs and cats has been shown to reach up to the T10 vertebra and provide sufficient anesthesia for a laparotomy, and pelvis, perineal area.

3. Dog: Penis, Prepuce, Urethra

Paraphimosis, balanoposthitis, ischemic priapism, fractured os penis, urethral obstruction and prostatitis are all painful conditions. Based on the nociceptive pathway, epidural analgesia/anesthesia can be obtained via lumbosacral epidural analgesia anesthesia. Refer to Chapter 30 case scenarios for analgesia, anesthesia and nursing care. Refer to [18] for medical and surgical management.

IV. Pelvis and Perineum [3, 5]

A. Pelvis

Pelvic fractures and repair may result in injury to the cauda equina within the lumbosacral canal and is composed of the:

- seventh lumbar (L7) nerve
- sacral nerve roots
- coccygeal nerve roots.

Injury of these roots causes deficits of sciatic, pudendal, pelvic, perineal and caudal rectal nerve function. At the pelvic outlet the pudendal nerve gives rise to the caudal rectal and perineal nerves, and nerves to the external genital organs.

Pudendal nerve entrapment in humans is a cause for chronic, disabling perineal pain (anorectal, urogenital, especially when sitting), urinary hesitancy, frequency, urgency, constipation/painful bowel movements and sexual dysfunction in both sexes.

B. Scrotum Cat and Dog, Penis Cat

Perineal sensations are via the pelvic nerve afferents, which enter the sacral spinal segments having a dermatomal distribution in the perineal area.

An enlarged scrotum may be due to scrotal dermatitis, edema, neoplasia, intrascrotal hemorrhage or testicular torsion. Testicular or epididymal enlargement may be due to a granulomatous, infiltrative or infectious cause. All are very painful and require specific therapy and multi-modal analgesia to resolve the pain [17, 18]. Surgical intervention for definitive management and elimination of pain is also required for some of these problems [18]. Urethral obstruction in the cat is a fairly common emergent condition, and is also very painful [18].

Epidural: sacrococcygeal (Chapter 14) is recommended to facilitate comfort when managing the above problems especially in cats with urethral obstruction during manipulation of the urethra. Proper technique blocks the sacral portion of the lumbosacral plexus, including the pelvic, pudendal and caudal nerves, providing anesthesia of the perineum, penis, urethra, colon, anus and tail.

C. Vulva

Vaginal hyperplasia and prolapse is painful and may result in urethral obstruction at the papilla. There are varying degrees of prolapse and subsequent injury requiring specific therapy based on severity in addition to multi-modal analgesia. Management and surgical procedures are outlined in [16]. The autonomic innervation is via the HGN and PN, while sensory impulses also pass through the pudendal nerve. Autonomic functions are via the HGN and PN.

D. Prolapsed Rectum, Perianal Fistulae and Anal Gland Abscess

Refer to abdomen, pelvis, perineum case scenarios for analgesic selection in Chapter 29 and Chapter 30.

Epidural: sacrococcygeal; Chapter 14 provides anesthesia of the perineum, penis, urethra, colon, anus and tail.

V. Visceral Pain Associated with Pelvis, Vertebral and Spinal Cord Injury or Illness

Extra-abdominal causes for pain to consider are vertebral and spinal cord illness or injury. In dogs and cats, the pelvis, lumbar and sacral vertebral fractures, intervertebral disc disease, abscess and discospondylitis, spinal neoplasia, retro-peritoneal abscess and hemorrhage may result in visceral pain. Humans with spinal cord injury resulting in partial to complete paraplegia may experience visceral pain, most often described as severe or excruciating, without identifiable GI, genitourinary or pelvic abnormalities that could account for visceral pain symptoms [19]. These may occur months to years after injury. The mechanisms of these are unknown. Theories are that visceral pain may be caused by: (1) a continuous slow fibre discharge caused by unrecognized alterations in visceral function, (2) a phenomenon occurring at the sympathetic chain ganglia or (3) a distortion of the afferent impulses from the viscera crossing the zone of injury in the vertebral column or spinal cord [19]. A question veterinarians may ask is: "Does visceral pain occur after these injuries or illness in our patients, and how would we know?"

VI. Modulatory Influences on Visceral Nociception

Pain in general can be **modulated by extra-nociceptive neuronal and non-neuronal influences.** These factors also influence visceral sensation. Several cortical and subcortical brain regions process central responses to external stressors. Visceral perception and pain can be influenced by three main effector mechanisms: (1) the descending spinal pathways, (2) the autonomic nervous system and (3) the hypothalamus–pituitary axis [2]. In veterinary medicine, evidence indicates that cats and dogs suffer from anxiety in certain situations and being hospitalized is definitely a situation that is associated with stress and anxiety [20, 21]. Stress is a component of inflammatory bowel disease in some cats and dogs [22]. Pain is often associated with gut motor abnormalities that generate exaggerated intraluminal pressures, and the high threshold baroreceptors of the gut wall are activated at lower, normally ineffective, intraluminal pressures. Idiopathic cystitis is another known cause of stress-induced pathology where some cats have benefitted from amitriptyline treatment for severe recurrent episodes [23]. This component of a potential cause for increased visceral pain in our patients is raised here to emphasize the importance of nursing care and environmental conditions of the hospital (e.g. avoid cats being close to dogs) to reduce the potential for inducing affective (emotional, anxiety) visceral co-morbidities. As the pathophysiology of affective visceral co-morbidities is assumed to be similar in cats and dogs as it is in the laboratory animal and human, information on pathophysiology in these species is presented for consideration in the cat and dog.

A. Pathophysiology of Affective Visceral Co-Morbidities: Review [2]

In humans, both acute stress and psychologic factors have important roles in chronic visceral pain conditions. Anxiety has also been shown to increase the "sensation" of intestinal gas and associated pain and to increase "unpleasantness" ratings to painful stimuli. These findings may be related to increased activity in the brain areas that are known to be associated with the affective-motivational component of pain processing. The connection between the visceral sensory experience and emotional state is explained by the function of the vagus in sensory feedback from the gut and integration with the limbic and para-limbic brain areas involved in homeostatic regulation, including pain modulation. Functional brain imaging studies indicate differences between somatic and visceral pain in "limbic cortex" activation as being responsible for the greater unpleasantness of visceral pain. On physical examination it is known that the human patient exhibits a greater response elicited by abdominal (visceral) palpation than the somatic response generated by a similar degree of pressure applied when examining a painful limb, other than that for fasciitis, for example. The complex network of brain structures modulates stress responses through an effector system referred to as the "emotional motor system", the main output components of which are descending spinal pathways, the autonomic nervous system and hypothalamus–pituitary axis.

Animal studies have demonstrated that experimentally induced stress in rats alters gut motility in a pattern similar to that seen in humans. An increase in abdominal cramps evoked by rectal distension in a rat model, without affecting rectal compliance, was induced by administration of corticotropin-releasing hormone (CRH) and subsequently blocked by a CRH antagonist, indicating a role of CRH in visceral hypersensitivity. The mast cell mediators also appear to be involved in the hypersensitivity response to rectal distension induced by stress as administration of a mast cell stabilizer suppressed stress and CRH-induced rectal hyperalgesia in this model. This effect has been reproduced in other laboratory studies.

Other animal studies have shown that responsiveness of these physiologic systems, and the ability to adapt, can be altered by adverse early life events increasing the susceptibility to the negative effects of stress in later life. Various human clinical studies have also demonstrated allodynia and hyperalgesia in juveniles and adults when inadequate pain management, or stressful situations, occurred when they were neonates, infants or juveniles. Anecdotally, this has been observed in dogs following tail docking and ear cropping. The importance of this is that these young animals feel pain as much as, and maybe even more than, we do, and administration of appropriate analgesia where indicated is essential. Refer to Chapter 25 for further discussion.

References

1 Joshi, S. K. and Gebhart, G. F. (2000) Visceral pain. *Current Review of Pain*, 4(6): 499–506.
2 Knowles, C. H. and Qasim, A. (2009) Basic and clinical aspects of gastrointestinal pain. *Pain*, 141: 191–209.
3 Bueno, L. (2000) Pathobiology of visceral pain: Molecular mechanisms and therapeutic implications: III: Visceral afferent pathways: A source of new therapeutic targets for abdominal pain. *Am J Physiol Gastrointest Liver Physiol*, 278: G670–G676.
4 Fass, J., Bares, R. and Hermsdorf, V. (1995) Effects of ketamine on gastrointestinal motility in dogs. *J Intensve Care Med*, 21(4): 584–589.
5 Sengupta, J. N. (2009) Visceral pain: The neurophysiological mechanism. In: Canning, B. J. and Spina, D. (eds.), *Sensory Nerves: Handbook of experimental pharmacology*. Springer Verlag, Berlin: 31–74.
6 White, M., Shah, N., Lindley, K., *et al.* (2006) Pain management in fulminating ulcerative colitis. *Pediatr Anesth*, 16: 1148–1152.
7 Groudin, S. B., Fisher, H A., Kaufman, R. P., Jr, *et al.* (1998) Intravenous lidocaine speeds the return of bowel function, decreases post-operative pain, and shortens hospital stay in patients undergoing radical retropubic prostatectomy. *Anesth Analg*, 86: 235–239.
8 Soleimanpour, H., Hassanzadeh, K., Mohammadi, D. A., *et al.* (2011) Parenteral lidocaine for treatment of intractable renal colic: A case series. *J Medical Case Reports*, 5: 256.
9 Boscan, P., Monnet, E., Mama, K., *et al.* (2011) Effect of maropitant, a neurokinin 1 receptor antagonist, on anesthetic requirements during noxious visceral stimulation of the ovary in dogs. *Am J Vet Res*, 72: 1576–1579.
10 Moshiree, B., Zhou, Q., Price, D. D., *et al.* (2006) Central sensitisation in visceral pain disorders. *Gut*, 55: 905–908.
11 Gebhart, G. F. (2000) Pathobiology of visceral pain: Molecular mechanisms and therapeutic implications: IV: Visceral afferent contributions to the pathobiology of visceral pain. *Am J Physiol Gatrointest Liver Physiol*, 278: G834–G838.
12 Ceyhan, G. O., Michalski, C. W., Demir, I. E., *et al.* (2008) Pancreatic pain. *Best Pract Res Clin Gastroenterol*, 22(1): 31–44.
13 Dimcevski, G., Sami, S. A., Funch-Jensen, P., *et al.* (2007) Pain in chronic pancreatitis: The role of reorganization in the central nervous system. *Gastroenterology*, 132(4): 1546–1556.
14 Buffington, C. A. T. (2011) Idiopathic cystitis in domestic cats: Beyond the lower urinary tract. *Vet Intern Med*, 25: 784–796.
15 Buffington, C. A. T. and Chew, D. J. (2013) Pandora syndrome: It's more than just the bladder. American Association of Feline Practitioners Conference September 26–29, Dallas, Texas.
16 Gartley, C. and Brisson, B. (2017) Chapters 97 and 98. In: Mathews, K. A. (ed.), *Veterinary Emergency & Critical Care Manual*, 3rd edn. LifeLearn, Guelph, Ontario, Canada.
17 Davidson, A. P. (2014) Reproductive system disorders. In: Nelson, R. W. and Couto, C. G. (eds), *Small Animal Internal Medicine*. Elsevier, St Louis, MO: 915–965.
18 Gartley, C., Defarges, A. and Bichot, S. (in press) Male urogenital emergencies. In: Mathews, K. A. (ed.), *Veterinary Emergency & Critical Care Manual*, 3rd edn. LifeLearn, Guelph, Ontario, Canada.

19 Kogos, S. C., Jr, Richards, J. S., Banos, J. H., *et al.* (2005) Visceral pain and life quality in persons with spinal cord injury: A brief report. *J Spinal Cord Med*, 28(4): 333–337.

20 Quimby, J. M., Smith, M. L. and Lunn, K. F. (2011) Evaluation of the effects of hospital visit stress on physiologic parameters in the cat. *J Feline Med Surg*, 13: 733–737.

21 Bragg, R. F., Bennett, J. S., Cummings, A. and Quimby, J. E. (2015) Evaluation of the effects of hospital visit stress on physiologic variables in dogs. *J Am Vet Med Assoc*, 246: 212–215.

22 Hall, E. J. and Day, M. J. (2017) Diseases of the small intestine. In: Ettinger, S. J., Feldman, E. C. and Cote, E. (eds), *Textbook of Veterinary Internal Medicine*, 8th edn. Elsevier, St Louis, MO.

23 Chew, D. J., Buffington, C. A. T., Kendell, M. S., *et al.* (1998) Amitriptyline treatment for severe recurrent idiopathic cystitis in cats. *J Am Vet Med Assoc*, 213: 1282–1286.

5

Physiology and Management of Cancer Pain

Karol Mathews and Michelle Oblak

As humans will testify, the pain induced by a neoplastic process is mild initially and commonly ignored. However, the pain level progresses over a variable period of time, appearing early when neural tissue is involved or is present in a "tight" environment (e.g. endosteal, periosteal, muscle or capsular organs). Clinical signs associated with the neoplastic process are associated with the pain experienced, type of cancer and anatomical structure involved. As an example, where the tumour involves innervation of/to the limbs, this is frequently misdiagnosed as osteoarthritis, as this cancer frequently occurs in older animals where an osteoarthritic lesion may be present. This misdiagnosis may result in delayed diagnosis of the tumour, contributing to the variable duration and severity of pain experienced. Cancer patients, either diagnosed or not yet diagnosed, may present as an emergency due to the final stage of associated illness or injury (e.g. pathologic fracture); at this stage, all are associated with pain. Due to the wind-up that has occurred prior to presentation, pain can be severe to excruciating (refer to Chapter 2 for details). When a patient presents with a diagnosed, or potential, neoplastic process, careful questioning to the owner is important to understand the course of progression. Questions of the owner must include asking for cues to insidious onset of pain, involving any anatomical area, and illness for all patients, but especially so for middle-aged and geriatric patients. Include questions of any previous history of pain or lameness, changes in play or exercise behaviours, changes in appetite or eating behaviours (i.e. dropping food and drooling more), sleeping patterns, or other behaviour, and any medications previously or currently administered.

Several distinct types of pain exist, classified as "nociceptive", "inflammatory" and "neuropathic" [1]. Cancer pain, in addition to the establishment of wind-up, most commonly comprises both inflammatory and neuropathic pain, which contributes to the high level of pain experienced. Refer to Chapters 2 and 3 for details. In all anatomical locations, inflammation due to tumour necrosis or direct pressure causes pain. Visceral pain, in addition to inflammation, arises from stretching and distension of the viscera and swelling of encapsulated organs. This pain is described by humans as cramping, aching, gnawing, deep and difficult to localize [2]. Refer to Chapter 4 for details. Somatic pain originates from lesions, or tissue that has been infiltrated, in bone, joints, muscle or skin and is described by humans as constant, sharp, aching, throbbing and is localized [2]. However, this pain may also originate from nerve sheath tumours, nerves, or nerve root compression. Some cancers such as lymphomas and leukemia have a lower incidence of pain experienced by humans; however, when present, the pain can be excruciating [2]. The incidence and severity of pain associated with various cancer types in animals is not well documented; however, one of the best documented is bone pain. This may be primary, as with osteosarcoma, or metastatic involvement of bone. The cause of pain for both results from direct

Analgesia and Anesthesia for the Ill or Injured Dog and Cat, First Edition. Karol A. Mathews, Melissa Sinclair, Andrea M. Steele and Tamara Grubb.
© 2018 John Wiley & Sons, Inc. Published 2018 by John Wiley & Sons, Inc.

invasion of the bone, microfractures, increased pressure of endosteum, distortion of the periosteum, or perilesional inflammation. In humans, the pain is described as dull, constant and gradually increasing in intensity; movement and pressure worsen it. Incident pain usually has a sudden onset, reaching peak pain intensity within a few minutes and is a cause of breakthrough pain in a large number of human patients [2]. In veterinary medicine, it is not unusual for the presentation to be one of acute-on-chronic pain and lameness due to a pathologic fracture. Another important mechanism in the genesis of bone pain is the release of chemical mediators such as amines, peptides, fatty acids, potassium and prostaglandins. Cancer pain, and bone pain in particular, is often associated with neuropathic-like clinical signs.

As always, it is essential to perform a thorough physical examination in all patients presenting with a medical problem as neoplasia may be the underlying cause of the clinical signs. Prior to handling the patient, evaluation of gait should be performed (Figure 5.1), which can help to indicate whether an abnormality is due to orthopedic or neurologic causes, or could identify an abnormal/hunched posture—an indication of abdominal or back pain. Since many of these patients can experience significant wind-up associated with their pain, evaluation prior to handling is important, as localization of the pain may become progressively more difficult as the exam progresses. Following gait assessment, physical examination should include both a neurologic and orthopedic assessment. In many cases these examinations are not mutually exclusive, but it is important to understand whether the patient's abnormalities are related to pain or neurologic deficiencies. If any bone pain is suspected, a gentle touch should first be employed during physical and orthopedic examination. In many cases, due to the severity of pain and chronic progression, these patients will require minimal manipulation to demonstrate the areas of pain. A slow increase in pressure, if required, should be used to identify areas of concern and level of pain. A thorough oral examination, and rectal where indicated, should be included. In many of these cases, wind-up, hyperalgesia and allodynia may exist. Therefore, a gentle touch could elicit a 10 out of 10 on the pain scale (refer to Chapter 2).

The orthopedic examination can provide significant insight into the overall condition of the patient and is likely to be more sensitive than other screening tests to identify potential bone or nerve lesions. Areas of concern identified on the orthopedic exam are then further examined with radiographs or computed tomography.

Removal of the underlying neoplastic process, where possible, is essential as even multi-modal analgesia may not "cure" the pain experienced. Limb amputation is frequently advised for patients with osteosarcoma. To reduce/eliminate the development of neuropathic pain following

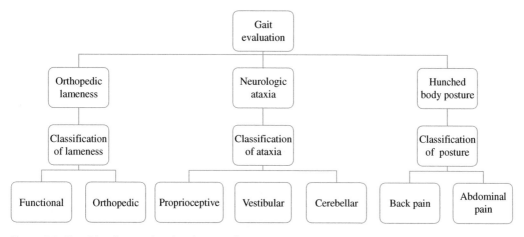

Figure 5.1 Algorithm for peripheral evaluation of patients presenting with gait abnormalities.

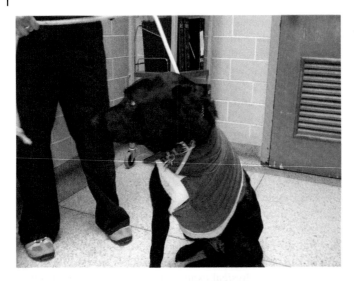

Figure 5.2a Post-operative forelimb amputation due to osteosarcoma. A wound diffusion catheter was placed during surgery as described in Chapter 14.

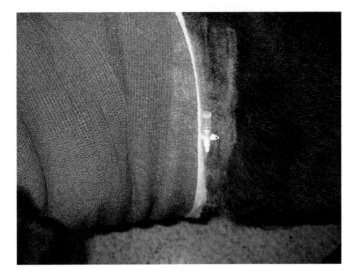

Figure 5.2b Access port to wound diffusion catheter.

amputation, a wound diffusion catheter is highly recommended (Figure 5.2a and b; refer to Chapter 14 for directions) [3]. Analgesia is also essential during diagnostic work-up and, where indicated, referral to a speciality practice for surgical and/or oncological (chemotherapy and radiotherapy) management. Based on the pathophysiology of cancer pain a multi-modal drug approach to the control of cancer pain is essential [2, 4, 5]. Non-steroidal anti-inflammatory drugs (NSAIDs) where there are no contraindications, opioids and adjunctive drugs, such as gabapentin, should be considered in the multi-modal regimen. A lidocaine patch placed over a located area of allodynia associated with a neuropathic component of cancer pain in human patients relieved the pain in 25% of these patients [6]. Due to the inconsistent absorption of lidocaine in cats and dogs, the success rate will probably be lower than in humans.

Integrative techniques should be used concurrently, where indicated, with the analgesics suggested above (refer to Chapter 15). The combination of acupuncture with drug therapy appears to be superior to either alone [7]. Other forms of adjunctive therapy, such as radiation therapy, tend to improve quality of life in cancer patients, although it is not known if they directly induce analgesia.

Refer to Chapter 8 and specific anatomic scenarios for analgesic guidance. Where there are no definitive treatment options refer to hospice and palliative care websites [8, 9].

References

1 Woolf, C. (2004) Pain: Moving from symptom control toward mechanism-specific pharmacologic management. *Annals of Internal Medicine*, 140: 441–451.

2 Gaynor, J. S. (2008) Control of cancer pain in veterinary patients. *Vet Clin North Am Small Anim Pract*, 38: 1429–1448.

3 Hansen, B., Lascelles, D. X., Thomson, A. and DePuy, V. (2013) Variability of performance of wound infusion catheters. *Vet Anaesth Analg*, 40: 308–315.

4 Trumpatori, B. and Lascelles, B. D. X. (2011) Relief of chronic cancer pain. In: Dobson, J. and Lascelles, B. D. X. (eds) *BSAVA Manual of Oncology*, 3rd edn. BSAVA Publications, Gloucester: 111–129.

5 Lascelles, B. D. X. (2012) Management of chronic cancer pain. In: Withrow, S., Vail, D. and Page, R. (eds) *Small Animal Clinical Oncology*, 5th edn. Saunders Elsevier, St Louis, MO.

6 Fleming, J. A. and O'Connor, B. D. (2009) Use of lidocaine patches for neuropathic pain in a comprehensive cancer centre. *Pain Res Manage*, 14(5): 381–388.

7 Choi, T. Y., Lee, M. S., Kim, T. H., *et al.* (2012) Acupuncture for the treatment of cancer pain: A systematic review of randomized clinical trials. *Support Care Cancer*, 20: 147–158.

8 International Association for Animal Hospice and Palliative Care (2017) https://www.iaahpc.org/resources-and-support/find-help-now.html.

9 Veterinary Society for Hospice and Palliative Care (2017) http://www.vethospicesociety.org/member-list/.

6

Movement-Evoked and Breakthrough Pain

Karol Mathews

Movement-evoked pain can be difficult to manage, especially when associated with nerve involvement. When increasing dosages of analgesics are given to stop movement-evoked pain, the patient may experience the adverse effects of the analgesic when at rest (i.e. dysphoria, panting with opioids) [1]. As movement is essential for a rapid recovery, delivery of local anesthetics (i.e. intrapleural, amputation site) or administration of two or more classes of analgesics (e.g. multi-modal therapy) is recommended. Other examples of stimulus-evoked pain could be related to pressing around the surgical wound to assess the presence of mechanical hyperalgesia. In a study, low-dose ketamine infusion reduced the intensity of mechanical hyperalgesia around the surgical wound for 24 h post-operatively [1]. Managing pain in situations other than when the patient is at rest can be challenging requiring analgesic protocols and procedures specifically prepared for the individual patient and their associated problem, and a search for a potential new underlying cause.

Breakthrough pain (BTP) is common in human patients who have cancer and in a variety of other problems causing pain. The reported incidence of BTP varies widely from 16 to 95% of those with persistent pain syndromes [2]. It is suggested that the variability may be due to lack of a clear consensus on the definition of BTP, but it is most commonly defined as an abrupt, short-lived and intense pain that "breaks through" the around-the-clock analgesia that controls persistent pain [2]. The three subtypes of BTP are incident, idiopathic and end-of-dose failure. BTP also is categorized as somatic, visceral, neuropathic or mixed [2].

BTP may occur in the post-operative setting or intermittently at home in animals on chronic pain medication for cancer or neuropathic pain. As described by the human patient, this pain is severe or excruciating, and of rapid onset which can disable or even immobilize the patient [2]. Should this occur in the hospital, intravenous administration of an opioid is the primary treatment, or add another class of fast-acting analgesic if an opioid has been administered. The analgesic protocol should then be re-assessed for duration and dose of prescribed medication, and to ensure that there is no underlying problem causing this pain. If the pain appears severe, this may be an indication of a neuropathic component. Careful observation as to the cause of BTP, such as a new problem, is required. It is essential to identify the source and severity of pain, as successful treatment is based on this. Therefore, careful ongoing observation is required while considering the severity of injury, invasiveness and anatomical area of surgery (assumed descending order of discomfort: oral cavity, rectum/vagina/testicles/penis, thorax, abdomen, pelvis, digits and limbs), the definite or potential involvement of neural tissue and the pain experienced prior to surgery. Medical inflammatory pain is also extremely painful requiring frequent, or preferred continuous rate infusion, dosing of analgesics until the illness

Analgesia and Anesthesia for the Ill or Injured Dog and Cat, First Edition. Karol A. Mathews, Melissa Sinclair, Andrea M. Steele and Tamara Grubb.
© 2018 John Wiley & Sons, Inc. Published 2018 by John Wiley & Sons, Inc.

subsides where the duration of analgesic administration can be increased. If there is no change in patient status, and a single analgesic agent is being used, consider a multi-modal analgesic regimen outlined in Chapters 3, 4, 8, 12 and 15 (see the list at the end of this chapter).

BTP is easily recognized in the acute pain setting in hospitalized animals; however, veterinarians may be unaware of the occurrence of BTP in patients with persistent chronic pain at home unless specific questions are asked of the client. Greater knowledge and awareness of BTP, especially when neuropathic pain may be occurring based on anatomic involvement of a lesion, or history of previous events predisposing to neuropathic pain, should lead to recognition, diagnosis and appropriate treatment of BTP in these patients. When BTP occurs at home, a careful history is required to obtain clues about the cause and pattern of BTP. It may be difficult to administer oral medication when animals exhibit excruciating pain. If the pain cannot be controlled, parenteral administration has to be considered. The dose and/or dosing frequency, of the around-the-clock analgesic, should be adjusted for patients with end-of-dose BTP. In addition to pharmacologic therapy, non-pharmacologic, integrative analgesic strategies (Chapter 15) are often helpful in alleviating pain and anxiety and should be considered on an individual patient basis as a supplement to pharmacologic intervention for BTP.

Refer to:

- Recognition, assessment and treatment of pain in dogs and cats, Chapter 8;
- Neuropathic pain, Chapter 3;
- Visceral pain, Chapter 4;
- Integrative techniques, Chapter 15;
- Adjunct analgesia, Chapter 12.

References

1 Stubhaug, A., Breivik, H., Eidei, P. K., *et al.* (1997) Mapping of punctuate hyperalgesia around a surgical incision demonstrates that ketamine is a powerful suppressor of central sensitization to pain following surgery. *Acta Anaesthesiol Scand*, 41: 1124–1132.
2 Payne, R. (2007) Recognition and diagnosis of breakthrough pain. *Pain Med*, 8(suppl. 1): S3–S7.

7

Pain: Understanding It

Karol Mathews

"Pain" (nociception) is defined as an unpleasant sensory and emotional experience associated with actual or potential tissue damage, **or described in terms of such damage** [1]. Nociceptive function is present in some form in all living organisms. This adaptive function is physiologically essential for protection, and when absent in any organism, the lifespan is shortened considerably [2]. Therefore, where tissue injury/inflammation (pain) exists, the nociceptive information is processed to the level of conscious perception making the organism aware of this and prompting some form of action to remedy it. In this context, this protective mechanism is present across species and the warning occurs at the same level of sensation for potential injury (e.g. heat, cold, pressure, sting, cut). This highlights the comparative component of pain – "that would hurt me" – assisting with the caregiver's appreciation of the pain the patient is likely experiencing with a given illness or injury.

The response to a painful (nociceptive) stimulus, be it traumatic, surgical or medical/inflammatory, has both physiological [2] and pathophysiological [3] components, whereas the "warning" scenario is a physiologic protective (adaptive) response where the individual experiences a noxious feeling and is able to remove themselves from the cause (e.g. touching a source of heat) prior to injury. The physiological response is protective – not only for the moment but also for awareness and memory – of potential future encounters. Therefore, the result is a complex multi-dimensional experience involving sensory and affective (emotional) components. Based on the central nervous system (CNS) pathways (refer to Chapter 2), one can see that the "programming" of the experience is intended to be protective, to make the experience unpleasant from many aspects and to embed it into memory so the causal situation is avoided in the future. Obviously, this is how all organisms survive. So, "pain is not just about how it feels, but how it makes you feel"; it is those unpleasant feelings that cause the suffering we associate with pain [4, 5]. We have all experienced pain – "the ouch feeling" – and this is our focus, but along with this is the emotional experience which contributes more to the offensive aspects of pain. The emotions include depression ("hangdog" look/feeling) and aggression, a reflex "slap" at anyone touching the painful area. A reflex slap for a dog is to bite, and/or scratch for a cat. This is a reminder for us all to approach and handle our patients carefully and with demonstrable care to make this a different experience from what the patient is currently undergoing. We know of the emotional aspect of pain, and a non-friendly environment contributes to the heightening of the pain experienced, again a reminder for the memory to avoid this in the future.

From our human interactions, we appreciate that pain is a uniquely individual experience, with some having what appears to be a higher tolerance, or a reduced perception, of the pain

Analgesia and Anesthesia for the Ill or Injured Dog and Cat, First Edition. Karol A. Mathews, Melissa Sinclair, Andrea M. Steele and Tamara Grubb.
© 2018 John Wiley & Sons, Inc. Published 2018 by John Wiley & Sons, Inc.

than others. Depending on where your thoughts are on the "how much it hurts scale", it may be difficult to appreciate how individuals feel, especially in non-verbal animals where we have to use behavioural signs and apply our expected or known knowledge of likely causes and degree of pain to guide its management. Furthermore, it is a subjective emotion that can be experienced even in the absence of obvious external noxious stimulation, and which can be modified by behavioural experiences including fear, memory and stress.

Pain is present in many medical, all traumatic and inflammatory conditions and, without appropriate analgesic management, all post-operative patients. The demonstration of pain is not always obvious; therefore, an animal should be assumed to be experiencing pain in any condition expected to produce pain in humans. Refer to Table 8.1 for expected degree of pain with various scenarios. Experimental animal models of pain show that the animal tries to escape from a noxious stimulus of about the same intensity that causes human subjects to first report pain. Increasing the intensity of the acute noxious stimulus such as an electric current, increases the vocalization, escape force and reflex force by the animal [6]. Veterinarians routinely witness this behaviour when our patients are exposed to an acute painful stimulus; however, this type of behaviour may not occur in animals with constant pain [7]. Many animals with severe pain may lie still to avoid enhanced movement-induced pain. Therefore, extrapolation, or to anthropomorphize, to a human situation may help to plan an analgesic regimen.

I.   Objective Markers of Pain

Unfortunately, there is no one objective clinical sign indicating a specific degree of pain. **Physiological parameters**, including heart rate, respiratory rate, blood pressure and temperature, are not consistent or reliable indicators of pain as they may be a reflection of the associated pathologic state [8–10], or stress in the hospital environment [11, 12]. However, these changes do occur in some painful states and, in the author's experience when markedly increased, and the patient has an underlying reason to be painful, these are associated with severe pain.

- **Heart rate:** There are some situations where heart rate can be normal or reduced in painful patients. Pain associated with the abdominal viscera (i.e. correction of portosystemic shunt and other surgical procedures involving bowel, viral diarrhea, inflammatory bowel disease) may produce a low to normal heart rate (personal observations) due to vagal activity. Pain persisting or recurring after opioid administration is frequently not diagnosed due to the emphasis placed on the low to normal heart rate. As the autonomic effects of opioids tend to persist beyond their analgesic effects, heart rate is frequently an insensitive indicator of pain. Pain assessment based on behaviour and interaction is required to confirm an analgesic state. Neuropathic, orthopedic pain and pain associated with bacterial fasciitis (e.g. *Streptococcal* fasciitis) are examples of severe to excruciating pain resulting in marked tachycardia. Tachycardia is also present in the trauma patient and may be associated with blood loss in addition to pain.
- **Respiratory rate**, but not heart rate, consistently correlated with visual analogue scores and numerical rating scales of pain assessment in one study [8]; however, this was not shown to be a useful indicator of pain in another study [10]. As with heart rate, respiratory rate can be affected by the associated pathologic state, making interpretation difficult. While the presence of an increased respiratory rate, including panting, does not indicate pain in every patient, the author has found this to be of value when assessing the degree of pain in some patients. This tends to be associated with moderate, severe or excruciating pain, which is

identified on physical examination and history. Continuous panting, without vocalization, was noted in a dog with neurofibroma extending through the intervertebral foramen at L1–L2 along the dorsal nerve root. This was identified on careful physical examination (refer to Chapter 3).

- **Pupillary dilation** is "loosely associated" with pain [10], but fear and stress without pain is a confounder. Pupils must be assessed prior to opioid administration as the opioid effect causes mydriasis in cats but miosis in dogs. Other medications (e.g. atropine) will also render pupil size inappropriate in assessment of pain.
- **Systolic hypertension** frequently correlates with pain where increased heart rate and respiratory rate are noted due to the sympathetic response associated with pain and the precipitating event. Systolic hypertension has been reported in cats receiving inadequate post-operative analgesia, which also correlated with increased serum cortisol concentration and behavioural changes associated with pain (withdrawn, remained still and vocalized when moved) [13].

As there are no objective parameters of pain that we can consistently rely on, we can make an assessment based on the condition known to cause pain and the behaviour the animal exhibits. The increased heart and/or respiratory rate and/or hypertension, if present, contribute to the assessment of pain. It is the author's opinion that the response to analgesic administration will aid in the assessment of pain. The higher the dose, and the requirement for two or more classes of analgesics to control the painful behaviour, the more severe the pain state (see Section V).

The analgesic regimen must be tailored to the individual's painful experience, personality and environmental needs. In addition to providing analgesics, reducing patient anxiety is an important aspect to pain management as anxiety lowers the threshold of pain perception. Sedatives may be required in some animals if anxiety is contributing to the pain experienced, or if **mild** dysphoric behaviour may be suspected after opioid administration. Reducing anxiety can also be met by maintaining a warm, clean, dry and comfortable environment. For cats, this is preferably away from barking dogs and by providing a "bed" where the cat can curl up, or a large towel rolled up and placed in a circle and taped. Individual nursing care for certain time periods during the day, especially while feeding the patient, reduces anxiety and often increases food intake. Refer to Chapter 17 for details on this very important aspect of pain management.

Confounding situations may exist when using behaviour to assess the degree of pain experienced.

- **Dysphoria:** Where opioids are administered at a dose for pain assessed higher than the patient's pain experience frequently results in dysphoria. Restlessness and "howling" during, or within a short time after, opioid administration is a dysphoric response associated with an overdose of opioid and may be perceived as worsening pain. Panting, nausea and vomiting may also occur.
- **Emergence delirium:** Similar behaviour to dysphoria and may occur post surgery when recovering from anesthesia where opioids were administered. This may also be assessed as pain.
- **Opioid-induced hyperalgesia** in the acute pain setting occurs in some human patients following opioid administration [14]. In this setting the patient experiences worsening pain rather than analgesia during administration of the opioid and is able to articulate what is happening [14]. This also occurs in the human chronic pain setting where opioids are used for pain management. While this has not been reported in veterinary medicine, the author has treated a patient recovering from lumbosacral stabilization, experiencing severe neuropathic pain prior to surgery and upon recovery. During morphine titration the dog barked louder, became very restless, started to "scream" and began to "flip out" in a violent

manner, which does not occur in dysphoria. This was interpreted as opioid-induced hyperalgesia. This, in combination with hyperalgesia associated with the neuropathic pain, would result in severe to excruciating pain. Ketamine was titrated to effect sleep; during injection, the dog became quiet and, at 4 mg/kg, finally slept. Multi-modal continuous rate infusions of low-dose opioid, ketamine and lidocaine were established, with slow weaning off lidocaine at 12–24 h and ketamine 24–36 h. Gabapentin was instituted when able to swallow. A non-steroidal anti-inflammatory analgesic (NSAIA) is also recommended in the multi-modal regimen for this degree of pain; however, corticosteroids had been administered.

II. Definitions of Pain Mechanisms

1. **Nociceptive pain** is an intense, noxious sensory response that may be short-lived or it can be ongoing pain which is present secondary to trauma, surgical incisions, inflammation of viscera, etc. [15]. To assess the presence and degree of pain in animals it is important to observe their behaviour at rest/in the cage prior to the patient being aware of your presence. Note respiratory rate and effort, body position, awake or asleep, looking/chewing at an area of potential pain, if awake, note facial expression. Also, note if pain is elicited when moving. With no external stimulus, the behaviour noted will relate to the presence or absence of nociceptive pain. Followed by this assessment, unless known to be sleeping, the caregiver must interact with the patient to further evaluate the absence or presence, and level of, pain following administration of an appropriate analgesic.

2. **Movement-evoked pain:** It is essential to interact with the patient to assess their response to you and to establish if, and how much, pain is detected when moving. It is obvious from personal experience that frequently our "injured or ill part" hurts more when we move, but may be minimally painful at rest. Should movement consistently result in vocalization or other signs of pain in the post-operative period, this will alert the clinician as to the potential for a surgical-associated problem, such as nerve entrapment. (Refer to Chapter 6.)

3. **Stimulus-evoked pain** [15] is also nociceptive, as described in point 1 above, and is an example of a "test" for the presence of pain when **gently** pressing around the surgical wound to assess the presence of mechanical hyperalgesia. The examination should extend to the area not resulting in pain to assess the boundaries of the painful area. Noting the presence of hyperalgesia, an exaggerated response to the pressure and location from the original source of pain, will indicate the degree of pain and guide the veterinarian to a modification in the analgesic regimen based on the patient's response.

4. **Touch-evoked pain is termed "allodynia"**, which is pain elicited with a light, non-noxious touch that, under normal conditions, would not cause pain. Allodynia is present in neuropathic pain conditions and may extend way beyond the origin of the problem. As an example in humans, lumbosacral disc herniation involving the sciatic nerve results in pain in any region of the limb where the "injured" segment of the nerve serves.

    Trials in human medicine suggest that pain assessment at rest should be assessed separately from several types of evoked pain. This is an important point to consider in veterinary medicine, where descriptors for assessing pain should be included in each scoring system and an "at rest" and "stimulus-evoked" component introduced. The algometer and thermal tests have been used in some veterinary studies as an objective measure for a "stimulus-evoked" assessment of pain.

5. **Breakthrough pain (BTP)** is an abrupt, short-lived and intense pain which breaks through the analgesia that controls the persistent pain in a "steady state" situation. BTP frequently occurs in conditions with a neuropathic component but may occur with all painful condi-

tions (e.g. acute medical, surgical or chronic). The three subtypes of BTP are incident, idiopathic and end-of-dose failure [16]. BTP also is categorized as somatic, visceral, neuropathic or mixed. It may be difficult to treat, as preventing the experience of this pain would potentially require extremely high dosages in a multi-modal analgesic protocol. However, the patient should be re-assessed by careful observation and examination to ensure there is no new underlying problem causing pain (refer to Chapter 6).

6. **Neuropathic pain** is defined as pain caused or initiated by a primary lesion, injury or dysfunction in the peripheral or central nervous system. Refer to Chapter 3 for details on pathophysiology, patient examination and treatment.

7. **Inflammatory pain** is the primary cause for most **medical pain** (i.e. inflammatory bowel disease, cystitis), post-surgical and traumatic pain. Infections also result in inflammation and can cause severe pain (i.e. *streptococcal* fasciitis). Inflammatory pain has a rapid onset and, in general, its intensity and duration are related directly to the severity and duration of tissue damage (i.e. burn injuries). Pain will persist until the inflammation/underlying problem is resolved.

8. **Medical pain** is frequently inflammatory, as noted above; however, there are many non-inflammatory conditions resulting in ischemia, distension of viscera, stretching of organ capsule due to acute enlargement (e.g. kidney) or urinary calculi, as examples, which cause severe pain.

9. **Surgical pain** is a "traumatic" injury resulting in a combination of inflammatory and potentially neuropathic pain should neural tissue be handled, injured or transected.

III. The Outcome of the Inappropriate Management of Pain

Hyperalgesia is an exaggerated and prolonged response of the CNS in response to a noxious stimulus – the "increasing the ring to do something about it" effect! This occurs where the level of pain in a patient is not recognized or appropriately assessed and treated; the neural bombardment results in a heightened pain state, hyperalgesia. Recognizing that physiologic, or adaptive, pain exists in all our trauma patients, and potentially exists in all medical illness to some degree, is key to protection from future pathologic or maladaptive pain.

Maladaptive pain is generated from a malfunction of neurologic transmission due to the ongoing "acute" pain and serves no physiological purpose [17, 18]. Of major concern is the link between acute pain and chronic pain, with the hypothesis that if the acute pain were better controlled the chronic pain would not develop [19]. In humans, this eventually becomes a chronic syndrome in which pain itself frequently becomes the primary disease. This maladaptive pain is also another essential factor to consider in animals. Another manifestation, especially where neural tissue is involved, is allodynia.

Allodynia is a pain response to a low-intensity, normally innocuous, stimulus such as light touch to the skin, putting on a shirt or gentle pressure and is elicited from non-injured tissue. The same effect occurs in animals. In humans, this experience also results in depression, which can become a significant chronic problem [20, 21]. Based on the physiologic/pathophysiologic similarities between humans and animals, we may assume that depression is a component of the present, and potentially past, untreated painful experience [19]. To fully understand the physiology of pain (Chapter 2), neuropathic pain (Chapter 3),visceral pain (Chapter 4), cancer pain (Chapter 5) and movement-evoked and breakthrough pain (Chapter 6) refer to the individual chapters for details. Refer to case scenarios throughout this book for individual patient pain management.

Above all, the humane factor must be considered with administration of analgesics and modalities to prevent and treat pain prior to the patient experiencing the noxious sensation.

IV.   Pain Scoring Systems

Pain assessment measures have been utilized by veterinary researchers as a way to quantify pain in various studies and to analyse data. These consist of verbal rating scales (VRS), simple descriptive scales (SDS), numerical rating scales (NRS) and the visual analogue scale (VAS). The VRS or SDS rate pain as none, mild, moderate or severe, and appear to be simple to use but may lack sensitivity as the small number of levels does not provide sufficient discrimination from one level to the next [22]. The NRS, where numbers are assigned to a level of activity within a given category of behaviour, may also lack sensitivity as frequently the categories are overly simplified [23]. One problem with simple descriptors heavily weighted in some NRS is also a lack of specificity. For example, vocalization may be associated with pain but could also be a manifestation of emergence delirium after anesthesia, dysphoria secondary to opioid administration, anxiety or fear. Therefore, vocalization can be one of the most difficult behaviours to interpret when assessing pain but can contribute to a high pain score if recorded. Defining vocalization may be more helpful (e.g. howling vs screaming vs barking vs whining). In one survey, veterinarians rated vocalization the highest as a sign of pain [24]. In contrast, the worst pain possible may occur in an immobile, quiet patient, and the absence of vocalization would decrease the total pain score [25] and personal observation. A pain scoring system for measurement of post-operative pain in dogs has addressed the issue of expanding descriptors to discriminate between some painful and non-painful behaviours [26].

The VAS is a ruler usually 100 mm in length with only a description of the limits of pain placed at either end of the scale: 0 = no pain and 100 = worst pain possible. The observer or patient is asked to mark anywhere along the scale where the perceived or experienced pain, respectively, would fall. This technique is widely used in human medicine and has been used in many veterinary analgesic studies. Potential drawbacks are that observers must be experienced in assessing pain and trained in the use of the VAS. A modification of the VAS, the DIVAS which, incorporates a dynamic and interactive assessment, has been reported [27]. It is suggested that the observer–patient interaction can more fully assess the overall state of the patient. In this study, an algometer was used to obtain nociceptive threshold values as an additional tool for assessing pain after ovariohysterectomy in dogs [27].

All measurement scales attach a number to our (individual) preconceived notions of what defines pain, which is influenced by gender, clinical experience and personal painful experiences. The individual's definition (or interpretation) of pain will differ as pain assessment is a subjective interpretation of an animal's behaviour, also the level of pain assessed by different individuals will vary. This is frequently the case when an individual attempting to identify pain by examining the subtle behavioural changes associated with mild to moderate pain is in conflict with someone relying on stereotypic signs of pain, such as crying, thrashing and other obvious signs of pain. An important factor to consider in the method of pain assessment is the variability amongst observers each method may produce. When a comparison of an SDS, NRS and VAS was evaluated, using dogs recovering from various procedures, significant variability amongst observers was reported with all three methods [28]. The conclusion of this study was that the NRS was the most suitable of the three scales studied for recording assessment of pain in dogs.

A pain scoring system to assess post-operative pain in dogs, adapted from a similar system developed in children (Children's Hospital of Eastern Ontario (CHEOP)) has demonstrated excellent agreement between evaluators [26]. This study was limited to healthy, normal dogs recovering from ovariohysterectomy and was therefore not tested through a wide range and degree of painful states. This study also included pre-operative behaviour as a comparison to post-operative behaviour, an aspect of pain evaluation not always available. However, this does raise another important issue on pain assessment and management. Familiarity with the personality of the animal is important when assessing pain and designing an analgesic regimen. The pet owner may be the best person to evaluate the level of anxiety or pain the patient may be experiencing. Treating anxiety, when this is a known characteristic of the patient, in addition to pain, improves patient comfort.

V.   Pain Assessment Scales Adapted for Veterinary Patients

A.   Simple Uni-Dimensional Scales

The NRS and VAS require the caregiver to record a subjective score for pain intensity, and the SDS to note the presence, and assessed level, of pain (No pain, Mild pain, Moderate pain, Severe Pain). The observer rating the level of pain is also influential in the evaluation. When using these scales, studies have shown that the observer's judgement can be affected by factors such as year of graduation from veterinary college, age, gender, personal health experiences and clinical experience. These factors introduce inter-observer variability and limit the consistent reliability of the scale. However, when used consistently, these are effective as part of a protocol to evaluate pain. Of these three types of scales, as noted above, the NRS on a 0–10 or 0–20 scale is recommended [29].

B.   Multi-Dimensional Composite Scales

Include the (1) **Glasgow Composite Measure Pain Scale** and its short form (CMPS-SF) for dogs only. The CMPS-SF, validated for use in measuring acute pain, and specifically surgical pain, is a clinical decision-making tool when used in conjunction with clinical judgement. This includes a series of questions relating to interactive and non-interactive behaviours. The score obtained can be used as a guide for the need for analgesic administration. Intervention level scores have been described (i.e. the score at which analgesia should be administered). The instrument is available to download online [30]. A similar scale for cats is available to download online [31].

The (2) **Colorado State University** (CSU) is designed as a teaching tool for assessment of acute pain for the dog. The scale combines aspects of the numerical rating scale along with composite behavioural observation, and it has been shown to increase awareness of behavioural changes associated with pain. It is not a validated assessment scale [32].

The (3) **University of Melbourne Pain Scale** is practical and combines physiologic data and behavioural responses [26]. As physiologic characteristics are not consistently associated with pain, this point should be taken into consideration when using this scale. This scale does not include suggested points for analgesic intervention. It is designed specifically for use in dogs.

The (4) **UNESP-Botucatu** English version, a scoring tool for use in assessing acute postoperative pain in **cats** undergoing ovariohysterectomy, provides useful information with respect to parameters to assess for ongoing pain [33]. Four factors were identified:

- psychomotor change (posture, comfort, activity, mental status and miscellaneous behaviours);
- protection of wound area (reaction to palpation of the surgical wound and palpation of the abdomen and flank);
- vocal expression of pain (vocalization);
- physiologic variables (systolic arterial blood pressure and appetite); however, as with other scoring systems, heart rate was not a consistent parameter, and neither was respiratory rate and pattern.

All of the composite scales above are easy to use and include interactive components and behavioural categories and are available online. See references [26, 28–33]. However, caution must be used when assessing pain using only scoring systems to assess pain. In a study assessing post-operative pain in children, many children who were lying in one position with a calm expression (resulting in a low score), at the same time, reported moderate to severe pain [25]. The acute pain scales were based on post-surgical assessment, frequently ovariohysterectomy; therefore, a more painful scenario including surgical, trauma and medical pain will require a more in-depth assessment. Assessing acute pain of all causes in both cats and dogs, including analgesic intervention, was developed for in-house use at the Ontario Veterinary College and is presented in the following chapter.

VI. Clinical Utility of Pain Assessment Methods

Many tools exist to assess pain in humans and a few have been used in veterinary medicine. There is no perfect method, primarily because of the subjective and unmeasurable nature of pain, even in people [34], and especially in veterinary patients where they cannot communicate verbally. Pain assessment methods are necessary to evaluate pain and its relief following administration of analgesics when performing studies requiring analysis and reporting.

As individual practitioners want to know what the best pain management strategy is for each patient, the number needed to treat (NNT) is proving to be a very effective alternative method of measuring the adequacy of pain management in human patients [35, 36]. An NNT of 1 describes an event which occurs in every patient given the treatment but in no patient in a comparative non-treated group. This would be the "perfect" result. There are few situations where the treatment is close to 100% effective and the control or placebo completely ineffective; therefore, an NNT of 2 or 3 often indicates an effective intervention. An NNT of 2 means that for every two patients treated with an analgesic for example one patient will obtain relief from pain as predetermined by the goals of the study. In people, this is usually defined as obtaining at least a 50% improvement in pain relief due to treatment. However, where severe to excruciating pain is experienced, a reduction greater than 50% is the goal, which requires a multi-modal regimen. As for unwanted effects, the NNT becomes the NNH (number needed to harm) which should be as large as possible when assessing the safety of the intervention. The details of calculating NNTs and NNHs is beyond the scope of this book; therefore, interested readers are referred to published articles on this topic [35, 36].

Veterinary technicians/nurses are the primary around-the-clock caregivers of patients in the hospital with a responsibility to assess and manage pain. A questionnaire was distributed to veterinary nurses across the United Kingdom to assess their attitudes towards the assessment and management of pain in practice. Of those asked, 80.3% of the veterinary nurses agreed that a pain scale was a useful clinical tool [37]. While pain scales are not consistently used, in a Canadian survey more than 95% of veterinary technicians/nurses informed the veterinarian when animals were in pain; analgesics were then administered [38].

VII. Misconceptions

Based on reputation, small and toy breeds ("white fluffies") may be inadequately treated for the pain experienced if the clinician assumes that their exaggerated demonstration of pain is merely a behavioural characteristic. Also, anecdotal reports from practitioners note that during post-operative follow-up the owners of the "white fluffies" seem to complain more than owners of other breeds that their pets are in pain. Of interest, pain in women with red hair was noted by a dentist and a study following up on this observation noted red hair colour in women was associated with increased sensitivity to thermal pain when compared to women with dark hair but not in baseline electrical pain thresholds [39]. It was also noted that redheads are more resistant to the analgesic effects of subcutaneous lidocaine and to volatile anesthetics [39]. The authors concluded that mutations of the melanocortin 1 receptor, or as a consequence of this, seem to modulate pain sensitivity. It remains unclear whether this modulation occurs at a central or peripheral level or both, but these differences seem to be most clearly defined in the presence of drugs (local anesthetic, volatile anesthetic) that suppress responses to noxious stimuli [39]. A similar finding has been reported in mice [40]. Based on these studies, the anecdotal observation of white-coat cats and dogs experiencing pain more or longer than other hair/fur colour may have a phenotypic basis not yet studied in cats and dogs. Key genes and phenotypic variants involved in nociception and response to acute pain and analgesics exist and potentially contribute to the individual or ethnic (humans) variability in the pain experience [41].

Pain may also be under-treated in some of the larger working breeds that have a reputation for being "stoic" or "able to handle pain", and cats and geriatric animals as they tend to withdraw when painful and may easily be ignored in a busy practice setting. On occasion, a dog may whine but will stop this behaviour when touched or spoken too. This is frequently interpreted as "attention seeking" and not pain, when in fact it may be the distraction from the pain which resulted in the dog becoming quiet. This can compare to the human situation where a distraction can produce a temporary reduction in pain perception.

Administration of opioid analgesics is frequently withheld in ill or injured animals as it is the belief that these drugs will "mask" the signs of deterioration. This is not so. In fact, the opposite occurs where alleviating pain and reducing the associated response of the sympathetic nervous system to pain will allow the practitioner to focus on other causes of tachycardia, tachypnea, pale mucous membranes and weak pulses. If hypovolemia or hypotension is not present, these parameters frequently return to normal after administration of analgesics.

In the past, veterinarians were reluctant to use analgesics in cats based on the adverse effects "reputation" bestowed on cats. The unique metabolism of some analgesics in cats, and previous reports of adverse behaviour associated with morphine administration, raised the veterinarians' concerns. However, since that time many studies assessing all different classes of analgesics in cats have been reported and, with appropriate dosing, these fears have been laid to rest. Pain management in cats is essential, as it is in dogs; analgesic regimens for acute pain encountered in the ill or injured cat is presented in the following chapter as are various scenarios throughout this book. For moderate to severe and excruciating pain, as with dogs, a multi-modal approach to pain management is essential in the cat. Careful pain assessment for this requirement – based on behaviour, response to examination, interaction and the underlying problem – will guide the veterinary technician/nurse and veterinarian in designing an individual protocol. Refer to Chapter 8 for details.

These examples highlight the importance of assessing pain in the individual patient and being aware of the subtle signs at rest and behavioural changes that may be elicited during interaction, regardless of "reputation". While the "reputation" aspect may be true for some patients, this should only be determined after a thorough assessment for the presence of pain.

Refer to Chapter 8 for key points and general considerations in assessment of pain in animals.

References

1 www.iasp-pain.org.
2 Woolf, C. J. (2004) Pain: Moving from symptom control toward mechanism-specific pharmacologic management. *Ann Intern Med*, 140441–140451.

3 Woolf, C. J. (2011) Central sensitization: Implications for the diagnosis and treatment of pain. *Pain*, 152, S2–S15.

4 Reid, J., Scott, M., Nolan, A., *et al.* (2013) Pain assessment in animals. *In Pract*, 35: 1–56.

5 Mathews, K. A., Kronen, P. W., Lascelles, B. D. X., et al. (2014) WSAVA Guidelines for Recognition, Assessment and Treatment of Pain. *Assessment and Treatment of Pain in Small Animals*, 55(6): E10–E68.

6 Vierck, C. J., Jr, Cooper, B. Y., Franzen, O., *et al.* (1983) Behavioural analysis of CNS pathways and transmitter systems involved in conduction and inhibition of pain sensations and reactions in primates. *Progress in Psychology, Physiology and Psychology*, 10: 113–165.

7 Morton, D. B. and Griffiths, P. H. M. (1985) Guidelines on the recognition of pain, distress and discomfort in experimental animals and hypothesis for assessment. *Vet Rec*, 116: 431–436.

8 Conzemius, M. G., Hill, C. M., Sammarco, J. L., *et al.* (1997) Correlation between subjective and objective measures used to determine severity of postoperative pain in dogs. *J Am Vet Med Assoc*, 210(11): 1619–1622.

9 Hansen, B. D., Hardie, E. M. and Carroll, G. S. (1997) Physiological measurements after ovariohysterectomy in dogs: What's normal? *Appl Anim Behav Sci*, 51: 101–109.

10 Holton, L. L., Scott, E. M., Nolan, A. M., *et al.* (1998) Relationship between physiological factors and clinical pain in dogs scored using a numerical rating scale. *J. Small Anim Pract*, 39: 469–474.

11 Quimby, J. M., Smith, M. L. and Lunn, K. F. (2011) Evaluation of the effects of hospital visit stress on physiologic parameters in the cat. *J Feline Med Surg*, 13: 733–737.

12 Bragg, R. F., Bennett, J. S., Cummings, A. and Quimby, J. E. (2015) Evaluation of the effects of hospital visit stress on physiologic variables in dogs. *J Am Vet Med Assoc*, 246: 212–215.

13 Smith, J. D., Allen, S. W., Quandt, J. E., *et al.* (1996) Indictors of postoperative pain in cats and correlation with clinical criteria. *Am J Vet Res*, 209: 1674–1678.

14 Laulin, J. P., Maurette, P. and Corcuff, J. B. (2002) The role of ketamine in preventing fentanyl-induced hyperalgesia and subsequent acute morphine tolerance. *Anesth Analg*, 94: 1263–1269.

15 Woolf, C. J. and Max, M. B. (2001) Mechanism-based pain diagnosis: Issues for analgesic drug development. *Anesthesioogy*, 95(1): 241–249.

16 Payne, R. (2007) Recognition and diagnosis of breakthrough pain. *Pain Med*, 8 (suppl. 1): S3–S7.

17 Bennett, G. J. (2012) What is spontaneous pain and who has it? *J Pain*, 13: 921–929.

18 Mogil, J. S. (2012) The etiology and symptomatology of spontaneous pain. *J Pain*, 13: 932–933; discussion: 934–935.

19 Kehlet, H. T., Jensen, T. L. and Woolf, C. J. (2006) Persistent post-surgical pain: Risk factors and prevention. *Lancet*, 367: 1618–1625.

20 Wang, J., Goffer, Y. and Xu, D. (2011) A single subanesthetic dose of ketamine relieves depression-like behaviors induced by neuropathic pain in rats. *Anesthesiology*, 115(4): 812–821; see reference [21] for editorial.

21 Romero-Sandoval, E. A. (2011) Depression and pain: Does ketamine improve the quality of life of patients in chronic pain by targeting their mood? *Anesthesiology*, 115: 687–688.

22 Ricard-Hibon, A., Chollet, C., Saada, S., *et al.* (1999) A quality control programme for acute pain management in out-of-hospital critical care medicine. *Ann Emerg Med*, 34: 738–744.

23 Grisneaux, E., Pibarot, P., Dupuis, J., *et al.* (1999) Comparison of ketoprofen and carprofen administered prior to orthopedic surgery for control of postoperative pain in dogs. *J Am Vet Med Assoc*, 215: 1105–1110.

24 Watson, A. D. J., Nicholson, A., Church, D. B., *et al.* (1996) Use of anti-inflammatory and analgesic drugs in dogs and cats. *Aust Vet J*, 74: 203–210.

25 Tessler, M. D., Holzemer, W. L. and Savedra, M. C. (1998) Pain behaviours: Postsurgical responses of children and adolescents. *J. Pedat Nurs*, 13: 41–47.

26 Firth, A. M. and Haldane, S. L. (1999) Development of a scale to evaluate postoperative pain in dogs. *J Am Vet Med Assoc*, 215: 651–659. (The University of Melbourne Pain Scale.)

27 Lascelles, B. D. X., Cripps, P. J., Jones, A. and Waterman-Pearson, A. E. (1998) Efficacy and kinetics of carprofen, administered preoperatively or postoperatively, for the prevention of pain in dogs undergoing ovariohysterectomy. *Vet Surg*, 27: 568–582.

28 Holton, L. L., Scott, E. M., Nolan, A. M., *et al.* (1998) Comparison of three methods used for assessment of pain in dogs. *J Am Vet Med Assoc*, 212: 61–66.

29 Jensen, M. P., Turner, J. A. and Romano, J. M. (1994) What is the maximum number of levels needed in pain intensity measurement? *Pain*, 58: 387–392.

30 Glasgow Composite Measure Pain Scale, short form CMPS-SF, http://www.gla.ac.uk/departments/painandwelfareresearchgroup/downloadacutepainquestionnair/.

31 Glasgow Composite Measure Pain Scale: CMPS – Feline, http://www.aprvt.com/uploads/5/3/0/5/5305564/cmp_feline_eng.pdf.

32 Colorado State University (CSU) Acute pain scale for the dog, http://csuanimalcancercenter.org/assets/files/csu_acute_pain_scale_canine.pdf.

33 Brondani, J. T., Mama, K. R., Luna, S. P., *et al.* (2013) Validation of the English version of the UNESP-Botucatu multidimensional composite pain scale for assessing postoperative pain in cats. *BioMed Central Veterinary Research*, 17: 143, doi: 10.1186/1746-6148-9-143.

34 Ahlers, S. J. G. M., van Gulik, L. and van der Veen, A. M. (2008) Comparison of different pain scoring systems in critically ill patients in a general ICU. *Critical Care*, 12: R15.

35 Cordell, W. H. (1999) Number needed to treat (NNT). *Annals of Emergency Medicine*, 33(4): 433–436.

36 McQuay, H. and Moore, A. (1998) *An Evidence-based Resource for Pain Relief*. Oxford University Press, New York.

37 Coleman, D. L. and Slingsby, L. S. (2007) Attitudes of veterinary nurses to the assessment of pain and the use of pain scales. *Vet Rec*, 160: 541–544.

38 Dohoo, S. E. and Dohoo, I. R. (1998) Attitudes and concerns of Canadian animal health technologists toward postoperative pain management in dogs and cats. *Can Vet J*, 39: 491–496.

39 Liem, E. B., Joiner, T. V., Tsueda, K., *et al.* (2005) Increased sensitivity to thermal pain and reduced subcutaneous lidocaine efficacy in redheads. *Anesthesiology*, 102(3): 509–514.

40 Xing, Y., Sonner, J. M., Eger, E. I., II, *et al.* (2004) Mice with a melanocortin 1 receptor mutation have a slightly greater MAC than control mice. *Anesthesiology*, 101: 544–546.

41 Shipton, E. A. (2011) Pharmacogenomics in acute pain: Review. *Trends in Anesthesia and Critical Care*, 117–122.

Further Reading

Bragg, R. F., Bennett, J. S., Cummings, A. and Quimby, J. E. (2015) Evaluation of the effects of hospital visit stress on physiologic variables in dogs. *J Am Vet Med Assoc*, 246: 212–215.

Mathews, K. A. (2000) Pain assessment and general approach to management. *Vet Clin North Am Small Anim*, 30(4): 729–755.

Quimby, J. M., Smith, M. L. and Lunn, K. F. (2011) Evaluation of the effects of hospital visit stress on physiologic parameters in the cat. *J Feline Med Surg*, 13: 733–737.

8

Recognition, Assessment and Treatment of Pain in Dogs and Cat

Karol Mathews

Continuing from the previous chapter, nociceptive function is a protective mechanism and the lowest, warning, level at which pain sensation (adaptive pain) is experienced is the same across species: the "What hurts me, will hurt them" rule. This highlights the comparative component of pain assisting with the assessment of the pain the patient is likely experiencing with a given illness or injury. Table 8.1 highlights perceived levels of pain with various illnesses or injuries to assist the practitioner in assessing the degree of pain where the patient's behaviour may be difficult to interpret. Table 8.2 lists many of the behavioural characteristics associated with pain in cats and dogs. Recognizing that physiologic or adaptive pain exists in all our trauma and surgical patients, and potentially exists in all medical illness to some degree, is key to protection from future pathologic or maladaptive pain.

If pain is not managed appropriately, maladaptive pain occurs, which leads to chronic pain syndromes where pain itself may become the primary disease [1, 2]. This is manifested as allodynia, a pain response to a low-intensity, normally innocuous stimulus such as light touch to the skin, or gentle pressure. This same effect occurs in animals. In humans, this experience also results in depression and can become a significant chronic problem. Based on the physiologic/pathophysiologic similarities between humans and animals, we may assume that depression is a component of the present, and potentially past, untreated painful experience [3, 4]. To fully understand the recognition of pain (previous chapter), the physiology of pain (Chapter 2), neuropathic pain (Chapter 3), visceral pain (Chapter 4), cancer pain (Chapter 5) and movement-evoked and breakthrough pain (Chapter 6) refer to the individual chapters for details. Refer to specific case scenarios throughout the book for individual patient pain management.

Of utmost importance for consideration is that a continual painful experience is detrimental to the overall healing process as well as the general well-being of any animal or person. Pain triggers the "stress response" with associated physiological changes (Table 8.2), and often results in prolonged hospital stay and increases the potential for secondary problems, such as hospital-associated infections, immune suppression and secondary illness, inappetence and cachexia. This is especially so in cats where hepatic lipidosis may occur due to inappetence and inadequate caloric intake. Based on all these potential problems, euthanasia is frequently considered due to added costs or interpretation of poor prognosis.

Analgesia and Anesthesia for the Ill or Injured Dog and Cat, First Edition. Karol A. Mathews, Melissa Sinclair, Andrea M. Steele and Tamara Grubb.

Table 8.1 A guide to pain assessment and analgesic selection.

The designation of conditions into categories below is intended to serve only as a guide. Pain may vary according to the patient and the condition. Each patient should be assessed individually.	
Severe-to-excruciating	
Fracture repair where extensive soft tissue injury exists Spinal surgery Ear canal ablation Burn injury Articular or pathological fractures Limb amputation Necrotizing pancreatitis or cholecystitis Thrombosis/ischemia	Bone cancer Hypertrophic osteodystrophy Aortic saddle thrombosis Neuropathic pain (nerve entrapment/inflammation, acute intervertebral disc herniation) Inflammation (extensive e.g. peritonitis, fasciitis – especially streptococcal, cellulitis)
Moderate-to-severe (varies with degree of illness or injury)	
Glaucoma Corneal abrasion/ulceration Uveitis Intervertebral disc disease Capsular pain due to organomegaly Hollow organ distension Traumatic diaphragmatic rupture Pleuritis Ureteral/urethral/biliary obstruction Mesenteric, gastric, testicular or other torsions Peritonitis with septic abdomen	Mucositis Oral cancer Mastitis Meningitis Dystocia Immune-mediated arthritis Panosteitis Trauma (i.e. orthopedic, extensive soft tissue, head) Frostbite Early or resolving stages of soft tissue injuries/inflammation/disease
Extensive resection and reconstruction for mass removal and corrective orthopedic surgery (osteotomies; cruciate surgery; open arthrotomies)	
Moderate	
Soft tissue injuries (i.e. less severe than above) Urethral obstruction Ovariohysterectomy	Cystitis Diagnostic arthroscopy and laparoscopy Osteoarthritis
Mild-to-moderate	
Dental disease Otitis Castration Mild cystitis	Abscess lancing Superficial lacerations
Chest drains (varies from none to moderate, patient and problem dependent)	

Source: Data adapted from [15]. With permission.

I. Key Points in Assessment of Pain in Animals

- Think in terms of the similarities of pain perception and anticipation in both humans and animals and treat with an analgesic regimen appropriate for the level of pain likely to be present **regardless** of whether or not you are convinced the animal is painful. Occasionally, animals will be less or more painful than expected for the injury, illness or surgical procedure they have.
- Adopt a specific approach in a consistent manner when assessing pain for the individual patient. Each painful condition and anatomical location results in differing levels of pain (e.g. a laceration on a limb may not be as painful as a similar injury on the prepuce, vulva or mouth).
- Acknowledge that invasive procedures, trauma and many medical illnesses cause pain that requires analgesic therapy.

- Frequent monitoring is essential as the textbook duration and dosing of analgesics may be inadequate for some conditions while being excessive for others.
- Age, as with humans, also contributes to certain behavioural patterns associated with pain. As with children, pediatric animals tend to be more vocal, whereas adults, especially geriatrics, tend to contain their emotions, thus making pain assessment more challenging.
- Recognize the subtle as well as the more obvious signs of behaviour associated with pain such as facial expressions. Facial expressions of the non-verbal human (e.g. infants and adults unable to communicate verbally) are used to identify the presence of pain [5]. Interestingly, non-verbal status of animals (e.g. mice, rats, rabbits, horses [6] and cats [7]) share the similarity of facial expression of pain in humans [8] providing evidence for evolutionary psychological accounts of pain communication, which is in agreement with Darwin's direct prediction of phylogenetic continuity of facial expression of emotions[5] (Figures 8.4–8.7). Keep in mind that cats, and many older animals, tend to withdraw and remain quiet through a wide range of painful experiences.
- Assess the behaviour from a distance without the patient's knowledge, if possible. Is it sleeping? Note respiratory rate and body position. Approach the patient and note interest or lack of. If sleeping, don't waken but reassess in 30 min.
- Interaction with the patient is necessary. Walking past the cage and noting that they are quiet, not sleeping, is an inadequate method to assess the presence and degree of pain.
- Response to appropriate analgesic therapy is the closest marker we have to a gold standard for diagnosing pain at the present time.
- Objective measurements such as heart rate, pupil size and respiratory rate have not been consistently correlated with signs of pain, as these are affected by emotional factors such as anxiety, stress and fear, lesion localization (e.g. vagal innervations may be associated with bradycardia) and drugs (e.g. opioid-associated bradycardia even with ineffective analgesia). Therefore, we depend on subjective evaluation based on behaviour.
- Opioid overdose should be considered where panting, nausea, vomiting or vocalization/dysphoria occurs immediately following opioid administration. Naloxone should be titrated cautiously should this occur (refer to Chapter 10).
- Opioid-induced hyperalgesia has rarely been witnessed by the author where pain appears to worsen with increasing, titrating dose of morphine. This pain behaviour is distinctly different from dysphoria and requires titration of ketamine to overcome this degree of pain.
- Painful sensations such as dull aching, sharp shooting, throbbing, stinging – we have all experienced these at some time – can be experienced in any individual as a single or multiple experience. A single patient can experience a combination of these painful sensations after trauma or after major orthopedic surgery. Combinations of different classes of analgesics are recommended in these animals, as one analgesic class alone is usually not adequate to control all types of pain.
- As a tip for the patient with a severe painful condition, ensure that an injection port on the IV line is outside the cage door. This ensures that if a patient should be aggressive when approached, analgesia can be administered through the IV line without concern for injury of the caregiver. This applies to both dogs and cats. This technique would have prevented a personal injury when assessing pain and accessing the injection port of the cat in Figure 8.7. The appearance of this cat indicated a lack of trust and pain prompting a photo opportunity, which was followed by a swift "nail bearing" paw, and incisor and canine teeth exposure, when attempting to assess the cat and access the intravenous (IV) line!

In considering these points, the veterinarian and veterinary technician/nurse (VT/N) will rapidly gain experience and confidence in assessing and treating pain in animals. A simple and effective way to gain skill in pain assessment is to observe the response to analgesic therapy in those equivocal situations where behavioural characteristics of pain are difficult to recognize. A return to more normal behaviour, such as eating and grooming, or a "more comfortable" appearance and sleep confirms the prior presence of pain, and ultimately their gratitude (Figure 8.1).

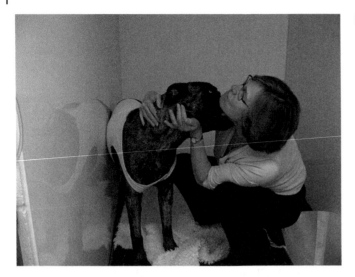

Figure 8.1 Gratitude.

When a determined effort is made on a daily basis to study the behaviour of cats and dogs, of different ages, with various traumatic injuries, after assorted surgical procedures or with medical problems, behavioural signs of pain are more readily detected. When assessing pain in animals, it is important to observe the behaviour and its response to analgesic therapy over time. The assessment must be appropriate for the age of the animal. Younger animals are much less tolerant of pain; refer to Chapter 25 for a physiologic explanation for this. This should not be interpreted as exaggerated "puppy or kitten behaviour", which may result in inadequate use of analgesics. Short-lived pain, such as vaccination, is obviously acceptable; however, it is essential to prescribe appropriate analgesia for longer-lasting pain.

Table 8.2 Behavioural characteristics associated with pain in CATS and DOGS.

Category of behaviour	Detailed description
Abnormal posture	Hunched up guarding/splinting of abdomen, Figure 8.2 "praying" position (forequarters on the ground, hind quarters in the air), Figure 8.3 Sit or lie in an abnormal position Not resting in a normal position (i.e. sternal or curled up)
Abnormal gait	Stiff No to partial weight bearing on injured limb Slight to obvious limp
Abnormal movement	Thrashing Restless No movement when not sleeping
Vocalization	Screaming Whining (intermittent\constant\when touched) Crying (intermittent\constant\when touched) None
Facial expression of emotions (proved to be important in non-verbal human patients)	Examples: Figures 8.4–8.7
Miscellaneous	Look, lick or chew at the painful area Hyperesthesia/hyperalgesia Allodynia

Table 8.2 (Continued)

Category of behaviour	Detailed description
Behavioural characteristics associated with pain in cats and dogs, but	**(1) may** also be associated with poor general health (medical problems) Restless/agitated Tremble/shake Tachypnea/panting Weak tail wag Low carriage of tail Depressed/poor response to caregiver Head hangs down Ears down, drawn back Not grooming Appetite decreased/picky/absent Dull Lie quietly and not move for hours\does not dream Stuporous Urinate\defecate and make no attempt to move Recumbent and unaware of surroundings Unwilling or unable to walk Bite\attempt to bite caregivers **(2) may** also be associated with apprehension/anxiety Restless\agitated Tremble\shake Tachypnea\panting Weak tail wag Low tail carriage Slow to rise Depressed (poor response to caregiver) Not grooming Bite\attempt to bite caregiver Ears pulled back Restless Remain in the back of the cage – dog and cat Barking\growling(intermittent\constant\when approached) dog Growl\hiss (intermittent\constant\when approached) cat Sit in the back of the cage\hide under a blanket – cat **(3) may** be normal behaviour Reluctant to move head (eye movement only) Stretch all four legs when abdomen touched Penile prolapsed when spoken to – dogs Cleaning (licking) a wound or incision
Physiological signs which can be associated with pain	The stress response – increased serum cortisol and epinephrine results in: • tachypnea/panting • tachycardia (mild, moderate severe) • hypertension • insulin resistance • hyperglycemia • neurtrophilia But severe stress results in general immunosuppression Dilated pupils may also be associated with opioid administration in cats (Figure 8.10a) These physiological signs are not all consistently present in painful states, and may also be present in any anxious or excited dog or cat Bradycardia may rarely be present in painful conditions associated with intrathoracic structures, abdominal pathology or post-laparotomy due to influence of the parasympathetic nervous system, or decompensated shock

Source: Data adapted from [15]. With permission.

Anecdotally, certain breeds of dogs, huskies or small and toy breeds ("white fluffies"), for example, may be inadequately treated for the pain experienced if the clinician assumes that their exaggerated demonstration of pain is merely a behavioural characteristic; although individual situations may be difficult to interpret. Of interest, hair colour has been associated with increased sensitivity to thermal pain [9]. Refer to Chapter 7 for the genetic mechanism for this. Based on these studies, the anecdotal observation of "white coat" cats and dogs experiencing pain more, or longer, than other hair colour may have a phenotypic basis not yet studied in cats and dogs. Pain may also be under-treated in some of the larger working breeds that have a reputation for being "stoic" or "able to handle pain". Similarly, cats and geriatric animals tend to withdraw when painful and may easily be ignored in a busy practice setting.

Geriatric veterinary patients frequently have chronic conditions such as osteoarthritis which may contribute to their acute pain should they be positioned abnormally in the cage or during procedures, even under general anesthesia where the result of painful manipulation may be present upon recovery. Always question the owner as to a pre-existing painful condition so appropriate handling can be planned.

On occasion, a dog may whine but will stop this behaviour when touched or spoken to. This is frequently interpreted as attention seeking and not pain when in fact it may be the distraction from the pain which resulted in the dog becoming quiet. This can compare to the human situation where a distraction can produce a temporary reduction in pain perception. Where gentle stroking of an area of (potential) pain reduces vocalization, this may be a reduction in the pain experienced due to the "gate effect" (refer to Chapter 2) and not attention-seeking, akin to humans rubbing an area following a bump.

These examples highlight the importance of assessing pain in the individual patient and being aware of the subtle signs at rest and behavioural changes that may be elicited during interaction, regardless of reputation. While the reputation aspect may be true for some patients, this should only be determined after a thorough assessment for the presence of pain.

As the focus of this book is acute pain, the pain scales described in the previous chapter are designed to assess acute pain. However, chronic pain is experienced by millions of dogs and cats, and many of these present with an acute problem or require surgical intervention for various ill or injury conditions. The insidious onset of signs, their similarity to those associated with the infirmities of age, makes owner recognition of their pet's pain more difficult. As chronic pain may result in hyperalgesia, the acute pain these patients experience may be worse than those with a similar condition without ongoing chronic pain. Osteoarthritis, and presumably other inflammatory states – such as otitis externa, cystitis, stomatitis and toothache – are common causes of chronic pain in animals. Careful questioning of the owner is required as many presume reduced activity to be associated with simple ageing. Although pain may be the cause of the ADR (ain't doin' right) animal, this must not be presumed, and other causes of this "syndrome" must not be overlooked. A complete history, physical examination and appropriate laboratory evaluation must be performed to elucidate potential illness. This approach will help avoid disasters, for example prescribing a non-steroidal anti-inflammatory analgesic (NSAIA) (Chapter 11) for "presumed pain", in an animal with liver or renal disease.

II. Clinical Utility of Pain Assessment Methods

Some common behavioural patterns, and response to caregivers during various activities, associated with various arbitrary levels of pain are listed in Table 8.3 and Table 8.6. The scale (0 to 10 with descriptors) is used as a teaching tool at the Ontario Veterinary College. The levels of pain were determined by the analgesic, the dose and the duration of action of the analgesic required to effectively control the animal's pain. The weakness in this scale is that not all possible combinations and permutations of behaviour associated with each potential level are documented and, therefore, it is incomplete, but this is also true for validated pain scales. An in-house study confirmed the efficacy of this system; however, this has not been published or validated by others.

A. Pain Measurement Tools

As pain is an individual experience, encompassing physical, emotional and previous painful experience, there is no gold standard for measurement, other than response to appropriate "analgesic" management. Many tools exist to assess pain in humans and a few have been validated in veterinary medicine [2, 10–12]. Refer to Chapter 7 for discussion and description of the various scales that may be used when assessing pain in our veterinary patients. No scale is perfect, primarily because of the subjective and unmeasurable nature of pain, even in humans [13] and especially in veterinary patients where they cannot communicate verbally.

Caution must be used when assessing pain using only scoring systems to assess pain. In a study assessing post-operative pain in children, many children who were lying in one position with a calm expression (resulting in a low score), at the same time, reported moderate to severe pain. Refer to Chapter 7 for details on the scoring systems given briefly below that may be used for assessing pain in your patient.

- **Simple uni-dimensional scales,** the numerical rating scale (NRS) and the visual analogue scale (VAS), require the caregiver to record a subjective score for pain intensity, and the simple descriptive scale (SDS) to note the presence, and assessed level, of pain (No pain, Mild pain, Moderate pain, Severe pain). Of these three types of scales, the NRS (0 to 10 or 20) is recommended due to its enhanced sensitivity over the SDS and increased reliability over the VAS [2].
- Multidimensional composite scales include:
  - **The Glasgow Composite Measure Pain Scale** and its short form (CMPS-SF). The CMPS-SF, validated for use in measuring acute pain in **dogs and CMPS-F in cats**, are clinical decision-making tool when used in conjunction with clinical judgement. Intervention level scores have been described (i.e. the score at which analgesia should be administered), thus it can be used to indicate the need for analgesic treatment. The instrument is available to download online [10].
  - **The University of Melbourne Pain Scale** combines physiologic data and behavioural responses in **dogs** and is available for download [11].
  - The **UNESP-Botucatu**, English version, is a tool for use in assessing acute postoperative pain in **cats** undergoing ovariohysterectomy and provides useful information with respect to parameters to assess [12]. Four factors are identified:
    - psychomotor change (posture, comfort, activity, mental status and miscellaneous behaviours);
    - protection of wound area (reaction to palpation of the surgical wound and palpation of the abdomen and flank;
    - vocal expression of pain (vocalization)
    - physiologic variables (systolic arterial blood pressure and appetite); however, heart rate was not a consistent parameter neither was respiratory rate and pattern in assessing the level/presence of pain.
  - **The Colorado State University (CSU) Acute Pain Scale for the Dog** combines aspects of the NRS along with composite behavioural observation, and is designed as a teaching tool to increase awareness of behavioural changes associated with pain; it is also available for download [1].

III. Assessing Pain

Response to analgesic administration (as with any other therapy-directed treatment of a problem) can guide the veterinarian in the management of pain (or presumed pain). The dose and classes of analgesic required to control pain will reflect the severity of pain experienced. Return to normal behaviour – including eating, sleeping, dreaming, yawning, "normal stretching", grooming and a general appearance of well-being – is the goal. General daily observations of behaviour of cats and dogs, with or without painful conditions, and those following analgesic administration, will also contribute to identifying the presence and degree of pain experienced by patients in the general population under various conditions.

A. In General

Dogs may continue to wag their tail in response to touch or commands even though they may be experiencing moderate to severe pain, although this is usually a weak "tail between the legs" wag. Therefore, a tail wag should not be used to judge a pain-free situation unless it is vigorous. Dogs may also remain quiet and motionless, but occasionally may growl, when in mild to moderate pain and may thrash, growl and scream when pain is severe. However, some will remain motionless, standing with elbows abducted as positioning to get down and lie down is too painful following laparotomy where abdominal and high abdominal pain exists (Figure 8.2). The praying position (Figure 8.3) is most commonly seen with abdominal pain; however, lower esophageal pain may also elicit this posture. Commonly, following orthopedic procedures where movement increases the severe pain experienced, others may remain in lateral recumbency. Interaction will identify this situation. The term "depressed" in this text means slow or a "hang-dog" response to a situation where the dog would normally act as described in pain level 0 in Table 8.3 if not painful. They may appear "tired", the palpebral fissures may be incompletely open, with a low carriage of the head and "sad" facial expression. Compare painful pancreatitis prior to analgesic administration (Figure 8.4), to that of post-analgesia (Figure 8.5). The level of depression may vary from that just described to poorly or non-responsive to the caregiver.

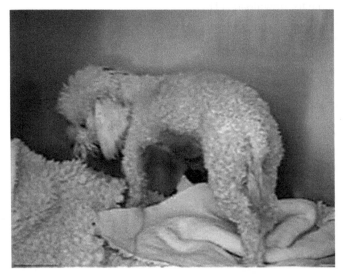

Figure 8.2 Post-laparotomy. Pain exhibited by slightly hunched back, elbows abducted due to high abdominal pain, hang dog look, low tail carriage and motionless standing. Slight touch on the abdomen resulted in splinting and vocalization. Appropriate monitoring and analgesic administration will avoid postoperative pain.

Figure 8.3 The "praying" posture due to pain resulting from a foreign body present in the stomach. A similar posture may be noted with distal esophageal pain/obstruction. Source: Courtesy Dr K Lamey.

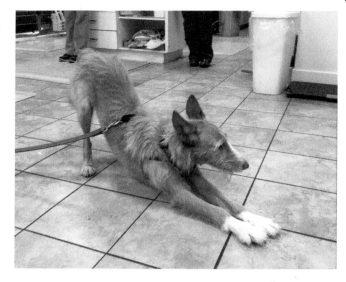

Figure 8.4 Acute pancreatitis prior to analgesic administration.

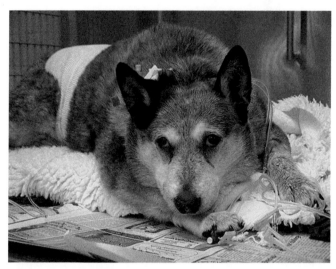

Figure 8.5 Acute pancreatitis post-analgesic administration.

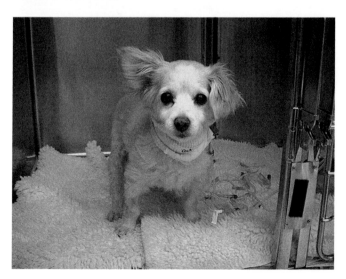

   Cats typically remain quiet and motionless, but occasionally may growl, when in mild to moderate pain, and may thrash, growl and scream when pain is severe. Cats may still purr when painful to any degree and, in fact, up until death. As with dogs, the term "depressed" in this text means slow or a "hang-dog" response to a situation where the cat would normally act as described in pain level 0, Table 8.6. The cat may remain in sternal with eyes closed (Figure 8.6), or partially open, not moving for several hours and remains in the back of the cage. The level of depression may vary from that just described to "poorly" or "non-responsive to caregiver". However, this appearance may also be associated with illness that may not necessarily be painful. On the other hand, note the ears pulled back and the pupils dilated, or on their way to becoming fully dilated (Figure 8.7, indicating an imminent attack! Therefore, knowing the underlying problem will assist with pain assessment. Most cats that are comfortable will curl up to sleep (Figure 8.8).

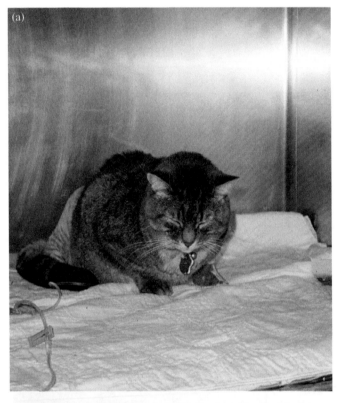

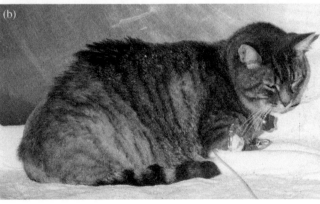

Figure 8.6 a and b Typical appearance of a painful cat; however, illness alone may be the problem. Careful examination and assessment for pain is required unless obvious trauma is present.

Figure 8.7 Recently admitted cat with fractured femur about to be assessed for analgesic efficacy and to obtain IV line access. Ears drawn back, pupils dilating moments prior to an "attack" on the caregiver.

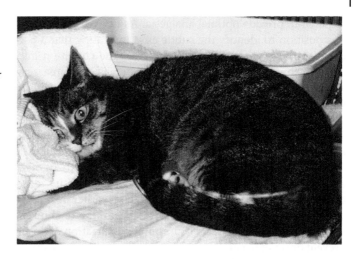

Figure 8.8 A happy cat.

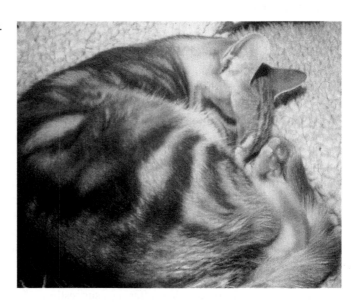

Following admission, stabilization and being placed in a cage, patients should be assessed on a regular basis to determine whether pain is adequately controlled, and, if it isn't, revise the established analgesic regimen. This also applies to those recovering from a surgical procedure, in the early recovery period. When pain is identified, ongoing assessment every 15–30 min is recommended until the patient is comfortable. Once effective analgesia is established, continue assessment on an hourly basis for the first 6–8 h. Thereafter, if pain is well controlled, assessment every 3–6 h is recommended. The exact time interval depends on the severity of the illness, injury and surgical procedure, the analgesic plan and other factors relating to the animal's physical status. If in doubt about pain status, re-assess the patient in 15 min. Where sleep is confirmed, do not wake the patient to assess pain.

To manage pain effectively, the team approach is essential especially where the case veterinarian is in surgery, in the emergency room or seeing appointments and is not available. During office hours and surgery, it is difficult for a veterinarian to observe patients with the frequency required to provide optimal analgesia. As the VT/N is the primary routine caregiver, they are in a position to identify the subtle cues indicating that a patient is more, or less, painful and trend pain and analgesic requirements as the condition improves or deteriorates. Reference [14] is recommended for the VT/N for details on pain assessment in cats. As pain is an individual and dynamic experience, analgesics must be administered as appropriate for that individual over time and it is the ongoing assessment for subtle changes in behaviour/attitude that the VT/N will notice, and be in a position to suggest a modification in the analgesic plan. These subtle changes should be discussed with the case veterinarian, as a patient's condition can rapidly change, causing a patient to be suddenly over- or under-dosed with an analgesic, or may be an indication of worsening of the underlying problem. In this context, the VT/N is the patient's advocate. Consider standing orders for analgesia using dose ranges and frequency with the option of PRN (as needed) dosing should an earlier dosing be required. Allowing the VT/N to intervene when they feel the patient is beginning to show signs of pain, or allowing them to modify the dose as needed, ensures individualization of dosing to the patient's needs. This will prevent onset of hyperalgesia should a more frequent dosing be required, and potential adverse effects (e.g. nausea, vomiting, dysphoria) with opioid excess. Where IV access is maintained, titrating an opioid slowly to effect is essential to avoid these adverse effects. Occasionally, adverse effects may occur, especially upon recovery from anesthesia where high dosages of opioid are administered. This will be recognized by the VT/N and reported to the veterinarian with recommendations for a titrated reversal with naloxone (0.1–0.25 mL of 0.4 mg/mL solution diluted in 5–10 mL saline, based on patient size, titrated in 1 mL increments to effect), analgesia is preserved using this technique. Ongoing observation may indicate a reduction in the opioid dose at the next administration or an increase in the dosing interval. An alternative to a pure mu-agonist (e.g. buprenorphine), as the patient's pain appears to be mild to moderate, may also be recommended. Or, where anxiety appears to be the problem, dexmedetomidine in the stable patient may be indicated. Patients should still be observed as frequently as possible, and the response to the analgesic noted at every opportunity.

Assigning the severity of trauma or degree of surgical invasiveness and tissue manipulation to a case may guide you as to which analgesic to use and how much to give, but even this has its variability. Surgical "trauma" (tissue handling) and duration of the surgical procedure will influence the degree of post-operative pain. For the more painful patient, a multi-modal approach must be considered. As an example, surgical procedures and injuries sustained to the abdomen, pelvis, hind limbs and soft tissue of the posterior portion of the body may benefit from epidural analgesia (Chapter 14) and/or adding a ketamine continuous rate infusion (CRI). The technician's ongoing contribution such as offering a suggestion – "can we try" or "can we add", and a reason for the suggestion – can help the veterinarian provide orders that may work better for that individual. Opioids cannot manage all types and degree of pain. A combination of opioid and an NSAIA will usually be adequate for pain assessed up to a level 7/10 for ≥ 7 pain levels multi-modal analgesia is essential and may also be beneficial at level 6.

As a cautionary note, when patients appear to be licking or chewing at the wound it is essential to closely observe the area that is being "attacked". As an example, the puppy in Figure 8.9 sustained a proximal femoral fracture, which was repaired using an intramedullary pin. Pain management was hydromorphone plus meloxicam. The patient was observed to be constantly "chewing the incision". An Elizabethan collar was placed. The puppy became extremely anxious and crying. When the collar was removed, he began licking what appeared to be the incision; however, on close examination, it was observed that he was licking slightly posterior to the incision. On gentle palpation of the area, the puppy cried, indicating potential "pin nerve impingement". Migration of the intramuscular (IM) pin was suspected and confirmed radiographically and at surgical exploration. Following correction, the puppy no longer showed signs of pain.

Figure 8.9 A 4-month-old puppy, post-femoral fracture repair, with Elizabethan collar placed in assumption that she was licking the surgical wound.

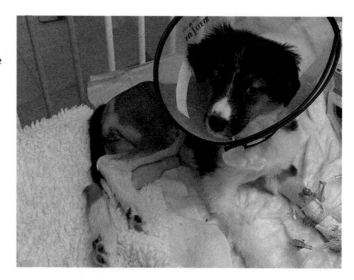

Figure 8.10a Attentive, non-painful cat after opioid administration. Note dilated pupils.

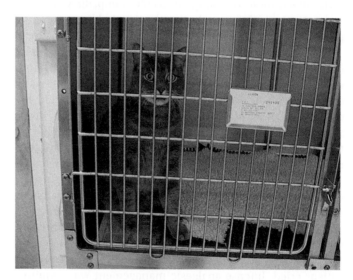

Figure 8.10b Pain-free cat responsive to presence of caregiver.

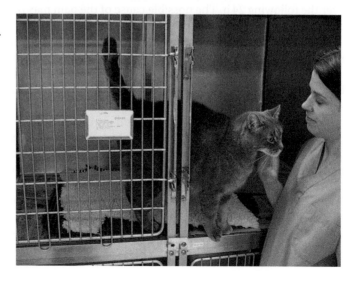

Other aspects of managing pain are: (1) to monitor for the effect of excess dosing of analgesics resulting in a "semi-comatose" state. Should high dosages/multimodal analgesia be required, it is essential that the owner be informed that this is drug-induced and not a deterioration in patient condition, to avoid the perception of worsening of the patient's condition and potential request for euthanasia, and (2) when to start weaning the patient off analgesics as the pain decreases and in preparation for discharge home. After 24h of comfort, where indicated, **slow weaning** (slight lowering of the dose q4h for moderate to excruciating pain) of analgesics is essential to avoid rebound hyperalgesia. In this context, the VT/N reports patient progress to the veterinarian with suggestion to start weaning. Should the patient appear painful after lowering the analgesic, return to the previous effective regimen. In preparation for home management, transition to oral meds (e.g. NSAIA, gabapentin, amantadine, oral transmucosal (OTM) buprenorphine – cats and small dogs) or transdermal fentanyl patch, when appropriate during weaning off IV analgesics. Another example of cautious assessment of post-operative behaviour is given in Chapter 32.

While the emphasis is on analgesics, a very important aspect of patient care and comfort is their immediate surroundings. As a cold, damp, dirty or noisy environment contributes to stress and anxiety, which in turn lowers the threshold to pain sensation, it is very important that the patient be made comfortable, clean, warm and dry (Chapter 17). Separate cats from dogs.

The behaviour associated with mild, moderate or severe pain (Table 8.1) may be similar (quiet, withdrawn, "hangdog expression", inappetent) and it is necessary to consider the underlying cause to ensure appropriate selection of the analgesic(s). The severity, acuity or chronicity of the surgical or medical problem should be evaluated when attempting to quantify the level of pain. Occasionally, pain is out of proportion to physical findings, such as the excruciating pain present with early presentation of an animal with *streptococcal* fasciitis (so-called flesh-eating disease) prior to obvious dermal lesions, or following a routine surgical procedure.

An example follows: a dog recovering from laparotomy for intestinal resection was extremely painful, tachycardic and hypertensive, remained in lateral recumbency and did not respond to the caregiver's voice. The only response was an increased respiratory rate, abdominal splinting and whining when touched. Epidural morphine, in combination with parenteral opioid, ketamine and lidocaine by CRI IV was required to control this dog's pain. Intermittent boluses of more opioid were administered for breakthrough pain when the patient cried. Intense analgesic management was required for 16h with a slow reduction over the following 24h. The possible cause of the pain may have been severe inflammation of the jejunum noted at laparotomy.

Pain is enhanced in the presence of inflammation, for example a cystotomy in an extremely inflamed bladder may be more painful than one performed in a normal bladder. Stretching and/or distension of viscera is also extremely painful but more so when the bowel is inflamed. Tissue handling also impacts on post-operative pain; surgical procedures performed by an experienced surgeon will result in less inflammation than that performed by an inexperienced surgeon.

Refer to the various scenarios presented in this book for initial management of acute pain. Refer to Chapter 9 (sedatives), Chapter 10 (opioids), Chapter 11 (NSAIAs) and Chapter 12 (adjunct analgesia) for details on the analgesics recommended for various levels of pain given in Table 8.3–8.8. In addition to analgesics, include integrative techniques where appropriate (Chapter 15).

Note 1: Where **NSAIAs** are recommended, it is assumed that there are **no contraindications** for their use (Chapter 11).

Note 2: Mu receptors on neural tissue are the target for the **mu opioid agonists**. However, while opioids preferentially bind the upregulated receptors on neural tissue when these are saturated the remainder of the opioid binds to other mu-receptors. These are present in the thermoregulatory centre, where they re-set the internal "thermostat" based on conditions the animal is experiencing. Should opioids bind these receptors, there is a lowering of the "thermostat"; the body is then "too hot" relative to the new setting, triggering panting to dissipate the heat. These receptors are also present in the area known to produce "euphoria". Excess opioid may stimulate the chemoreceptor trigger zone resulting in nausea and vomiting. Depending on the opioid dose administered, these adverse effects may be mild or dramatic (Figure 8.11a). Therefore, **when titrating opioids to effect, the goal is to achieve** a restful appearance without an increase in respiratory rate, signs of nausea, restlessness or beginning of vocalization. Should these signs start to appear, further opioid dosing will enhance these adverse effects and potentially jeopardize the health of the patient. Should pain still be noted, add another analgesic class. While vocalization may be associated with dysphoria, should the patient appear more painful (crying and thrashing distinct from dysphoria) opioid-induced hyperalgesia (OIH) may have occurred. Ketamine to effect is the treatment of choice for this.

The importance of opioid titration, where possible, is demonstrated in a case example of bolus administration of an opioid. A greyhound referred for radial fracture repair. A fentanyl patch was present upon admission; however, the dog was still assessed as painful and he was uncooperative for IV catheter placement. Hydromorphone was administered IM at a dose estimated to manage pain and facilitate IV catheter placement. As the opioid became effective, the dog's respiratory rate increased to the point of panting (Figure 8.11a and b). IV access was established and 0.25 mL naloxone (0.4 mg/mL) diluted with 10 mL saline was slowly titrated until the adverse effects were reversed and the patient was comfortable (Figure 8.11c). This technique frequently results in sleep. A reversal dose of naloxone cannot, and should not, be assumed. Do not administer a pre-determined dose of naloxone in a patient experiencing a painful condition as this may be an "overdose" resulting in peracute hyperalgesia (screaming, "freaking out"). In humans, this massive sympathetic response has resulted in massive venous return, pulmonary overload and flash pulmonary edema.

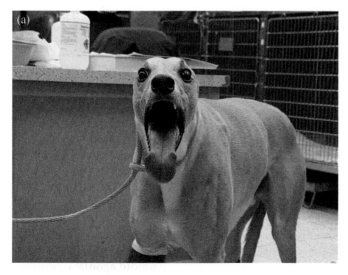

Figure 8.11 (a) Excessive panting due to opioid overdose.

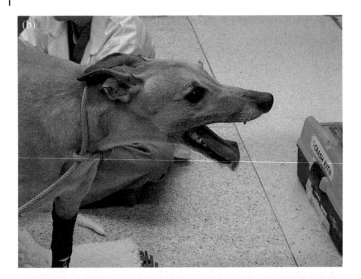

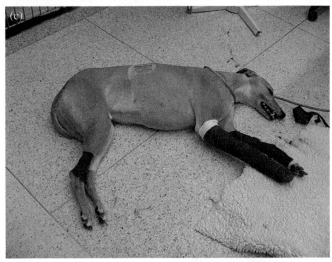

Figure 8.11 (Cont'd) (b) Opioid overdose. (c) Naloxone reversal.

IV. Dogs: Assessing Pain Behaviours

Opioids titrated IV to effect, or halted at the very early onset of nausea, increased respiratory rate or dysphoria. One-quarter of the effective opioid dose may be used as an hourly CRI for all except fentanyl, where the effective dose is used as a 1 h CRI. Should the patient still appear painful, add an NSAIA where not contraindicated, or ketamine. The effective titrated dose of ketamine may also be used as a 1 h infusion. Ketamine relies on hepatic metabolism in dogs; therefore, the duration of action may be prolonged in dogs with hepatic dysfunction. Refer to Chapter 19 for details on the preparation and delivery of analgesics.

Table 8.3 DOGS Suggested analgesic regimens based on behaviour associated with pain severity in dogs. Note: all suggested dosages are based on ideal body weight in the overweight or obese

Assessed level of pain	Pain Description and suggested analgesic regimen
0	**No pain** **Observing the patient**. Sleeping comfortably with dreaming. Grooming normally and not focusing on surgical/injured area. Sitting normally or in sternal recumbency observing the surroundings and activities. Normal respiratory rate. Food has been eaten **When approaching the cage/patient** there is a normal, affectionate response to the caregiver **Out of the cage** patient is walking normally and may be bouncy/jumping **Physical examination** reveals normal heart rate, but if elevated, it is due to excitement. Minimal/no response to palpation of surgical/injured/medical area. A minimal response is expected when the pathological site is gently palpated around the area, but pain does not persist. This "incident" pain cannot be eliminated, we have all experienced this **Behaviour different from this**, known not to be associated with pain, may be associated with apprehension or anxiety. Apprehension/anxiety can be a feature of hospitalized patients OR, there may be systemic illness associated with various medical problems e.g. renal failure No pain medication required **Dexmedatomidine§ below**
1	**Probably no pain** **Observing the patient**. Patient appears to be normal as in 0 above, but interest in food may be decreased **When approaching the patient** there is a lack of enthusiasm Heart rate should be normal, or slightly increased due to excitement **Where a potentially painful** condition exists in the naïve patient with potential for progression, administer an injectable **NSAIA** (Chapter 11) where not contraindicated or opioid based on the underlying condition causing pain Reassess q15–30 min and see scores below
2	**Mild discomfort** Patient will still eat or sleep but may not dream. May limp slightly or resist palpation of the surgical wound, but otherwise shows no other signs of discomfort. Not depressed. There may be a slight increase in respiratory rate; heart rate may or may not be increased. Dogs may continue to wag their tail vigorously **Treat** as in 1. Above, reassess q15–30 min
3	**Mild pain or discomfort** **Observing the patient**, frequently remains in the back of the cage. Looks a little depressed. Respiratory rate may be increased and a little shallow, slight pant. Cannot get comfortable. May tremble or shake. May or may not be interested in food, may still eat a little, but somewhat picky **When approaching the patient**, there is reluctance to move towards the caregiver and get out of the cage. Head hangs down. There may be a tail wag with tail between the legs **Physical examination**. Heart rate may be increased or normal, depending on whether an opioid was given previously. Opioids can reduce heart rate while pain still present. Guards incision, or the abdomen may be slightly tucked up if abdominal surgery was performed. Palpation of the injured/surgical area elicits a twitch with attempts to move away **When out of the cage**, the patient's limp may be more noticeable if there is an orthopedic problem. You may notice a change from being comfortable to becoming restless, as though the analgesia is wearing off. **Needs analgesia.** The analgesic selected will depend on whether (i) it is a repeat in a patient with moderate to severe pain (fracture repair) or (ii) the patient has a problem resulting in mild to moderate pain which is not expected to worsen

(Continued)

Table 8.3 (Continued)

Assessed level of pain	Pain Description and suggested analgesic regimen
3	**Analgesia:** • **If (i),** an injectable **NSAIA** (see Table 11.1) is highly recommended for **orthopedic procedures**, if not contraindicated) Then continue with • **fentanyl** 2–6 µg/kg titrated to effect IV followed by the effective dose as an hourly CRI, **or** sufentanil or alfentanil (refer to Chapter 10 for dosing), **or** • **methadone** 0.2 mg/kg IV, IM q3–6 h, **or** • **hydromorphone** or **oxymorphone** 0.05 mg/kg IV, IM, SC, q3-6 **or** • **morphine** IM, SC: 0.2 mg/kg q3-6 h Where administered IV, titrate to effect; other than fentanyl, the effective dose is used to maintain analgesia as a CRI for the following 4 h (1/4 effective dose mg/kg/h) Where the problem being treated is expected to generate pain ≥ 7, addition of **ketamine** 0.25–1.0 mg/kg/h, titrate to effect followed with effective dose as hourly CRI, to the existing regimen is suggested For GI problems, **lidocaine** 1–2+ mg/kg followed by 1–2+ mg/kg/h may be of benefit (refer to Chapter 12) • **If (ii),** an **NSAIA** where appropriate and no contraindications (refer to Chapter 11), or • **butorphanol** 0.1–0.4 mg/kg IV, IM, or • **buprenorphine** 0.01 mg/kg, IV, IM **or** if no IV access, buprenorphine slow release (SR) SC 0.03–0.06 mg/kg If this is a mild pain situation (e.g. selected biopsy procedure), pure mu-agonists are not necessary, as the patient may become dysphoric. However, it is essential that butorphanol or buprenorphine not be administered prior to the potential need for pure mu-agonists. Where this is the case, administer a low dose of the pure mu-agonist **Dexmedetomidine§ see below**
4	**Mild to moderate pain** **Observing the patient.** The patient may sit or lie in an abnormal position and is not curled up or relaxed. May tremble or shake. May or may not appear interested in food. May start to eat and then stop after one or two bites. Respiratory rate may be increased or shallow. May look, lick or chew, at the painful area **Approaching the patient.** Will be somewhat depressed with reduced response to caregiver **Physical examination.** Patient resists touching of the operative site, injured area, painful abdomen, or neck, etc. There is guarding or splinting of the abdomen or may stretch all four legs when abdomen palpated. Heart rate may be increased or normal. Pupils may be dilated but may be affected by administered drugs **When out of the cage.** May whimper, be slow to rise and, hang the tail down. There may be no weight bearing or a toe touch on the operated limb due to movement-evoked pain **Analgesia.** An NSAIA, or **buprenorphine**, as for 3 above for mild to moderate pain For continuing analgesia where the expected potential level of pain is ≥ 7, and the patient has already received an NSAIA and an opioid, consider addition of **ketamine or lidocaine** as for 3 above **Dexmedetomidine§ see below**
5	**Moderate pain.** As for 4 above but pain is worsening. Patient may be reluctant to move, depressed, inappetent and may bite or attempt to bite when the caregiver approaches the painful area. Trembling or shaking with head down may be a feature, depressed. The patient may vocalize when caregiver attempts to move them or when it is approached. There is definite splinting of the abdomen if affected, e.g. pancreatitis, hepatitis, incision) or the patient is unable to bear weight on an injured or operative limb. The ears may be pulled back. The heart and respiratory rates **may** be increased; however, opioids can reduce heart rate while pain is still present. Pupils may be dilated; however, miosis is opioid-dose-related. The patient is not interested in food, will lie down but does not really sleep and may stand in the praying position if there is abdominal pain

Table 8.3 (Continued)

Assessed level of pain	Pain Description and suggested analgesic regimen
5	**Analgesia.** An injectable **NSAIA** (see Table 11.1, Chapter 11), either alone or as adjunct to opioids, if orthopedic and soft tissue surgery or injury, where there are no contraindications, **and/or** • **fentanyl** 3–5 µg/kg titrate IV to effect followed by effective dose as hourly CRI or Using effective dose as a 4 h infusion: • **methadone** 0.2–0.5 mg/kg, **or** • **oxymorphone or hydromorphone** 0.05–0.1 mg/kg, **or** • **morphine** 0.2–0.4 mg/kg, For medical (e.g. pancreatitis) pain **buprenorphine** 0.02–0.04 mg/kg q4–6 IV, where pain is not anticipated to worsen Where NSAIAs are contemplated in combination with an opioid, the opioid dose may be reduced **Dexmedatomidine§ see below**
6	**Increased moderate pain. As above (5)**, but patient **may** vocalize or whine frequently, without provocation and when attempting to move. Heart rate may be increased or within normal limits if an opioid was administered previously. Respiratory rate may be increased with an abdominal lift. Pupils may be dilated **Analgesia.** Injectable **NSAIA**(see Table 11.1,), where no contraindications, **or** add if needed: Titrate IV opioid, listed in order of preference, to effective dose: • **fentanyl** 6–8 mg/kg IV to effect followed by effective dose as an hourly CRI, **or** Follow with effective dose as a CRI over 4 h for: • **methadone** 0.3–0.5 mg/kg, **or** • **hydromorphone or oxymorphone** 0.05– 0.1 mg/kg, **or** • **morphine** 0.1–0.2 mg/kg, slowly titrate over 3 min. If **butorphanol** or buprenorphine was given within the last 20 min, and the condition is still painful, then a higher dose of pure mu-agonist is usually required due to the antagonistic effects of butorphanol and buprenorphine **Dexmedatomidine§ see below**
7	**Moderate to severe pain** (include signs from 5 and 6 above). The patient is depressed and frequently is not concerned with its surroundings but usually responds to direct voice (this may be a stop in whining, turning of the head or eyes). The patient may urinate and defecate (if diarrhea) without attempting to move, will cry out when moved or will spontaneously or continually whimper. Occasionally, an animal doesn't vocalize. Heart and respiratory rates may be increased. Hypertension may also be present. Pupils may be dilated. However, heart rate and pupil size may appear normal if an opioid has been administered. Pupil size in cats are dilated, but constricted in dogs, with opioid administration **Analgesia:** An **NSAIA**(see Table 11.1,), especially if orthopedic/traumatic/inflammatory pain, and no contraindications Patients require the higher dose (6 above) of fentanyl, methadone oxymorphone, hydromorphone or morphine; select one of these opioids and titrate to effect, **halt with early signs of adverse effects***. Continue with effective dose as 4 h CRI Addition of **ketamine** 0.5–1 mg/kg followed with a CRI of 0.25–2 mg/kg/h is also of benefit for improved bronchodilation Also consider adding **lidocaine** 1–2 mg/kg bolus followed with 1+ mg/kg/h CRI for 9-24h, especially for associated visceral pain. Epidural and/or local analgesia/anesthesia should be considered where indicated. Both parenteral and epidural routes of a local anesthetic should not be administered simultaneously. **Dexmedatomidine§ see below**

(Continued)

Table 8.3 (Continued)

Assessed level of pain	Pain Description and suggested analgesic regimen
8	**Severe pain.** Signs as above (7). Vocalizing may be more of a feature, the patient is so consumed with pain that the patient will not notice your presence and just lie there. The patient may thrash around in the cage intermittently. If it is traumatic or neurologic pain, the patient may scream when being approached. Tachycardia, ± tachypnea with increased abdominal effort and hypertension are usually present even if an opioid was previously given, although these can be unreliable parameters if not present **Analgesia:** An **NSAIA** (see Table 11.1,) especially if orthopedic/traumatic/inflammatory pain, and no contraindications **High dose titrate to effect, halt with early signs of adverse effects*** • **fentanyl** 8–10+ µg/kg followed by hourly CRI, **or** **Follow** effective dose as 4 h CRI of: • **methadone** 0.5+ mg/kg, **or** • **oxymorphone or hydromorphone** 0.1–0.2 mg/kg, **or** • **morphine** 0.5+ mg/kg titrate over 3 min Add **ketamine** 1+ mg/kg IV followed by 0.5–2 mg/kg/h CRI ± **lidocaine** 1–2 mg/kg bolus (dogs only) followed with 1–2 mg/kg/h CRI for 9-24 h. **Epidural and/or Local analgesia/anesthesia** should be considered where indicated Chapter 14 and individual scenarios in this book. Both parenteral and epidural routes should not be administered simultaneously. **Dexmedatomidine§ see below**
9	**Severe to excruciating.** As above (8), but patient is hyperesthetic. The patient will tremble involuntarily when any part of the body in close proximity to wound, injury, etc., is touched. Neuropathic pain (entrapped nerve or inflammation around the nerve) or extensive inflammation anywhere (i.e. peritonitis, pleuritis, fasciitis, myositis, severe necrotizing pancreatitis) **Analgesia:** Requires multi-modal analgesia. Intubation and ventilation may be required Injectable **NSAIA** (see Table 11.1) especially if orthopedic and inflammatory pain, where no contraindications **Requires high dose opioids. Titrate to effect, halt with early signs of adverse effects*:** • **fentanyl** 10+ µg/kg follow with hourly CRI, **or** Followed by a 4-hour CRI of effective dose of • **methadone** 0.5–1+ mg/kg, **or** • **hydromorphone** 0.1–0.2 mg/kg, **or** • **morphine** 0.5–1 mg/kg *At this point, ADD **ketamine** 0.6–2+ mg/kg IV titrated to effect followed by the effective dose as hourly CRI; ± **lidocaine** 2 mg/kg slowly titrated followed by a 0.5–2 mg/kg/h CRI. Lidocaine by this route cannot be used if local anesthetics are being administered via another route as the dose of lidocaine will likely exceed the safe limit. May be beneficial for abdominal pain. Nausea may be noted at 12-24 hours, wean off should this occur. Tachycardia may persist and may be impossible to control the pain Consider combining analgesics with **epidurally placed analgesics or local blocks**. If not successful, anesthetize the patient, see 10 below, while attempting to find or treat the inciting cause. Remove the inciting cause immediately. **This degree of pain can cause death. Continue all analgesics as a CRI with frequent monitoring** Dexmedatomidine§ below
10	**As above (9), but patient emitting piercing screams or almost comatose.** The patient is hyperesthetic/hyperalgesic and pain is elicited wherever you touch the patient **Analgesia:** • As for (9), increase ketamine dose to facilitate intubation and continue to maintain general anesthesia **or** supplement with **propofol** 2–6 mg/kg, IV to effect, **or** • **Alfaxalone** 1–3 mg/kg, IV to effect general anesthesia, **or** • Maintain anesthesia with an inhalant while attempting to find or treat the inciting cause **This degree of pain can cause death**

Source: Data adapted from [16]. With permission.

In general, if the pain is not being managed, increase analgesia to effect (opioids and ketamine). *Opioids alone cannot manage severe to excruciating pain. If early adverse effects of opioids are noted (i.e. nausea, increased respiratory rate, vocalization) this indicates saturation of mu-receptors but not necessarily an indication of adequate analgesia, as pain is also mediated via other mechanisms. This indicates that a higher dose of an opioid will not be effective in alleviating pain if the animal still appears painful, and will increase the adverse opioid effects. A different class of analgesic must be administered in addition to the opioid.

For the restless patient where appropriate analgesia has been provided but anxiety is also contributing to the painful experience, addition of §**Dexmedetomidine** bolus 2 µg/kg IV followed by 0.5–2.0 µg/kg/h CRI may be considered. Dexmedetomidine has both analgesic and sedative effects and may facilitate lowering of the opioid and other classes of analgesics; therefore, frequent assessment is required. Only use in otherwise healthy dogs. If used prior to induction of general anesthesia, titrate induction agent with one-quarter increments of usual dose.

Neuropathic pain may be associated with a variety of surgical procedures or medical conditions.

Gabapentin is a useful adjunct to opioids for managing pain associated with neuritis, nerve entrapment secondary to trauma, cervical or thoracolumbar disc disease or post-laminectomy. Gabapentin can be used in combination with opioids. Post-seizure or CPR vocalization, if relentless, may also be managed with gabapentin. Suggested dose range is 5–25 mg/kg q8h for pain. This author starts at 10 mg/kg q8h for dogs and cats increasing the dose if no effect seen in ~4 h. Sedation/sleep is the limiting factor; however, when in hospital this is usually desirable. There may be a requirement for up to 12 mg/kg q6h for post-seizure or post-CPR vocalization and thrashing. Wean off slowly; otherwise, the patient will experience worse pain. Increase duration of dosing interval, and potential reduced dosing, in hepatic insufficiency. Where indicated (see Chapter 3, 12 and case scenarios in this book), commence therapy prior to discharge home where it can be continued.

Table 8.4 Suggested Analgesia for Various Levels of *Ongoing Pain* in DOGS NOTE: The drugs and doses given are suggestions. If the pain is not being managed, then increase to effect (not NSAIAs). If administered IV, morphine must be administered slowly to prevent hypotension in all animals. Ketamine 1-2+ mg/kg IV, or 10 mg/kg **per os (fractious dogs)**, may be an alternative to control pain quickly if opioids are not available and hypertrophic cardiomyopathy is not a concern. General anesthesia is another alternative (refer to Pharmacologic and Clinical Application of Anesthetics Chpt13).

NOTE: ALL DOSAGES ARE BASED ON IDEAL BODY WEIGHT IN THE OVERWEIGHT OR OBESE DOGS. Opioids, ketamine, lidocaine as a CRI can be combined in IV crystalloid fluids (lactated Ringer's or Ringer's may not be compatible due to calcium content). For Preparation and Delivery of Analgesics by CRI refer to Chpt 18 for details. Where available, syringe pumps with individual analgesics may also be used.
Severe to Excruciating Pain   **Requires multimodal analgesia. Higher dose opioids, titration to effect is essential, halt with early signs of adverse effects*.At this point, ADD ketamine**   **Opioids** in order of preference: • **fentanyl** 10+ µg /kg (refer to Opioids Chpt 10 for sufentanil, alfentanil dosing), continue the effective dose as an hourly CRI. OR   • **methadone** up to 1mg/kg OR   • **hydromorphone or oxymorphone** 0.1mg/kg and titrate up to 0.2 mg/kg; OR,   • **morphine** 0.5+mg/kg, titrate over **3 minutes to avoid hypotension**. For all mu opioids (except fentanyl, or sufentanil) use the effective dose divided by 4 to establish an hourly IV CRI.

(Continued)

Table 8.4 (Continued)

NSAIA (Table 1 Chpt 11) add where not contraindicated.

Ketamine 1–4 mg/kg combined with the opioid above, titrated to effect, followed by this dose as an hourly CRI
Lidocaine 0.5–2 mg/kg slow push to effect followed by this dose as an hourly CRI for 9–24 hours. May be beneficial where abdominal pain is present. This should not be included if local anesthetics have been administered via a different route. Do not overdose with local anesthetic.

Consider combining the above analgesics with **epidurally placed analgesics or local blocks (Chpt 14)**,

Tachycardia may persist. It may be impossible to control the pain. It may be necessary to anesthetize the patient by increasing the ketamine dose to facilitate intubation and continue to maintain general anesthesia OR add **propofol** 2–6 mg/kg, IV to effect OR **alfaxalone** 1–3 mg/kg, IV to effect general anesthesia, OR maintain **anesthesia with an inhalant** while attempting to find or treat the inciting cause (refer to Anesthesia Chpt 13 and individual scenarios in this book for guidance. Remove the inciting cause immediately. **This degree of pain can cause death.**

Moderate to Severe Pain

SELECT ONE ANALGESIC FROM WITHIN EACH CLASS

Analgesic	Dosing	Frequency
Fentanyl *OR*	4–10 + µg /kg IV Administer intermittently or follow with a CRI using effective dose /h	q 15–20 min CRI
Sufentanil, Alfentanil *OR*	Refer to Opioids Chapt 10 for dosing	
Methadone preferred *OR Morphine* *OR*	0.3–1 mg/kg IV Administer intermittently or follow with effective dose as a CRI over dosing interval	2–4 h 4h
Hydromorphone or *Oxymorphone*	0.05–0.2 mg/kg IV Administer intermittently or follow with effective dose as a CRI over dosing interval	2–4 h 4h
#Ketamine combined *with an opioid or sedative*	0.5–2+ mg/kg/h IV 0.5–2+mg/kg IV	Titrate to effect use this as Hourly CRI
*Injectable NSAIA(Table 1 *Chpt 11) where no* *contraindications*	As per label instructions for dosing, contraindications and drug combination warnings	As per label instructions
Bupivacaine 0.5%	Interpleural and Interperitoneal use: Using 0.5% bupivacaine (5mg/mL) Administer bupivacaine at 1 mg/kg (0.2 mL/kg) based on ideal body weight. Use sodium bicarbonate (1 mEq/ml) to buffer 0.5% bupivacaine at a 20 : 0.1 ratio (~0.2mL bupivacaine and 0.001mL sodium bicarbonate/kg BW). For instillation volumes add bupivicaine dose to 6–12mL sterile water for larger dogs (relative to size of dog); 3 mLs for tiny dogs. Warmed to body temperature prior to administration. (Buffering is not required when administered under anesthesia or for repeat instillation as the previous bupivicaine should still be effective. Chapter 14)	4–6 h

Table 8.4 (Continued)

In preparation for discharge, to manage ongoing pain, consider placement of a fentanyl patch while weaning off an IV opioid		
Fentanyl patch	<8kg: 12.5 µg /h 8–10kg: 25 µg /kg 10–20kg – 50 µg /h 20–30kg – 75 µg /h >30kg – 100 µg /h	12–24 hours to effect; Replace q 48–72 h

Mild to Moderate Pain

Opioids above OR	Low dosages	Titrate down to lowest effective dose
Buprenorphine	0.02–0.04 mg/kg IV, IM	4–8h
OR		
Butorphanol **Mild pain only or mild gastrointestinal pain** OR	0.1–0.4 mg/kg IV, IM Administer intermittently or follow with a CRI with effective dose over dosing interval	2 h
Meperidine (pethidine)	5–10 mg/kg IM, SC for short duration analgesia or prior to obtaining IV access especially where vomiting is a concern	20–30 minutes
Injectable NSAIA* **(Table 1 Chpt 11)**	Low dosages. As per lable instructions for contraindications and drug combination warnings	Low dosages. As per lable instructions

Sedatives to combine with opioids where indicated, select one

Midazolam	0.1–0.5 mg/kg IV, IM	up to 6h
Diazepam	0.1–0.5 mg/kg IV	up to 6h
Acepromazine	0.01–0.05 mg/kg IV 0.02–0.1 mg/kg IM, SC	1–2 h 2–6 h
Dexmedetomidine§	2–4 ug/kg IM, SC 0.5–2 ug/kg/h	CRI

*Refer to the individual COX-2 Preferential/selective NSAIA labeling for duration of use and for safety information. Refer to Non-steroidal Anti-inflammatory Analgesics Chpt 11 for further information. It is not always necessary to administer the recommended loading dose. The dose is determined based on the degree of pain assessed. It is advised that a dose as low as possible be used to manage the varying degrees of pain. This will reduce the potential for adverse effects.

#Not first line but may be beneficial in difficult to manage cases.

§**Dexmedetomidine** has both analgesic and sedative effects. Only use in otherwise healthy dogs. If used prior to induction of general anesthesia, titrate induction agent with one-quarter increments of usual dose.
Data adapted from Mathews KA[15]. Pain assessment and general approach to management. Vet Clin North Am. Sm Anim.2000;30(4). With Permission

Table 8.5 Adjunctive analgesics suggested dosages based on ideal body weight in overweight or obese dogs

Analgesic	Dosage	Route of Administration	Duration
Ketamine	0.2–2 mg/kg (may need up to 4 mg/kg for excruciating pain or opioid-induced hyperalgesia)	IV	Bolus for control followed by CRI depending on severity of pain
Lidocaine	0.5–2 mg/kg 1–3 mg/kg/h	IV IV	Bolus followed by CRI depending on severity of pain Limit to 9 <24 h to avoid nausea
Gabapentin	5–25 mg/kg up to 12 mg/kg	PO PO	q8h for pain q6h for post-seizure or post-CPR vocalization and thrashing Wean off slowly
Amantadine	3–5 mg/kg	PO	q12–24 h
Amitriptyline	1–2 mg/kg	PO	q12–24 h

V. Cats: Assessing Pain Behaviours

Ketamine and lidocaine are contraindicated in cats with hypertrophic cardiomyopathy. Refer to Chapter 12 for lidocaine guidelines. Morphine is indicated only where other pure mu-opioids are not available as onset of action is slow. As with dogs, slow titration is essential to avoid hypotension

Table 8.6 CATS Suggested analgesic regimens associated with behaviour in cats all dosages are based on ideal body weight in the overweight or obese

Assessed level of pain	Pain description and suggested analgesic regimen
0	**No pain.** Patient is playing, jumping, sitting or walking normally. Sleeping comfortably curled up. Normal, affectionate response to caregiver; will rub their face on the caregiver's hand or cage, may roll over and purr. Heart rate should be normal, but if elevated, it is due to excitement. Cats will groom themselves when free of pain. Appetite is normal. Behaviour different from this, not associated with pain, may be associated with a medical illness, apprehension or anxiety. Apprehension/anxiety can be a feature of hospitalized patients
1	**Probably no pain.** Patient appears to be normal but condition is not as clear-cut as above. Heart rate should be normal, or slightly increased due to excitement. Cats may still purr. Reassess in 15–30 min
2	**Mild discomfort.** Patient will still eat or sleep but may not curl up. May limp slightly or resist palpation of the surgical wound, but otherwise shows no other signs of discomfort. Not depressed. There may be a slight increase in respiratory rate; heart rate may or may not be increased and may still purr. Reassess at 15–30 min; give an analgesic if condition appears worse. Refer to 3 (i) below.

Table 8.6 (Continued)

Assessed level of pain	Pain description and suggested analgesic regimen
3	**Mild pain or discomfort.** Patient will limp or guard incision or the abdomen may be slightly tucked up if abdominal surgery was performed. Looks a little depressed. Cannot get comfortable. May tremble or shake. May remain sternal with eyes closed, or partially open, not moving for hours and remains in the back of the cage. Appears to be interested in food when offered and may still eat a little but somewhat picky. This could be a transition from 2 above, so you notice a change from being comfortable to becoming restless, as though the analgesia is wearing off. Respiratory rate may be increased and a little shallow. Heart rate may be increased or normal, depending on whether an opioid was given previously. The cat may continue to purr even when in pain; therefore, disregard this as a consistent indicator of comfort. **Needs analgesia.** The analgesic selected will depend on whether **(i)** it is a repeat in a patient with moderate to severe pain (e.g. fracture repair) or **(ii)** the patient has a problem resulting in mild to moderate pain **Analgesia:** **If (i)**, add an NSAIA if not already (see Table 11.1) administered, where no contraindications, especially for orthopedic pain then continue with **fentanyl** 2–5 µg/kg titrate IV to effect followed by the effective dose as an hourly CRI, **or** sufentanil or alfentanil (refer to Chapter 10 for dosing), **or** Where administered IV, titrate to effect. The effective dose is used to maintain analgesia as a CRI for the following 4 h (1/4 dose mg/kg/h) • **methadone** 0.2+ mg/kg IV, IM q4–6h, **or** • **hydromorphon**e 0.05 mg/kg IV, IM, SC q4–6h, **or** • **oxymorphone** 0.05+ mg/kg IV, IM SC q4–6h, **or** • **morphine**^ IM, SC : 0.1 mg/kg **If (ii) NSAIA** (see Table 11.1) where appropriate where no contraindications If intestinal pain, **butorphanol** 0.1–0.4 mg/kg may be of value, **or** **buprenorphine** 0.005–0.02 mg/kg, IV, IM or OTM (0.04 mg/kg) **or buprenorphine slow release** (SR) 0.03–0.12 mg/kg If the underlying problem may become more painful, it is essential that butorphanol or buprenorphine not be administered prior to the potential need for a pure mu-agonist. Where this is the case, administer a low dose of the pure mu-agonist. If this is a mild pain situation (e.g. selected biopsy procedure), pure mu-agonists are not necessary as the patient may become dysphoric
4	**Mild to moderate pain** with the patient resisting touching of the operative site, injured area, painful abdomen, etc. Guarding or splinting of the abdomen. The patient may sit crouched (especially medical pain or abdominal/thoracic surgery) or lie in an abnormal position (relative to injury) and is not curled up or relaxed. May or may not appear interested in food. May start to eat and then stop after one or two bites. Respiratory rate may be increased or shallow. Heart rate may be increased or normal. Pupils may be dilated. May cry occasionally, be slow to rise and hang the tail down. There may be no weight bearing or a toe touch on the operated limb. Will be somewhat depressed with reduced response to caregiver. Often, cats may lie quietly and not move for prolonged periods in the back of the cage **Analgesia.** As for 3 above. **Opioids: If (i)** requires higher dosage or decreased duration between dosages. Consider an **NSAIA** if has not been given and no contraindications
5	**Moderate pain.** As above but condition progressing from above. Patient may be reluctant to move, usually remaining in a crouched position, depressed, inappetent and may bite or attempt to bite when the caregiver approaches the painful area. The patient may vocalize when caregiver attempts to move them or when it is approached. There is definite splinting of the abdomen if affected (i.e. peritonitis, pancreatitis, hepatitis, incision), or the patient is unable to bear weight on an injured or operative limb. The ears may be pulled back. The heart and respiratory rates **may** be increased. **Rule out hyperthermia due to opioid**. Pupils may be dilated. The patient is not interested in food, will lie down but does not really sleep. Frequently, cats may remain sternal and hunched and not move **Analgesia.** An injectable **NSAIA** (see Table 11.1) where there are no contraindications, either alone or as adjunct to opioids, especially if orthopedic and soft tissue surgery/injury or integument injuries. Lower dosages of opiate are required when combined with an NSAIA.

(Continued)

Table 8.6 (Continued)

Assessed level of pain	Pain description and suggested analgesic regimen
5	• **Buprenorphine** 0.02–0.04 mg/kg, is the preferred opioid if pain is not expected to increase. Or, if pain has the potential to increase: **Titrate opioid analgesics to effect**, halt at the early signs of adverse effects: • **fentanyl** 2–3+ µg/kg followed with hourly CRI, **or** One of the following, and where administered IV, titrate to effect. The effective dose is used to maintain analgesia as a CRI for the following 4 h (1/4 dose mg/kg/h) • **methadone** 0.2–0.5 mg/kg IV, IM q4–6h, **or** • **oxymorphone** or **hydromorphone** 0.05– < 0.1 mg/kg IV, IM q4–6h **or** • **morphine**^ 0.1–0.2 mg/kg, IM q3–6 h
6	**Increased moderate pain. As above (5)**, but patient **may** vocalize without provocation and when attempting to move. Heart rate may be increased or within normal limits if an opioid was administered previously. Respiratory rate may be increased with an abdominal lift. **Rule out hyperthermia due to opioid** [hydromorphone esp]. Pupils may be dilated due to pain or previous dose of opioid **Titrate opioid analgesics to effect**, halt at the early signs of adverse effects **Analgesia.** Administer an injectable **NSAIA** (see Table 11.1) where no contraindications, especially if the pain is associated with orthopedic or inflammatory pain • **fentanyl** 3–5 µg/kg IV to effect, effective dose followed as an hourly CRI, **or** One of the following titrated to effect with the effective dose continued as a 4-hour infusion (1/4 effective dose/h) • **methadone** 0.3–0.5 mg/kg, or • **oxymorphone** or **hydromorphone** 0.05 < 1 mg/kg, **or** • **morphine**^ 0.1–0.2 mg/kg IM, SC q3–6 h or 3 min slow push IV A lower dosage of opiate is required with co-administration of an NSAIA
7	**Moderate to severe pain** (include signs from 5 and 6 above). The patient is very depressed and is not concerned with its surroundings but usually responds to direct voice (this may be turning of the head or eyes). The patient will urinate and defecate (if diarrhea) without attempting to move, will cry out when moved or spontaneously. Occasionally an animal doesn't vocalize. Heart and respiratory rates may be increased. Hypertension may also be present. Pupils may be dilated due to pain or opioid mydriasis **Analgesia:** An **NSAIA** (see Table 11.1) if no contraindications present, especially if orthopedic or inflammatory pain. **Titrate opioid analgesics to effect**, halt at the early signs of adverse effects. • **fentanyl** 5+ µg/kg, continue with hourly CRI, **or** Titrate to effect one of the following and opioids and continue with effective dose as a CRI over 4 h (1/4 effective dose/h) • **methadone** 0.3–0.5 mg/kg, **or** • **oxymorphone** or **hydromorphone** maximum 0.1 mg/kg, **or** • **morphine**^ 0.1–0.2 mg/kg Addition of **ketamine, titrate IV** 0.5–2 mg/kg and CRI of 0.25–2 mg/kg/h should be considered if pain is not controlled **Epidural and/or local analgesia/anesthesia** should be considered where indicated
8	**Severe pain.** Signs as above (7). Vocalizing may be more of a feature, or so consumed with pain the patient will not notice your presence and just lie there but trembling. The patient may thrash around in the cage intermittently. If it is traumatic or neurologic pain, the patient may scream when being approached. Tachycardia, ± tachypnea with increased abdominal effort and hypertension are usually present even if an opioid was previously given, although these can be unreliable parameters if not present **Analgesia:** An injectable **NSAIA** (see Table 11.1) especially if orthopedic or inflammatory pain (e.g. burn), with no contraindications. **Titrate opioid analgesics to effect**, halt at the early signs of adverse effects. **Multi-modal analgesia is essential** • **fentanyl** 5–10 µg/kg and maintain te effective dose as an hourly CRI, **or** Titrate to effect one of the following opioids and continue with the effective dose as a CRI over 4 h (1/4 effective dose/h): • **high dose methadone 0.4–0.5+ mg/kg**, or • **oxymorphone** or **hydromorphone up to** 0.1 mg/kg to effect and • Add **ketamine** titrate 1–2+ mg/kg followed by 0.5–2 mg/kg/h CRI **Lidocaine for infusion** refer to Chapter 12 for guidelines. Not to be administered if local or epidural analgesia is used **Epidural and/or local analgesia/anesthesia** should be considered where indicated

Table 8.6 (Continued)

Assessed level of pain	Pain description and suggested analgesic regimen
9	**Severe to excruciating.** As above (8), but patient is hyperesthetic, will tremble involuntarily when any part of the body in close proximity to wound, injury, etc., is touched. Neuropathic pain (entrapped nerve or inflammation around the nerve) or extensive inflammation anywhere (i.e. peritonitis, pleuritis, fasciitis, myositis, especially when caused by a streptococcal organism; severe necrotizing pancreatitis). **Rule out hyperthermia due to opioid** **Titrate opioid analgesics to effect**, halt at the early signs of adverse effects. Multi-modal analgesia is essential **Analgesia:** An **NSAIA** (see Table 11.1) where not contraindicated in addition to **fentanyl** 5–10 μg/kg may require higher dosages requiring intubation; or alfentanil or sufentanil Chapter 10 for dosing, or high dose **methadone, oxymorphone** or **hydromorphone** continue with one-quarter effective dose as an hourly CRI Add **ketamine** 1–2+ mg/kg titrated IV followed by 2–4 mg/kg CRI Consider **epidurally placed analgesics or local blocks** (Chapter 14 and chapter of appropriate scenario) If pain is managed appropriately and the cat appears restless, consider addition of **Dexmedetomidine**§ see below **Where indicated, anesthetize** the patient: • **propofol** 2–6 mg/kg, IV **or** • **alfaxalone** 1–3 mg/kg, IV to effect intubation ± ventilation while attempting to find or treat the inciting cause. Remove the inciting cause immediately. **This degree of pain can cause death**
10	**As above (9), but patient emitting piercing screams, thrashing or almost comatose.** The patient is hyperesthetic/hyperalgesic, pain is elicited wherever you touch the patient **Analgesia:** As (9) above Very high doses of opioids do not relieve this pain; however, you must **titrate fentanyl** 10 μg/kg and maintain at 10 μg/kg/h, **or** sufentanil, alfentanil (refer to Chapter 10 for dosing), **or** • **methadone** up to 0.5 mg/kg at least, **or** • **oxymorphone** or **hydromorphone** <0.1 mg/kg • **Add ketamine,** titrate 1–2+ mg/kg followed by 1–2+ mg/kg/h CRI **Lidocaine for infusion**, refer to Chapter 12 for guidelines. Not to be administered if local or epidural analgesia is used This combination of analgesics may result in anesthesia requiring intubation ± assisted ventilation. It may be necessary to anesthetize the patient: • **propofol** 2–6 mg/kg, IV **or** • **alfaxalone** 1–3 mg/kg, IV to effect intubation ± ventilation while attempting to find or treat the inciting cause. Where applicable, remove the inciting cause immediately. **Epidural and/or local analgesia/anesthesia** (Chapter 14) should be considered where indicated **This degree of pain can cause death**

Source: Data adapted from [16]. With permission.

^Morphine may have a slow onset of analgesic action; therefore, fentanyl, methadone, oxymorphone or hydromorphone are preferred if available.

For orthopedic pain, neuropathic pain and pain associated with myositis, fasciitis, burns, etc., an NSAIA (Chapter 11) should be administered where no contraindications for their use are present. If the pain is not being managed, increase analgesic to effect (opioids and ketamine), or add another class. In the author's experience, there have been minimal or no side effects with high-dose opioids when titrated to effect in painful animals while stopping at the onset of side effects. However, for a pain score of > 6, multi-modal analgesia is necessary.

§**Dexmedetomidine** bolus 2 μg/kg IV followed by 0.5–2.0 μg/kg/h CRI may be considered for the **restless patient** appropriately treated for pain. Dexmedetomidine has both analgesic and sedative effects. Only use in otherwise healthy cats. If used prior to induction of general anesthesia, titrate induction agent with one-quarter increments of usual dose.

Neuropathic pain may be associated with a variety of surgical procedures or medical conditions. Gabapentin is a useful adjunctive analgesic for pain associated with neuritis, nerve entrapment secondary to trauma, cervical or thoracolumbar disc disease or post-laminectomy and chronic pain, especially acute on chronic. Gabapentin can be used in combination with opioids and NSAIAs. Post-seizure or CPR vocalization, if relentless, may also be managed with gabapentin. Suggested range in cats is 5–35 mg/kg q12h, for pain. This author starts at 10 mg/kg and increase if no effect seen in 4h. Wean analgesics off slowly; otherwise, the patient will experience worse pain. Reduce in renal insufficiency. Usually the limit of dosing is reached when the animal is sedated. Refer to Chapter 3 for further details on managing pain.

Table 8.7 CATS Suggested analgesia for various levels of ongoing pain in cats. Note: all suggested dosages are based on ideal body weight in the overweight or obese cat. Opioids, ketamine, as a CRI can be combined in IV crystalloid fluids (lactated Ringer's or Ringer's may not be compatible due to calcium content). For Preparation and delivery of analgesics by CRI refer to Chapter 18 for details. Where available, syringe pumps with individual analgesics may also be used. Titrate analgesics to effect.

Severe to excruciating pain
Requires multi-modal analgesia titrated to effect: Opioids alone will not be effective; therefore, careful titration while observing for early signs of adverse effects or worsening of pain (hyperalgesia) and halting titration at this point. An **NSAIA** (see Table 11.1) where not contraindicated **Opioids:** Titrated slowly IV to prior to adverse effects: • **fentanyl** (the author's preference for cats)10 to 15 µg/kg with titrated dose used for hourly CRI, **or** Continue titrated dose of one of the following as a 4 h CRI: • **methadone up to 0.6 mg/kg, or** • **oxymorphone or hydromorphone** <0.1 mg/kg (**suggest titrating up to this dose IV to effect over 1–3 min, caution with hyperthermia**) • Add **Ketamine** 1– 2+ mg/kg combined with the opioid above slowly titrated and followed with a 1–2 mg/kg/h CRI is advised to lower the opioid requirements • **Dexmedetomidine** [§] **see below** It may be impossible to control the pain. Consider anesthetizing the patient **with propofol** 2–6 mg/kg, IV or **alfaxalone** 1–3 mg/kg, IV to effect intubation ± ventilation while attempting to find or treat the inciting cause. Remove the inciting cause immediately where applicable. Consider combining the above analgesics with **epidurally placed analgesics or local neural blockade** (Chapter 14)**This degree of pain can cause death**

Moderate to severe pain		
Select one analgesic from each class		
Analgesic	*Dosing*	*Frequency*
Fentanyl (author's choice), **or**	2–10+ µg/kg IV bolus 2–10+ µg/kg/h	15–20 min CRI
Sufentanil, Alfentanil	Chapter 10 for dosing	
Methadone **or**	0.1–0.5+ mg/kg IM, SC or titrate to effect over 3–5 min if given IV Addition of a sedative may be required Administer intermittently or follow with a CRI with effective dose over 4 h	4 h
Morphine Onset of action is slower than other mu-agonists; therefore, suggest other mu-agonists	0.1–0.2 mg/kg As above for methadone	4 h
Oxymorphone **or** Hydromorphone	0.05–0.1 mg/kg IV, IM, SC Administer intermittently, or follow with a CRI of the effective dose obtained by titration, over the 4 h dosing interval. Hydromorphone may cause hyperthermia, temperature monitoring essential	4 h
#Ketamine combined with an opioid or sedative	0.5–2+ mg/kg titrate bolus IV, SC 0.2–2+ mg/kg/h IV	1 h CRI
Injectable NSAIA* (see Table 11.1)	As per label instructions for contraindications and drug combination warnings Titrate down to lowest effective dose	As per label instructions
Bupivacaine 0.5%	Interpleural and interperitoneal use: as for dogs Table 8.4.	6 h

Table 8.7 (Continued)

Mild to moderate pain		
Opioids above **or**	Lower dosages than above	Titrate to lowest effective dose
Fentanyl patch (only where other opioid modalities not available, preparing for discharge home) **or**	12.5 µg/h	12 h to effect; and may last up to 5 days but unpredictable
Buprenorphine preferred **or**	0.02–0.04 mg/kg IV, IM 0.02–0.04 mg/kg OTM, **or** SC buprenorphine (Simbadol®, Zoetis)	4–8 h 7 h q24h for up to 3 days
Butorphanol	0.1–0.4 mg/kg IV, IM, SC Administer intermittently or follow with a CRI with effective dose over dosing interval	2 h
Meperidine (pethidine) for short duration analgesia or administered at time of NSAIA injection for interim analgesia	5–10 mg/kg IM, SC	20–30 min
NSAIA* (see Table 11.1)	Low dosages As per label instructions for contraindications and drug combination warnings	Titrate down to lowest effective dose As per label instructions
Bupivacaine 0.5%	Interpleural and interperitoneal use: as for dogs Table 8.4.	6 h
Sedatives to combine with opioids		
Midazolam	0.1–0.5 mg/kg IV, IM	Can be > 6 h
Diazepam	0.1–0.5 mg/kg IV	Can be > 6 h
Acepromazine	0.01–0.05 mg/kg IV 0.02–0.1 mg/kg IM, SC	1–2 h 2–6 h
Dexmedetomidine§	0.005–0.020 mg/kg IM, SC, IV 0.001–0.003 mg/kg/h IV	PRN CRI

Source: [15]. With permission

*Review prescribing label information for the individual NSAIA preparations for dosing, duration, contraindications for NSAIA administration and for safety information.** It is not always necessary to administer the recommended loading dose (see Table 11.1), as lower dosages may be effective. It is advised that a dose as low as possible is used to manage the varying degrees of pain to reduce the potential for adverse effects.

§**Dexmedetomidine** has both analgesic and sedative effects. Only use in otherwise healthy cats. If used prior to induction of general anesthesia, titrate induction agent with one-quarter increments of usual dose. The sedative effects outlast the analgesic effects.

#**Ketamine** is not a first line analgesic.

^Morphine may have a slow onset of analgesic action; therefore, fentanyl, methadone, oxymorphone or hydromorphone are preferred if available.

Note: The drugs and dosages given are suggestions. If the pain is not being managed, increase to effect (not NSAIAs). If administered IV, morphine must be administered slowly to prevent hypotension in all animals. Caution in cats due to slow onset of action. Ketamine 0.5–1 mg/kg IV (or 10 mg/kg **per os fractious cat with no IV access**), may be an alternative to control pain quickly if opioids are not available and renal function or hypertrophic cardiomyopathy is not a concern. Ketamine (100 mg/ml) and diazepam (5 mg/ml) or midazolam (5 mg/ml) mixed 1:1 and administered at 0.05–0.15 mL/kg to effect, should also be considered as general anesthesia may be required. Ketamine is renaly excreted in cats; therefore, duration of action may be prolonged in cats with renal dysfunction.

Table 8.8 CATS Adjunctive analgesics suggested dosages for cats based on ideal body weight in the overweight or obese.

Analgesic	Dosage	Route of administration	Duration
Ketamine	0.5–2 mg/kg/h 0.5–2 mg/kg/h	IV	Slow push for control followed by CRI depending on severity of pain
Lidocaine	Refer to Chapter 12		
Gabapentin	5–35 mg/kg (start at 10 mg/kg)	PO	q12h Wean off slowly
Amantadine	3–5 mg/kg	PO	q12–24 h
Amitriptyline	2.5–12.5 mg/cat	PO	q24h

References

1 Reid, J., Scott, M., Nolan, A., *et al.* (2013) Pain assessment in animals. *In Pract*, 35: 1–56.

2 Mathews, K. A., Kronen, P. W., Lascelles, B. D. X., *et al.* (2014) WSAVA Guidelines for Recognition, Assessment and Treatment of Pain. *Assessment and Treatment of Pain in Small Animals*, 55(6): E10–E68.

3 Wang, J., Goffer, Y. and Xu, D. (2011) A single subanesthetic dose of ketamine relieves depression-like behaviors induced by neuropathic pain in rats. *Anesthesiology*, 115(4): 812–821. (See [4] for editorial.)

4 Romero-Sandoval, E. A. (2011) Depression and pain: Does ketamine improve the quality of life of patients in chronic pain by targeting their mood? *Anesthesiology*, 115: 687–688.

5 Chambers, C. T. and Mogil, J. S. (2015) Ontogeny and phylogeny of facial expression of pain. *Pain*, 156: 98–799.

6 Dalla Costa, E., Minero, M., Lebelt, D., *et al.* (2014) Development of the Horse Grimace Scale (HGS) as a pain assessment tool in horses undergoing routine castration. *PLoS One*, 9: e92281.

7 Holden, E., Calvo, G., Collins, M., *et al.* (2014) Evaluation of facial expression in acute pain in cats. *J Small Anim Pract*, 55: 615–621.

8 Grunau, R. V. and Craig, K. D. (1987) Pain expression in neonates: Facial action and cry. *Pain*, 28: 395–410.

9 Liem, E. B., Joiner, T. V., Tsueda, K., *et al.* (2005) Increased sensitivity to thermal pain and reduced subcutaneous lidocaine efficacy in redheads. *Anesthesiology*, 102(3): 509–514.

10 The Glasgow Acute Pain Scale, http://www.newmetrica.com/.

11 Firth, A. M. and Haldane, S. L. (1999) Development of a scale to evaluate postoperative pain in dogs. *J Am Vet Med Assoc*, 214: 651–659.

12 Brondani, J. T., Mama, K. R., Luna, S. P., *et al.* (2013) Validation of the English version of the UNESP-Botucatu multidimensional composite pain scale for assessing postoperative pain in cats. *BioMed Central Veterinary Research*, 17, 9: 143, doi: 10.1186/1746-6148-9-143.

13 13http://csuanimalcancercenter.org/assets/files/csu_acute_pain_scale_canine.pdf.0000

14 Barratt, L. (2013) Feline pain assessment and scoring systems. *The Veterinary Nurse*, 4(8): 470–477.

15 Mathews, K. A. (2000) Pain assessment and general approach to management. *Vet Clin North Am Small Anim*, 30(4): 729–755.

16 Mathews, K. A. (2017) Pain assessment and management in dogs and cats. In Mathews, K. A. (ed.), *Veterinary Emergency & Critical Care Manual*, 3rd edn. LifeLearn, Guelph, Ontario, Canada.

Further Reading

Epstein, M. E., Rodan, I. and Griffenhagen, G. (2015) AAHA/AAFP Pain Management Guidelines for Dogs and Cats. *J Feline Med Surg*, 17: 251–272.

J Pain. A new evidence-based clinical practice guideline that includes 32 recommendations related to post-operative pain management in children and adults has been released by the American Pain Society (APS), 2016, 17: 131–157.

9

Pharmacologic and Clinical Application of Sedatives

Melissa Sinclair

Sedation and analgesia on its own during the initial evaluation of a critical patient is always warranted. Diagnostic tests, wound management and surgery often become necessary once these patients are stabilized, which requires general anesthesia or heavy sedation. Knowledge of specific drug pharmacology, indications and contraindications is imperative especially in this patient population with multiple co-morbidities and painful conditions. The veterinary team requires an understanding of the appropriate sedative analgesic and anesthetic agent for a given patient with underlying diseases and trauma.

Currently available sedatives result in dose-related negative cardiovascular and respiratory depression necessitating knowledge and familiarity of each class of drug and their expected effects. The administration of alpha$_2$ agonists, opioid single boluses or continuous rate infusions (CRIs), lidocaine single bolus or CRIs and local anesthetic techniques will beneficially reduce the amount of the anesthetic agent required. The following outlines the specific pharmacology and techniques for the most commonly used sedative agents. The reader is also referred to the next three chapters for details on opioids and adjunct analgesia, which are frequently combined with sedatives peri-operatively.

Sedation prior to performing a procedure, or before general anesthesia and surgery, is always recommended. Some sedative agents also offer analgesia. However, not all sedatives have analgesic actions. The aim of sedation is to provide pre-emptive analgesia, reduce anxiety of the patient, facilitate handling thereby reducing the chance of injury to personnel, counter the effects of other agents and smooth out the anesthetic induction, endotracheal intubation, maintenance and recovery phases, which is especially beneficial in critically ill or trauma patients.

Evaluation of critical patients on presentation will result in some sort of intervention necessitating sedation and analgesia (catheterization, radiographic positioning of forelimb fracture, abdominal ultrasound positioning of a trauma case, etc.). In many critical cases, the sedation level achieved with the opioid analgesic will be sufficient on its own and so additional sedatives (acepromazine or benzodiazepines) may not be required. When sedatives (acepromazine, benzodiazepines) are required, they are typically combined with an analgesic class of drug (opioid, alpha$_2$ agonist) as indicated for the patient's condition. With the combinations, the overall doses of each are reduced which ultimately may reduce the negative effects of the agent or the duration of any side effects.

Sedative agents may be given by intravenous (IV), intramuscular (IM), subcutaneous (SC) and oral routes based on their pharmacokinetic profiles. In the critical or ill veterinary patient population, an IV catheter will most likely be in place, facilitating IV administration of sedative

Analgesia and Anesthesia for the Ill or Injured Dog and Cat, First Edition. Karol A. Mathews, Melissa Sinclair, Andrea M. Steele and Tamara Grubb.
© 2018 John Wiley & Sons, Inc. Published 2018 by John Wiley & Sons, Inc.

agents, which will aid in using lowered doses of these drugs. An IV access may not be present in some situations on admission and IM or SC administration will be necessary. Certain sedatives (alpha$_2$ agonists) will be more beneficial in aggressive animals until IV access can be established.

I. Acepromazine

A. General Considerations for Use

Acepromazine is a dopamine receptor antagonist that provides sedation, anxiolysis and MAC reduction; however, it is not an analgesic. It exerts its effects by depressing the reticular activating system of the brain. It is warranted in certain critical cases to reduce the stress and anxiety of the patient pre- or post-operatively. It has anti-emetic properties and can reduce the incidence of opioid associated vomiting, but only when administered 20 min prior to the opioid, not when given concurrently. It is Schedule F2 and does not require drug recording.

Acepromazine provides dose-dependent sedation and anxiolysis from 0.01–0.05 mg/kg. However, increasing the dose higher than 0.05 mg/kg is unlikely to increase sedative effects in this patient population, but merely increases the duration of negative side effects. Giant breed dogs require lowered doses of acepromazine. This is in part due to an overdose based on the surface area, and giant breeds appear to be more sensitive to the sedative effects of acepromazine, hence total doses should be reduced regardless of the animal's weight. Even once stabilized a giant breed dog is unlikely to require >1–1.5 mg of acepromazine.

Acepromazine should not be administered until the animal is fully evaluated and stabilized. After evaluation, acepromazine is commonly given with an opioid to improve sedative reliability with lowered acepromazine doses and reduce the incidence, or treat, any dysphoria associated with a pure mu opioid agonist administration. It is commonly used in the post-operative period to minimize dysphoria and excitement. In feline cases, hyperthermia associated with hydromorphone use can be treated or minimized with acepromazine sedation.

While not recommended, if acepromazine is contemplated in the ill or compromised patients for anxiolysis, the doses are generally low (0.01–0.02 mg/kg).

B. Cardio-Respiratory Effects

The main adverse effect of acepromazine is vasodilation from alpha$_1$ receptor antagonism. This results in lowered arterial blood pressures that may produce hypotension, or worsen it, in an unstable, critical patient. The realization of a significant or disastrous hypotension is likely with inhalant anesthesia in a sick animal that has received acepromazine as a sedative, hence acepromazine is typically withheld from this patient population until the recovery phase. Vasodilation also promotes heat loss from the periphery and the development of hypothermia. There is no available antagonist to reverse any negative effects. Treatment is supportive for hypotension and it should be taken into account that the response to sympathomimetics is less effective when acepromazine has been used; therefore, higher supportive doses may be required.

Minimal respiratory depression is encountered; however, where high doses are used in combination with opioid administration, moderate to marked respiratory depression may occur. Monitoring of respiratory function is based on additional medications and co-morbidities of the patient.

C. Contraindications

Acepromazine administration should be withheld if an animal is in shock, weak, dehydrated, severely debilitated, has undergone major trauma to the head or chest or there is evidence of advanced kidney, liver or cardiovascular disease. The true effect of acepromazine on the seizure threshold is still debated in the veterinary literature with most authors suggesting that acepromazine should be withheld if there is a past history of seizures. However, scientific references for this recommended avoidance are lacking. In a situation of trauma and emergency stabilization in a patient with a seizure history prior to referral, acepromazine will be withheld for other hemodynamic reasons. Once stabilized, a stressed or dysphoric patient with a distant seizure history may be given a low dose of acepromazine for sedation if a clear benefit of anxiolysis can be justified. In a previous retrospective study [1], dogs with a previous history of seizures admitted to a veterinary hospital for a secondary condition were administered acepromazine (0.006–0.04 mg/kg) for sedation, anxiolysis or pre-anesthetic medication, and no seizures were noted. In people, the incidence of seizure prevalence for those receiving a psychotropic medication (phenothiazine) has been associated with their underlying disease and dosage of the phenothiazine itself. It is unknown if dosage plays a role in veterinary medicine; however, lowered doses of acepromazine should be used in animals with a history of seizures.

Previous reports of seizing following myelography in dogs with metrizamide contrast agent have been reported and it was speculated that acepromazine increased the incidence of seizures. A retrospective study in dogs pre-medicated with acepromazine methadone or methadone alone, induced with propofol and maintained on isoflurane for a myelogram using iohexol as the contrast agent did not associate the risk of seizures with acepromazine pre-medication [2].

Acepromazine should not be used as the main sedative agent in Boxer dogs, especially if they are critically ill or injured. It has been reported to unmask cardiac problems in Boxers resulting in arrhythmias and hypotension, although these reports are anecdotal without clear scientific evidence or references. Low doses (0.01–0.02 mg/kg) of acepromazine in young healthy Boxers have been utilized; however, the veterinarian should be aware of the potential issues in Boxers.

> **Dose:**
> **Dog or Cat: 0.01–0.05 mg/kg, IV, IM or SC**
> Should not be administered to compromised patients.
> For stable, non-compromised patients, administer after inhalational anesthesia in the recovery and post-operative phase where indicated.

II. Alpha$_2$ Adrenergic Receptor (Alpha$_2$) Agonists

A. General Considerations for Use

The beneficial effects of alpha$_2$ adrenoceptor agonists (alpha$_2$ agonists) include reliable sedation, analgesia, muscle relaxation, anxiolysis, reversibility as well as a decrease in the anesthetic requirements of injectable and inhalant agents. The most commonly used alpha$_2$ agonists in small animals are medetomidine and dexmedetomidine. Currently, dexmedetomidine is marketed for use in cats and dogs. They are not controlled substances. Unfortunately, the negative cardiovascular effects – including bradycardia and associated arrhythmias, hypertension and reduced cardiac output – are a cause for concern related to their use as sedatives or pre-anesthetics in critically ill or compromised patients. These drugs should be avoided in severely compromised patients and those with urinary obstruction due to the increase in urine production. With stability, lowered doses as CRIs may be advantageous to complement analgesia with opioids.

B. Dexmedetomidine

Dexmedetomidine is the active dextro-isomer of the previous medetomidine formulation. The latter contains both the dextro- and levo-isomer forms. Hence doses of dexmedetomidine are half that of medetomidine and should be considered as such throughout in subsequent chapters.

1. Sedation

The dose recommendations on the bottle are based on surface area, while doses below are in μg/kg. In general, higher doses are indicated to achieve sedation in smaller dogs and cats and lower doses for larger dogs. Doses can be given IM or IV, but the animal should be left undisturbed for 15 min for sedation to take effect. When administered IV at larger doses, the initial increase in blood pressure will be more dramatic and the significance of this should be considered on a case-by-case basis.

Decreased doses of dexmedetomidine (compared to the recommended label dose) can be considered in combination with opioid analgesics to enhance sedation and analgesia even in this patient population. It is important to remember that lowered doses will reduce the duration of the negative cardiovascular side effects, but will not prevent them. Hence, these drugs should only be used in cases where the cardiovascular effects are not contraindicated. The aggressive critical patient may require dexmedetomidine sedation to facilitate handling and examination. In these situations, monitoring and availability of the reversal agent is important.

Sedative Dose
Dogs: 1–10 μg/kg
Cats: 5–20 μg/kg
Analgesic Dose
Dogs or cats: CRI: 1–3 μg/kg/h
To be used in combination with an opioid in stable patients, where lower opioid dosages are required (e.g. meningitis), or difficult to manage painful patients.

Urinary catheterization and oxygen supplementation should be considered with prolonged infusions.

2. Anti-Nociception

Anti-nociception with alpha$_2$ agonists likely involves spinal and supra-spinal mechanisms [3]. However, to date the exact defined mechanisms are unclear, although it is clear that, due to the widespread location of alpha$_2$ receptors, their effects could promote analgesia at many levels of the pain pathway. Alpha$_2$ agonists bind to receptors in the substantia gelatinosa, suggesting a direct spinal action. Other effects include inhibiting neurotransmitter release from the primary afferent fibres to second-order neurons, affecting modulation segmentally in the spinal cord, effects on descending modulatory mechanisms from the brainstem or changing ascending modulation to the brain. The analgesic effects are shorter acting than the sedative effects; therefore, sedation should not be assessed as analgesia when single doses are used.

3. Cardio-Respiratory Effects

Hypoventilation occurs with dexmedetomidine sedation in dogs; however, respiratory depression becomes most significant when given in combination with other sedative or injectable agents. Oxygen administration is recommended with heavy sedation when combined with opioids.

The typical negative cardiovascular effects produced with other alpha$_2$ agonists (bradycardia, bradyarrhythmias, reduced cardiac output, hypertension) are also produced with dexmedetomidine limiting its use in sick patients [3].

Sedative doses of dexmedetomidine typically raise the blood pressure in dogs due to the effect on peripheral α_2-adrenoceptors. This spike is most dramatic with IV bolus doses compared to IM administration. In general, hypotension (MAP < 80 mmHg) has not been documented in the research literature to date using medetomidine or dexmedetomidine in veterinary medicine in healthy animals. This increase in blood pressure does not seem as dramatic in cats, but it should still be considered. Anticholinergic pre-medication with alpha$_2$ agonists to prevent bradyarrhythmias does not prevent the reduction in cardiac output produced by these agents and can actually exacerbate it, since the anticholinergic induced increase in heart rate potentiates the alpha$_2$ agonist mediated hypertension and may increase myocardial oxygen tension, demand and workload, affecting the cardiac output, and is likely to be more significant in a geriatric or compromised patient. Overall, reversal with the specific antagonist atipamezole is recommended when significant cardiorespiratory complications occur.

4. Other Effects

Other physiologic effects of dexmedetomidine administration include vomiting, increased urine volumes, changes to endocrine function and uterine activity, decreased intestinal motility, decreased intra-ocular pressure and potentially hypothermia. Dexmedetomidine reduces endogenous insulin release resulting in a transient hyperglycemia. Use of these agents should be avoided in diabetic patients. Despite the reduction in cardiac output, dexmedetomidine has not been found to reduce liver blood flow in dogs, however its use should be based on the animals overall condition. Due to the potential to induce vomiting, dexmedetomidine should be avoided if vomiting is a concern (noted in the various case scenarios throughout this book). Dexmedetomidine and medetomidine are contraindicated in cases with a urinary obstruction.

Veins and arteries may become more difficult to access in animals sedated with dexmedetomidine due to peripheral vasoconstriction. Monitoring with pulse-oximetry or oscillometric blood pressure devices may be unsuccessful due to vasoconstriction and bradyarrhythmias. The Doppler signal will sound faint initially due to the initial hypertension.

5. Reversal

Dexmedetomidine sedation and analgesia are rapidly reversed with atipamezole. Prior to reversal, analgesia should be supplemented with an alternative agent.

Atipamezole is licensed for IM administration only and recoveries from sedation with IM doses are typically smooth. Full reversal with atipamezole IV boluses may result in rapid arousal and excitement, and should not be performed unless it is an emergency. An equal volume of atipamezole as the sedative volume of dexmedetomidine should be administered IV in any emergency situation. Bradycardia and bradyarrhythmias can also be reversed with lowered volumes of atipamezole compared to the sedative volume of dexmedetomidine, mixed in saline; however, note that the sedative and analgesic effects will also be reversed.

Dose

Emergency

Equal volume of atipamezole (5 mg/mL) to sedative volume of dexmedetomidine (0.5 mg/mL)

This equates to 10 times the dose of dexmedetomidine used

Partial reversal: 5–20 μg/kg, IV to effect

This atipamezole dose can be mixed with saline and administered slowly IV, 0.5 mL/min, to offset bradycardia, bradyarrhythmias and dramatic increases in arterial blood pressure.

Attention to anesthetic depth is imperative.

III. Benzodiazepines

A. General Considerations for Use

Diazepam and midazolam are most commonly used as sedatives or as co-induction agents in small animal practice. In people, benzodiazepines cause greater sedation or even unconsciousness as a sole agent. However, they are not always good sedatives in healthy or young cats and dogs and even have the potential to cause excitement. Sedation may be more likely in geriatric or sick animals. Excitement may appear to be due to disinhibition when given as the sole sedative agent in healthy cats or dogs. Due to this potential, benzodiazepines are commonly administered with another sedative, such as an opioid in sick patients, to reduce the risk of excitement. It is recommended that benzodiazepines not be administered to patients with severe liver dysfunction, with or without hepatic encephalopathy. Where hepatic function is questionable, flumazenil should be available for reversal if needed.

1. Sedation

Benzodiazepines exert sedation through depression of the limbic system and interaction with the GABA receptor complex, which is the major inhibitory neurotransmitter system in the CNS. Both diazepam and midazolam can be used IV. Midazolam has the benefit of being water-soluble allowing IM injection without pain and irritation. Diazepam is insoluble in water, is usually prepared with propylene glycol, which may cause pain on IV injection, and makes IM injection painful with unpredictable absorption. Both are metabolized in the liver. Metabolites with midazolam are inactive, but diazepam has active metabolite formation. Both are reversible with flumazenil if sedative effects are slow to wane, or in patients suspected of liver disease after administration.

Dose
Cat or Dog
Diazepam: 0.1–0.4 mg/kg, IV
Midazolam: 0.1–0.5 mg/kg, IV, IM

2. Cardio-Respiratory Effects

In critically ill or compromised patients, the main benefit of using a benzodiazepine as a sedative is that they have minimal to no negative cardio-respiratory effects. This makes them ideal as pre-medicants or as co-induction agents in cardiovascular compromised animals.

B. Co-Induction with Injectable Anesthetics

Benzodiazepines can be administered as part of the induction phase with propofol or alfaxalone versus the sedative phase. The main reasons for using a co-induction agent with an injectable anesthetic agent are to smooth the overall induction process enabling endotracheal intubation without swallowing or coughing, minimize the negative side effects of propofol or alfaxalone (cardiovascular and respiratory), minimize the dose of injectable drug administered and thereby lower the overall cost and promote a smoother transfer to the maintenance phase of anesthesia. The main advantage of using the different types of drugs together during the induction of anesthesia in cardiovascular compromised or critical patients is the lowered dose of the primary anesthetic induction agent (propofol or alfaxalone) and enhanced cardio-respiratory stability, muscle relaxation and ease of endotracheal intubation.

Dose

Cat or Dog

Diazepam: 0.1–0.4 mg/kg, IV

Midazolam: 0.1–0.5 mg/kg, IV

Midazolam shows the most consistent injectable dose reduction, typically at a bolus dose of 0.2–0.4 mg/kg, IV for co-induction administered after the initial bolus of propofol or alfaxalone.

Diazepam has less consistent results especially at higher doses or when administered prior to the initial injectable bolus dose of propofol or alfaxalone.

However, either benzodiazepine can be used as a co-induction agent.

1. Reversal

Both are benzodiazepines are reversible with flumazenil. The dose is 0.01–0.03 mg/kg, IV for flumazenil. It is generally recommended to reverse slowly to prevent excitement and remove only to the level of awareness optimal for the patient. A 0.01 or 0.02 mg/kg dose can be diluted in 3–6 mL of saline, giving 0.25–0.5 mL/min, IV until the desired effect is achieved.

References

1 Tobias, K. M., Marioni-Henry, K. and Wagner, R. (2006) A retrospective study on the use of acepromazine maleate in dogs with seizures. *J Am An Hosp Assoc*, 42: 283–289.
2 Drynan, E. A., Gray, P. and Raisis, A. L. (2012) Incidence of seizures associated with the use of acepromazine in dogs undergoing myelography. *J Vet Emerg Crit Care*, 22(2): 262–266.
3 Murell, J. C. and Hellebrekers, L. J. (2005) Medetomidine and dexmedetomidine: A review of cardiovascular effects and antinociceptive properties in the dog. *Vet Anaesth Analg*, 32: 117–127.

10

Pharmacologic and Clinical Application of Opioid Analgesics
Melissa Sinclair

Analgesia on its own during the initial evaluation of a critical patient is always warranted. Diagnostic tests, wound management and surgery often become necessary once these patients are stabilized, which requires general anesthesia or heavy sedation. Knowledge of specific drug pharmacology, indications and contraindications is imperative, especially in this patient population with multiple co-morbidities and painful conditions. The veterinary team requires an understanding of the appropriate anesthetic and analgesic agent for a given patient with underlying diseases and trauma.

Currently available sedatives and analgesics result in dose-related negative cardiovascular and respiratory depression necessitating knowledge and familiarity of each class of drug and expected effects. The administration of alpha₂ agonists, opioid single boluses or continuous rate infusions (CRIs), lidocaine single bolus or CRIs, and local anesthetic techniques, will beneficially reduce the amount of the anesthetic agent required. The following outlines the specific pharmacology and techniques for the most commonly used opioid analgesic agents, which are also applied to anesthetic procedures. The reader is also referred to Chapter 9 (application of sedatives), Chapter 12 (adjunct analgesia) and Chapter 13 (general anesthetics).

I. Opioid General Considerations

Opioid receptors (mu, kappa, delta) are present in many tissues and their distribution and proportions vary according to the tissue and species. The mu and delta opioid receptors gate potassium ions hyperpolarizing the cell membrane, making it resistant to excitation, whereas the kappa opioid receptor blocks calcium flux across the cell membrane, thereby decreasing neurotransmitter release [1, 2].

In general, opioid receptors are located in the nervous system and peripheral organs; therefore, their actions impact the brain, spinal cord, heart, lungs, gastrointestinal system, liver, musculoskeletal and reproductive organs. Of interest for this review are the actions of opioids as anti-nociceptive (analgesic) and sedative drugs, as well as their associated adverse effects on different organs [3].

A. Sedation

Sedation from opioids is believed to be the result of disrupted sleep patterns by decreasing REM sleep, in both animals and humans. In this state, arousal mechanisms and content

Analgesia and Anesthesia for the Ill or Injured Dog and Cat, First Edition. Karol A. Mathews, Melissa Sinclair, Andrea M. Steele and Tamara Grubb.
© 2018 John Wiley & Sons, Inc. Published 2018 by John Wiley & Sons, Inc.

processing are functional but attenuated, which affects the level of consciousness, making the patient drowsy and less aware of their environment [4].

The sedative effects of opioids can be disassociated from their anti-nociceptive effects; anti-nociception can be achieved with lower doses than those inducing sedation, which is important because of the likelihood of excitatory and dysphoric effects associated with higher doses of opioids in some animal species; therefore, analgesia is possible without the need for higher doses that can transition from sedation to adverse excitatory effects.

B. Anti-Nociception

Anti-nociception from endogenous and exogenous opioids can be achieved by three mechanisms, which are interlinked from periphery to the brain [1]. In the periphery, opioids depress pre-synaptic and post-synaptic membrane potentials from nociceptive fibres. At the spinal cord level, opioid receptors are present in high concentrations in lamina I and II of the dorsal horn, where opioids directly inhibit the firing of nociceptive signals to the brain from dorsal horn neurons. Lastly, in the brain stem, opioids activate descending pain modulatory pathways that originate within neurons of the periaqueductal gray matter and that project to the nucleus raphe magnus located in the medulla, which in turn sends projections to the spinal cord inhibiting dorsal horn neurons in lamina I, II and V.

The binding of opioids to their receptors inhibits the release of Substance-P (S-P) from C nociceptive fibres and to a lesser extent A-delta fibres, which prevents signalling from these fibres to the brain. Nociceptive C fibres are slow conducting and their activation results in dull, burning or aching pain, which is the type of pain experienced with inflammation and post-surgical; therefore, opioids are very effective against this type of pain. A-delta fibres are responsible for fast pricking or sharp pain, which is the type of pain experienced during surgery; therefore, opioids are not completely effective against surgical pain, but they play an important role in exerting inhibitory mechanisms that modulate dorsal horn neuronal excitability after repetitive noxious inputs, preventing the development of spinal neuronal sensitization (windup) [5].

Most of the opioids used in veterinary medicine are targeted at mu-receptors and include morphine, hydromorphone, oxymorphone, fentanyl, meperidine, methadone, remifentanil and buprenorphine. Buprenorphine is the only one that is not a full mu-receptor agonist (partial mu-agonist); therefore, maximum efficacy, such as anti-nociception, is not achieved with this opioid, but it can still be considered adequate for conditions where pain is not severe and that is compatible with the mechanism of action of the opioid (C fibre) [6]. It is essential that pain be appropriately assessed, because increasing the dose of buprenorphine above that recommended will not improve analgesia. Should a pure mu-agonist be required, it will be very difficult to overcome the buprenorphine bound to the mu-receptors. Therefore, the clinician should decide if buprenorphine would be acceptable for pain control; if this is questionable, a full mu-agonist should be chosen instead.

The rest of the mu-agonists are full agonists and maximum efficacy is achieved from their actions as long as the type of pain treated is compatible with the mechanism of action of the opioid. Butorphanol is also commonly used and is a kappa-receptor agonist and mu-receptor antagonist, so it may interfere with the actions of other opioids that are mu-receptor agonists when administered close together. The kappa-receptor actions also confer anti-nociception, but in general mu-receptor agonists are considered better analgesics. There are no delta-specific opioid agonists in use in veterinary medicine.

The anti-nociceptive and sedative effects of opioids contribute to a sparing effect of inhalational anesthetics when they are used as part of the pre-medication or when given intraoperatively. This allows for a reduction in the minimum alveolar concentration of inhalants necessary for adequate anesthetic depth, which can result in better cardio-respiratory function under anesthesia. Mu-agonist opioids have more profound sparing effects than kappa-agonists or partial mu-agonists.

C. Cardiovascular

In regards to cardiovascular effects, most opioids exert a dose-dependent bradycardia from enhanced parasympathetic tone. The exception is meperidine, which can maintain or increase heart rate through an atropine-like effect.

Bradycardia should be treated if it compromises blood pressure and/or cardiac output. This occurs more frequently in the anesthetized patient, where autonomic responses are blunted by inhalant and other injectable anesthetics. In the sedated patient, bradycardia is usually not accompanied by impaired cardiovascular function as occurs under general anesthesia. Anticholinergics, such as atropine (0.02–0.04 mg/kg) or glycopyrrolate (0.005–0.01 mg/kg), intravenously (IV) or intramuscularly (IM), may be used pre-emptively or as treatment to counteract the bradycardia.

Some opioids, such as fentanyl or remifentanil, can increase vascular resistance slightly and blood pressure, but the slower heart rate results in a concomitant decrease in cardiac output that eventually can lead to lower blood pressures, despite preservation of cardiac contractility. Other opioids, such as morphine and meperidine, can elicit the release of histamine resulting in vasodilation and subsequent to hypotension, especially if administered IV and rapidly. Meperidine is associated with profound hypotension when administered IV and, therefore, is not recommended via this route. However, morphine can be given slowly IV to minimize the transient hypotension.

D. Respiratory

Respiratory adverse effects of opioids are dose-dependent but are less profound in animals than people [7]. However, this adverse effect is not clinically relevant if opioids are administered within the dose range and the patient is healthy. More so, the presence of pain can reverse opioid-induced respiratory depression through stimulation of breathing, since respiration is also mediated through S-P and NK-1 receptors in the respiratory centre and central chemoreceptors, as well as peripheral chemoreceptors; however, if multi-modal analgesia is used, the balance between pain and breathing can be altered and respiratory depression ensue. GABA agonists – such as benzodiazepines, propofol and inhalant anesthetics – can have additive or synergistic effects with opioids and enhance their effects on respiratory depression.

The respiratory rate can decrease with high or cumulative doses and apnoea is uncommon unless the patient is critically ill. Panting is observed frequently after sedative doses in dogs, and because of dead space ventilation it does not necessarily result in hypocapnia but hypercapnia. More frequently, regardless of the breathing pattern that results from opioid administration, PaO_2 values remain within acceptable levels and $PaCO_2$ increases slightly in healthy patients. Noteworthy is that under general anesthesia, the influence of opioids upon the respiratory depression caused by inhalant anesthetics can be additive and therefore close monitoring is recommended.

E. Antitussive

Opioids have antitussive effects, which are the result of actions on receptors within the central nervous system (CNS) and in some degree to peripheral receptors [8]. The central action is associated with mu-receptors in the nucleus tractus solitarius (NTS), considered the cough centre due to the sensory input from the lower airway and its stimulation causing cough-like responses. In the NTS, mu-receptors are more abundant than kappa-receptors, although stimulation of both receptors is believed to have antitussive effects. Peripheral actions are associated with mu-receptors located in the airway vagal sensory neurons, where inhaled opioids have been shown to inhibit tachykinergic transmission of excitatory non-adrenergic non-cholinergic nerves and cholinergic contraction of smooth muscle.

This antitussive action is beneficial when coughing during endotracheal intubation or extubation is to be avoided (e.g. patients with increased intracranial or intraocular pressure).

F.   Vomiting

Vomiting is the result of opioid stimulation of the chemoreceptor trigger zone (CTZ), which is a structure partially outside the blood–brain barrier and under the control of the vomiting centre within the blood–brain barrier. If opioids reach the CTZ before the vomiting centre, vomiting occurs, whereas if opioids reach the vomiting centre first, there is an inhibitory action on the CTZ. Therefore, opioids that are lipid soluble have the ability to penetrate the blood–brain barrier and inhibit their own emetic actions on the CTZ; these include fentanyl, remifentanil, meperidine, buprenorphine, butorphanol and to a lesser degree methadone and oxymorphone. Non-lipid soluble opioids, which include morphine and hydromorphone, cause vomiting frequently because of their difficulty in reaching the vomiting centre and the ease with which they reach the CTZ.

G.   Dysphoria

Dysphoria consists of CNS behavioural excitatory changes that include vocalization, unawareness and lack of interaction with the surroundings. These signs are more common in patients overdosed with opioids or administered recommended high-end doses without concomitant use of tranquilizers or sedatives when analgesia is not required. In the recovery period from anesthesia, it can be confused with emergence delirium, and it is important to differentiate them to dispense proper treatment. Dysphoric animals remain unaware of the surroundings for a longer time than a patient in delirium; the latter tends to settle with time and become more interactive with the surrounding. A dysphoric animal will respond to reversal of the opioid with naloxone, whereas pain recurrence is of concern in a patient in delirium that has its analgesic effects reversed. If in doubt, it is best to titrate the dose of naloxone over time to recognize which condition is present in the patient and to be able to reverse the excitement without completely reversing the analgesia (see Section I.K.1). In dogs overdosed with opioids, pupil size tends to be decreased (miosis), whereas in cats it increases (mydriasis); however, the effects of other anesthetic drugs on pupil size (ketamine, anticholinergics) needs to be considered. An alternative treatment that benefits both conditions is to administer a tranquilizer, such as acepromazine, to counteract either excitatory condition.

H.   Increased Sphincter Tone and Constipation

Mu-agonists can increase sphincter tone and decrease gastrointestinal propulsion, which promotes fluid absorption from the gastrointestinal tract and results in constipation. These effects are mediated centrally and peripherally, via mu-receptors, and therefore can result from systemic and spinal administration [9]. Constipation is not common from a single administration of mu-agonists but should be considered as a potential serious adverse effect in patients receiving chronic administration of opioids. This tends to be more of a problem in humans than animals. The use of laxatives and gastrointestinal stimulants should be considered in these situations.

I. Urinary Retention

Mu-agonists may cause detrusor atony and increased sphincter tone, resulting in urinary retention. This may occur in any patient receiving epidural opioids or higher opioid dosages during and after anesthesia/surgery. Bladder assessment where no urinary catheter is in place is essential as the discomfort associated with this can be interpreted as pain resulting in an increase in opioid dosing. Careful naloxone titration can reverse this. Refer to Chapter 3 for details on neuropathic pain management, especially for the patient with spinal trauma.

J. Hyperthermia

Mu-receptor activation can result in hyperthermia in laboratory rodents and clinically in cats, but it is not seen in dogs. In cats hyperthermia has been associated with the use of hydromorphone, morphine and buprenorphine, and even with butorphanol (kappa-agonist) [10]. Conversely, kappa-receptor activation is associated with hypothermia in laboratory rodents. The hyperthermia is usually self-limiting but can make patients uncomfortable, and cooling management may be necessary in some cases. Without adequate assessment, the behaviour may be mistaken for pain, so monitoring temperature in cats is essential prior to repeating the opioid.

K. Reversal of Opioids

Opioids are effectively reversed with naloxone, which is a full antagonist to mu-, kappa- and delta-agonists. Other reversal drugs are available but less commonly used than naloxone and include naltrexone, which is also a full antagonist at the three receptors; nalbuphine, a mixed agonist-antagonist that acts as a mu-antagonist and kappa-agonist; and butorphanol, also a mixed agonist-antagonist that can antagonize mu-agonists and acts as a kappa-agonist.

Reversal is most commonly used in human anesthesia to counteract excessive respiratory depression; however, in veterinary medicine it is also used to counteract dysphoria, nausea and vomiting, excessive persistent panting, hyperthermia and (rarely) constipation in dogs and cats. The major uses are to shorten the duration of action of opioids in animals that have been sedated for diagnostic procedures, and for dysphoria in animals that have received a dose of opioids in excess of their requirements for analgesia or for sedation without a concomitant tranquilizer (acepromazine) or sedative drug (dexmedetomidine).

Naloxone is effective at reversal of both opioid agonists and agonist/antagonist drugs by competitive inhibition at the three different receptor types. Full or partial reversal is possible, which is achieved by titration of naloxone (see point 1 below), which is useful for eliminating adverse effects while preserving analgesia, since sedation and dysphoria require higher doses of the agonist than anti-nociception. Remifentanil is unlikely to require reversal, which is an advantage.

1. Naloxone

The recommended dose (lower volumes of naloxone, and saline for cats and small dogs) and mode of administration of naloxone involves dilution of 0.1–0.25 mL of 0.4 mg/mL of naloxone in 5–10 mL of saline and slowly titrating to effect by IV administration of volumes of 0.5–1.0 mL each minute until the adverse effect (respiratory depression, excessive sedation, panting, nausea or dysphoric behaviour) begins to subside and then discontinue administration. Because the duration of action of naloxone is shorter (60 min) than the opioid, it may be necessary to repeat the naloxone administration if adverse signs reappear; however, this is rarely required.

Buprenorphine reversal usually requires higher doses of naloxone because of its high affinity for the mu-receptor. Reversal of butorphanol's kappa-agonist effects may also require higher doses of naloxone. Previously, reversal of mu-agonists with butorphanol, by titrating to effect increments of 0.1 mg/kg every 2–5 min until the undesired effect is eliminated, or for up to four doses, was suggested; however, this is not recommended as this may/does compound the problem in many instances.

Careful and correct administration of naloxone with slow administration and monitoring is important to prevent complete withdrawal of analgesia. By this method an ideal state of analgesia will be maintained. Overdosing, such as occurs with bolus administration of naloxone to a painful patient, may result in hyperalgesia with subsequent restlessness, pain, nausea, diarrhoea, tachycardia, vasoconstriction, hypertension and even flash pulmonary oedema.

II. Mu-Agonists

All mu-agonists are schedule N drugs (narcotics), for which records of administration must be kept due to the higher potential for abuse and dependence (US Schedule II, Canada Schedule I).

Potency is related to dose. The more potent the opioid is compared to morphine, the lower the dose required to induce the effect. Potency of opioid analgesics when compared to morphine is given in Table 10.1.

A. Morphine

Morphine is the opioid to which other opioids are compared. It is a hydro-soluble opioid that, because of this property, provides prolonged analgesia (12–24 h) when administered by the epidural route, due to entrapment in the cerebrospinal fluid and contact with the spinal cord opioid receptors once it traverses the arachnoid membrane. Because of its low solubility, a low dose is administered epidurally when compared to parenteral doses. The hydro-soluble property impairs its passage through the blood–brain barrier when administered parenterally (IM, IV, subcutaneously (SC)) and favours stimulation of the CTZ frequently resulting in vomiting (75%). Oral liquid and sustained release formulations of morphine are not effective in cats and dogs.

Morphine is used for sedation and analgesia of 3–4 h duration in conditions where moderate or severe pain is present. IV administration should be slow and cautious as bolus administration can result in 5–10 min periods of lowered blood pressure even in healthy animals due to histamine release and vasodilation; therefore, blood pressure monitoring is recommended if given IV. Ill or compromised patients are more likely to have more severe and lasting hypotension from IV dosing of morphine. Due to this, a main disadvantage of morphine is the inability to give it rapidly IV in seconds as a rescue analgesic in patients experiencing extreme pain. However, it may be given over 1–5 min IV if it is the only opioid available.

Table 10.1 Potency of opioid analgesics compared with morphine.

Morphine	Oxymorphone	Hydromorphone	Fentanyl	Remifentanil	Meperidine	Tramadol	Methadone	Butorphanol	Buprenorphine
1	7–10	5	50–100	100–200	1/5	1/10	1–2	5–6	40

Morphine, by parenteral or epidural administration, can result in a sparing effect of inhalant anesthetics (decreased minimum alveolar concentration, or MAC). Morphine is metabolized in the liver. The two main metabolites of morphine are morphine-3-glucuronide (M3G) and morphine-6-glucuronide (M6G). Only M6G gives analgesia, while M3G contributes to side effects and tolerance. In cats, the analgesia from morphine is less predictable due to deficient glucuronidation and less biotransformation to the active analgesic metabolite M6G and some cats may not benefit from morphine administration.

Morphine had initial reports of causing constriction of the sphincter of Oddi, leading to spasm of the common bile duct [11]. This has led to the recommendation of avoiding morphine in cases with hepatobiliary disease; however, there is no clear evidence in veterinary patients of this occurrence. In general, with cholecystitis, it is advisable to avoid morphine; however, in cases without hepatobiliary disease morphine may be used if it is the only opioid available for analgesia.

Dose

Dogs: 0.3–0.5 mg/kg IM, SC (higher dose for restraint)

Cats: 0.1–0.2 mg/kg IM, SC

CRI

Loading dose: 0.3–0.5 mg/kg, IM or slow IV to effect (another mu-agonist can also be used for loading dose)

Infusion rate: 0.1–0.4 mg/kg/h, IV (can be added to the hourly fluids) for mild, moderate and severe pain. Or, the effective IV dose can be used as a 4 h infusion (1/4 of the effective loading dose/h)

Epidural use

0.1 mg/kg

B. Hydromorphone

Similar to morphine, hydromorphone is hydro-soluble and shares most of the properties in regards to prolonged epidural analgesia (12–16 h), activation of the CTZ and vomiting (50%). Because of its low solubility, a dose lower than the parenteral dose can be administered epidurally.

Hydromorphone is used for sedation and analgesia of 3–4 h duration in conditions where moderate or severe pain is present. Unlike morphine, the release of histamine from hydromorphone is less and hypotension is uncommon after IV bolus administration. Hyperthermia in cats has been more commonly reported with hydromorphone, and hence doses lower than 0.1 mg/kg are recommended with less frequent dosing (>6 h), unless extreme pain exists. Combining hydromorphone with a sedative, such as acepromazine, will minimize hyperthermia in cats.

Dose

Dogs: 0.03–0.1+ mg/kg IM, IV, SC (higher dose may be required for restraint). For larger dogs (>25 kg) 0.05 mg/kg is considered a higher end dose, gives adequate sedation and may result in less dysphoria upon recovery after shorter procedures. A maximum dose of 3 mg should be sufficient in giant breed dogs (>60 kg) for pre-medication; however, analgesia requirements should be monitored when administered in intermittent boluses in animals with more severe pain. In toy breed dogs, 0.1 mg/kg hydromorphone results in pleasant sedation with less dysphoria. Where IV access is available, it is recommended to titrate slowly to effect to avoid adverse effects due to an overestimation of pain, resulting in "overdose" of the opioid.

Cats: 0.05–0.1 mg/kg IM, IV, SC.

CRI

Loading dose: 0.03–0.1 mg/kg IM, or preferred, titrated to effect IV (another mu-agonist can also be used for loading dose).

Infusion rate: 0.01–0.02 mg/kg/h, IV (can be added to the hourly fluids) for mild, moderate and severe pain. Or, an hourly rate may be based on the loading dose required to achieve a comfortable analgesic state. Assuming the loading dose will last 4 h, administer one-quarter of this per hour.

Epidural use

0.02 mg/kg

C. Oxymorphone

Oxymorphone is used for sedation and analgesia of 3–4 h duration in conditions where moderate or severe pain is present. Histamine release is of no concern after IV bolus administration. Dysphoria can be noted after higher end dosing or too frequent administration of analgesic doses.

Oxymorphone is less hydro-soluble, and more lipid soluble, than either morphine or hydromorphone, but it is still associated with some vomiting (<30%) after parenteral administration. Epidural administration results in a 6–10 h duration of analgesia, which is less than the hydro-soluble opioids. Hence, when administered epidurally, oxymorphone requires a similar dose to that administered parenterally.

The main disadvantage of oxymorphone is the relatively higher cost in most areas of North America compared to similar effective analgesics, such as morphine, hydromorphone or methadone.

Dose

Dogs: 0.02–0.2 mg/kg IM, IV, SC (higher dose for restraint). Similar to hydromorphone, a dose of 0.05 mg/kg is a sufficient starting dose in larger dogs, with a maximum of 3 mg initially in giant breed dogs (>60 kg). In toy dogs, 0.1 mg/kg is recommended

Cats: 0.05–0.1 mg/kg IM, IV, SC

CRI

Loading dose: 0.02–0.1 mg/kg IM, or preferred, titrated to effect IV (another mu-agonist can also be used for loading dose)

Infusion rate: 0.01–0.02 mg/kg/h, IV (can be added to the hourly fluids) for mild, moderate and severe pain. Or, as with hydromorphone, one-quarter of the loading dose/h may be more accurate for the individual patient

Epidural use

0.1 mg/kg

D. Fentanyl

Fentanyl is a synthetic mu-agonist of rapid onset and short duration. Its use as an adjunct in general anesthesia results in a significant inhalant (MAC) sparing effect, which is facilitated by its pharmacokinetic properties that facilitate rapid plasma concentrations when used as a CRI. Fentanyl does not cause vomiting when given intravenously because its high lipid solubility facilitates rapid access to the inhibitory zone of the vomiting centre blocking the CTZ emetic action. This is an advantage in cases where vomiting must be prevented (increased intracranial or intraocular pressure).

Fentanyl is metabolized in the liver mainly to norfentanyl, which is inactive, but the pharmacokinetics of fentanyl appear to be marginally impacted by liver disease, hence reversal with naloxone may be required in liver disease patients if side effects are encountered.

Low doses of this opioid (<5 µg/kg, IV) result in short duration of analgesic effects (<30 min) because of rapid lowering of the plasma therapeutic analgesic concentrations, but higher doses can prolong the analgesia to >1 h with a single bolus. Bradycardia or associated bradyarrhythmias (sinus arrhythmia and/or first- and second-degree atrioventricular heart block) can be observed in dogs after IV bolus administration, and is likely with higher doses (>5 μg/kg, IV). To avoid adverse effects from higher intermittent single doses, titrate the initial dose to effect and continue with this dose as an hourly CRI.

Epidural use of fentanyl offers no advantage over parenteral use, except for a more specific spinal action, but the duration of analgesia is usually < 1 h. So it is not used frequently in veterinary medicine for long-term analgesia by the epidural route. Systemic administration is more typical. CRIs are generally reserved for use during anesthetic management or moderate to severe post-operative or medical pain either alone or in a multi-modal regimen.

Because of its lipo-solubility and pharmacokinetic properties, fentanyl can be administered via a transdermal patch, which facilitates a slow and continuous release of fentanyl for systemic analgesia. Fentanyl transdermal patches may not always result in consistent therapeutic levels in the individual animal as the epidermal structure differs from humans. Therapeutic blood levels are not reached prior to 24 h in most patients, and sometimes longer. Frequent pain assessment is essential as systemic analgesia is required, with gradual reduction as transdermal blood levels rise.

Dose
Dogs: 3–10 μg/kg IM, IV, SC (higher dose for restraint)
Cats: 3–10 μg/kg IM, IV, SC (higher dose for restraint)
CRI
Loading dose: 3–10 μg/kg IM, SC or (preferred) titrated IV to effect (another mu-agonist can also be used for loading dose)

Infusion rate: 5–15 μg/kg/h IV (can be added to the hourly fluids) for mild, moderate and severe pain. Or, take the effective titrated loading dose and administer as an hourly CRI to meet the individual's analgesic requirements
Fentanyl transdermal patches in 25, 50, 75 and 100 μg/h dosage
Patches can be used alone or with supplemental analgesia, and can provide three days, rarely five days, of analgesia when optimal plasma levels are attained. Application of fentanyl patches just prior to general anesthesia and surgery should not be relied upon as an analgesic. Systemic administration will be necessary. It is recommended to place fentanyl patches after general anesthesia and surgical recovery.

Therapeutic plasma concentrations are achieved with a 75 and 100 μg/h patch in dogs ~20 kg but requires 12–24 h to reach therapeutic levels. More importantly, great individual animal variability has been noted with many not able to reach therapeutic levels and so remain in pain. The fentanyl patch, therefore, may be a poor choice for cats and dogs due to the difference in epidermis from humans resulting in inconsistent absorption of fentanyl. Smaller animals require the smaller size patch (25 μg/h patch resulting in approximately 4 μg/kg/h). Cats achieve analgesia in 6–12 h with the 25 μg/h patch. If a low dose is required, only part of the seal can be removed and exposed to the skin. **Do not cut** the patch itself. Place the patch between, and on the cranial aspect of, the scapulae to avoid the potential of the patch lying on a warm area (e.g. heating pad) as there will be increased absorption and subsequent overdose. The patch can be removed at any time adverse effects are noted and the reversal is generally fairly rapid (2–3 h). The skin requires shaving but not cleaning unless seborrhoea is noted. However, once cleaned with warm water, the skin should be allowed to dry prior to patch application. No other solutions should be used. Skin that has abrasions or openings will have enhanced absorption. Mild contact dermatitis may occur in around 50% of patients and resolves in 24 h after patch removal.
Transdermal (Recuvyra®, Elanco)
Designed for a **single** transdermal dose lasting for 72 h; has been discontinued. It is not known whether this will be reinstated.

E.   Sufentanil/Alfentanil/Remifentanil

These drugs are derivatives of fentanyl. All are short-acting opioids and hence require administration as a CRI. The main disadvantage of these drugs is cost. Remifentanil is the newer fentanyl derivative and has the fastest titratability and rapid offset of this group due to its pharmaco-dynamic characteristics. It has the fastest recovery in people, regardless of high dose or duration of the CRI. While remifentanil's anti-nociceptive effects are useful in anesthetized patients due to rapid plasma concentrations without a loading dose, and without accumulation in tissues or blood from a CRI, regardless of the duration of infusion, this also means that this drug confers no analgesic effects once it is discontinued. In fact, it has been reported in humans that tolerance and hyperalgesia have been noted even with short-term infusions of remifentanil [12]. This is supported by studies on animal models, human volunteers and clinical studies [13]. A systematic review of human studies showed an association between intraoperative remifentanil use and increased post-operative pain intensity at rest, and also higher morphine consumption in the first 24 h after surgery. Remifentanil was also associated with measurable hyperalgesia as assessed by a decreased nociceptive threshold [13]. Where remifentanil is used intraoperatively, it is essential to administer a different opioid, or different class of analgesic, post-operatively along with careful assessment of pain. To date, no veterinary studies have reported this; however, in the post-operative setting the pain assessed may be interpreted as that associated with the procedure and not remifentanil use. Until studies investigating this are performed, the authors of this book advise against remifentanil administration.

The main advantages of these drugs are a rapid onset of action; remifentanil has a very rapid onset of 1–2 min, compared to fentanyl of 4–6 min; a loading dose is not essential to achieve remifentanil's steady-state concentrations; and the context-sensitive half-life (the time necessary to achieve a 50% decrease in blood or plasma) is only 3 min, independent of infusion duration.

Remifentanil is 100–200 times more potent than morphine, and approximately twice as potent as fentanyl; however, due to the establishment of hyperalgesia as the analgesic effects wear off, it is not recommended for use. Doses listed below are for completeness. Sufentanil is 5–7 times more potent than fentanyl, 3–4 times more potent than remifentanil and 500–1000 times more potent than morphine, while alfentanil is 10–20 times more potent than morphine, 15–30 times less potent than remifentanil and 5–10 times less potent than fentanyl. Both sufentanil and alfentanil have similar effects and metabolism to fentanyl. Remifentanil is metabolized by non-specific tissue and plasma esterases to non-toxic, inactive metabolites, which makes it useful for patients with liver or renal failure.

Dose
Sufentanil: Loading dose: 0.2–0.5 µg/kg, IV
CRI: 0.3–0.6 µg/kg/h, IV
Alfentanil: Loading dose: 20–50 µg/kg, IV
CRI: 30–60 µg/kg/h, IV
Remifentanil:
Dog: Loading dose: Not required
CRI: 6–18 µg/kg/h, IV
18 µg/kg/h, IV, intraoperatively results in a MAC reduction of 60%. Higher doses do not increase the sparing effect [14, 15]
Cat: Loading dose: Not required
CRI: 15–30 µg/kg/h, IV, intraoperatively results in a MAC reduction of 23 and 30%, respectively. Same doses are effective in conscious cats for analgesia. Higher doses do not increase the sparing effect of inhalants and also result in dysphoria in conscious cats [16, 17].

F. Meperidine

Meperidine is an opioid of very short analgesic duration (30 min to 1 h) that is used frequently in geriatrics, brachycephalic breeds and in conditions where only mild levels of pain are anticipated. It is highly lipid soluble and therefore does not cause vomiting and does not generally result in panting or excessive sedation, hence this drug's main advantage is for sedation and mild pain control to permit IV catheterization and initial examination in patients where vomiting, excessive sedation or panting might be a contraindication (head trauma, severe depression). It is not reported to cause bradycardia as other mu-agonists do, which may be another advantage in certain cases. As a mu-agonist, a more potent and longer duration opioid may be administered once the patient is stabilized without the fear of receptor interactions.

The main contraindication to meperidine is IV administration and histamine release, hence it is contraindicated to use meperidine IV in any situation due to the potential to induce a cardiovascular arrest. Careful labelling of syringes is required.

Dose
Dogs: 3.0–5.0 mg/kg IM, SC (>200 mg rarely needed)
Cats: 5.0–10.0 mg/kg IM, SC

G. Methadone

Methadone is a mu-agonist that also has antagonistic actions at the N-methyl-D-aspartate (NMDA) receptor, which confers its activity against intraoperative surgical pain because of the actions on A-delta fibres, in addition to actions on C fibres from opioids in general. Lipid solubility is less than for fentanyl and meperidine, so signs of nausea/salivation can be observed in some cases; however, vomiting is not common. It is not associated with histamine release, so IV bolus administration is without complications. Bradycardia is noted with IV bolus dosing.

Methadone's potency is similar to morphine, but because of different solubility its epidural dose is similar to its parenteral doses, despite greater analgesic effects reported for the epidural route.

Methadone is used for sedation and analgesia of 3–4 h duration in conditions where moderate or severe pain is present and, because of its NMDA actions, is very effective for intraoperative analgesia.

Dose
Dogs: 0.3–0.5 mg/kg IM, SC or titrated to effect IV (higher dose for restraint)
Cats: 0.3–0.5 mg/kg IM, SC or titrated to effect IV (higher dose for restraint)
CRI
Loading dose: 0.1–0.3 mg/kg IM, SC or preferred, titrated to effect IV, (another mu-agonist can also be used for loading dose)
Infusion rate: 0.12 mg/kg/h IV (can be added to the hourly fluids) for mild, moderate and severe pain. Or, take one-quarter of the effective IV loading dose/h
Epidural use
0.1–0.5 mg/kg

III.   Partial Mu-Agonists

A. Buprenorphine

Buprenorphine is a mu-receptor agonist with a high affinity to the receptor, but it has limited efficacy, classifying it as a partial mu-agonist. It is also a kappa-antagonist. Any clinical effect achieved is always inferior to the effects of a pure mu-agonist, and the effects elicited by buprenorphine will not reach 100% efficacy. Due to this, it is not commonly used as a CRI. The partial agonism of buprenorphine confers an advantage related to its ceiling effect for any adverse effects as well, which will limit the degree of respiratory depression. Use of this class of drug should be limited to cases where only mild to moderate pain exists.

Buprenorphine is lipid soluble and as such it does not cause vomiting or nausea, which is an advantage. However, despite this lipid solubility, there is a delay from administration to the desired analgesic effect. Research in rats has indicated that this delay may be related to distribution of buprenorphine into the CNS and not necessarily due to slow receptor binding. Clinically, animals appear to have signs of sedation with a bolus dose IV; however, the delay in achieving analgesia limits its effectiveness for rescue analgesia, and its limited mu-agonism and efficacy makes it unsuitable as an analgesic in severely painful patients.

With buprenorphine, the duration of analgesia by the parenteral route is reported as 4–6 h, and sedative effects are less evident than for full mu-agonists, which may be an advantage in certain critical patients. It also has the advantage of efficacy for sublingual or oral transmucosal administration in cats. Oral transmucosal in dogs may also be effective but is restricted to small dogs based on volume required. Buprenorphine has similar epidural analgesic effects to morphine for quality and duration probably because of receptor occupancy at the spinal level. A subcutaneous formulation – Simbadol® 1.8 mg/mL (Zoetis), 0.25 mg/kg lean body mass, q24h for up to 72 h – is now available. Owners are advised to return to the clinic for each injection.

Dose
Dogs: 5–20 µg/kg IM, IV, SC
Cats: 10–20 µg/kg IM, IV, SC or 20–50 µg/kg transmucosal
Epidural use
4 µg/kg

IV. Kappa-Agonist, Mu-Antagonist

A. Butorphanol

Butorphanol is a mixed agonist-antagonist. Its kappa-agonistic actions confer analgesic and sedative effects as well, but it antagonizes the actions of mu-agonists if administered concomitantly. A pure mu-agonist can be administered for supplemental analgesia an hour after butorphanol administration; however, when administered together, the mu-antagonist effects of butorphanol will minimize the analgesic benefit of the pure mu-agonist.

Because of its kappa actions, there is less concern for drug abuse, and less strict record keeping in the US is required – although it is recommended and is classified as schedule G (US and Canada Schedule IV). The analgesia is less effective than for mu-agonists and can be used for mild pain only and has a maximum duration of action of only 1–2 h. In combination with tranquilizers or sedatives, it causes very reliable and profound sedation and can be administered by the IV route without resulting in histamine release.

Butorphanol is lipid soluble and does not cause nausea or vomiting. It is commonly reported to have good antitussive effects. It has been used epidurally at doses similar to parenteral doses with a longer duration of effect (5–8 h), but it is still only effective for milder pain conditions.

Dose
Dogs: 0.1–0.4 mg/kg IM, IV, SC (higher end of dose range for restraint)
Cats: 0.2–0.6 mg/kg IM, IV, SC (higher end of dose range for restraint)
Epidural use
4 µg/kg

V. Oral Opioid Drugs

A. Tramadol

Tramadol is classified as an atypical opiate and has one-tenth the potency of morphine. It is not controlled by the scheduling and drug enforcement agencies in Canada and the US, making it an easily obtainable analgesic for use at home; however, in some countries it is controlled similar to other opioids. It is commonly prescribed for use in chronic pain states, although efficacy for acute surgical conditions or severe pain is questionable.

Tramadol is metabolized in the liver via N- and O-demethylation and glucuronidation or sulfation with only 30% excreted unchanged in the urine. Naloxone only reverses some of the adverse effects if an overdose is encountered, but its use may precipitate seizures.

Both the parent drug and active metabolite (M_1 or O-desmethyl-tramadol) bind the mu-receptors but with weak activity. The M_1 metabolite has a much higher affinity for the mu-receptors than the parent compound in humans, but this metabolite is only produced in small amounts in dogs. The analgesic efficacy in dogs is questionable and probably any analgesia achieved is associated with the parent drug, not M_1 [18]. Inhibition of noradrenaline and serotonin reuptake (similar to antidepressants) or some alpha$_2$ effects may be responsible for part of the analgesia that is purported with tramadol. Few randomized controlled studies are available to clearly define the analgesic use for painful conditions in dogs and cats. Owners should be aware that additional analgesic medication may be required, and they should consult with the veterinarian as needed. It is not approved for veterinary use but has been used for the moderate pain associated with chronic conditions such as osteoarthritis and cancer. It has also been prescribed for mild post-operative surgical pain.

Adverse effects reported in humans are: dizziness, nausea, vomiting, constipation, diarrhoea, headache, somnolence, pruritus, asthenia, dyspepsia, dry mouth and CNS stimulation. CNS stimulation has been reported more frequently in cats than dogs; however, it does occur in dogs. Anecdotal owner reports indicate these adverse effects occur frequently. A combination of tramadol with deracoxib resulted in duodenal perforation in a case report of three dogs [19].

Dose

Tramadol is available in 50 mg tablets. It may be compounded into an injectable form and an oral solution

Dogs: 1–4 mg/kg IV or PO q6h is suggested for management of severe pain. 1–2 mg/kg PO q12h is suggested for osteoarthritis

Doses of 1–4 mg/kg have also been used IV without major adverse effects but nausea, salivation and sedation have been observed

Cats: 1–2 mg/kg PO q12–24h

Codeine is structurally similar to morphine and is classified as a mu opioid agonist. It can be administered IV slowly, IM, SC or orally in cats and dogs. It is generally recommended as an oral analgesic; however, limited data does not demonstrate analgesic efficacy in dogs, and studies are not available for cats. Codeine may be formulated with acetaminophen, and this combination should never be administered to cats. There is poor oral bioavailability of codeine in Beagle dogs at a dose of 1.85 mg/kg of only 6–7% compared to 60% in humans [20]. In addition, the oral administration of codeine in people results in 10% of the dose being metabolized to morphine and morphine metabolites [21]; however, there is no detectable morphine in dogs after oral administration [22]. Considering this, oral administration of codeine in cats and dogs is expected to have minimal analgesic efficacy. With IV and oral administration, large amounts of codeine-6-glucuronide is formed in dogs [22], while norcodeine is the main metabolite in cats [23]. While these metabolites may offer some analgesic effect, the efficacy in dogs of codeine (1 mg/kg, SC) offered less effective and shorter duration of analgesia compared to morphine (0.2 mg/kg, SC) under experimental conditions of dental pulp stimulation [24]. No clinical studies are available for the efficacy of codeine in dogs or cats for analgesia, and, considering this, it is not recommended for analgesic therapy at this time.

Hydrocodone is a mu opioid agonist that is available as oral combination preparations. The drug combinations that can be administered to dogs include hydrocodone with homatropine and hydrocodone with acetaminophen. The drug combination that can be administered to cats is hydrocodone with homatropine. The interest in hydrocodone is related to the metabolism of oral hydrocodone to hydromorphone, which has been demonstrated in dogs [25]. Unfortunately, there is limited data on the efficacy of hydrocodone in veterinary medicine experimentally or clinically, hence strong recommendations cannot be made to use oral hydrocodone for analgesia.

References

1 Feng, Y., He, X., Yang, Y., *et al.* (2012) Current research on opioid receptor function. *Curr Drug Targets*, 13: 230–246.
2 Vanderah, T. W. (2010) Delta and kappa opioid receptors as suitable drug targets for pain. *Clin J Pain*, 26(suppl. 10): S10–S15.
3 Lötsch, J. (2005) Pharmacokinetic-pharmacodynamic modeling of opioids. *J Pain Symptom Manage*, 29: S90–S103.
4 Young-McCaughan, S. and Miaskowski, C. (2001) Definition of and mechanism for opioid-induced sedation. *Pain Manag Nurs*, 2: 84–97.
5 Guan, Y., Borzan, J., Meyer, R. A. and Raja, S. N. (2006) Windup in dorsal horn neurons is modulated by endogenous spinal μ-opioid mechanisms. *J Neurosci*, 26: 4298–4307.
6 Yassen, A., Olafsen, E. and Dahlhof, M. (2005) Pharmacokinetic-pharmacodynamic modeling of the anti-nociception effect of buprenorphine and fentanyl in rats role of receptor equilibration kinetics. *J Pharm Exp Ther*, 313: 1136–1149.
7 Pattison, K. T. S. (2008) Opioids and the control of respiration. *Br J Anesth*, 100: 747–758.
8 Takahama, K. and Shirasaki, T. (2007) Central and peripheral mechanisms of narcotic antitussives: Codeine-sensitive and -resistant coughs. *Cough*, 3: 8, doi: 10.1186/1745-9974-3-8.
9 Mori, T., Shibasaki, Y., Matsumoto, K., *et al.* (2013) Mechanisms that underlie μ-opioid receptor agonist-induced constipation: Differential involvement of μ-opioid receptor sites and responsible regions. *J Pharmacol Exp Ther*, 347: 91–99.
10 Posner, L. P., Pavuk, A. A., Rokshar, J. L., *et al.* (2010) Effects of opioids and anesthetic drugs on body temperature in cats. *Vet Anesth Analg*, 37: 35–43.
11 Flancbaum, L., Alden, S. M. and Trooskin, S. Z. (1989) Use of cholescintigraphy with morphine in critically ill patients with suspected cholecystitis. *Surgery*, 106: 668–673.
12 Ramaswamy, S. and Langford, R. M. (2017) Antinociceptive and immunosuppressive effect of opioids in an acute postoperative setting: An evidence-based review. *British J Anesthesia Education*, 17(3): 105–110.
13 Fletcher, D. and Martinez, V. (2014) Opioid-induced hyperalgesia in patients after surgery: A systematic review and a meta-analysis. *Br J Anesth*, 112: 991–1004.
14 Michelsen, L. G., Salmenperä, M., Hug, C. C. Jr, *et al.* (1996) Anesthetic potency of remifentanil in dogs. *Anesthesiology*, 84, 865–872.
15 Monteiro, E. R., Teixeira-Neto, F. J., Campagnol, D., *et al.* (2010) Effect of remifentanil on the minimum alveolar concentration of isoflurane in dogs. *Am J Vet Res*, 71: 150–156.

16 Brosnan, R. J., Pypendop, B. H., Siao, B. S., *et al.* (2009) Effect of remifentanil on measures of anesthetic immobility and analgesia in cats. *Am J Vet Res*, 70: 1065–1071.

17 Ferreira, T., Aguar, J. A., Valverde, A., *et al.* (2009) Effect of remifentanil hydrochloride administration via a constant rate infusion on the minimum alveolar concentration of isoflurane in cats. *Am J Vet Res*, 70: 581–588.

18 KuKanich, B. and Papich, M. G. (2011) Pharmacolinetics and antinociceptive effects of oral tramadol hydrochloride administration in greyhounds. *Am J Vet Res*, 72: 256–262.

19 Case, J. B., Fick, J. L. and Rooney, M. B. (2010) Proximal duodenal perforation in three dogs following deracoxib administration. *J Am Anim Hosp Assoc*, 46: 255–258.

20 Findlay, J. W., Jones, E. C. and Welch, R. M. (1979) Radioimmunoassay determination of the absolute oral bioavailabilies and O-demethylation of codeine and hydrocodone in the dog. *Drug Metabolism Disposition*, 7: 310–314.

21 Kirchheiner, J., Schmidt, H., Tzvetkov, M., *et al.* (2006) Pharmacokinetics of codeine and its metabolite morphine in ultra-rapid metabolizers due to CYP2D6 duplication. *The Pharmacogenomics Journal*, 7: 257–265.

22 KuKanich, B. (2010) Pharmacokinetics of acetaminophen, codeine, and the codeine metabolites morphine and codeine-6-glucuronide in healthy Greyhound dogs. *J Vet Pharmacol Ther*, 33: 15–21.

23 Yeh, S. Y. and Woods, L A. (1971) Excretion of codeine and its metabolites by dogs, rabbits and cats. *Arch Int Pharmacodyn Ther*, 191: 231–242.

24 Skingle, M. and Tylers, M. B. (1980) Further studies on opiate receptors that mediate antinociception: Tooth pulp stimulation in the dog. *British Journal of Pharmacology*, 70: 323–327.

25 KuKanich, B. and Spade, J. (2013) Pharmacokinetics of hydrocodone and hydromorphone after oral hydrocodone in healthy Greyhound dogs. *Veterinary Journal*, 196: 266–268.

11

Pharmacologic and Clinical Application of Non-Steroidal Anti-Inflammatory Analgesics

Karol Mathews

The indications, adverse effects and contraindications for all non-steroidal anti-inflammatory analgesics (NSAIAs) are similar. Where there are unique differences, these will be noted as related to each drug. Only veterinary-approved NSAIAs should be administered to dogs and cats when NSAIAs are recommended in this book, unless a non-approved type is suggested. As all animals discussed are ill or injured with intravenous (IV) access, and some may not be able to take medications per os, only injectable NSAIAs will be highlighted.

I. Pharmacology

NSAIAs are, with varying differences, inhibitors of cyclooxygenase enzyme 1 (COX-1), COX-2, or both, or COX-3, resulting in reduced prostaglandin (PG) synthesis. In addition to the anti-inflammatory analgesic action, a significant part of the NSAIAs' anti-nociceptive effect is exerted at the spinal cord and supraspinal levels where both COX-1 and COX-2 isoenzymes function in nociceptive transmission independent of inflammation, which is the peripheral action [1–7]. The supraspinal actions, in addition to pain relief, may account for the observed overall well-being and improved appetite of patients receiving injectable NSAIAs for relief of acute pain (personal observations).

Associated with the use of NSAIAs is the risk of perturbation of the constitutive functions of COX-1 and COX-2 resulting in potential organ dysfunction. Therefore, contraindications for their use must be considered in all patients prior to administration. However, in this regard, not all NSAIAs are created equal, as the COX-1, COX-2 and COX-3 enzymes variably control these functions.

A. Cyclooxygenase-1

Cyclooxygenase-1, in addition to the inflammatory and spinal nociceptive transmitter functions, may also generate PGs at sites of inflammation (e.g. joints); it is present within the central nervous system and active in transmission of pain, especially visceral nociception. COX-1 is also a constitutive enzyme, converting arachidonic acid into thromboxane, prostacyclin and prostaglandins (PGE_2, PGF_2 and PGD_2) which are involved in many homeostatic functions throughout the body [6]. Some examples that are extremely important to note in the ill or injured patient are regulation of vascular and bronchial smooth muscle tone, renal blood flow

Analgesia and Anesthesia for the Ill or Injured Dog and Cat, First Edition. Karol A. Mathews, Melissa Sinclair, Andrea M. Steele and Tamara Grubb.

regulation, tubular function and fluid balance, platelet function (thromboxane A_2), gastric cytoprotection, mucous production, mucosal repair and blood flow. As urine volume is frequently measured in our patients, it is important to note the PG functions that may alter urine production independent of kidney function. As an example, renal water reabsorption depends on the action of antidiuretic hormone (ADH), which is mediated by cyclic adenosine monophosphate (cAMP), with PGs exerting a negative feedback action. Inhibition of PG synthesis may lead to increased levels of cAMP with a potential for enhanced ADH activity. Urine volume may be decreased and specific gravity increased through this mechanism but without renal injury [6, 8, 9].

B. Cyclooxygenase-2

Cyclooxygenase-2 is also inducible and synthesized by macrophages and inflammatory cells, potentially increasing by twentyfold over baseline, especially in injured tissue and inflammatory conditions, where these compounds serve as mediators of inflammation and amplifiers of nociceptive input and transmission in both the peripheral and central nervous systems [2]. By this mechanism, COX-2 is responsible for a significant amount of pain and hyperalgesia experienced after tissue injury. COX metabolites have been implicated in functional and structural alterations in glomerular and tubulo-interstitial inflammatory disease [9]. Because COX-2 expression is also increased in glomerulonephritides, such as lupus nephritis, it is possible that COX-2 inhibitors may also alter the natural history of glomerular inflammatory lesions [9]. COX-2 is glucocorticoid sensitive, in that it is reduced following administration of glucocorticoids, which may partially explain the anti-inflammatory and analgesic effects of this class of medications.

As with COX-1, COX-2 also has important constitutive functions [7, 10]. There is a protective role for COX-2 in the maintenance of gastrointestinal integrity and ulcer healing [11]. In addition, there is constitutive activity associated with nerve, brain, ovarian and uterine function and bone metabolism [8, 12]. COX-2 has constitutive functions in the kidney, which differ from those of COX-1. COX-2-derived metabolite production is regulated and localized to the structures in the kidney that play an essential role in renal blood flow associated with renin activity and fluid-electrolyte homeostasis [9, 13, 14]. COX-2 is important in nephron maturation [9, 13]. The canine kidney is not fully mature until three weeks after birth, or optimally functional until six weeks after birth [13]; continual administration of an NSAIA during this time, or prior to birth for both the dam and queen, or during lactation, may cause a permanent nephropathy (refer to Chapter 24 for specific information). Most important is the dual role of the PGs as inflammatory and anti-inflammatory mediators, where COX-2-derived PGs also function in resolution of inflammation [7].

C. Cyclooxygenase-3

Cyclooxygenase-3, characterized as generated from COX-1, is expressed in the brain and brain microvasculature in dogs and has been proposed to be a target of the analgesic/antipyretics acetaminophen and metamizole [6, 15, 16]. Both acetaminophen and metamizole/dipyrone have minimal effect on COX-1 and COX-2 [6] and are frequently used to reduce fever in animals with little gastrointestinal or renal adverse effects. Acetaminophen is toxic to cats. Metamizole/dipyrone is not approved for cats but has been used in this species [17].

The COX-3 isoenzyme is more susceptible to NSAIAs that are analgesic and antipyretic but have low anti-inflammatory activity. As the COX-3 isoenzyme genetic profile is derived from the COX-1 gene, this suggests that the COX-1 gene plays an integral role in pain and/or fever depending on the physiologic context [4].

D. EP4 Receptor

The EP4 receptor, one of the four PGE_2 receptors, has a primary function of mediating the PGE_2-elicited sensitization of sensory neurons and PGE_2-elicited inflammation resulting in inflammatory pain. Piprants are prostaglandin receptor antagonists (PRAs), a new class of analgesic agents. The EP4 receptor has been associated with osteoarthritis (OA) in rodents, dogs and cats [18]. Grapiprant (Galliprant®, Aratana Therapeutics), an EP4 PGE_2 receptor antagonist, has recently been approved for OA in dogs. In a field study, grapiprant 2 mg/kg PO q24h improved pain scores when compared to placebo (48.1% vs 31.3%). Based on the specific receptor target, grapiprant was well tolerated with occasional vomiting (17% of dogs) throughout the 28-day study [19]. However, long-term studies are required to further assess safety. Studies examining analgesic efficacy for other sources of pain have not been performed; however, grapiprant is included here based on the potential safety profile and if considered in the "discharge home" analgesic plan. Appropriate patient selection and monitoring, as with other NSAIDs, is advised. Only tablets are available for dogs only. Studies in cats are underway.

E. 5-Lipoxygenase (5-LOX) Pathway

Most NSAIAs that inhibit COX have been shown to result in diversion of arachidonate to the 5-LOX pathway. This results in an excessive production of leukotrienes (LT), which have been implicated in many pathologic states, including hyperalgesia and the creation of NSAIA-induced ulcers [6, 20, 21]. As with the prostanoids, it is impossible to list all the activities of the LTs as these are also dependent on organ involvement. An in-depth discussion of dual inhibitors is available elsewhere [7, 21–24].

II.   Veterinary-Approved NSAIAs

There are several veterinary-approved NSAIAs with specific instructions for dosing and administration. The package insert must be reviewed prior to administration as all NSAIAs differ in some respects; age, below which should not be used and dosing. Also, drug combinations and contraindication warnings are listed. **Table 11.1 lists in bold veterinary-approved injectable NSAIAs**, under their cyclooxygenase inhibitory properties with **dosages given, based on lean weight in obese patients and actual weight for those below or at ideal body weight**, for those appropriate for conditions presented in this book.

III.   Indications

The NSAIAs are effective in controlling surgical and non-surgical acute and chronic painful conditions associated with inflammation. In many painful situations some may be superior to opioids in efficacy. The NSAIAs act synergistically in combination with other modalities of pain management, including all opioids, local anesthetics and various sedatives. In the postoperative setting, and any other moderate to severe painful condition, an opioid should be administered concurrently to ensure adequate analgesia until the NSAIA becomes effective. NSAIAs usually take 30–60 min for a full analgesic effect to be recognized when administered by the oral and IV routes, and longer when given subcutaneously. This combination confers excellent analgesia in patients with moderate to severe pain. As these two groups of analgesics modulate nociceptive input through different mechanisms, their combination may require reduced dosing of the opioid in mild to moderate, but not in severe, pain states. This combination

Table 11.1 Veterinary-approved injectable NSAIAs.

	Dogs	Cats
COX-1 and COX 2 inhibitors		
Ketoprofen	1.0 mg/kg IV < SC < IM q24h	1.0 mg/kg IV, IM, SC q24h
COX-2 preferential (weak COX-1 inhibition)		
Carprofen	2 mg/kg q12h IV, PO	1–2 mg/kg IV **once**
Meloxicam	0.1 mg/kg IV, SC medical/soft tissuesurgical pain q24h or 0.2 mg/kg IV, SC once for orthopedic/moderate to severe pain, then 0.1 mg/kg q24h	0.1–0.2 mg/kg* IV, SC **once**, then 0.1 mg/kg IV, PO q24h up to 2 days, then 0.05 mg/kg IV, PO q24h for 4 days then 0.025 mg/kg every other day
COX-2 specific inhibitor		
Robenacoxib	2 mg/kg SC once 1 mg/kg, PO q24h	2 mg/kg SC once 1 mg/kg, PO q24h 6 days
COX-3 inhibitor		
Metamizole/Dipyrone dogs only	25–50 mg/kg IV, q8–12h ~3–5 days IM is painful	

* Clinical studies do not support the USA label 0.3 mg/kg once, dose.

facilitates sleep and profound analgesia. However, in some severe pain states adjunct analgesia will be required (refer to Chapter 12).

Prior to administration of an NSAIA, all contraindications must be ruled out. To avoid potential adverse effects, dosing of any NSAIA must be based on the patient's ideal body weight, and not on actual weight, in overweight/obese patients until clinical studies prove otherwise. However, actual weight dosing is indicated for the below ideal weight patients. It is also essential that veterinarians become familiar with all the potential adverse effects and contraindications. Contraindications are discussed in Section V.

For a review of the clinical use of the NSAIAs in greater depth the reader is encouraged to read reviews of published veterinary studies [25–29].

A. Trauma and Post-Operative Pain

NSAIAs are recommended for orthopedic and selected soft tissue surgical procedures, especially where extensive inflammation or soft tissue trauma is present. Opioid administration is preferred immediately after any surgical procedure due to the sedative/analgesic effects and to ensure a smooth recovery. However, the injectable NSAIAs, (carprofen, ketoprofen, meloxicam, robenacoxib) can be co-administered with an opioid initially and subsequently used alone. Selection is based on the underlying problem and concern for adverse effects associated with either the COX-1 or COX-2 preferential/selective NSAIA (see Section V). The initial dose of NSAIAs depends on the expected severity of pain. Assuming a difficult fracture repair would require the recommended loading dose, then a laparotomy without complications may be successfully treated with half this dose. When combination opioid and NSAIAs are used, it is wise to reduce any repeat opioid dose to avoid potential dysphoria or panting that might occur due to a "relative" opioid overdose in patients with mild to moderate pain. This very rarely occurs for a short period of time when therapeutic blood levels of both analgesics exist and the degree of pain does not warrant this level of analgesia.

B. Inflammatory Conditions Associated with Illness

For pain due to meningitis, bone tumours (especially after biopsy), soft tissue swelling (mastitis), polyarthritis, cystitis, otitis, severe inflammatory dermatologic diseases or injury (e.g. degloving, animal bites), combination opioids and low-dose NSAIAs are effective.

C. Miscellaneous Conditions

Other indications for the use of NSAIAs are panosteitis, hypertrophic osteodystrophy (HOD), cancer pain, (especially of bone) and dental pain. COX-1 selective NSAIAs (e.g. ketoprofen, aspirin) may cause hemorrhage when used with dental extractions, or other areas of non-compressible hemorrhage. Thromboxane activity may be unaltered with COX-2 preferential NSAIA administration. Some dogs will present with acute, severe pain associated with pan-osteitis or HOD where the loading dose of an NSAIA is required to see an effect. The HOD of Weimaraners is poorly responsive to NSAIA therapy and is better treated with high-dose, short-term, corticosteroids provided infectious disease has been ruled out and clinical signs are consistent with HOD alone (refer to Chapter 31). Irish setters and Great Danes are also prone to refractory HOD and have responded well to corticosteroids.

D. Pyrexia

Most NSAIA have antipyretic activity and can be used for this purpose. The antipyretic activity of ketoprofen and meloxicam has been studied in cats. In the author's experience, half, and sometimes less, of the analgesic dose of meloxicam or ketoprofen is adequate for this effect. Aspirin or acetaminophen frequently requires the recommended dose for the antipyretic effect in dogs only. Metamizole/Dipyrone is an excellent antipyretic and is available as tablets, and injectable solution, which must be given IV to avoid the pain/irritation when given intramus-cularly (IM). The analgesia produced is inadequate for severe pain. Gastric ulceration or nephrotoxicity with metamizole is not a concern in the short term even in critically ill dogs.

E. Osteoarthritis

The NSAIAs concentrate in inflamed joints and tissues, likely contributing to duration of effect, which varies between 12 and 24 h [30]. Acute on chronic pain may occur in patients with OA, resulting in severe lameness. As many patients with OA are geriatric, a rapid reduction of the dose to effect a comfortable state is advised to reduce potential toxicity. Some geriatric patients may have renal insufficiency and yet be in a great deal of pain, While renal insuffi-ciency is a relative contraindication for NSAIA administration, the consideration of the "risk vs benefit" of therapy with an NSAIA for these dogs and cats frequently proves to be of benefit in improving the quality of life. Reports of dogs and cats with renal insufficiency have improved quality of life, while maintaining a stable baseline of creatinine, after administration of meloxicam or carprofen.

IV. Safety

In the majority of cases, the adverse effects appear minimal, predominantly associated with the gastrointestinal tract. However, gastric and duodenal perforation have been reported to occur with co-administration of two NSAIAs or corticosteroids, co-administration of a COX-2 pref-erential NSAIA and tramadol [31] and when given to patients where NSAIAs are contraindicated.

If an individual patient requires a persistent high dose of a particular NSAIA to manage their pain, prescribing a different NSAIA may be more effective due to individual variation in response to the different analgesics. Where the adverse effects of an NSAIA is a concern (see Section V and VI), reducing the dose and adding an opioid (e.g. buprenorphine for cats, amantadine for dogs or gabapentin for cats and dogs; refer to Chapter 12) may be as effective for chronic severe pain. Other important therapies to consider are the various integrative modalities (refer to Chapter 15).

During NSAIA therapy all patients should be monitored for inappetence, hematochezia or melena, vomiting, increased water consumption and a non-specific change in demeanour. If this occurs, the owner should be instructed to stop the medication and call the office. Intermittent monitoring of creatinine and alanine aminotransferase (ALT) is recommended when NSAIAs are prescribed chronically to identify potential toxicity. Where an increase in creatinine and ALT is present in the geriatric patient with chronic pain, and other classes of analgesics are ineffective, prescribing an NSAIA may be considered. Discuss with the owner the potential adverse effects but that alleviating pain will improve the animal's quality of life. With the use of any NSAIA, the drug should be decreased to the lowest possible dose that will confer a comfortable state. This may reduce the potential for toxicity, especially with long-term use. When given per os, NSAIAs must be given with food to protect the gastric mucosa. If food is not present in the stomach, the contact area of the tablet/liquid on the mucosa results in a highly localized concentration of the drug increasing the potential for localized ulcer formation. Potential for generalized gastric ulceration exists with all NSAIAs regardless of the route of administration.

V. Contraindications [32]

- NSAIAs should never be administered to patients in shock, or trauma cases upon presentation. After a traumatic incident, the patient must be stable with no evidence of blunt abdominal trauma/hemorrhage (it may take several hours to determine this) and maintained on IV crystalloid therapy until adequate fluid intake has been guaranteed. Opioids should be administered in the interim.
- Patients in renal or hepatic failure.
- Where dehydration, hypotension and other conditions associated with low "effective circulating volume" (e.g. congestive heart failure, ascites, diuretics in the acute setting) are present.
- Coagulopathies (e.g. thrombocytopenia, von Willebrand disease, factor deficiencies) or where hemorrhage is evident (e.g. epistaxis, hemangiosarcoma, head trauma).
- Concurrent use of other NSAIAs (i.e. all human or veterinary NSAIAs, homeopathic compounds including willow bark) or corticosteroids.
- Evidence of gastric irritation or ulceration (vomiting with or without the presence of "coffee ground material", melena) or gastrointestinal disorder of any kind.
- As intervertebral disc disease can be considered a "spinal injury", NSAIAs are contraindicated in severe cases due to potential hemorrhage after acute herniation (with subsequent worsening of neurologic function), and prior to laminectomy as bleeding may be increased in this difficult-to-compress area. The COX-2 preferential/selective NSAIAs may not cause, or worsen, hemorrhage in spinal injury; however, at this time, it is not known whether this may be a problem. A COX-2 preferential/selective NSAIA is recommended for the less neurologic and more stable dogs where corticosteroids have not been administered.
- Humans with severe or poorly controlled asthma, or other moderate to severe pulmonary disease, may deteriorate with COX-1 NSAIA use due to potential for antagonism of PG-mediated smooth muscle relaxation. However, this has not been reported in veterinary patients. COX-2 preferential/selective NSAIAs may be suitable in these conditions.

- Toxicity of NSAIAs may be increased with co-administration of aminoglycosides, furosemide, cyclosporine, heparin, gingko, garlic, ginger and ginseng cisplatin. However, toxicity of these and other medications may also be increased with co-administration of an NSAIA [33]. For the individual NSAIA, caution may be advised with angiotensin-converting enzyme inhibitors, and highly protein-bound agents (e.g. phenobarbital, digoxin, chemotherapeutic agents) due to competition for binding sites, although unbound may be eliminated faster.
- As COX-2 induction is necessary for ovulation and subsequent implantation of the embryo, NSAIAs should be avoided in breeding females during this stage of the reproductive cycle if possible. However, pain management should take precedence over breeding. Pregnant animals, puppies and kittens (until proven otherwise) less than 6 weeks old should not receive NSAIAs. Continual administration of an NSAIA to the dam/queen during this time (as the drug may pass into the milk) may cause a permanent nephropathy, with the exception of carprofen which appears safe in lactating dogs for six days following C-section (refer to Chapter 23).

VI. Comments and Other Considerations

The NSAIAs are highly protein bound. While this may not be of importance in most instances (since increases in free drug that result from protein binding interactions are offset rapidly by increased clearance of the extra free drug), concomitant drug interactions may occur and should be considered. Caution here would apply to patients with even mild or potential organ dysfunction, hypoalbuminemia and in those receiving medication, which are also highly protein bound, and those with a narrow therapeutic index. Should pain be the primary concern, frequent monitoring is advised until safety is established.

NSAIA-induced acute kidney injury is usually temporary and reversible with drug withdrawal and administration of IV fluids [34]. Accidental ingestion of NSAIAs should be managed with gastric lavage followed by administration of activated charcoal and gastric protectants. IV fluid therapy should continue for a minimum of 24h. Therapy beyond this period will depend on the renal and gastric status of the individual patient, severe injury may require 1–2 weeks to return to normal renal function. If evidence of gastric irritation/ulcers exist, omeprazole and sucralfate, 1–2+ h following omeprazole, therapy is necessary. Recently in human medicine it has been reported that chronic use of proton pump inhibitors (PPIs) is associated with chronic kidney disease (CKD). A disturbing fact is that patients did not recognize any symptoms of acute kidney injury, and so continued with the PPI with subsequent development of CKD. It is important to evaluate the ongoing necessity for patient PPI use in light of the potential for CKD. A short course is not a problem; however, those who do need PPIs should be aware that acute kidney injury may not occur as a warning sign for those at risk for adverse renal outcomes. Pantoprazole and omeprazole are effective in reducing gastric acid secretion; however, ranitidine is not [35].

References

1 Chopra, B., Giblett, S., Little, J. G., *et al.* (2000) Cyclooxygenase-1 is a marker for a subpopulation of putative nociceptive neurons in rat dorsal root ganglia. *Eur J Neurosci*, 12: 911–920.
2 Malmberg, N. B. and Yaksh, L. (1992) Antinociceptive actions of spinal nonsteroidal anti-inflammatory agents on the formalin test in the rat. *J Pharmacol Exp Ther*, 263: 136–146.

3 McKormack, K. (1994) Non-steroidal anti-inflammatory drugs and spinal processing. *Pain*, 59: 9–43.

4 McKormack, K. (1994) The spinal actions of non-steroidal anti-inflammatory drugs and the dissociation between their anti-inflammatory and analgesic effects. *Drugs*, 47 (suppl. 15): 28–45.

5 Yaksh, T. L., Dirig, D. M. and Malmberg, A. B. (1998) Mechanism of action of nonsteroidal anti-inflammatory drugs. *Cancer Invest*, 16: 509–527.

6 Vane, J. R. and Botting, R. M. (1995) New insights into mode of action of antiinflammatory drugs. *Inflamm Res*, 44: 1–10.

7 Khanapure, S. P., Garvey, D. S., Janero, D. R. and Letts, L. G. (2007) Eicosanoids in inflammation: Biosynthesis, pharmacology, and therapeutic frontiers. *Curr Top Med Chem*, 7: 311–340.

8 Dubois, R. N., Abramson, S. B., Crofford, L., *et al.* (1998) Cyclooxygenase in biology and disease. *FASEB J*, 12: 1063–1073.

9 Harris, R. C. (2000) Cyclooxygenase-2 in the kidney. *J Am Soc Nephrol*, 11: 2387–2394.

10 Lipsky, P. E., Brooks, P., Crofford, L. J., *et al.* (2000) Unresolved issues in the role of cyclooxygenase-2 in normal physiologic processes and disease. *Arch Intern Med*, 160: 913–920.

11 Schmassmann, A., Peskar, B. M. and Stettler, C. (1998) Effects of inhibition of prostaglandin endoperoxide synthase-2 in chronic gastro-intestinal ulcer models in rats. *Br J Pharmacol*, 123: 795–804.

12 Strauss, K. I. (2008) Antiinflammatory and neuroprotective actions of COX2 inhibitors in injured brain. *Brain Behav Immun*, 22: 285–298.

13 Horster, M., Kember, B. and Valtin, H. (1971) Intracortical distribution of number and volume of glomeruli during postnatal maturation in the dog. *J Clin Invest*, 50: 796–800.

14 Imig, J. D. (2000) Eicosanoid regulation of the renal vasculature. *Am J Physiol Renal Physiol*, 279: F965–F981.

15 Botting, R. (2003) COX-1 and COX-3 inhibitors. *Thromb Res*, 110(5–6): 269–272.

16 Chandrasekharon, N. V., Dai, H., Roos, K. L., *et al.* (2002) COX-3, a cyclooxygenase-1 variant inhibited by acetaminophen and other analgesic/antipyretic drugs: Cloning, structure and expression. *Proc Natl Acad Sci USA*, 99(21): 13926–13931.

17 Ottenjann, M., Weingart, C. and Arndt, G. (2006) Characterization of the anemia of inflammatory disease in cats with abscesses, pyothorax, or fat necrosis. *J Vet Intern Med*, 20: 1143–1150.

18 Shaw, K. K., Rausch-Derra, L. C. and Rhodes, L. (2016) Grapiprant: An EP4 prostaglandin receptor antagonist and novel therapy for pain and inflammation. *Vet Med Sci*, 2: 3–9.

19 Rausch-Derra, L., Huebner, M. and Wofford, J. (2016) A prospective, randomized, masked, placebo-controlled multisite clinical study of grapiprant, an EP4 prostaglandin receptor antagonist (PRA), in dogs with osteoarthritis. *Vet Intern Med*, 30: 756–763.

20 Leone, S., Ottani, A. and Bertolina, A. (2007) Dual acting anti-inflammatory drugs. *Curr Top Med Chem*, 7: 265–275.

21 Bertolini, A., Ottani, A. and Sandrini, M. (2001) Dual acting anti-inflammatory drugs: A reappraisal. *Pharmacol Res*, 44(6): 437–450.

22 Kirchner, T., Argentieri, D. C. and Barbone, A. G. (1997) Evaluation of the antiinflammatory activity of a dual cyclooxygenase-2 selective/5 lipoxygenase inhibitor RWJ 63556, in a canine model of inflammation. *J Pharmacol Exp Ther*, 282: 1094–1101.

23 Gonzalez-Periz, A. and Claria, J. (2007) New approaches to modulation of the cyclooxygenase-2 and 5-lipooxygenase pathways. *Curr Top Med Chem*, 7: 297–309.

24 Clark, T. P. (2006) The clinical pharmacology of cyclooxygenase-2-selective and dual inhibitors. *Vet Clin North Am Small Anim Pract*, 36: 1061–1085.

25 Aragon, C. L., Hofmeister, E. H. and Budsberg, S. C. (2007) Systematic review of clinical trials of treatments for osteoarthritis in dogs. *J Am Vet Med Assoc*, 230: 514–521.

26 Papich, M. (2008) An update on nonsteroidal antiinflammatory drugs (NSAID) in small animals. *Vet Clin North Am Small Anim Pract*, 38(6): 1243–1266.

27 Johnston, S. A., McLaughlin, R. M. and Budsberg, S. C. (2008) Management of osteoarthritis in dogs. *Vet Clin North Am Small Anim Pract*, 38(6): 1449–1470.

28 Lascelles, B. D, Court, M. H. and Hardie, E. M., *et al.* (2007) Nonsteroidal anti-inflammatory drugs in cats: A review. *Vet Anaesth Analg*, 34(4): 228–250.

29 Robertson, S. A. (2008) Managing pain in feline patients. *Vet Clin North Am Small Anim Pract*, 38(6): 1267–1290.

30 Lees, P., May, S. A. and McKellar, Q. A. (1991) Pharmacology and therapeutics of nonsteroidal anti-inflammatory drugs in the dog and cat: 1: General pharmacology. *J Small Anim Pract*, 32: 183–193.

31 Case, J. B., Fick, J. L. and Rooney, M. B. (2010) Proximal duodenal perforation in three dogs following deracoxib administration *J Am Anim Hosp Assoc*, 46: 255–258.

32 Mathews, K. A. (2000) Non-steroidal anti-inflammatory analgesics: Indications and contraindications. *Vet Clin North Am Small Anim Pract* (review), 30(4): 783–804.

33 Trepanier, L. A. (2005) Potential interactions between NSAIDs and other drugs. *J Vet Emerg Crit Care*, 15(4): 248–253.

34 Mathews, K. A. (2017) Management of acute kidney injury/failure. In: Mathews, K. A. (ed.), *Veterinary Emergency & Critical Care Manual*, 3rd edn. LifeLearn, Guelph, Ontario, Canada.

35 Bersenas, A. M. E., Mathews, K. A., Allen, D. G. and Conlon, P. D. (2005) The efficacy of gastric-acid lowering therapy in the dog. *Am J Vet Res*, 66(3): 425–431.

Further Reading

Bergh, M. S. and Budsgerg, S. C. (2005) The coxib NSAIDs: Potential clinical and pharmacologic importance in veterinary medicine. *J Vet Intern Med*, 19: 633–643.

Carroll, G. L., Howe, L. B. and Peterson, K. D. (2005) Analgesic efficacy of preoperative administration of meloxicam or butorphanol in onychectomized cats. *J Am Vet Med Assoc*, 226(6): 913–919.

Dobbins, S., Brown, N. O. and Shofer, F. S. (2002) Comparison of the effects of buprenorphine, oxymorphone hydrochloride, and ketoprofen for postoperative analgesia after onychectomy or onychectomy and sterilization in cats. *J Am Anim Hosp Assoc*, 38(6): 507–514.

Gassel, A. D., Tobias, K. M., Egger, C. M. and Rohrbach, B. W. (2005) Comparison of oral and subcutaneous administration of buprenorphine and meloxicam for preemptive analgesia in cats undergoing ovariohysterectomy. *J Am Vet Med Assoc*, 227(12): 1937–1944.

Grisnaux, E., Pibarot, P. and Dupuis, J. (1999) Comparison of ketoprofen and carprofen administered prior to orthopedic surgery for control of postoperative pain in dogs. *J Am Vet Med Assoc*, 215: 1105–1110.

Gunew, M. N., Menrath, V. H. and Marshall, R. D. (2008) Long-term safety, efficacy and palatability of oral meloxicam at 0.01–0.03 mg/kg for treatment of osteoarthritic pain in cats. *J Feline Med Surg*, 10(3): 235–241.

Johnston, S. A., Conzemius, M. G., Cross, A. R., *et al.* (2001) A multi-center clinical study of the effect of deracoxib, a COX-2 selective drug, on chronic pain in dogs with osteoarthritis (abstract). *Vet Surg*, 30: 497.

Lascelles, B. D. X., Cripps, P. J., Jones, A., *et al.* (1998) Efficacy and kinetics of carprofen, administered preoperatively or postoperatively, on the prevention of pain in dogs undergoing ovariohysterectomy. *Vet Surg*, 27: 568–582.

Mathews, K. A. and Dyson, D. (2001) *The Safety and Efficacy of Pre-operative Administration of Meloxicam or Carprofen to Dogs or Cats Undergoing Various Orthopedic Procedures.* 26th Congress of the World Small Animal Veterinary Association, Vancouver, British Columbia, 11 August 2001.

Mathews, K. A., Paley, D. M., Foster, R. F. *et al.* (1996) A comparison of ketorolac with flunixin, butorphanol, and oxymorphone in controlling postoperative pain in dogs. *Can Vet J*, 37: 557–567.

Mathews, K. A., Pettifer, G., Foster, R. and McDonell, W. (2001) A comparison of the safety and efficacy of meloxicam to ketoprofen or butorphanol for control of post-operative pain associated with soft tissue surgery in dogs. *Am J Vet Res*, 62(6): 882–888.

Punke, J. P., Speas, A. L., Reynolds, L. R. and Budsberg, S. C. (2008) Effects of firocoxib, meloxicam, and tepoxalin on prostanoid and leukotriene production by duodenal mucosa and other tissues of osteoarthritic dogs. *Am J Vet Res*, 69(9): 1203–1209.

Slingsby, L. S. and Waterman-Pearson, A. E. (1998) Comparison of pethidine, buprenorphine and ketoprofen for postoperative analgesia after ovariohysterectomy in the cat. *Vet Rec*, 143: 185–189.

Slingsby, L. S. and Waterman-Pearson, A. E. (2002) Comparison between meloxicam and carprofen for postoperative analgesia after feline ovariohysterectomy. *J Small Anim Pract*, 43: 286–289.

Wood, A. J. J. (2001) The coxibs, selective inhibitors of cyclooxygenase-2 (review). *N Engl J Med*, 345(6): 433–442.

12

Pharmacologic and Clinical Principles of Adjunct Analgesia
Karol Mathews and Tamara Grubb

Analgesia, usually provided by opioids and non-steroidal anti-inflammatory analgesics (NSAIAs), can be enhanced by other classes of medication that have a different primary role but with a pharmacological mechanism of action that supports their analgesic actions [1, 2]. The integrative techniques are also important in the management of pain. Refer to Chapter 15 for details. There are several mechanisms of nociceptive transmission and the opioid receptors, and NSAIA "targets" are not the only "targets" that can be blocked to reduce the pain experience. Refer to Chapters 2–4 for further information. As the mechanisms and, therefore, targets to block nociceptive transmission differ with each of these medications, these are discussed under each drug. Adjunct analgesic methods/medications added to standard opioid and NSAIA analgesia has gained popularity in veterinary medicine; however, there are few veterinary clinical trials assessing efficacy [3, 4]. Adjunctive analgesics are frequently used in combination with other analgesics to confer a synergistic effect in a multi-modal regimen or to facilitate lower drug dosages to reduce adverse effects. As an example, lidocaine, ketamine or gabapentin may be used to reduce the opioid requirement, and/or complement the regimen, by blocking nociception at different sites, resulting in a synergistic effect [1]. Case reports, clinical experience and understanding the mechanism of action, supports their role as adjuncts to the opioids and NSAIAs. In addition to the known or potential benefit, these drugs have a minimal adverse effect profile. Magnesium has been reported to be a potential adjunct; however, based on human clinical reports, this has not proved to be clinically effective and, in fact, is associated with adverse effects (see Section VI).

As oral drugs may have to be compounded to facilitate appropriate dosing, enquire as to whether xylitol is used in preparation as some compounded drugs for human patients contain xylitol (e.g. gabapentin). Xylitol can be toxic to dogs and cats, especially when administered on a continuing basis, or with multiple products containing xylitol. Discuss the potential of another compounding agent with the pharmacist. As an example, where less than the smallest capsule of 100 mg of gabapentin is required, ask the compounding pharmacy to suspend gabapentin 200 mg/mL in an oil base chicken flavour. Dogs and cats really like chicken flavour. Also, with this high concentration, the dose volume is very small.

(Dr. Robin Downing Personal communication with KM)

Analgesia and Anesthesia for the Ill or Injured Dog and Cat, First Edition. Karol A. Mathews, Melissa Sinclair, Andrea M. Steele and Tamara Grubb.
© 2018 John Wiley & Sons, Inc. Published 2018 by John Wiley & Sons, Inc.

Table 12.1 Adjunct Analgesics.

Drugs currently used as adjuncts	Primary function
Lidocaine systemically	Regional and local anesthetic
Alpha$_2$-adrenergic agonists	Sedative analgesic
Ketamine low dose	General anesthetic
Gabapentin	Anticonvulsant
Amitriptyline	Antidepressant
Amantadine	Antiviral and dopaminergic (Parkinson therapy)

I. Injectable Adjunctive Analgesics

A. Lidocaine

Lidocaine is primarily used for local anesthetic blocks (refer to Chapter 14). However, it is also used as an infusion during anesthesia to reduce the inhalant required to maintain anesthesia. The infusion is also efficacious in a multi-modal analgesic regimen in non-anesthetic situations. It may be necessary to discontinue at, or before, 24 h as nausea has been observed at this time. Conversely, the infusion is often administered for several days in dogs with ongoing pain that have no adverse effects from the infusion.

1. Indications

In addition to the local anesthetic effects, lidocaine has been shown to alleviate neuropathic pain and hyperalgesia and to reduce opioid requirements following surgery when administered as a continuous rate infusion (CRI) [5]. A CRI can be used intraoperatively to reduce the inhalant requirements or post-operatively in combination with opioids and ketamine for the severely painful patient. One veterinary study reports lidocaine 1.0 mg/kg IV (intravenous) bolus followed by 0.025 mg/kg/minute (1.5 mg/kg/h) IV CRI administered to dogs intra- and post-operatively, having similar efficacy to morphine 0.15 mg/kg IV bolus followed by 0.1 mg/kg/h IV CRI [6]. In a more recent study where lidocaine was used alone, 40 healthy dogs undergoing soft tissue or orthopedic procedures were equally divided between two groups, one receiving lidocaine and the other saline placebo [7]. Following buprenorphine and acepromazine premedication, propofol induction and maintained with isoflurane, an initial 2 mg/kg lidocaine dose administered over 5 min, was followed by 50 μg/kg/min infusion, increasing up to 100 or 150 μg/kg/min for dogs undergoing soft tissue procedures and up to 200 μg/kg/min for dogs undergoing orthopedic procedures. Intraoperative fentanyl was required in 4/20 dogs receiving lidocaine compared with 11/21 dogs in the control group. These lidocaine dosages did not result in clinically significant hemodynamic instability. Isoflurane was maintained at 1.15 ± 0.1 vol% in all cases [7]. However, in this study enrolling healthy dogs, the indirect blood pressure measurement was lower (70 mmHg) and heart rate higher in the lidocaine group at the 200 min point and is assumed to be at the highest lidocaine dose. While not noted in this report, at the higher intraoperative dosages, the author has noted nausea and vomiting in the post-anesthetic setting. Therefore, based on current recommendations, the benefits of lidocaine are best demonstrated at lower dosages than those reported in this study and in a multi-modal regimen, including an opioid with ketamine where indicated.

Lidocaine CRI has an isoflurane minimum alveolar concentration (MAC) sparing effect in dogs; however, in cats laboratory studies have not shown benefit with tail clamp and thermal threshold as a nociceptive stimulus at dosages not associated with adverse effects. See Section I.A.5.

A recent review of human patients receiving lidocaine administered at doses ~1.5 mg/kg^{-1} of body weight as bolus and ~2 mg/kg^{-1}/h^{-1} as continuous infusion intraoperatively did not produce relevant clinical side effects in the investigated cohort of participants; however, no conclusions could be made regarding the tolerability in patients with compromised liver or renal function [8]. The review demonstrated that patients undergoing any elective surgery under general anesthesia who received perioperative IV lidocaine have slightly lower pain scores at 1–4 h after surgery compared with those receiving a control treatment, despite having received the same post-operative access to opioid analgesia. A slowly declining benefit occurred over the following 24 h. At 48 h after surgery, there was no benefit with respect to pain relief. A subgroup analysis suggested that best benefit in the level of pain reduction and the duration of pain relief is for patients undergoing laparoscopic and open abdominal surgery. In addition, opioid requirements and opioid-related side effects (nausea, vomiting) during the postoperative phase were lower among patients who received IV lidocaine intraoperatively. From a gastrointestinal (GI) perspective, the other positive effects of systemic lidocaine were a reduction of postoperative ileus, time to first flatus and bowel movement/sounds; however, the time to first defecation was no different between groups [8].

In addition to the analgesic effects, lidocaine may be useful in managing patients in the following situations, while also conferring some associated analgesia:

- Lidocaine may be useful in managing head trauma patients during periods of increasing intracranial pressure (ICP), such as occurs during vomiting or "gagging". Lidocaine has been reported to lower ICP during endotracheal intubation. Refer to Chapter 3, Section VIII.
- Lidocaine has been shown to be neuroprotective following a cerebral ischemic event in laboratory animals by limiting the expansion of infarction. Refer to Chapter 3, Section VIII.
- Lidocaine 1.5 mg/kg/h (25 μg/kg/minute) may be used as an adjunctive analgesic where bowel motility is a concern. Refer to Chapter 4.
- The pain of renal colic in human patients was relieved more effectively with lidocaine 1.5 mg/kg than morphine. Refer to Chapter 4.
- Lidocaine also has some anti-inflammatory and anti-microbial effect.

2. Mode of Action

When lidocaine is applied to nerves voltage-gated sodium channels, present in nociceptive fibres (A-delta and C fibres), are blocked, whereas lidocaine administered IV causes a selective central blockade of C fibre activity, because the concentration of lidocaine is proportionally less when administered IV than when it is infiltrated near a nerve. Other mechanisms for the analgesic action involves antagonistic actions at the muscarinic and N-methyl-D-aspartate (NMDA) receptor, inhibition of glycine, reduction in the production of excitatory amino acids, neurokinins and thromboxane A2, release of endogenous opioids and adenosine triphosphate [9], which makes lidocaine effective for treatment of several types of pain, including neuropathic pain. While it focuses on horses, Doherty's article is an excellent overview on the mechanism of action and clinical use [9].

3. Adverse Effects

The author (KM) has noted nausea in some dogs at 18–24 h of infusion at dosages recommended below. Therefore, careful observation is required in order to reduce, or discontinue, the infusion where the very early signs are noted. Lidocaine overdose may predispose to seizure activity. In anesthetized dogs, higher doses than those used in conscious states can be used because general anesthesia is protective against central nervous system (CNS) excitation from local anesthetics. In cats, the risk of toxicity is higher, which is probably related to altered liver metabolism of lidocaine and direct action on the CNS and cardiovascular system [10].

Cardiovascular effects may also occur in both cats and dogs, which include prolonged conduction of cardiac impulse, bradycardia and other arrhythmias; therefore, lidocaine is contraindicated in patients with third-degree atrioventricular (AV) block. Hypotension and potentially asystole may also occur. Rapid IV administration of local anesthetics frequently decreases vascular tone and myocardial contractility, resulting in the acute onset of hypotension.

Human patients reported adverse effects, potentially associated with lidocaine, including tingling or paresthesia, blurred vision and visual hallucinations. Symptoms resolved spontaneously or with dose reduction; none of the adverse effects resulted in discontinuation of the infusion [11]. Desensitization of the mouth and pharyngeal area has also been reported. In veterinary patients, strange behaviour may be reflective of a similar experience.

4. Administration to Dogs

Lidocaine has a short elimination half-life which requires a CRI for effective steady plasma concentrations. For prolonged infusions of more than 8–12 h, it is recommended to lower the CRI to avoid toxicity from accumulation, nausea and vomiting, and the potential signs noted above in humans.

- Dogs: 1–2 mg/kg, IV (give over 2–5 min) followed by 1 up to 3 mg/kg/h in combination with an opioid ± ketamine.

5. Administration to Cats

Lidocaine is used as a treatment for ventricular tachycardia (VT), with specific criteria, in both cats and dogs. Recommendations for cats, with VT: a lidocaine slow push 0.25–1 mg/kg (over 5 min), repeat if needed then, if lidocaine responsive, establish a CRI of 10–20 μg/kg/min. However, when used systemically for analgesic purposes, lidocaine infusion in cats is controversial with the suggestion that it is appropriate at the **dosages** used below in a standard multimodal regimen [12], and evidence shows that adverse effects at higher bolus (~3 mg/kg) dosages required to reduce MAC under isoflurane anesthesia may limit its use [10, 13, 14].

Laboratory studies investigating efficacy and safety indicate that lidocaine 2 mg/kg in **healthy** isoflurane-anesthetized cats had a minimal MAC sparing effect in a thermal test model [10]. In another study, a lidocaine plasma-target infusion administered to healthy cats that reached a high concentration equivalent to a bolus of ~3.4 mg/kg had an isoflurane MAC sparing effect. However, the adverse cardiovascular effects, including a low cardiac output and increase in vascular resistance associated with this high MAC reduction dosage, provided no benefit for the use of lidocaine [13]. As the goal for balanced anesthesia is improved hemodynamics, based on the cardiovascular effects noted in this study, the conclusions were that the use of lidocaine for balanced anesthesia in cats is not recommended. However, Dr Bruno Pypendop (KM, personal communication) notes that the **dosages** given below are appropriate for a multimodal regimen and adverse effects may not be experienced.

In a conscious **healthy** cat model, lidocaine 2 mg/kg administered IV did not affect thermal anti-nociception and, therefore, was not effective in this model [14]. There are no studies assessing the efficacy of lidocaine administered to conscious cats in the clinical setting.

Dosing is based on ideal body weight in the overweight patient. While there are no clinical studies assessing efficacy of lidocaine in cats, anecdotally its benefits have been recognized when combined with an opioid and ketamine for severe painful procedures or medical conditions. In this setting, the author (TG) administers an initial lidocaine 0.25 mg/kg bolus, then continues with 10–20 μg/kg/min in combination with other drugs (e.g. opioids, ketamine) for selective, painful surgical procedures and for GI pain in select patients.

Dr Bonnie Wright (personal communication with KM) notes that lidocaine is a valuable analgesic across species, but in deference to the data that shows reduced cardiac function when used during anesthesia at the bolus dosing to reduce MAC, and a lack of solid evidence of the level of benefit that it provides when used alone, it is only utilized as an add-on to very difficult feline cases, rather than as a standard intraoperative protocol. More commonly it is used in a multi-modal regimen in the awake cat, where pain is difficult to control, with a combination of opioid, NSAIA and ketamine, and/or where GI motility is poor; although Dr Wright notes that eating is a stronger modifier of motility where the cat has an interest in eating. Also noted is that lidocaine IV appears to inhibit appetite in some cases. In summary, Dr Wright states that, in her experience, lidocaine 1 mg/kg loading, and generally 25 µg/kg/min (1.5 mg/kg/h) as a CRI can be used in cats following which the analgesic effect is noted, but it should be a deliberate, thoughtful and careful addition, with a good understanding of the drug and involve monitoring of the patient.

Dr Bob Stein uses similar dosing, 0.6 mg/kg/h in combination with fentanyl, and ketamine at 1 mg/kg/h CRI, for essentially all feline surgical patients. For the more painful surgical procedures, the lidocaine infusion is commenced at 3 mg/kg/h for the intraoperative period with dose reduction to 1–1.5 mg/kg/h for up to 9 h of **total** use. At these dosages, in cats with no cardiovascular concerns, no adverse effects have been noted over a period of more than 12 years, and the overall clinical benefit associated with these regimens appears to have been very good.

The author (KM) has added lidocaine 0.25–0.5 mg/kg slow push followed by this dose as an hourly CRI for 6–8 h added to fentanyl, ± ketamine, in traumatic brain-injured cats as a neuroprotectant and to lower opioid use to reduce ileus and vomiting. In this setting it is essential to ensure that CO_2 remains within normal limits.

Based on the mechanism of action of lidocaine noted above, and these anecdotal reports, there appears to be a potential benefit for lidocaine administration in cats, but at this time it has not been confirmed in clinical trials and the adverse cardiovascular effects are concerning. However, while monitoring for potential adverse effects, should lidocaine facilitate a lowering of an opioid, improve intestinal motility, be of benefit where abdominal pain exists, hopefully, future studies will be conducted to confirm this.

Keeping in mind that pain is an individual experience, as are drug effects, the importance of monitoring the individual patient for both should be emphasized.

6. Lidocaine Patches

Pharmacokinetic studies in dogs indicate potential as an adjunct to an opioid and/or an NSAIA [15].

B. Ketamine [16–18]

1. Indications

Ketamine is an adjunctive analgesic recommended for use in a multi-modal regimen for treatment of severe pain. The analgesic dose is much lower than that used for anesthesia (refer to Chapter 13). Ketamine has been reported to effectively reduce the requirements for opioids post-operatively, reducing potential adverse effects associated with higher dosages of this class of analgesics when managing severe pain. Dosages are based on severity of pain and titrated to effect after an opioid, ± an NSAIA, has proved insufficient, or may be used in any painful setting to reduce the dosages of opioids and NSAIAs and, therefore, their associated adverse effects. While opioid requirements may not be reduced, two veterinary studies have shown improved behaviour following surgery. During and following forelimb amputation, dogs receiving an IV bolus of 0.5 mg/kg prior to surgery, 0.6 mg/kg/h during surgery and 0.12 mg/kg/h for 18 h following surgery had significantly lower pain scores and were more active on day three [19]. Female dogs undergoing mastectomy showed improved eating behaviour after receiving an

IV bolus of 0.15 mg/kg or 0.7 mg/kg followed by 0.6 mg/kg/h CRI [20]. While not used as an analgesic in this setting, ketamine 5 mg/kg can be sprayed onto the mucous membranes of the mouth of the "bad", that is unapproachable, cat. Warning: humans report a terrible taste! This will slow down but not anesthetize the cat so as soon as the cat can be handled, administer an opioid or sedative as the situation requires.

2. Mode of Action

The main mode action of ketamine as an analgesic, or anti-hyperalgesic, is due to:

- antagonism of the NMDA receptor. The NMDA receptor is activated by excitatory amino acids, such as glutamate and aspartate, which leads to an increase in intracellular calcium and activation of second messengers, which stimulate protein kinases and modify neuronal excitability, leading to central sensitization, acute opioid tolerance and opioid-induced hyperalgesia. In addition to NMDA receptor antagonism, ketamine may also abolish established central sensitization [21]. Ketamine's dose-based differences in the mechanism of NMDA receptor blockade demonstrate the analgesic (and also in humans and laboratory animals anti-depressant) properties of ketamine at low levels, both of benefit for many ill or injured patients, and the anesthetic effects at much higher dosages.
- Ketamine also has a direct weak affinity for the opioid receptors, $\mu < \kappa < \delta$, contributing some weak analgesia via this mechanism [21].
- Other analgesic actions are related to enhancement of descending inhibitory systems by inhibition of re-uptake of norepinephrine and serotonin, as well as inhibition of nitric-oxide synthase [22].
- The activity of the inhibitory pathway is approximately 50% lower in animals with neuropathic lesions when compared to normal controls, with reduced opioid receptor function and efficacy of both intrathecal or IV administered morphine. Reduced inhibition increases the likelihood that the dorsal horn neuron will fire spontaneously or more energetically to primary afferent input [22]. The decreased responsiveness to morphine was prevented by pre-treatment of laboratory animals with an NMDA-receptor antagonist, such as ketamine.

3. Additional Properties of Ketamine that Indirectly Contribute to Patient Comfort

- Bronchodilation and diminishing vagal tone due to ketamine's interactions with cholinergic receptors [23].
- The anti-inflammatory action [16] of ketamine is of importance in the ill or injured patient, where inflammation can be a major component of ongoing pain. Ketamine has anti-pro-inflammatory effects, preventing exacerbation of inflammation, but also modulating inflammation when already initiated. The immunomodulatory effects of ketamine are only described in "the presence of immune-stimulation without being immunosuppressive". In the absence of a stress situation, ketamine has no effect on cytokine balance. Ketamine's anti-inflammatory effects include reducing release of TNF-α, interleukin 6 (IL-6) and IL-8, suppressing NF-κβ expression and stabilizing neutrophil activation. These actions have been observed in vitro, in animal models and in human patients. The survival rate of patients with septic shock in the intensive care unit was improved when they received ketamine as a sedative. These properties make ketamine a very useful adjunctive analgesic for surgical procedures and for painful conditions associated with inflammation (e.g. pancreatitis and trauma). These anti-pro-inflammatory effects noted at dosages of 0.25 mg/kg, occurred without impeding the local healing processes.
- Ketamine is also reported to alleviate visceral inflammatory pain in human pediatric patients with fulminating ulcerative colitis where opioids and NSAIAs were contraindicated [24].
- Gastric emptying and intestinal motility in dogs enrolled in a laboratory study were not affected by ketamine 3 to < 30 mg/kg/h. This is in contrast to the opioids where GI motility is affected to some degree [25].

- Ketamine's sympathomimetic effects may be of benefit in some critical cases to aid in the maintenance of heart rate and cardiac output.
- Neuroprotection is another potential benefit of ketamine administration as it is safe and, as a non-competitive inhibitor of the NMDA receptor, may actually protect against further ischemic and glutamate-induced injury when managing pain in a head-injured patient. Earlier studies have reported increased ICP following ketamine administration in patients with reduced intracranial compliance; however, this has since been re-evaluated identifying an increased CO_2 as the cause of increased ICP [26]. Refer to Chapter 3 for details.
- Ketamine's anti-hyperalgesic property [21] is also used to treat opioid-induced hyperalgesia reported in humans but not yet in veterinary patients. However, the author (KM) has noted this in a dog with severe pre-operative neuropathic pain compounded by spinal surgery. The crying progressed to thrashing during careful titration of morphine to manage the pain. This was a very different reaction from a dysphoric response. Careful titration of ketamine, to effect a comfortable plane of analgesia, facilitated sleep.

4. Adverse Effects

Ketamine also has a sympathomimetic action with the potential for increasing heart rate. Should a cat with hypertrophic cardiomyopathy experience a ketamine-induced tachycardia, there is potential for left ventricular outflow tract obstruction. Patients with cardiac tachyarrhythmia may also experience a further increase in heart rate. However, at the low analgesic dosages, this may not occur and heart rate monitoring will identify a potential problem. The ketamine-induced impact on seizures is still somewhat unclear. Ketamine may rarely exacerbate certain types of seizures through sympathetic nervous stimulation but does not precipitate spontaneous seizure activity and is used in humans to treat refractory seizure activity. This has also proven effective in dogs [27]. While a history of seizures in a patient may preclude ketamine use at anesthetic doses, the low dosages used in a CRI are unlikely to be a problem and are commonly used by the author (TG) in patients with seizure history. The sympathetic stimulation produced by ketamine may induce hyperglycemia, potentially making glucose monitoring difficult in diabetic patients. For patients with kidney, liver and cardiac dysfunction, and in severe pain, it may be essential to include low-dose ketamine CRI, in addition to an opioid, to control pain. Frequent assessment and tailoring the ketamine dose based on the individual patient's response and analgesic requirement will reduce the potential for adverse effects.

5. Dosing

Ketamine 0.2–1.0 mg/kg titrated to effect, followed by the effective dose as an hourly CRI. Where severe pain/hyperalgesia is present, higher dosages will be required; therefore, titration to effect is necessary to deliver the appropriate dose. From experience, this mg/kg "effective dose" can be used as an hourly infusion to maintain the analgesic effect. Ketamine has a relatively short elimination half-life (1–1.6 h) [28]; therefore, the analgesic effect of a single low dose will be short-lived, requiring a CRI to maintain analgesia. Depending on duration of the infusion, weaning over 12–24 h is essential to prevent rebound hyperalgesia.

As ketamine is eliminated via the kidney in cats and the liver in dogs, caution is required when administering to cats with kidney dysfunction and dogs with liver dysfunction.

In addition to IV, ketamine administration in human patients may be administered by intramuscular (IM) (93% bioavailability (BA)), rectal (25% BA), subcutaneous, transdermal and oral (20% BA) and intranasal (50% BA) routes for treatment of chronic pain, or in battlefield emergencies.

Where NMDA receptor blockade is required for ongoing pain management at home, amantadine (see Section II.A) can be administered during weaning down of ketamine. Refer to Chapter 3 for further details.

C. Alpha$_2$ Adrenergic Agonists (Alpha$_2$ Agonists)

Drugs in this group of sedative analgesics are frequently used for chemical restraint, sedation, pre-medication and as adjuncts in managing pain in veterinary patients to reduce opioid requirements. Medetomidine was the primary alpha$_2$ agonist used for several years; however, dexmedetomidine is currently most commonly used. Refer to Chapter 9 for further details.

1. Dexmedetomidine

i. Indications

In this context, it is administered where an opioid-sparing effect is required, as examples:

- Traumatic brain injury (TBI), meningitis, spinal injury, especially where frequent neurologic assessment is required, in otherwise healthy animals [29, 30]. Refer to Chapter 3 for details on use and benefits.
- Always use the lowest effective dose.
- Where additional sedation is required for cats and dogs.
- Particularly useful in anxious painful patients.
- As a routine premedicant or sedative in patients undergoing painful procedures. The analgesic and sedative effects are synergistic with those provided by opioids.

ii. Mode of Action

As agonists of alpha$_2$-adrenergic receptors in the dorsal horn of the spinal cord and locus coeruleus in the brain stem.

iii. Dose

Can be given IM or IV and requires 15 min for the drug to reach the peak effect (leave the animal undisturbed). The drug produces a more consistent effect when it is administered IV with an opioid

- As an adjunct, dexmedetomidine 0.5–1 µg/kg is administered as a 15 min loading dose IV followed by 0.5–1 µg/kg/h CRI, conferring good analgesia with minimal cardiovascular effects at these doses and rates in stabilized patients.
- CRI: 1–3 µg/kg/h combined with an opioid in stable but difficult to physically manage painful animals.
- For other scenarios, refer to Chapter 9 or see the dosing chart in the dexmedetomidine product insert.

iv. Adverse Effects

Vasoconstriction causes increased cardiac work, making the use of this drug class contraindicated in patients with most forms of cardiac disease. Also, due to increased urine volumes, do not use in patients with ureteral/urethral obstruction and cystic calculi unless a urinary catheter can be placed to allow elimination of urine. When used in diabetic patients, frequent glucose monitoring is required. Changes to uterine activity, decreased intestinal motility, decreased intraocular pressure may occur, although these effects rarely, if ever, cause a clinical impact. As with most sedatives and anesthetic drugs, alpha$_2$ agonists can contribute to hypothermia.

Notes on using alpha$_2$ agonists
- Alpha$_2$ agonists commonly cause bradycardia. Bradycardia can be treated with an anticholinergic if the patient is bradycardic AND hypotensive. However, do not treat the bradycardia noted (35–55 bpm commonly) with an anticholinergic unless the bradycardia is contributing to hypotension, as vasoconstriction plus tachycardia will increase cardiac work. If you are

concerned about the bradycardia in a sedated (non-anesthetized) animal that is normotensive, reverse the dexmedetomidine.

- Animals that appear to be very sedated may (rarely)become 'vicious' if suddenly approached or if a painful procedure is initiated (eg, painful ear cleaning). Approach and handle the patient carefully and assess the "sedation" to make sure it is real.
- Intermittent spastic jaw tone, muscle twitching and tail wagging can make some procedures more difficult.
- Veins and arteries may be more difficult to access in some animals due to the alpha$_2$-induced vasoconstriction. Monitoring with pulse oximetry and blood pressure equipment may also be difficult due to the vasoconstriction.
- Gray mucus membranes are often produced due to vasoconstriction and venous desaturation secondary to low cardiac output and to an over-abundance of alpha$_2$ receptors in the skin and mucous membranes, resulting in localized but profound vasoconstriction and reduced blood flow in these areas. Oxygen supplementation is advised.
- Vomiting can occur following administration; however, in the author's experience, this has not been a concern with such small doses.

Caution: When used at higher dosages than those recommended or in normal dosages in patients with cardiovascular disease, profound cardiac output depression, bradycardia and vasoconstriction can occur, and cause impaired perfusion.

v. Reversal

Atipamezole (one-half of or the same volume as dexmedetomidine used) administered IM, SC or very slow titration IV to effect for a desired level of reversal. Where a reversal agent is not used, animals appear to recover from the sedative effects in 2h and eat and act normally at this time. However, the analgesic effect is much shorter than the sedative effect, approximately 1h.

D. Maropitant

Maropitant is a central anti-emetic indicated for the prevention and treatment of acute canine and feline vomiting, which is a feature of many illnesses and a potential problem upon anesthetic induction and recovery alone, or following surgery. Based on the mechanism of action, maropitant also has some anti-nociceptive properties. Maropitant administered as an infusion decreased the anesthetic requirements during visceral stimulation of the ovary and ovarian ligament in dogs, suggesting the potential role for neurokinin-1 (NK-1) receptor antagonists to manage ovarian and visceral pain [31].

Also, the stress associated with nausea and vomiting contributes to the pain experience.

1. Indication

Anti-emetic prophylaxis, and treatment for nausea and vomiting. Should not be used as an analgesic but to be aware that there is some anti-nociceptive action which may contribute to some degree of analgesia, especially in patients with GI pain.

2. Mode of Action

Blocks NK-1 receptors in the emetic centre of the brain, the chemoreceptor trigger zone (CTZ) and the vagal afferents. The analgesic effects of maropitant work through a blockade of Substance-P binding to the NK-1 receptor, which is involved in pain processing throughout the peripheral and central nervous systems (refer to Chapter 2). However, the complete pain-modifying effect of maropitant remains uncertain but appears to have some effect on visceral pain (refer to Chapter 4).

3. Dosing

- Dogs: 1–2 mg/kg IV **very slowly** or SC q24h for up to five consecutive days.
- Cats: 1 mg/kg SC q24h up to five consecutive days.
- Use with caution, or not at all, in patients with hepatic dysfunction.

4. Adverse Effects

- Histological evidence of bone marrow hypoplasia was seen at higher frequency and greater severity in puppies younger than 11 weeks of age treated with Cerenia® than in control puppies. In puppies 16 weeks and older, bone marrow hypoplasia was not seen.
- Rarely, diarrhea, hematochezia.

II. Oral Adjunctive Analgesics

The reader is directed to an excellent in-depth review of this topic by KuKanich [2].

A. Amantadine

Amantadine has been used clinically in humans for the treatment of Parkinson disease, as an antiviral drug and antidepressant, especially when associated with neuropathic pain.

1. Indications and Considerations

Amantadine is not an effective analgesic when used alone. Amantadine's role is in the patient with established pain and is used in combination with NSAIAs, opioids or gabapentin/pregabalin, where it appears to enhance their analgesic effects. It can be incorporated into a chronic pain management regimen or, where acute or chronic neuropathic pain exists/suspected, it can be introduced during weaning of ketamine in the acute setting in preparation for discharge home with an NSAIA and/or gabapentin, and where TBI exists [32]. Refer to Chapter 3 for further information.

Comments: Amantadine 3–5 mg/kg q24h added to meloxicam in dogs with osteoarthritis noted a significant improvement at 21 days [3]. A degree of improvement likely occurred prior to the 21-day assessment. Based on the 5 h half-life, recommendations for q12h dosing is recommended for both cats [33] and dogs [34] which may result in noticeable analgesia earlier.

No controlled clinical trials are available for amantadine use in cats; however, where chronic pain exists dosing is similar to that for dogs [35].

2. Mode of Action

Mode of action is an NMDA antagonist that stabilizes these channels in the closed state rather than block as ketamine does, thus conferring its safety profile. Due to amantadine's similar mechanism of action to that of ketamine, it has potential for preventing the adverse effects of NMDA receptor activation. Amantadine also increases CNS dopamine concentration; it is this aspect of the drug that is prescribed for Parkinson disease.

- In dogs, amantadine 2.8–5 mg/kg appears to be well absorbed with approximately 10% metabolized to N-methyl-amantadine, with a terminal half-life of 5 h and completely eliminated within 24 h. No reports are available assessing the potential activity of the metabolite [36].
- In cats, after 5 mg/kg, there is a high oral BA and a half-life of approximately 5.5 h [33].

3. Adverse Effects

Adverse effects from amantadine in humans include dry mouth, drowsiness, hallucinations, excitation, irritation, dizziness, dyskinesia and loss of hair. High anxiety, restlessness and dry mouth may occur up to 6 mg/kg or, if there is renal impairment, at lower dosages. Potential adverse effects are agitation and diarrhoea during the initial use of the drug. As amantadine is > 90% eliminated via the kidney, any reduction in renal function may lead to adverse effects [36]. Obstructive uropathy, associated with seizure activity, with amantadine overdose has been reported in a human [37]. Combination with other drugs will also influence toxicity of amantadine; therefore, interactions with current prescribed drugs must be investigated prior to recommending amantadine. Behavioural effects in dogs and cats have been reported at 15 mg/kg [38].

Clinical safety studies have not specifically been reported for amantadine in dogs or cats; therefore, dosages should not be increased above those below until further studies in the clinical setting have been performed.

4. Dosing

3–5 mg/kg q12–24h both cats and dogs. It is recommended that dosages higher than this not be used until further studies can establish safe limits at higher dosing in the clinical setting. Amantadine is excreted via the kidneys requiring careful monitoring and potential extended duration between dosing when used in animals with decreased renal function. The palatability of amantadine has a reputation of being "awful", so trying to administer a second dose is almost impossible. Compounding with a chicken-flavoured vehicle may help for dosing when the dose required is less than available in capsule form.

B. Gabapentin

Gabapentin's primary mode of action is as an anticonvulsant but it also has anti-nociceptive and anti-hyperalgesic properties [1, 2]. Gabapentin is prescribed for chronic neuropathic pain and fibromyalgia in humans [39]. The perioperative administration of gabapentin in humans is effective in reducing pain scores, opioid requirements and opioid-related adverse effects in the first 24h after surgery [40, 41]. The addition of gabapentin appears to be of greater benefit in those with severe pain and high opioid requirements [42], which is an appropriate use for adjunctive analgesic drugs [1]. Also, in human patients, it has a well-established role in the treatment of chronic pain, in particular for neuropathic pain of all causes, including diabetic neuropathy. Refer to Chapter 3. Gabapentin shows no significant benefit in situations of mild pain [42]. Also, gabapentin is not expected to be effective in preventing acute, rapidly transient pain; therefore, the lack of analgesic efficacy in the acute thermal experimental models cannot be extrapolated to lack of efficacy for clinical use. In addition to the model, or clinical problem, an appropriate dose must be used. In addition to the analgesic properties, gabapentin is effective for the treatment of itching produced by burns and wound healing in children [43].

Gabapentin is being used to manage pain more frequently in veterinary patients as case reports [44, 45] and the anecdotal benefits are being realized [35].

1. Indications

Anecdotal evidence appears to indicate its value in managing chronic and neuropathic pain in dogs and cats in a multi-modal regimen and continued as a sole analgesic in some patients. Follow-up assessment is essential to ensure it is effective and to manage the dose to avoid adverse effects. Case reports have suggested that gabapentin produced desirable effects in managing traumatic and orthopedic pain in cats [44]. Conditions where gabapentin is indicated:

- In dogs and cats suffering from neuropathic pain secondary to cervical or thoracolumbar intervertebral disc disease, or spinal column or pelvic trauma. The chronic neuropathic pain associated with feline onychectomy appears to be responsive to high dosages of gabapentin (Dr K. St. Denis, personal communication with KM). Initially, gabapentin is administered in combination with an opioid and/or an NSAIA, but gradually these drugs can be tapered off and gabapentin may remain the sole method of analgesia. There is an extremely wide dose range for gabapentin and it should be given to effect. The dose limiting effect generally observed is sedation, which tends to subside after a period of time. Frequently, some animals need several weeks or even months, if ever, for resolution of their pain requiring continuing analgesia.
- Peri-operative in addition to an opioid, ± an NSAIA, where neural tissue is involved or chronic pain/ hyperalgesia is established prior to surgery.
- Following cardiopulmonary arrest or seizures for animals that are extremely restless, disoriented, vocalizing and/or manic, the author (KM) has found gabapentin useful in treating these patients. Dosing to effect and resolution of these signs is the goal. Sedation in this instance is appropriate! Careful lowering of the drug is recommended.
- The discomfort of pruritus associated with burn wounds is reported to be alleviated following the addition of gabapentin at dosages given below, usually starting at 10 mg/kg q8h [42].

2. Mode of Action

Gabapentin reduces the stimulated release of excitatory neurotransmitters by binding at calcium channel alpha$_2$-delta (Ca-a$_2$δ) proteins blocking the development of hyperalgesia and central sensitization [46]. The Ca-a$_2$δ nomenclature is used to avoid confusion with unrelated adrenergic alpha-receptors. As an example, prolonged central sensitization manifesting as hyperalgesia does occur after surgical trauma. When administered pre-operatively, gabapentin reduces hyper-excitability of secondary nociceptive neurons in the dorsal horn preventing central sensitization.

3. Adverse Effects

Adverse effects of gabapentin can include sedation and ataxia, which are more likely to occur when administered at higher dosages or when combined with other drugs that produce similar adverse effects. This tends to subside over time. As with any chronically administered analgesic, tapering off is essential to avoid a rebound hyperalgesia. If the patient was receiving gabapentin as an anti-epileptic, rebound seizures could occur. It is suggested to taper the dose over the course of at least one week, and potentially longer following prolonged administration.

Comments: As pain is an individual experience, as is the underlying cause, it is expected that pain experienced from direct involvement of neural tissue is extremely painful requiring a higher dosage of gabapentin initially than recommended for non-neural involvement. Clinical usage and experience with various scenarios and pharmacokinetic studies are assisting with recommendations for prescribing. As examples,

- a study of post-limb amputation in dogs showed no benefit with a dose of gabapentin 5 mg/kg q12h for three days [47].

- Another canine study examining efficacy of gabapentin 10 mg/kg q12h added to an opioid post intervertebral disc surgery, reported no detectable reduction in pain behaviour compared to the control group receiving opioid analgesia alone, although a trend to lower pain levels was present.
- However, a case series reported significant improvement with gabapentin 6.5 mg/kg q12h for long-term management of musculoskeletal pain, or following head trauma, in three cats [44].

These reports highlight the need for individual dosing based on the underlying cause of pain. With more information from pharmacokinetic studies, the dosing and frequency must be increased for the neuropathic pain associated with these conditions.

4. Dosing

The terminal half-life of gabapentin in dogs is 3–4 h [48] and cats ~3 h [49]. In general, to maintain therapeutic levels dosing at least every 8 h is required to confer efficacy. A dosage of 10–20 mg/kg every 8 h maintains targeted concentrations in dogs and cats [2]. However, as analgesics are given to effect, and to avoid the potential sedative effects at higher unnecessary dosages, gabapentin's dose will depend on the individual's requirement and should be based on this. Gabapentin exhibits less than proportional increases in plasma concentrations with increasing doses following oral administration because of saturation of active transporters in the GI tract [2]. Dietary macronutrient composition (i.e. protein) may favourably influence gabapentin oral absorption [50].

- Dogs and cats: 5–25+ mg/kg PO, for pain, usually starting at 10 mg/kg q8h. Taper dose and duration up or down to effect. Wean off slowly.
- Post-seizure or post-CPR vocalization and thrashing up to 12 mg/kg PO q6h. Taper dose and duration up or down to effect. Wean off slowly.

   Titration of dosages up to 30 mg/kg q8h have been required to manage arthritic pain, post-onychectomy neuropathic pain and interstitial cystitis in cats, resulting in greater activity and what appears to be pleasant sleep (Dr K. St. Denis, personal communication with KM).

   In the dog, ~40% hepatic metabolism occurs prior to renal elimination, whereas in other species gabapentin is excreted unchanged in the urine [1]. Metabolism/excretion has not been studied in the cat. As dosing to effect is the method by which the appropriate dose is selected, once this effect is reached dosing frequency (q8h or q12h) should be judged in the individual patient with hepatic or renal dysfunction.

   Tapering the dose down is important, as stopping the drug abruptly may lead to rebound pain, which may be severe.

C. Pregabalin

The mechanism of action and adverse effects are similar to those of gabapentin. In addition, visual disturbances including blurred vision, peripheral edema unrelated to changes in blood pressure and angioedema have also been reported in humans. Pharmacokinetic studies suggest a dosage of 4 mg/kg by mouth every 12 h in dogs. No case reports, experimental data or clinical efficacy data are available in dogs or cats [2]. Pregabalin should **not** be administered to pregnant or nursing animals.

III. Tricyclic Antidepressants, Selective Serotonin Reuptake Inhibitors, Monoamine Oxidase Inhibitors

A. Mode of Action

- Tricyclic antidepressants (TCAs), block reuptake of norepinephrine and serotonin at presynaptic membranes, e.g. amitriptyline (Elavil®) and clomipramine (Clomicalm®).
- Selective serotonin reuptake inhibitors (SSRIs) – block reuptake of serotonin at postsynaptic membrane; increase brain serotonin levels, e.g., fluoxetine (Prozac®), paroxetine (Paxil®), sertraline (Zoloft®).
- Monoamine oxidase inhibitors (MAOIs) normally function in the catabolism of CNS neurotransmitters, such as serotonin, dopamine and norepinephrine. The main effect may also be on dopamine in the CNS, e.g. selegiline (Anipryl®), phenelzine (Nardil®).
- Atypical antidepressants – mechanism varies, alteration of neurotransmitter in the CNS, e.g. bupropion (Wellbutrin®), buspirone (Buspar®).

Comments: Abrupt discontinuation of a serotonin reuptake inhibitor (SRI), norepinephrine reuptake inhibitor (NERI) or tricyclic antidepressant (TCA) usually leads to withdrawal, or "discontinuation syndrome", which could include states of anxiety and other symptoms. Tapering is essential.

B. Adverse Effects

Are rare but can occur with a high dose or, more frequently, with combinations of drugs. Combinations of serotonergic drugs acting by different mechanisms are capable of raising intrasynaptic serotonin to a level that is life threatening. The combination that most commonly does this is an MAOI drug combined with any SRI [51].

The mechanism of action varies but the clinical signs are similar; at low doses lethargy is seen, while at higher doses CNS stimulation may occur.

- **TCAs** have a very narrow therapeutic range; signs can be seen at therapeutic doses.
- **SSRIs** may cause mild depression at lower doses; tremors, cardiac effects and or serotonin syndrome possible (see below) at high dosages.
- **MAOIs** may cause vomiting, diarrhea, lethargy, pacing, agitation, seizures and hyper-salivation. Stereotypical behaviour possible after a therapeutic dose, and seen with 3 mg/kg selegiline.
- **Bupropion**: vomiting and depression at 5 mg/kg.

SSRIs and TCAs, in particular, may cause serotonin syndrome, which is manifested as central, autonomic and neuromuscular signs. In descending order of occurrence they include: vomiting, diarrhea, myoclonus, hyper-reflexia, seizures, hyperthermia, hyperesthesia, depression, mydriasis, vocalization, blindness, hyper-salivation, tachycardia, tachypnea, dyspnoea, ataxia/paresis, disorientation, coma and death. Clinical signs can occur within 30 min to several hours, if extended release products are consumed. They can last for 12–72 h in severe cases [51].

Several other medications have similar actions including serotonin re-uptake inhibition; however, not all have been shown to contribute to serotonin syndrome in veterinary patients but if used in combination at high dosages, may occur:

- **Amitriptyline** – weak SRI, NERI

- **First-generation antihistamines that are also SRIs**
  - chlorpheniramine (Chlor-Trimeton, etc.)
  - diphenhydramine (Benadryl, etc.)
  - mepyramine/pyrilamine (Anthisan, etc.)
  - tripelennamine (Pyribenzamine, etc.)
- **The phenylpiperidine series opioids**
  - tramadol – weak SRI, NERI. The author (KM) has witnessed serotonin syndrome in a dog following tramadol dosed at the high end of the normal range.
- **The following** are mentioned in the phenylpiperidine series of opioids but due to the VERY weak SRI effect are rarely implicated in the serotonin syndrome in humans and is associated with high or chronic usage, and combination, with a TCA, SRI or MAOI
  - meperidine (pethidine) – very weak SRI.
  - methadone – very weak SRI.
  - fentanyl – very weak SRI.
- **Morphine, codeine, oxycodone and buprenorphine** have no serotonin re-uptake inhibition and, therefore, do not precipitate serotonin toxicity with TCAs, SRIs or MAOIs. However, codeine is not metabolized to the active component, morphine, in dogs and is therefore, not an effective analgesic.
- **Gabapentin** – NERI as measured in CSF.

It is essential that drugs in the following section not be co-administered. Should serotonin syndrome be observed, symptomatic treatment including treating/preventing hyperthermia and administration of a muscle relaxant (e.g. a benzodiazepine) is essential for duration of clinical signs. There are no reversal agents.

C. Amitriptyline

Amitriptyline is a TCA that produces analgesia at supraspinal, spinal and peripheral sites. Analgesia can be achieved faster, and at lower doses, than those required for the antidepressant effect and can provide analgesia in patients with and without depression [52]. From a systematic review in humans, TCAs are in general effective in diabetic neuropathy and post-herpetic neuralgia, and there is some indication of effectiveness for central pain [52]. As is the case for other adjunctive analgesics, the usefulness of amitriptyline is variable in clinical trials, but it has been shown to be effective in at least one-third of the patients with neuropathic pain in humans [52]. Amitriptyline is the TCA most consistently reported to produce analgesic effects in human neuropathic pain.

1. Indications
There are no prospective studies assessing efficacy in ill or injured veterinary patients. However, as with human patients, neuropathic pain may be an indication. A case series of three dogs reported either a dramatic improvement or a full resolution of neuropathic pain following administration of amitriptyline or gabapentin [53]. Prior to this the dogs were treated, unsuccessfully, with NSAIAs or glucocorticoids and opiate agonists, with minimal or no response.

2. Mode of Action
Block re-uptake of norepinephrine and serotonin (5-HT), which enhances descending inhibitory actions in the spinal cord. It also has direct and indirect actions on opioid receptors, inhibits histamine, cholinergic, serotonin and NMDA receptors, inhibits ion channel activity (Na^+, Ca^{2+} and K^+ channels) and blocks adenosine uptake [54]. There is evidence for a local anesthetic

effect, when applied transdermally to rats with the combined application of amitriptyline and capsaicin resulting in prolonged cutaneous analgesia compared with amitriptyline alone, suggesting that the activation of the transient receptor potential vanilloid – 1 (TRPV1) channel by capsaicin facilitates the passage of amitriptyline into nociceptors [55]. This transdermal patch achieves far longer cutaneous analgesia than currently available patch applications such as EMLA® cream [55]. This makes it potentially useful to treat chronic pain, such as neuropathic pain and neuralgia, and to prevent pain in procedures such as venipuncture [55]. However, plasma concentrations of a pluronic lecithin organogel formulation of amitriptyline placed in the pinna of cats resulted in low and undetectable concentrations, suggesting it was not a reasonable vehicle for, or route of, administration [56].

3. Dosing Currently Recommended
- Dogs: 1–2 mg/kg PO q12–24h with food.
- Cats: 1–1.5 mg/kg PO q12h with food.

Based on pharmacokinetic studies in dogs, 3–4 mg/kg q12h PO would maintain plasma concentrations of amitriptyline, without nortriptyline, in the range shown to be clinically effective in humans [57]. Pharmacokinetics in fasted dogs resulted in a low BA; therefore, administration with food is advisable [57].

Cats administered doses of 1.3–1.4 mg/kg PO achieved amitriptyline and metabolite(s) concentrations of 61 ng/mL within 2 h and declined to 20 ng/mL by 12 h, which is at or below optimum levels conferring analgesia in humans [58].

Based on the pharmacokinetic studies noted above, the following dosing may be more appropriate; however, no clinical studies or reports are published using these dosages, and therefore potential adverse effects associated with these dosages are not known.

- Dogs: 3–4 mg/kg PO q12h – unfasted.
- Cats: 2.5–12.5 mg/cat PO q24h – unfasted, 1–1.5 mg/kg PO q12h.

4. Adverse Effects
Due to the multiple mechanisms of action and receptor interactions of amitriptyline, adverse effects reported in humans, in addition to those above, include drowsiness, dry mouth, blurred vision, constipation, urinary retention, polyuria, polydipsia, hyponatremia, bradycardia and heart blocks. These may potentially occur in cats and dogs.

D. Venlafaxine

Venlafaxine is a serotonin and norepinephrine reuptake inhibitor (SNRI). It is also a TCA and has very similar effects to amitriptyline, which is also shown to be effective in at least one-third of human patients with neuropathic pain [52].

As for several other adjunctive analgesics, there is no knowledge of plasma concentrations that are effective for analgesia in dogs or cats; plasma concentrations for venlafaxine and its predominant metabolite, O-desmethylvenlafaxine (ODV), of up to 400 µg/L are considered effective in humans as antidepressants [59]. The metabolite ODV was not detected in dogs; therefore, the pharmacologic effects are produced by the parent drug [60].

The pharmacokinetics of venlafaxine have not been reported in cats.

There are no clinical studies reported in cats and dogs receiving venlafaxine.

1. Adverse Effects
As noted above, the combination of some analgesics or adjunctive analgesic agents with SRI capability may induce serotonin toxicity. This may be more of a concern when the patient is

also receiving selective SRIs (e.g. fluoxetine (Reconcile, Prozac)), TCAs, and/or MAOIs (e.g. selegiline (L-deprenyl, Anipryl)) prescribed for anxiety in dogs.

E. Duloxetine

Duloxetine is a mixed SRI and NRI that is approved in humans for the treatment of diabetic neuropathy [61]. It has been noted that the unfavourable pharmacokinetic profile of duloxetine favours venlafaxine for further assessment in dogs at this time [2].

IV. Corticosteroids (Prednisone, Dexamethasone, Prednisolone, Methylprednisolone)

Corticosteroids should not be used as analgesics but, when used to treat the appropriate underlying problem, they do contribute to managing the associated pain. Among other actions, corticosteroids inhibit cyclooxygenase -2 (COX-2) gene expression, which is upregulated in inflammatory states, reduces aberrant firing originating from nerve injury and reduces inflammation at the site of injury. Corticosteroids should not be administered with NSAIAs. Ascertain no infection present prior to starting a course of corticosteroid therapy.

A. Prednisone

1. Indications
Immune-mediated disease or as part of the regimen for the treatment of certain neoplastic diseases. As an example of corticosteroids relieving pain associated with inflammation, large breed dogs (e.g., Weimaraner) with hypertrophic osteodystrophy may be presented as an emergency due to severe pain and have been managed successfully using the following dosing regimen.

2. Dosage
- Prednisone 0.75 mg/kg PO q12h for 4–5 days, extending to no more than seven days if signs persist.
- Gradually wean off over a 4-week period, reducing the total daily dose by one-half each week, then administer final reduced dose every other day for an additional 1–2 weeks.
- In all cases, also administer 3 V Caps (or Derm Caps) and either Glyco-Flex or Multi-source Glucosamine.
- Supportive care should be provided as needed.

3. Contraindications
Do not administer concurrently with or immediately following NSAIA administration. Gastric ulceration/perforation may occur.

V. Magnesium

In the CNS, magnesium exerts depressant effects, acting as an antagonist at the NMDA glutamate receptor and an inhibitor of catecholamine release. Magnesium is mentioned here as it is reported as a potential adjunct in managing pain; however, there are mixed reports [62]. The dosing and effectiveness of this use for magnesium is still under investigation. Caution should be exercised to monitor carefully for side effects and interactions with other medications that act on neuromuscular transmission (e.g. neuromuscular blocking agents whilst under general anesthesia), as severe weakness has been noted upon recovery requiring mechanical ventilation. The adverse effects outweigh any benefit of adding magnesium to an analgesic or MAC-sparing regimen (Dr L. Porayko, personal communication with KM).

VI. Non-Pharmacologic Modalities for Pain Management

Refer to Chapter 15 for procedures that will enhance the pharmacologic management of pain and also assist with recovery from illness and injury.

VII. Case Example of Utilizing Adjunctive Analgesics

A dog presented with forelimb lameness. This was diagnosed as a primary cervical disc prolapse with referred pain to the limb. Following surgery, a small amount of irretrievable disc remained and the patient was extremely painful and assessed as a 10/10 on the pain scale. Fentanyl, ketamine, lidocaine and an NSAIA were administered; however, pain was still present. Gabapentin was added. As the patient improved, amantadine was introduced and he was gradually weaned off lidocaine at 24 h, and fentanyl and ketamine over 72 h. The dog still had mild forelimb lameness when discharged home on an NSAIA q24h, gabapentin 10 mg/kg q8h and amantadine 3 mg/kg q24h. Forelimb lameness resolved two weeks after discharge. The NSAIA was slowly discontinued. Lowering of amantadine followed two weeks later. Amantadine was gradually weaned off with gabapentin as the sole analgesic. When changing gabapentin to q12h, the lameness recurred. Gabapentin at q8h was reinstituted. Gradual lowering over the following six months was required as on occasion lameness recurred. Increasing the gabapentin dose to the previous level resolved the lameness. At six months, the lameness resolved.

References

1 Lamont, L. A. (2008) Adjunctive analgesic therapy in veterinary medicine. *Vet Clin North Am Small Anim Pract*, 38: 1187–1203.

2 KuKanich, B. (2013) Outpatient oral analgesics in dogs and cats beyond nonsteroidal antiinflammatory drugs: An evidence-based approach. *Vet Clin North Am Small Anim Pract*, 43: 1109–1125.

3 Lascelles, B. D., Gaynor, J. S., Smith, E. S., *et al.* (2008) Amantadine in a multimodal analgesic regimen for alleviation of refractory osteoarthritis pain in dogs. *J Vet Intern Med*, 22: 53–59.

4 Aghighi, S. A., Tipold, A., Piechotta, M., *et al.* (2012) Assessment of the effects of adjunctive gabapentin on postoperative pain after intervertebral disc surgery in dogs. *Vet Anesth Analg*, 39: 636–646.

5 Leng, T., Gao, X., Dilger, J. P., *et al.* (2016) Neuroprotective effect of lidocaine: Is there clinical potential? *Int J Physiol Pathophysiol Pharmacol*, 8(1): 9–13.

6 Smith, L. J., Bentley, E., Shih, A., *et al.* (2004) Systemic lidocaine infusion as an analgesic for intraocular surgery in dogs: A pilot study. *Vet Anaesth Analg*, 31: 53–63.

7 Ortega, M. and Cruz, I. (2011) Evaluation of a constant rate infusion of lidocaine for balanced anesthesia in dogs undergoing surgery. *Can Vet J*, 52: 856–860.

8 Weibel, S., Jokinen, J. and Pace, N. L. (2016) Efficacy and safety of intravenous lidocaine for postoperative analgesia and recovery after surgery: A systematic review with trial sequential analysis. *Br J Anaesth*, 116(6): 770–783.

9 Doherty, T. J. and Seddighi, M. R. (2010) Local anesthetics as pain therapy in horses. *Vet Clin Equine*, 26: 533–549.

10 Pypendop, B. H. and Ilkiw, J. E. (2005) Assessment of the hemodynamic effects of lidocaine administered IV in isoflurane-anesthetized cats. *Am J Vet Res*, 66: 661–668.

11 Soleimanpour, H. R., Hassanzadeh, K., Mohammadi, D. A., *et al.* (2011) Parenteral lidocaine for treatment of intractable renal colic: A case series. *J Medical Case Reports*, 5: 256.

12 Muir, W. W. (2007) *Small Animal: Anesthesiology: Lidocaine for every surgery patient.* Proceedings of the North Am Veterinary Congress, Orlando, Florida.

13 Pypendop, B. H. and Ilkiw, J. E. (2005) The effects of intravenous lidocaine administration on the minimum alveolar concentration of isoflurane in cats. *Anesth Analg*, 100: 97–101.

14 Pypendop, B. H., Ilkiw, J. E. and Robertson, S. A. (2006) Effects of intravenous administration of lidocaine on the thermal threshold in cats. *Am J Vet Res*, 67(1): 16–20.

15 Ko, J., Weil, A., Maxwell, L., *et al.* (2007) Plasma concentrations of lidocaine in dogs following lidocaine patch application. *J Am Anim Hosp Assoc*, 43(5): 280–283.

16 Loix, S., De Kock, M., Henin, P. (2011) The anti-inflammatory effects of ketamine: State of the art. *Acta Anaesth Belg*, 62: 17–58.

17 Bhutta, A. T. (2007) Ketamine: A controversial drug for neonates. *Semin Perinatol*, 31: 303–308.

18 Himmelseher, S. and Durieux, M. E. (2005) Ketamine for perioperative pain management. *Anesthesiology*, 102: 211–220.

19 Wagner, A. E., Walton, J. A., Hellyer, P. W., *et al.* (2002) Use of low dosages of ketamine administered by constant rate infusion as an adjunct for postoperative analgesia in dogs. *J Am Vet Med Assoc*, 221: 72–75.

20 Sarrau, S., Jourdan, J., Dupuis-Soyris, F., *et al.* (2007) Effects of postoperative ketamine infusion on pain control and feeding behaviour in bitches undergoing mastectomy. *J Small Anim Pract*, 48(12): 670–676.

21 Lee, M., Silverman, S. M., Hansen, H. R., *et al.* (2011) Comprehensive review of opioid-induced hyperalgesia. *Pain Physician*, 14: 145–161.

22 Sleigh, J., Harvey, M., Voss, L. and Denny, B. (2014) Ketamine: More mechanisms of action than just NMDA blockade. *Trends Anaesth Crit Care*, 4: 76–81.

23 Pabelick, C. M., Jones, K. A., Street, K., *et al.* (1997) Calcium concentration-dependent mechanisms through which ketamine relaxes canine airway smooth muscle. *Anesthesiology*, 86: 1104–1111.

24 White, M., Shah, N., Lindley, K., *et al.* (2006) Pain management in fulminating ulcerative colitis. *Pediatr Anesth*, 16: 1148–1152.

25 Fass, J., Bares, R., Hermsdorf, V., *et al.* (1995) The effects of intravenous ketamine on gastrointestinal motility in dogs. *Intensive Care Med*, 21: 584–589.

26 Himmelseher, S. and Durieux, M. E. (2005) Revising a dogma: Ketamine for patients with neurological injury? *Anesth Analg*, 101: 524–34.

27 Serrano, S., Hughes, D. and Chandler, K. (2006) Use of ketamine for the management of refractory status epilepticus in a dog. *J Vet Intern Med*, 20: 194–197.

28 Pypendop, B. H. and Ilkiw, J. E. (2005) Pharmacokinetics of ketamine and its metabolite, norketamine after intravenous administration of a bolus of ketamine to isoflurane-anesthetized dogs. *Am J Vet Res*, 66: 2034–2038.

29 Kamtikar, S. and Nair, A. S. (2015) Advantages of dexmedetomidine in traumatic brain injury: A review. *Anaesth Pain & Intensive Care*, 19(1): 87–91.

30 Tang, J. F., Chen, P., Tang, E. J., *et al.* (2011) Dexmedetomidine controls agitation and facilitates reliable, serial neurological examinations in a non-intubated patient with traumatic brain injury. *Neurocritical Care*, 15(1): 175–181.

31 Boscan, P., Monnet, E., Mama, K., *et al.* (2011) Effect of maropitant, a neurokinin 1 receptor antagonist, on anesthetic requirements during noxious visceral stimulation of the ovary in dogs. *Am J Vet Res*, 72: 1576–1579.

32 Giacino, J. T., Whyte, J., Bagiella, E., *et al.* (2012) Placebo-controlled trial of amantadine for severe traumatic brain injury. *N Engl J Med*, 366: 819–826.

33 Siao, K. T., Pypendop, B. H., Stanley, S. D. and Ilkiw, J. E. (2011) Pharmacokinetics of amantadine in cats. *J Vet Pharmacol Ther*, 34: 599–604.

34 Norkus, C., Rankin, D., Warner, M. and KuKanich, B. (2015) Pharmacokinetics of oral amantadine in greyhound dogs. *J Vet Pharmacol Therap*, 38: 305–308.

35 Epstein, M. E., Rodan, I. and Griffenhagen, G. (2015) AAHA/AAFP pain management guidelines for dogs and cats. *J Feline Med Surg*, 17: 251–272.

36 Ing, T. S., Daugirdas, J. T., Sound, L. S., *et al.* (1979) Toxic effects of amantadine in patients with renal failure. *Can Med Assoc J*, 120: 695–698.

37 Nakai, K., Takeda, K. and Kimura, H. R. (2009) Obstructive acute renal failure related to amantadine intoxication. *Am J Emerg Med*, 27(3): 371.

38 Gaynor, J. S. (2009) Other drugs used to treat pain. In: Gaynor, J. S. and Muir, W. W. (eds), *Handbook of Veterinary Pain Management*, 2nd edn. Mosby Elsevier, St. Louis, MO: 266–267.

39 Moore, R. A., Wiffen, P. J., Derry, S., *et al.* (2014) Gabapentin for chronic neuropathic pain and fibromyalgia in adults. *Cochrane Database of Systematic Reviews* 4 (Art. No.: CD007938), doi: 10.1002/14651858.CD007938.pub3.

40 Clarke, H. R., Pereira, S., Kennedy, D., *et al.* (2009) Gabapentin decreases morphine consumption and improves functional recovery following total knee arthroplasty. *Pain Res Manage*, 14(3): 217–222.

41 Ho, K.-Y., Gan, T. J. and Habib, A. S. (2006) Gabapentin and postoperative pain: A systematic review of randomized controlled trials. *Pain*, 126: 91–101.

42 Doleman, B., Heinink, T. P., Read, D. J., *et al.* (2015) A systematic review and meta-regression analysis of prophylactic gabapentin for postoperative pain. *Anaesthesia*, 70: 1186–1204.

43 Mendham, J. E. (2004) Gabapentin for the treatment of itching produced by burns and wound healing in children: A pilot study. *Burns*, 30: 851–853.

44 Lorenz, N. D., Comerford, E. J. and Iff, I. (2013) Long-term use of gabapentin for musculoskeletal disease and trauma in three cats. *J Feline Med Surg*, 15: 507–12.

45 Vettorato, E. and Corletto, F. (2011) Gabapentin as part of multi-modal analgesia in two cats suffering multiple injuries. *Vet Anaesth Analg*, 38: 518–520.

46 Wagner, A. E., Mich, P. M., Uhrig, S. R., *et al.* (2010) Clinical evaluation of perioperative administration of gabapentin as an adjunct for postoperative analgesia in dogs undergoing amputation of a forelimb. *J Am Vet Med Assoc*, 236(7): 751–756.

47 Taylor, C. P. (2009) Mechanisms of analgesia by gabapentin and pregabalin – Calcium channel a2-d [Cava2-d] ligands. *Pain*, 142: 13–16.

48 KuKanich, B. and Cohen, R. L. (2011) Pharmacokinetics of oral gabapentin in Greyhound dogs. *Vet J*, 187: 133–135.

49 Siao, K. T., Pypendop, B. H. R. and Ilkiw, J. E. (2010) Pharmacokinetics of gabapentin in cats. *Am J Vet Res*, 71: 817–821.

50 Gidal, B. E., Maly, M. and Kowalski, J. W. (1998) Gabapentin absorption: Effect of mixing with foods of varying macronutrient composition. *Ann Pharmacother*, 32(4): 405–409.

51 Gillman, P. K. (2005) Monoamine oxidase inhibitors, opioid analgesics and serotonin toxicity. *B J Anaesthesia*, 95(4): 434–441.

52 Saarto, T. and Wiffen, P. J. (2007) Antidepressants for neuropathic pain. *Cochrane Database of Systematic Reviews* 4 Art. No.: CD005454), doi: 10.1002/14651858.CD005454.pub2.

53 Cashmore, R. G., Harcourt-Brown, T. R., Freeman, P. M., *et al.* (2009) Clinical diagnosis and treatment of suspected neuropathic pain in three dogs. *Australian Veterinary Journal*, 87(1–2): 45–50.

54 Sawynok, J., Esser, M. J. and Reid, A. R. (2001) Antidepressants as analgesics: An overview of central and peripheral mechanisms of action. *J Psychiatry Neurosci*, 26: 21–29.

55 Haderer, A., Gerner, P., Kao, G., *et al.* (2003) Cutaneous analgesia after transdermal application of amitriptyline versus lidocaine in rats. *Anesth Analg*, 96: 1707–1710.

56 Murdan, S. (2005) A review of pluronic lecithin organogel. *Hospital Pharmacist*, 12: 267–270.

57 Norkus, C., Rankin, D. and KuKanich, B. (2015) Pharmacokinetics of intravenous and oral amitriptyline and its active metabolite nortriptyline in Greyhound dogs. *Vet Anaesth Analg*, 42: 580–589.

58 Mealey, K. L., Peck, K. E., Bennet, B. S., *et al.* (2004) Systemic absorption of amitriptyline and buspirone after oral and transdermal administration to healthy cats. *J Vet Intern Med*, 18: 43–46.

59 Charlier, C., Pinto, E., Ansseau, M. and Plomteux, G. (2002) Venlafaxine: The relationship between dose, plasma concentration and clinical response in depressive patients. *J Psychopharmacol*, 16: 369–372.

60 Howell, S. R., Hicks, D. R., Scatina, J. A., *et al.* (1994) Pharmacokinetics of venlafaxine and O-desmethylvenlafaxine in laboratory animals. *Xenobiotica*, 24: 315–327.

61 Patel, D. S., Deshpande, S. S., Patel, C. G., *et al.* (2011) A dual action anti-depressant. *Indo Global J Pharm Sci*, 1: 69.

62 Lysakowski, C., Dumont, L. and Czarnetzki, C. (2007) Magnesium as an adjuvant to postoperative analgesia: A systematic review of randomized trials. *Anesth Analg*, 104: 1532–1539.

Further Reading

Eriksson, A. S., Sinclair, R., Cassuto, J. and Thomsen, P. (1992) Influence of lidocaine on leukocyte function in the surgical wound. *Anesthesiology*, 77: 74–78.

Gianotti, G., Valverde, A., Johnson, R., *et al.* (2014) Influence of prior determination of baseline minimum alveolar concentration (MAC) of isoflurane on the effect of ketamine on MAC in dogs. *Can J Vet Res*, 78: 207–213.

Murrough, J. W. (2012) Ketamine as a novel antidepressant: From synapse to behavior. *Clinical Pharmacology & Therapeutics*, 91: 303–309.

Jones, C. K., Peters, S. C. and Shannon, H. E. (2005) Efficacy of duloxetine: A potent and balanced serotonergic and noradrenergic reuptake inhibitor, in inflammatory and acute pain models in rodents. *JPET*, 312: 726–732.

Kaka, J. S. and Hayton, W. L. (1980) Pharmacokinetics of ketamine and two metabolites in the dog. *J Pharmacokinet Biopharm*, 8: 193–202.

Lois, F. and De Kock, M. (2008) Something new about ketamine for pediatric anesthesia? *Current Opinion in Anaesthesiology*, 21: 340–344.

Mion, G. and Villevieille, T. (2013) Ketamine pharmacology: An update (pharmacodynamics and molecular aspects, recent findings). *CNS Neurosci Therapeut*, 19: 370–380.

Radulovic, L. L., Turck, D., Von Hodenberg, A., *et al.* (1995) Disposition of gabapentin (Neurontin) in mice, rats, dogs, and monkeys. *Drug Metab Dispos*, 23: 441–448.

Valverde, A., Doherty, T. J., Hernández, J. and Davies, W. (2004) Effect of lidocaine on the minimum alveolar concentration of isoflurane in dogs. *Vet Anaesth Analg*, 31: 264–271.

13

Pharmacologic and Clinical Application of General Anesthetics

Melissa Sinclair

The choice of available anesthetic agents on the market has increased with improvements in each class of drugs. However, currently available induction and inhalant anesthetics, and combined sedatives and analgesics, still result in dose-related negative cardiovascular and respiratory depression necessitating knowledge and familiarity of each class of drug and its expected effects. The administration of alpha$_2$ agonists, opioid single bolus or continuous rate infusions (CRIs), lidocaine single bolus or CRIs and local anesthetic techniques will beneficially reduce the amount of the anesthetic agent required. The veterinary team requires an understanding of the appropriate anesthetic and analgesic agent for a given patient with underlying diseases and trauma. The following will outline the specific pharmacology and techniques for the most commonly used anesthetic agents. Refer to Chapter 9 (sedatives), Chapter 10 (opioid analgesics) and Chapter 12 (adjunct analgesia) for details on individual agents.

I. Injectable Anesthetics

A. General Considerations

Small animal practices typically induce unconsciousness in small animal veterinary patients with injectable anesthetic agents intravenously (IV). Propofol and alfaxalone are two common and readily available injectable induction agents, which are licensed for use in dogs and cats in South Africa, Australia, Canada, the United States and Europe. Ketamine mixed with a benzo-diazepine is also used.

Information available on induction anesthetic drugs is usually the result of research investigations conducted on healthy patients. Doses recommended from such studies are based on the requirements of those patients to achieve unconsciousness and cardio-respiratory effects reported are representative of a healthy research animal. Patients that are sick and debilitated – with less than ideal cardio-respiratory function from hypovolemia, shock, central nervous system (CNS) depression, cardiovascular disease and other concomitant diseases – will require lower doses of anesthetic induction agents. The cardiovascular and respiratory depressant effects of these drugs can be exacerbated, even with lower doses, in a sick animal. For this reason, doses suggested below for each induction drug should always be carefully titrated to obtain the desired induction effect, especially in the compromised patient. Stabilization of the animal is always required to reduce the chance of a major morbidity or mortality on induction. Monitoring pulse rate, quality, respiratory rate, mucous membrane colour and depth will be key in the compromised animal.

Analgesia and Anesthesia for the Ill or Injured Dog and Cat, First Edition. Karol A. Mathews, Melissa Sinclair, Andrea M. Steele and Tamara Grubb.

B. Propofol

1. Dosing and Cardio-respiratory Effects

Propofol primarily acts on $GABA_A$ receptors, as well as $alpha_2$ adrenoceptors, NMDA receptors and glycine receptors to induce their anesthetic effects.

Propofol can be used at low doses (0.5–1 mg/kg) IV to achieve sedation. This may be advantageous in many situations of critical case management.

For anesthesia, the induction dose of propofol ranges in the literature from 2–6 mg/kg, IV in dogs and cats. The appropriate induction dose depends largely on the level of sedation of the animals achieved with pre-medication, overall alertness, and health status of the animal. In both species with stabilization, the appropriate starting dose or propofol is 2 mg/kg. After the initial bolus volumes, signs of depth are monitored and incremental additional boluses every 6–12 s of 0.5 or 0.75 mg/kg can be given until endotracheal intubation is achieved. In very critical cases, anesthetic doses of propofol should be used cautiously until the animal is examined and fluid resuscitation has been initiated. Sick, depressed or heavily sedated animals may require a lowered initial dose of propofol of 0.5–1 mg/kg.

Even though the induction quality of propofol in dogs is generally reported as satisfactory, excitement, dystonia, involuntary muscle contraction, paddling and potentially even opisthotonus and hyperextension are reported. These side effects are postulated to be caused by antagonism of inhibitory glycine receptors at the subcortical level and imbalance between inhibitory dopamine receptors and excitatory cholinergic receptors in the basal ganglia, especially during rapid brain concentration changes. These effects are not true seizures.

Propofol has negative cardiovascular effects in cats and dogs when used for anesthetic induction. It directly and indirectly reduces cardiac contractility and causes vasodilation. These effects, in combination with the fact that the baroreceptor reflex sensitivity is reset by propofol, result in a dramatic decrease in arterial blood pressure when propofol is used for anesthetic induction.

Propofol has well-documented respiratory depression and commonly results in post-induction apnea, which is both rate and dose-dependent, hence, titrating propofol to effect for induction or the level of sedation you require is important to minimize these negative cardio-respiratory effects and intervene as appropriate.

2. Advantages

Recovery from propofol is rapid following induction or maintenance with a CRI due to rapid redistribution and excellent metabolism. Propofol can be used safely in patients with liver disease. The ability to titrate to effect with propofol minimizes overdose and allows appropriate dosing for the individual animal minimizing the potential for adverse cardiovascular/respiratory effects.

3. Concerns

Propofol should be used with caution in debilitated patients due to the resultant cardiovascular and respiratory depression until the patient is stabilized. Pre-operative stabilization, monitoring during induction and minimizing the total induction dose with appropriate titration will reduce the chance of a major negative cardiovascular event. Pre-oxygenation is also of benefit in the compromised animal during induction. Propofol contains no preservative, so it must be used on the day that the vial is opened.

C. Alfaxalone

1. Dosing and Cardio-respiratory Effects

Alfaxalone, the pharmacologically active substance within the earlier induction agent Althesin, is formulated with 2-hydroxypropyl-beta-cyclodextrin. It can be used for chemical restraint as a general anesthetic for short procedures, or as a CRI. It is generally not given as an IV sedative at very low doses, as can be done with propofol. It can be used intramuscularly (IM) as a sedative in cats. It is licensed as an IV induction agent in dogs and cats and company doses of 2–3 mg/kg in dogs and 5 mg/kg in cats are listed. These doses are higher than what is required clinically. It is not licensed for IM use in Canada, as it is in Australia and New Zealand, but may be used by this route in cats.

Alfaxalone causes a dose-dependent minimal to moderate reduction in systemic vascular resistance (66–101%) and mean arterial pressure (73–95%), and minimal to mild increases in heart rate (109–125%) and cardiac index (100–115%), in both sedated and unsedated healthy dogs, at clinically relevant induction doses (1.5–4.15 mg/kg, IV).

Alfaxalone has been shown to induce dose-dependent respiratory depression characterized by a reduction in respiratory rate and minute volume to even complete apnea at various doses ranging from 2 to 40 mg/kg, IV, in dogs aged 8 months to 10 years old.

Reported side effects in dogs include excitement, paddling or muscle twitching. Pre-medication is strongly recommended by the pharmaceutical manufacturer (Jurox Pty Ltd, Australia) and listed within the product monograph to prevent excitement and rough recoveries in dogs. Because alfaxalone is rapidly re-distributed, the company recommends an initial dose of 2–3 mg/kg in dogs to prevent arousal during the induction phase and/or transfer to inhalational anesthesia. However, these doses are not always necessary.

In compromised patients, with appropriate sedation, these higher doses may not be required, especially if a co-induction agent is also administered. General guideline doses are 2 mg/kg for dogs and 3 mg/kg in cats. Hence for both sick or compromised dogs and cats an initial starting bolus dose of 1–1.5 mg/kg, IV is appropriate with titration to effect with additional doses of 0.3–0.4 mg/kg, IV to achieve intubation.

2. Advantages

The recovery with alfaxalone is rapid, even following extended administration, due to rapid redistribution and excellent metabolism. Induction of anesthesia with alfaxalone can be titrated to effect to minimize the adverse cardiovascular/respiratory effects.

3. Concerns

The cardio-respiratory effects of alfaxalone are more likely to be significant in debilitated patients. Titration to effect is advised to minimize this, in addition to pre-oxygenation and co-administration with midazolam during induction. Alfaxalone contains no preservatives, so it must be used within 24 h of opening.

D. Ketamine with Diazepam or Midazolam

1. Dosing and Cardio-respiratory Effects

Diazepam or midazolam in combination with ketamine can be prepared by mixing the two drugs in a 1:1 or 2:1 volume ratio. Usual concentrations of diazepam and midazolam are 5 mg/mL and of ketamine is 100 mg/ml. The use of a larger volume of the benzodiazepine (2:1 ratio) may be used in very sick patients due to the fact that benzodiazepines cause minimal to no negative effects on the cardiovascular system. In general, ketamine–benzodiazepine combinations will result in maintenance or an increase in arterial blood pressure and cardiac output on induction and an increase in heart rate.

The usual IV recommended dose that allows induction of healthy patients is 0.1–0.15 mL/kg of the combined ketamine–benzodiazepine drug volumes. This volume mixture results in doses of ketamine of 5–7 mg/kg and diazepam or midazolam dose of 0.25–0.3 mg/kg. The dose should be titrated to effect in more critical animals with an initial starting bolus of 0.05–0.1 mL/kg, IV. Low doses (approximately 0.05 mL/kg) can produce sedation or profound restraint.

2. Advantages

This combination maintains good cardiovascular stability, which is related to ketamine's sympathetic stimulation and minimal negative cardiovascular effects from the benzodiazepine. This combination can be given as a sedative and has minimal risk of causing excitement on induction compared to other induction agents.

3. Concerns

Normal renal function is required in cats for elimination and recovery from ketamine. With significant chronic kidney disease, cats may have a delayed recovery. In dogs, normal liver function is required for ketamine elimination. Liver disease will impact the biotransformation of benzodiazepines in both species, and flumazenil should be available if used in patients with liver disease.

Ketamine's sympathomimetic effects may be of benefit in some critical cases to aid in the maintenance of heart rate and cardiac output. However, an increase in the sympathetic activity may be a concern in the following situations:

- Cats with hypertrophic cardiomyopathy due to ketamine-induced tachycardia and the likelihood of left ventricular outflow tract obstruction.
- Tachycardia may happen and persist for the initial 20 min of anesthesia in patients with previously normal heart rates. Patients with cardiac tachyarrhythmia may have further exacerbation when ketamine is used for induction and so it should be avoided.
- Head trauma due to associated increases in cerebral blood flow, cerebral oxygen consumption and increased intracranial pressure. However, recent evidence suggests that ketamine's administration in combination with benzodiazepines is safe in patients with head trauma if mechanical ventilation is also provided to maintain normocapnea. In addition, ketamine has neuroprotective effects in these types of cases.
- History of seizures in patients may preclude ketamine use due to the possible association of increased metabolic rate. However, ketamine does not precipitate seizure activity.
- Diabetes, the sympathetic stimulation of ketamine may induce a hyperglycemia, making further glucose monitoring difficult during anesthesia.

E. Etomidate

1. Dosing and Cardio-respiratory effects

Etomidate at doses of 1-3 mg/kg causes minimal to no cardiovascular effects.

2. Advantages

Etomidate may be a good option in unstable patients considering the lack of significant cardiovascular effects.

3. Concerns

Etomidate causes adrenocortical suppression, and its use in septic patients is controversial. Etomidate should never be used without adequate pre-anaesthetic sedation as it commonly causes muscle rigidity, muscle twitching and vocalization in unsedated patients.

F. Co-Induction Agents

Co-induction agents are administered with propofol or alfaxalone to promote a smooth induction to unconsciousness and endotracheal intubation, and to minimize the dose of the primary anesthetic induction agent, potentially reducing negative cardiovascular effects. The co-induction agents reported in veterinary medicine are fentanyl (2–5 µg/kg, IV), diazepam (0.2–0.4 mg/kg, IV), midazolam (0.2–0.4 mg/kg, IV) and lidocaine (1–2 mg/kg, IV in dogs).

These agents are given just before or after the initial bolus of propofol or alfaxalone. The benefit in healthy research dogs is debatable within the literature. However, in compromised or critical patients the benefits of dose reduction and the potentially negative cardiovascular effects of the induction agent should be considered.

With benzodiazepines, the ability to prove a dose reduction with propofol or alfaxalone is influenced by the order of administration of the midazolam or diazepam relative to the primary injectable induction agent. Other factors impacting the benefits of the benzodiazepine in dogs include the dose of the co-induction agent and speed of injection, speed of injection of the induction agent, the bolus dose of the induction agent, assessment methods of the study and the sedation level of the dog prior to induction. The benzodiazepines are commonly administered as co-induction agents in cats as well.

Consistent dose reduction, improved induction quality and ease of endotracheal intubation are most commonly achieved with midazolam of 0.2–0.4 mg/kg, IV, after the initial IV bolus of propofol or alfaxalone versus diazepam. In healthy research dogs, there is no cardiovascular benefit with the dose reduction of propofol or alfaxalone.

II. Inhalational Anesthesia

A. General Considerations

Critical patients requiring diagnostic, medical or surgical interventions are most commonly maintained on inhalant anesthetics for long procedures. Inhalant anesthesia is delivered in oxygen through an endotracheal tube. Endotracheal intubation will aid in preventing aspiration of refluxed material, but it is not 100% protective. The main disadvantages of inhalant anesthesia are the need and cost of equipment (machine and vaporizer) and dose-dependent cardiopulmonary depression. Monitoring and adjustment of depth to the lowest level possible is important, especially in the critically ill patient. Attention and support of cardio-respiratory parameters is indicated to minimize post-operative morbidities.

B. Cardiovascular Effects

Inhalant anesthetics cause dose-dependent cardiovascular depression. According to the potency of inhalant anesthetics, determined as the minimum alveolar concentration (MAC), the higher the MAC delivered to the patient, the more pronounced the cardiovascular depression.

In general, decreases in cardiac output, stroke volume and blood pressure are common to all inhalant anesthetics. Mechanical ventilation can exacerbate these changes, due to increases in intrathoracic pressure that exert a negative effect on venous return and to a lowering of arterial CO_2, which blunts the sympathetic actions of this gas.

The cardiovascular effects of both isoflurane and sevoflurane are similar. The decrease in blood pressure is the result of vasodilatory actions (decreased vascular resistance) and is less related to contractility.

C. Respiratory Effects

Similar to cardiovascular effects, respiratory function is affected in a dose-dependent fashion. Respiratory rate decreases progressively with increasing doses of isoflurane or sevoflurane; tidal volume can also be reduced from muscle relaxation, all of which results in higher $PaCO_2$

levels than normal. Hence, in conditions where hypercarbia is detrimental to the patient (head trauma, increased intracranial pressure), $ETCO_2$ should be monitored and ventilation assisted.

D. Biotransformation

Respiration is responsible for eliminating most of the inhalant anesthetic in the body. The remaining anesthetic in the body is eliminated mostly through liver metabolism. Isoflurane and sevoflurane are metabolized by liver metabolism by 0.2 and 3–5%, respectively; therefore, both are considered very safe for patients with liver or kidney disease.

E. Potency

Inhalant anesthetics are compared by their potency (MAC), defined as the alveolar concentration that prevents movement in 50% of subjects in response to a noxious stimulus. This value is decreased by most sedatives, tranquilizers and analgesics, which allows for lower requirements of the inhalant and potentially better cardio-respiratory function from less dose-dependent effects of the inhalant; however, the effects of any of the injectable anesthetic drugs can be synergistic or additive to those of the inhalant and not lessen or improve the effects of the inhalant anesthetic.

MAC of isoflurane
Dog: 1.27–1.68%
Cat: 1.2–2.2%
MAC of sevoflurane
Dog: 1.86–2.36%
Cat: 2.5–3.95%

Further Reading

Grimm, K. A., Lamont, L. A., Tranquilli, W. J., *et al.* (eds) (2015) *Veterinary Anesthesia and Analgesia*, 5th edn. Wiley-Blackwell, Ames, IA.

14

Local Anesthetic Techniques

Alexander Valverde

Local anesthetics can be infiltrated in close proximity to peripheral nerves or nerve endings, applied on the skin as transdermal patches or cream, injected into the epidural/spinal space, and injected into the systemic circulation of an area confined by a tourniquet. The local anesthetic acts on sodium channels of nociceptive fibres (A-delta and C) by blocking influx and therefore preventing the generation of an action potential (blockade of transduction) and its propagation to the spinal cord along the nerve (blockade of transmission).

Lidocaine and bupivacaine are the most commonly used local anesthetics in small animals, and the choice of drug is often based on its speed of onset and duration of action. Lidocaine has a shorter action than bupivacaine due to a lower binding to the receptor. Receptors are proteins, and plasma protein binding can be used to reflect receptor binding. Lidocaine's plasma protein binding is 65% versus bupivacaine's 95%. Lidocaine is faster in onset than bupivacaine because the dissociation constant (pKa) is closer to plasma's pH, which facilitates passage through cell membranes to reach the sodium channels of the nociceptive fibres. Lidocaine's pKa is 7.9 versus bupivacaine's 8.1. In general, lidocaine's onset can occur in 1–5 min with a duration of action of 1–2 h, whereas bupivacaine's onset of action is 5–10 min with a duration of 2–4 h.

Bupivacaine is commonly dosed at 2 mg/kg in dogs and 1.0–1.5 mg/kg in cats. Lidocaine is dosed at 4.0–6.0 mg/kg in dogs and 2.0–4.0 mg/kg in cats. However, at many injection sites, the volume of local anesthetic achieved using those dosages is unnecessarily large. Thus, the volume of local anesthetic that should be injected is listed in the description of each block below.

The concentration of lidocaine recommended in the blocks described in this chapter is 2% for lidocaine and for bupivacaine is 0.5%, unless stated otherwise. The volumes of local anesthetic recommended are based on these concentrations for dogs, reduce by one-third for cats. The dosages of local anesthetics achieved by the volumes listed in this chapter do not exceed the clinical dosages listed above.

I. Toxicity of Local Anesthetics

Local anesthetics can affect the central nervous system (CNS) and the cardiovascular system. Toxicity of local anesthetics is related to their plasma concentration and depends on dose, speed of absorption from the site of injection and efficiency of elimination for the species. In general, peak plasma concentrations for routes other than intravenous (IV) are achieved faster for

Analgesia and Anesthesia for the Ill or Injured Dog and Cat, First Edition. Karol A. Mathews, Melissa Sinclair, Andrea M. Steele and Tamara Grubb.
© 2018 John Wiley & Sons, Inc. Published 2018 by John Wiley & Sons, Inc.

intercostal, which is > epidural, which is > brachial plexus, which is > subcutaneous injections. It is unlikely that adverse effects would arise from toxic doses of local anesthetic, unless an accidental IV injection had occurred, since the rate of absorption from infiltration techniques tends to be slow and resultant plasma concentrations are of less magnitude per unit of time.

In general, doses that cause adverse effects to the cardiovascular system are usually higher than those required to cause adverse effects to the CNS, except for bupivacaine, which has a profound cardiotoxic effect that can occur at doses closer to those affecting the CNS. General anesthesia has a protective effect against CNS signs, and doses that cause toxicity in conscious patients do not affect anesthetized patients. Therefore, it is important to keep track of the total dose of local anesthetic used in the anesthetized patient and be observant during their return to consciousness in recovery, since the lack of adverse CNS effects during anesthesia may become obvious if overzealous administration occurred. In contrast, cardiovascular signs can occur in conscious and anesthetized patients with similar doses.

Cats are considered more sensitive to the toxic effects of local anesthetics and the doses reported below for dogs should be decreased by at least 30%. Should toxicity occur, intravenous lipid emulsion (e.g. 20% Intralipid®) has been established as first-line therapy for local anesthetic toxicity [1]. A bolus of 1.5 to 4 mL/kg (0.3–0.8 g/kg), IV, over 1 min, followed by a continuous infusion of 0.25 mL/kg/min for 30–60 min is recommended. Check serum every 2 h for fat clearance. Repeat as needed once serum has cleared, up to three times. If no effect, discontinue.

A. Lidocaine

The reported toxic dose for CNS signs, such as convulsions, in conscious dogs after sequential IV doses of lidocaine of 1 mg/kg, 3 mg/kg, 5 mg/kg, 10 mg/kg and 15 mg/kg at 30 min intervals is approximately 22 mg/kg, and was achieved at 90–100 min; however, signs of tremors, sedation, salivation, rigidity, and convulsions can be observed with single IV doses of < 10 mg/kg [2]. The reported single IV dose that causes cardiovascular collapse in the anesthetized dog is 28 mg/kg. However, signs of hypotension, decreased cardiac output and alterations in heart rate occur at lower doses [3].

B. Bupivacaine

The dose that causes convulsions after sequential IV doses of bupivacaine of 1 mg/kg, 3 mg/kg and 5 mg/kg at 30 min intervals in conscious dogs is 5 mg/kg and was achieved in 30–40 min. Tremors, salivation, rigidity and convulsions can be observed with doses of 3 mg/kg [2]. The single IV dose that causes cardiovascular collapse in anesthetized dogs is 11 mg/kg. However, signs of hypotension, decreased cardiac output, dysrhythmias and bradycardia occur at lower doses [3]. Bupivacaine is considered very cardiotoxic due to the frequency of dysrhythmias associated with IV use and should never be administered by this route.

II. Preparation for Blocks

Comfort of the patient is important for performing any local anesthetic block. Although some blocks can be performed in conscious patients, it is more common to perform blocks in sedated or anesthetized patients, due to anxiety and pain. The site of injection does not always need to be clipped; however, some of the blocks are invasive and in close proximity to tissues where the risk of sepsis cannot be tolerated, so clipping and full surgical preparation with aqueous-based iodophors (safe for mucosal membranes) or alcohol-based solutions is always recommended. The use of sterile gloves is also recommended for most blocks.

In general, it is important to check for negative blood aspiration before injection of the local anesthetic and that there is no resistance upon injection. Resistance is usually the result of a needle against a bony structure or of an intraneural injection; in either situation, it is recommended to reposition the needle to facilitate the ease of injection and avoid trauma.

III. Head Blocks

The trigeminal nerve (cranial nerve V) is responsible for all sensory input of the head. This includes the three branches of the trigeminal nerve, (1) the ophthalmic nerve supplies the eye once it emerges through the orbital fissure and provides sensation to the cornea, ciliary body, lacrimal glands, conjunctiva, nasal mucosa and the skin of the nose, eyelid and forehead; (2) the maxillary nerve emerges through the round foramen and supplies sensation to the middle third of the face, the side of the nose and nasal passages, the lower eyelid, maxilla and maxillary teeth and the oral maxillary mucosa; and (3) the mandibular nerve emerges through the oval foramen and supplies sensation to the lower third of the face, the anterior two-thirds of the tongue, the mandible and mandibular teeth and the oral mandibular mucosa (Figure 14.1 and Figure 14.2) [4–6].

Noxious stimuli are transmitted from any of the three branches of the trigeminal nerve to the trigeminal ganglion, which is located on the anterior surface of the petrous part of the temporal bone in the trigeminal impression. Each branch of the trigeminal nerve enters the cranial cavity through their respective foramens to reach the trigeminal ganglion and from there the trigeminal fibres enter the pons to descend to the medulla and synapse in the spinal trigeminal nucleus, where they cross midline and ascend as the trigeminothalamic tract, which is a neospinothalamic tract. The A-delta fibres go to the ventral thalamus and from there to the somatosensory cortex for awareness of the exact location where pain is originating from, and the C fibres terminate in the parafasciculus and centromedian thalamus (intralaminar nuclei) to finally ascend to the somatosensory cortex.

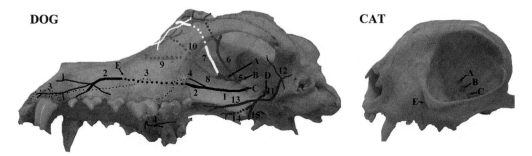

Figure 14.1 Nerves originating from the trigeminal nerve and providing sensory input to the head. (A) Optic canal; (B) Orbital fissure; (C) Round foramen in rostral alar canal; (D) Oval foramen; (E) Infraorbital foramen. The maxillary nerve (1) divides into the (i) infraorbital nerve (2), which enters the infraorbital canal through the maxillary foramen and branches the incisivomaxillary nerve (3) before exiting through the infraorbital foramen, and (ii) the greater palatine nerve (4), which enters the posterior palatine foramen to exit in the palate through the anterior palatine foramen. The ophthalmic nerve (5) divides into the lacrimal nerve (6), frontal nerve (7) and nasociliary nerve (8). The latter divides into the ethmoidal nerve (9) and the infratrochlear nerve (10). The mandibular nerve (11) divides into the auriculo-temporal nerve (12), the buccal nerve (13), the lingual nerve (14) and the inferior alveolar nerve (15), which enters the mandibular foramen.

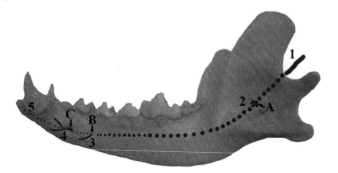

Figure 14.2 Lateral view of the mandible of the dog. The mandibular nerve (1) continues as the inferior alveolar nerve (2), which enters the mandibular foramen (A) on the medial aspect and emerges from the mandibular canal as the caudal mental nerve (3) through the caudal mental foramen (B) on the lateral aspect, the middle mental nerve (4) through the middle mental foramen (C) on the lateral aspect and the incisive nerve (cranial mental nerve) (5) at the cranial mental foramen on the cranial aspect (not shown).

A. Maxillary Block

The maxillary nerve can be blocked near its site of emergence from the round foramen using a transcutaneous approach or an intraoral approach [5, 6]. A third option has been described of an infraorbital approach and advancement of a catheter to the level of the lateral canthus within the infraorbital canal [5].

Deposition of local anesthetic at any of these locations blocks the maxillary nerve and its branches, the infraorbital nerve and the greater palatine nerve caudal to the second maxillary molar, providing a block of the whole ipsilateral maxilla, including molars and premolars, and associated bone and soft tissue, the soft palatal mucosa, hard palatal mucosa and bone, the canine and incisor teeth, the upper lip, nose, roof of the nasal cavity and skin as far caudal as the infraorbital foramen.

1. Transcutaneous Maxillary Approach

The maxillary nerve courses perpendicular to the palatine bone, between the maxillary foramen and the round foramen. A spinal needle, 20- or 22-gauge, 1.5–2.5 in is preferred over a regular needle and can be inserted through the skin at a 90° angle, in a medial direction, ventral to the border of the zygomatic arch and about 0.5 cm caudal to the lateral canthus, and then advanced towards the pterygopalatine fossa. Frequently, the needle will contact the ramus of the mandible, and it can be walked off the ramus cranially and then directed slight caudal immediately after until it comes in contact with the fossa and then withdrawn a short distance and the local anesthetic slowly injected after an aspiration test to rule out blood (Figure 14.3). A volume of 2–4 mL of local anesthetic, lidocaine or bupivacaine, is appropriate for a 20–30 kg patient. The location of the tip of the needle is in close proximity to the oval foramen (mandibular nerve) and orbital fissure (ophthalmic nerve); therefore, the volume of injectate can also affect these nerves. **There is a risk of puncturing the maxillary artery**, so gentle manipulation of the needle is recommended and aspiration before injection.

In cats, a 22-gauge, 1.5 in spinal needle can be used and a volume of 0.5 mL is appropriate.

Clipping: Recommended
Surgical preparation: Yes
Sterile gloves: Yes

(A)

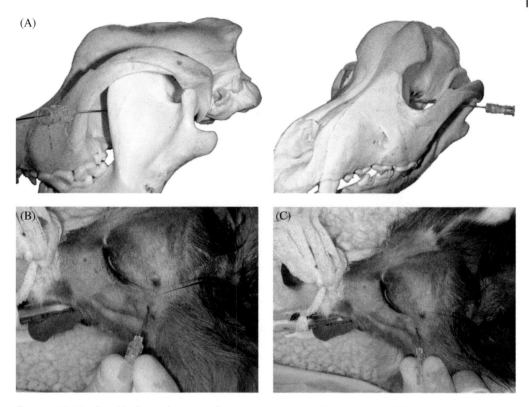

Figure 14.3 Maxillary block in a dog using the transcutaneous maxillary approach. (A) A spinal needle is inserted through the skin at a 90° angle, ventral to the border of the zygomatic arch and caudal to the lateral canthus, advanced towards the pterygopalatine fossa, avoiding the ramus of the mandible, and directed caudal immediately after until it comes in contact with the fossa, near the round foramen in the rostral alar canal. The needle should then be withdrawn a short distance and the local anesthetic slowly injected after an aspiration test to rule out blood. (B) Needle placement for the maxillary block with the needle directed caudally. (C) Needle placement for an eye block with the needle directed cranially.

2. Oral Maxillary Approach

The patient's mouth is opened and the lip's commissure retracted caudally. A 22- or 23-gauge, 1 in needle is advanced in a dorsal perpendicular direction to the plane of the palate, penetrating the mucosa directly behind the palatal and distobuccal roots of the maxillary second molar tooth, next to the maxillary tuberosity. Depending on the patient's size, the needle is advanced for no more than 5 mm beyond the mucosa. This approach blocks the greater palatine nerve in close proximity to the maxillary tuberosity, and the maxillary nerve closer to the maxillary foramen, before it becomes the infraorbital nerve. A volume of 1–2 mL of local anesthetic is appropriate for a 20–30 kg patient.

In cats, a 23- or 25-gauge, 1 in needle can be used and a volume of 0.25–0.5 mL is appropriate.

Clipping: No
Surgical preparation: Recommended
Sterile gloves: No

3. Infraorbital Injection in Infraorbital Canal

The infraorbital foramen is located approximately halfway between the medial canthus and the base of the maxillary canine, above the third premolar tooth. For a maxillary block using this approach, it is necessary to introduce a 22- or 20-gauge, 1–1.88 in catheter into the infraorbital

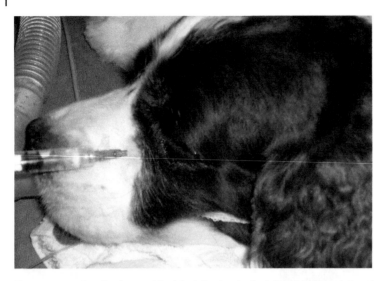

Figure 14.4 Infraorbital nerve block by injection in the infraorbital canal. A catheter is threaded into the infraorbital canal until the tip of the catheter reaches an imaginary line drawn perpendicular to the lateral canthus. The catheter can be introduced through the mucosa by elevating the upper lip and locating the infraorbital foramen or through the skin without elevation of the skin. Alternatively, the block can be done with a needle introduced into the infraorbital canal through the infraorbital foramen to the level of the first maxillary molar and the local anesthetic injected while gentle digital pressure is applied to the infraorbital foramen in order to force the local anesthetic into the canal and a large volume of local anesthetic is injected to reach the maxillary nerve within the orbit.

canal through the infraorbital foramen until the tip of the catheter reaches an imaginary line drawn perpendicular to the lateral canthus [5]. The catheter can be introduced through the mucosa by elevating the upper lip and locating the infraorbital foramen or through the skin without elevation of the skin (Figure 14.4 and Figure 14.5). A volume of 0.5 mL of methylene blue provided good stain of the nerve in skulls of 10–20 kg dogs. A volume of 1 mL of local anesthetic for dogs of 10–20 kg is probably appropriate.

A variation of this block is to use a 22- or 23-gauge, 1 in needle introduced into the infraorbital canal through the infraorbital foramen to the level of the first maxillary molar, and once aspiration is performed, to avoid intravascular injection, gentle digital pressure is applied to the infraorbital foramen in order to restrict the local anesthetic to the canal and a larger-than-usual volume than for an infraorbital block is used, so that the amount in excess of local anesthetic travels retrograde into the canal and reaches the maxillary nerve and surrounding tissue. A volume of 3–4 mL of local anesthetic is appropriate for a 20–30 kg patient.

In cats, the length of the infraorbital canal is very short (2–3 mm), and it is safer to not introduce needles into it due to the proximity of the eye dorsal to it. So this approach is not recommended (see Figure 14.1).

Clipping: Yes for catheter
Surgical preparation: Yes
Sterile gloves: Yes

B. Rostral Maxillary or Infraorbital Block

The rostral maxillary block provides blockade to the infraorbital nerve and the incisivomaxillary nerve within the infraorbital canal. The latter leaves the canal to enter the incisivomaxillary

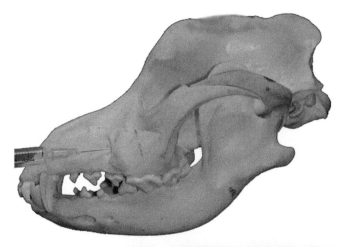

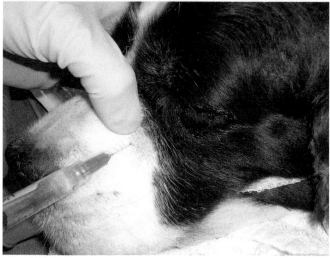

Figure 14.5 Rostral maxillary or infraorbital block in a dog. The infraorbital foramen is located approximately halfway between the medial canthus and the base of the maxillary canine, above the third premolar tooth. The needle is introduced slightly through the infraorbital foramen into the canal to facilitate the spread of the local anesthetic along the nerve.

foramen to innervate the canine and incisor teeth, which are therefore blocked. The infraorbital nerve is sensory to the upper lip, nose, roof of the nasal cavity and skin as far caudal as the infraorbital foramen. The first three premolar teeth, as well as the maxillary bone and surrounding soft tissue, are affected.

The block is performed as described above for the infraorbital injection in the infraorbital canal, through the mucosa or skin, except that the 22- or 23-gauge, 1 in needle does not need to be introduced in the infraorbital canal for more than 2–5 mm (Figure 14.5). A volume of 1 mL is appropriate for dogs of 10–20 kg.

In cats, the needle should not be introduced into the infraorbital canal, since this canal is only 2–3 mm long and it travels into the orbit from its opening ventral to the medial canthus at the junction of the maxilla and zygomatic bone. Instead, the needle is directed dorsally from above the second premolar to the site of the foramen or ventrally aligned with the

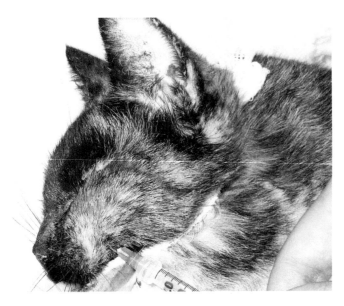

Figure 14.6 Rostral maxillary or infraorbital block in a cat. The needle is directed dorsally from above the second premolar to the site of the foramen or ventrally aligned with the second premolar, and the anesthetic volume injected in the surrounding area.

second premolar, and the anesthetic volume injected in the surrounding area (Figure 14.6). A volume of 0.25–0.5 mL is appropriate for adult cats.

Clipping: Not necessary
Surgical preparation: Yes
Sterile gloves: Not necessary

C. Mandibular Block

The mandibular nerve originates several sensory nerves, in addition to its motor involvement via the masseteric nerve. For the sensory involvement, it branches shortly after emerging from the oval foramen, into the buccal nerve, which supplies the cheek skin and oral mucous membrane (see Figure 14.1). Another branch is the auriculotemporal nerve, which descends laterally to the middle meningeal artery and then passes posteriorly to the temporomandibular joint (TMJ) and reaches the temporal region supplying the skin of this area, ear and TMJ. The lingual nerve passes inferiorly between the lateral and medial pterygoids and reaches the pterygomandibular space, ending in the anterior part of the mucous membrane of the floor of the mouth, from where it supplies the submandibular and sublingual glands, the anterior two-thirds of the tongue and the lingual gingiva of all mandibular teeth. The inferior alveolar nerve enters the mandibular foramen and travels along the mandibular canal to divide into a mental nerve and an incisive nerve at the level of the inferior premolar teeth. The mental nerve leaves the mandibular canal through both the caudal mental foramen and middle mental foramen, to supply the skin and mucous membrane of the lower lip, skin of the chin and vestibular gingiva of the mandibular incisive and canine teeth. The incisive nerve travels within the mandibular canal and ends at the level of the mandibular symphysis, and one of its branches exits through the cranial mental foramen.

The ideal block of the mandibular nerve is to block the inferior alveolar nerve, which, by blocking the mental and incisive nerve, facilitates involvement of the sensory supply to the alveolar process in the mandibular premolar, molar, canine and incisive teeth region, the periosteum of the mandible body, as well as the vestibular gingiva of all teeth, skin of the chin and the lower lip, without affecting sensory innervation to the tongue (unless desired) to avoid self-inflicted bites.

An intraoral or transcutaneous approach can be used for the inferior alveolar nerve.

1. Transcutaneous Approach to the Inferior Alveolar Nerve

The location of the mandibular foramen can be determined by drawing an imaginary line midway between the angular process of the mandible and the last molar tooth, approximately halfway on the medial side of the mandible. Alternatively, it can be located by dropping a plumb line from the lateral canthus to the ventral edge of the mandible at the point of maximum concavity, just rostral to the angular process (Figure 14.7). A 22- or 23-gauge, 1 in needle is introduced perpendicular and medial from the ventral edge of the mandible for a distance of 1–2 cm in a 20–30 kg patient and a volume of 1–3 mL is appropriate.

For a more accurate location, the hand can be introduced into the oral cavity and the mandibular foramen palpated underneath the mucosa and the needle introduced transcutaneously to that depth for the injection.

Clipping: Not necessary
Surgical preparation: Yes
Sterile gloves: Not necessary

2. Oral Approach to the Inferior Alveolar Nerve

For the oral approach, the hand is introduced in the oral cavity and the mandibular foramen located to allow for the other hand to place a 23-gauge, 1 in needle behind the last molar on the medial surface of the mandible and through the mucosa. A volume of 1–3 mL is appropriate in a 20–30 kg patient.

Clipping: No
Surgical preparation: Recommended
Sterile gloves: No

D. Alveolar or Mental or Rostral Mandibular Block

The caudal mental and middle mental nerve are branches of the mental nerve (branch of the inferior alveolar) and leave the mandibular canal through the caudal mental foramen and middle mental foramen, respectively. The most common block is the middle mental block, which desensitizes most of the area that involves the mandibular incisors, the canine and the first three premolars and the adjacent bone and soft tissues rostral to the foramen. The middle

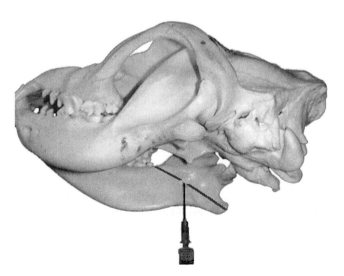

Figure 14.7 Transcutaneous inferior alveolar block in a dog. The mandibular foramen is midway between the angular process of the mandible and the last molar tooth, halfway on the medial side of the mandible. It can also be located above the point of maximum concavity of the mandible, just rostral to the angular process. A needle is introduced perpendicular and medial from the ventral edge of the mandible, where the concavity can be palpated.

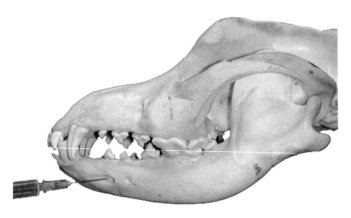

Figure 14.8 Rostral mandibular block in a dog. The needle is located at the middle mental foramen, ventral to the second premolar, to block the middle mental nerve. It can also include the caudal mental nerve by aiming the needle at the caudal mental foramen, ventral to the third premolar. Not shown is the incisive nerve (cranial mental nerve), which exits the mandible at the cranial mental foramen, located on the cranial aspect of the mandible, under the first incisor, just lateral to the symphysis.

foramen is located and can be palpated on the lateral aspect of the mandible and ventral to the second premolar (Figure 14.8). A 22- or 23-gauge, 1 in needle is introduced through the mucosa or skin towards the foramen in a cranial to caudal direction, although it is often very difficult to be able to introduce the needle in the foramen. A volume of 0.5–1 mL is appropriate for a 20–30 kg patient.

The caudal mental nerve can also be blocked to assure involvement of all premolars and is located on the lateral aspect of the mandible, under the third premolar (Figure 14.8). The same technique described for the middle mental nerve is used for this block.

The incisive nerve (cranial mental nerve) is also a branch of the inferior alveolar nerve and provides sensation to incisors and mucosa of the area and it exits the mandible at the cranial mental foramen, located on the cranial aspect of the mandible, under the first incisor, just lateral to the symphysis. The same technique described previously for the other mental nerves can be used for this nerve.

Clipping: Not necessary
Surgical preparation: Yes
Sterile gloves: Not necessary

E.   Eye Block

The ophthalmic nerve reaches the orbital cavity through the superior orbital fissure and is responsible for most sensory innervation to the eye and surrounding orbit (see Figure 14.1). The ophthalmic nerve divides into the lacrimal nerve, the frontal nerve and the nasociliary nerve. The lacrimal nerve arises from the ophthalmic nerve at its origin and supplies the lacrimal gland, part of the upper eyelid and skin of the temporal region. The frontal (supraorbital) and nasociliary (palpebronasal) nerves branch shortly after the ophthalmic nerve emerges into the orbit. The frontal nerve supplies the skin of the forehead region and upper eyelid, forming a plexus with the lacrimal and auriculopalpebral nerve. The nasociliary nerve provides the long sensory root to the ciliary ganglion and also originates two nerves: (1) the ethmoidal nerve to supply the mucous membrane of the nasal septum and dorsal turbinate and (2) the infratrochlear nerve, which supplies the conjunctiva, third eyelid and lacrimal ducts and sac.

Blocks to the eye and eyelids can be performed with different infiltration approaches and, most commonly, in combination with general anesthesia to provide more complete analgesia. Analgesia to the cornea is also possible by direct instillation of 1–2 drops of proparacaine (0.5%).

1. Eyelid Block

The sensory innervation to the upper eyelid is blocked through a frontal nerve block, which can be performed by infiltrating the upper eyelid along its length. This approach also blocks innervation from the lacrimal nerve. A 23- or 25-gauge, 1 in needle is introduced through the skin and a volume of 1 mL of local anesthetic, infiltrated subcutaneously, is appropriate for a 20–30 kg patient. Besides the sensory innervation, this approach also blocks the zygomatic branches of the auriculopalpebral nerve, which provide motor innervation to the eyelids; therefore, akinesia is also obtained. Akinesia without sensory blockade can be accomplished by blocking the auriculopalpebral nerve, a branch of the facial nerve, although this block is not commonly performed in small animals, but if akinesia is all that is desired, it can be elicited by inserting a 23-gauge, 1 in needle through the skin on the dorsal aspect of the zygomatic arch, just behind the lateral canthus and into the temporal fossa. A total of 0.5–1 mL of local anesthetic can be injected at different subcutaneous planes in a 20–30 kg patient (Figure 14.9).

Clipping: Not necessary
Surgical preparation: Yes
Sterile gloves: Not necessary

2. Eye Block

The ophthalmic nerve emerges through the orbital fissure with three other nerves: the oculomotor, abducens and trochlear. Therefore, in addition to sensory innervation to the eye and surrounding structures (cornea, ciliary body, lacrimal glands, conjunctiva, third eyelid, nasal mucosa and the skin of the nose, eyelid and forehead), all muscles to the eye are affected if the local anesthetic infiltration is performed near the orbital fissure, including the rectus lateralis and retractor muscle of the eyeball supplied by the abducens nerve, the rectus dorsalis, levator palpebrae superioris, rectus medialis and rectus ventralis supplied by the oculomotor nerve, and the dorsal oblique muscle of the eyeball supplied by the trochlear nerve.

There are two main options for performing an eye block.

i. Transcutaneous Maxillary Approach

The same technique used for the maxillary block can be used for an eye block due to the close proximity between the round foramen (maxillary nerve) and the orbital fissure. This also includes the oval foramen (mandibular nerve).

Figure 14.9 Motor blockade of the eyelid in a dog is achieved by blocking the auriculopalpebral nerve (2), a branch of the facial nerve (1), which emerges from the stylomastoid foramen. The block is performed on the dorsal aspect of the zygomatic arch, just behind the lateral canthus and into the temporal fossa, near the auriculopalpebral division into the auricular (3) and palpebral (4) branches. Sensory blockade is achieved injecting anesthetic along the eyelids to include the branches of the frontal nerve (5), a branch of the ophthalmic nerve that emerges from the cranium at the orbital fissure.

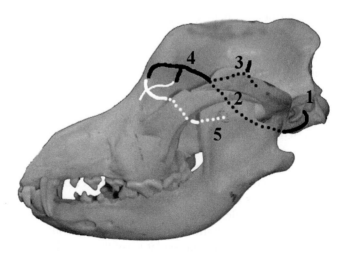

To prevent inclusion of the other nerves with this block, the maxillary approach can be modified. The spinal needle, 20- or 22-gauge, 1.5–2.5 in, is inserted at a 90° angle through the skin, ventral to the border of the zygomatic arch and about 0.5 cm caudal to the lateral canthus, and then advanced towards the pterygopalatine fossa. Once in contact with the ramus of the mandible, it's walked off the ramus cranially and kept with that cranial angle instead of directing it caudally, so that the needle is directed towards the back of the eyeball until it comes into contact with the bone at the back of the orbit (Figure 14.3C). Then the needle is withdrawn a short distance and the local anesthetic slowly injected after an aspiration test to rule out blood. A volume of 2–4 mL is appropriate for a 20–30 kg patient. In cats, a 22-gauge, 1.5 in spinal needle can be used and a volume of 0.5 mL is appropriate.

It is important to monitor heart rate while doing this block, since the volume of injectate can cause pressure on the muscles of the eye and stimulate the oculocardiac (trigeminovagal) reflex.

The advantage of this block is that the approach to the eye is from behind the globe and there is less risk of perforation.

Clipping: Recommended
Surgical preparation: Yes
Sterile gloves: Yes

ii. Retrobulbar Approach

A spinal needle, 20- or 22-gauge, 1.5–2.5 in, can be curved to follow the shape of the orbit and inserted into the orbit at any of these positions: medial canthus, lateral canthus, dorsal eyelid or ventral eyelid. A single position is usually sufficient, but two opposite positions can also be used in larger animals. The needle is inserted through the eyelids if preferred or through the conjunctiva at the same time that the globe is deflected away from the needle, with the curvature of the needle following the orbit to the back of the globe where 1–3 mL of local anesthetic can be injected for a 20–30 kg patient, after avoidance of intravascular injection by aspiration. In cats a volume of 0.5 mL is usually sufficient.

Proptosis indicates a successful block from blockade of the muscles of the eye, supplied by the oculomotor, trochlear and abducens. The block also involves the ophthalmic nerve for sensory innervation and the optic nerve.

Disadvantages of this technique include trauma of the optic nerve; therefore, it is only recommended for enucleation. In addition, the needle could pierce the meninges surrounding the optic nerve and enter the cerebrospinal fluid. The globe can also be perforated as well as there is risk of retrobulbar hemorrhage and initiation of the oculocardiac reflex.

Clipping: Recommended
Surgical preparation: Yes
Sterile gloves: Yes

IV. Thoracic Limb Block

The brachial plexus is the most important nerve structure for the thoracic limb. The brachial plexus is located in the axilla, cranial to the first rib and on the medial aspect of the shoulder joint and supplies the whole thoracic limb, from scapula to digits; however, only five out of 11 nerves are specific to the limb itself from below the location of the plexus. These include the axillary, musculocutaneous, radial, median and ulnar nerve; whereas the other six nerves innervate the surrounding musculature of the scapula, pectoral region and musculature over the back of the thorax and include the long thoracic, lateral thoracic, cranial pectoral, suprascapular, subscapular and thoracodorsal nerve. All of these nerves originate from ventral rami of spinal nerves C6 through T1 (C6, C7, C8, T1), which are contributors to the brachial plexus in the majority of dogs, although in some instances C5 and T2 may also contribute (Figure 14.10) [7, 8].

The axillary nerve originates from C7 and provides innervation to the subscapularis, teres major, teres minor and deltoideus muscles and contributes to flexion of the shoulder. The musculocutaneous nerve is composed of two filaments of C7. It descends from the plexus to the medial surface of the thoracic limb and divides to provide innervation to the biceps brachii and brachialis muscles to flex the elbow joint. The radial nerve is formed from C8 and small contributions of C7 and T1, and occasionally T2. This nerve provides innervation to the extensor muscles of the forearm through the coracobrachialis muscle, triceps brachii muscle and the forelimb extensors (ulnaris lateralis, lateral digital extensor, common digital extensor, extensor carpi radialis and extensor carpi obliquus) and provides sensory innervation to the craniolateral aspect of the forearm, carpus and paw. The median and ulnar nerves travel to the level of the brachial plexus within a common sheath and are formed from C8 and T1 with occasional contribution from T2, and both nerves provide innervation to the digital flexors. The median nerve innervates the flexor carpi radialis, superficial digital flexor and deep digital flexor. The

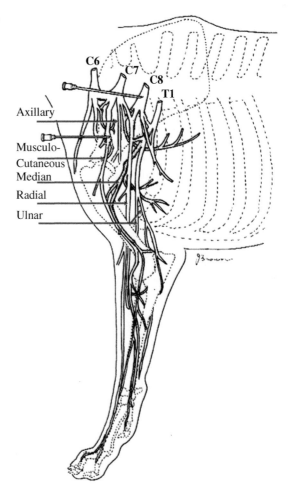

Figure 14.10 Medial aspect of the right forelimb of a dog depicting the nerves to the brachial plexus and limb.

ulnar nerve innervates the flexor carpi ulnaris and deep digital flexor. The ulnar nerve provides sensory innervation to the skin on the caudal aspect of the forearm, carpus and paw.

Blockade of the brachial plexus can be performed to provide analgesia/anesthesia and muscle relaxation for patients undergoing procedures of the thoracic limb to improve pain relief intra- and post-operatively. Since some nerves innervate their corresponding structures from below the plexus (axillary, musculocutaneous, radial, median and ulnar nerve), and some also do it from above the plexus (long thoracic, lateral thoracic, cranial pectoral, suprascapular, subscap- ular and thoracodorsal nerve), the site where the block is performed will influence which nerves are affected and the extent of the block. The options are to block the brachial plexus directly via an axillary approach or to block the ventral rami of cervical and thoracic contribu- tors to the brachial plexus via a paravertebral approach. Alternatively, some nerves can be blocked below the plexus individually or in combination, along their paths, to provide specific analgesia/anesthesia of the forelimb.

A. Brachial Plexus Block via Axillary Approach

The traditional approach for a brachial plexus block is performed by positioning the patient in lateral recumbency with the leg to be blocked uppermost and at a standing angle. The lateral tuberosity of the humerus (point of the shoulder joint) is identified and the needle is advanced from this point along the medial aspect of the scapula, in a parallel fashion to both the spine and costochondral joints, for a distance that places the tip of the needle slightly cranial to the first rib (Figure 14.11). This block has recently been further examined and simplified by identi- fying three specific landmarks: the transverse process of C6, the point of the shoulder joint and the first rib. The needle point should be positioned at the level midway between the transverse process of C6 and the point of the shoulder and advanced to the cranial aspect of the first rib, where the needle makes contact with the first rib and is then withdrawn slightly to inject cra- nial to it, at the specific location of the brachial plexus [9]. A volume of 0.2 mL/kg of local anesthetic is injected. A spinal needle, 20- or 22-gauge, 1.5–2.5 in, is used in a 20–30 kg dog and a volume of 0.2–0.3 mL/kg of local anesthetic is appropriate. This block is specific for the axil- lary, musculocutaneous, radial, median and ulnar nerves, so that the anesthesia/analgesia obtained is specific from the humerus to distal.

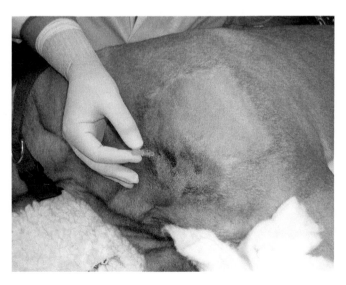

Figure 14.11 Brachial plexus block via axillary approach. The lateral tuberosity of the humerus (point of the shoulder joint) is identified and the needle is advanced from this point along the medial aspect of the scapula, in a parallel fashion to both the spine and costochondral joints, for a distance that places the tip of the needle slightly cranial to the first rib.

Figure 14.12 Brachial plexus block via a perpendicular approach caudal to the shoulder joint. With this approach, the needle is introduced perpendicularly to the skin caudal to the shoulder joint, to a depth above the thoracic wall at the level of the brachial plexus and cranial to the first rib.

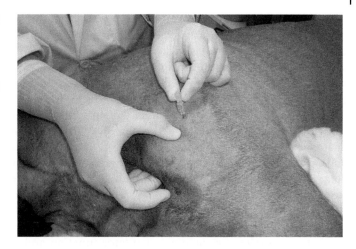

Alternatively, this approach can be modified to inject perpendicularly from the lateral to medial aspect of the limb by placing the needle caudal to the shoulder joint so that the tip of the needle is above the brachial plexus once it is introduced to a depth above the thoracic wall and cranial to the first rib (Figure 14.12) [9].

The axillary approach can be improved by use of ultrasound or electrostimulation or a combination of the two [8]. The use of ultrasound allows direct visualization of the nerves and needle position, decreasing the risk of intravascular injection and reducing the amount of required volume of local anesthetic. To perform this technique for the traditional approach, dogs are placed in dorsal recumbency with the thoracic limbs in a naturally flexed position and the transducer is placed in a parasagittal plane in the fossa between the manubrium and scapula, so that the axillary artery and vein can be identified below the brachial plexus. The needle is advanced craniocaudally, just dorsal to the identified axillary artery and vein, and visualized as it comes into proximity of the individual C6 to T1 nerves, where the local anesthetic is injected. With electrostimulation, a peripheral nerve stimulator applies an electric current to the peripheral nerve that will result in a corresponding muscle contraction if the proximity is appropriate so that the exact location of the nerve is identified and the injection of local anesthetic completed. The use of special needles with insulation is needed to permit current only at the tip of the needle, where the injection occurs. The nerve stimulator is set at an initial current of 0.8–1 mA, and once muscle contraction is elicited, the current is decreased to 0.2–0.4 mA to pinpoint that the muscle contraction is due to specific nerve stimulation; at this point, the injection is performed and the muscle will stop contracting. The procedure is repeated for the remaining nerves in the plexus.

Clipping: Yes
Surgical preparation: Yes
Sterile gloves: Yes

B. Brachial Plexus Block via a Paravertebral Approach

The paravertebral technique can provide analgesia/anesthesia of all 11 nerves associated with the brachial plexus (long thoracic, lateral thoracic, cranial pectoral, suprascapular, subscapular, axillary, musculocutaneous, thoracodorsal, radial, median and ulnar). The patient is placed in lateral recumbency and the limb to be blocked is uppermost, then the transverse process of C6 is identified as the largest process in front of the scapula and a spinal needle, 20- or 22-gauge, 1.5–2.5 in, is inserted in a dorsoventral direction until it contacts the dorsal aspect of the transverse process of C6, then the needle is walked off the cranial and caudal margins of the transverse process to block the ventral branch of C6 cranially and the ventral branch of C7 caudally. For C8, the needle is walked off the caudal margin of the transverse process of C7. For T1, the head of the first rib is palpated and the needle directed towards the cranial border of the proximal third of the rib where the nerve tends to emerge on its way to the plexus and the injection can be performed at this site (Figure 14.13) [6].

The technique allows for more precise deposition and a lower volume of local anesthetic (0.5–1.0 mL per nerve in a 20–30 kg dog) over the traditional approach; however, correct anatomical landmark identification and expertise are mandatory for a successful block. In addition, inadvertent puncture of the thoracic cavity, and resultant pneumothorax, intravascular injection of the vertebral arteries and epidural migration are potential complications associated with this technique. In dogs and cats, the phrenic nerve arises from C5 to C7; therefore, the paravertebral block can result in some risk of hemidiaphragmatic paralysis by blocking C6 and C7. However, compensation from the contralateral phrenic nerve and inspiratory muscles can maintain ventilator function and the block should never be performed bilaterally.

Clipping: Yes
Surgical preparation: Yes
Sterile gloves: Yes

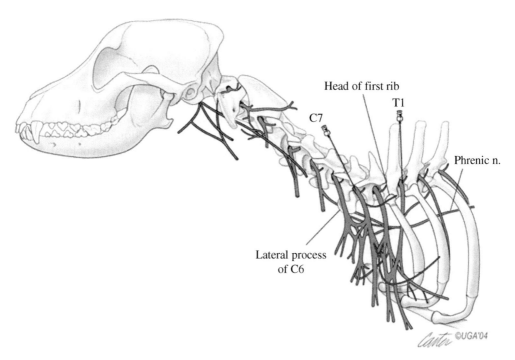

Figure 14.13 Brachial plexus block via a paravertebral approach. The transverse process of C6 is identified as the largest process in front of the scapula and a needle is inserted in a dorsoventral direction until it contacts the dorsal aspect of the transverse process of C6, then the needle is walked off the cranial and caudal margins of the transverse process to block the ventral branch of C6 cranially and the ventral branch of C7 caudally. For C8, the needle is walked off the caudal margin of the transverse process of C7. For T1, the head of the first rib is palpated and the needle directed towards the cranial border of the proximal third of the rib where the nerve tends to emerge on its way to the plexus and the injection can be performed at this site.

C.   Axillary, Musculocutaneous, Median, Radial, Ulnar Blocks

These nerves can be blocked at any location along their paths throughout the limb, if a more specific and localized block is desired for the required procedure. A more common approach is described below for a higher and general block of the limb.

1.   Axillary Block

The axillary nerve provides sensory innervation to the caudal aspect of the shoulder joint and craniolateral aspect of arm and forearm. The close proximity of the axillary nerve to the brachial plexus and its short path to the muscles that flex the shoulder make an isolated block of this nerve difficult without including the plexus itself, so it's rarely done individually.

2.   Musculocutaneous, Median and Ulnar Block

The musculocutaneous nerve provides sensory innervation to the craniomedial aspect of the forearm and elbow. The median nerve provides sensory innervation to the medial aspect of elbow joint, and the medial and palmar aspects of the forearm and paw. The ulnar nerve provides sensory innervation to the caudal aspect of the elbow joint and the caudolateral aspect of forearm and paw. On leaving the brachial plexus these three nerves run very closely to each other on the medial aspect of the humerus towards the elbow joint and can be blocked at this location. The patient is positioned with the leg to be blocked down to facilitate palpation of the nerves halfway or distally on the medial aspect of the humerus, between the biceps and triceps muscles, where the musculocutaneous nerve is cranial and the median and ulnar nerves are caudal to the brachial artery. They can be blocked as a group by injecting 0.1–0.15 mL/kg of local anesthetic using a 22- or 23-gauge, 1 to 1.5 in needle. The use of a nerve stimulator and insulated needle is also possible to locate the nerve according to the muscle contraction elicited, as described in Section IV.A.

Clipping: Yes
Surgical preparation: Yes
Sterile gloves: Yes

3.   Radial Block

The radial nerve provides sensory innervation to the craniolateral aspect of the forearm, carpus and paw and runs distal from the brachial plexus on the lateral aspect of the humerus towards the elbow joint. The patient is positioned with the leg to be blocked uppermost and the nerve is blocked halfway or distally on the humerus, between the biceps and triceps muscles. A volume of 0.1 mL/kg of local anesthetic is injected using a 22- or 23-gauge, 1–1.5 in needle. The use of a nerve stimulator and insulated needle is also possible to locate the nerve according to the muscle contraction elicited, as described in Section IV.A.

Clipping: Yes
Surgical preparation: Yes
Sterile gloves: Yes

V.   Thoracic Block

The most common blocks performed in the thorax include the intercostal, interpleural and epidural blocks [6, 10, 11]. The principle of all of them is to block the input from the intercostal nerves to the spinal cord, which can be done at different levels, including the sensory endings (interpleural block), the conduction along the nerve (intercostal nerve) or the discharge at the spinal cord level (epidural).

The thoracic nerves have a dorsal and ventral branch. The dorsal branch divides into a medial and lateral branch to supply muscles along the back of the trunk. The ventral branches constitute the intercostal nerve, and in the first two intercostal nerves (T1 and T2) additional ventral branches are contributors to the brachial plexus and nerves to the limb. Ventral branches of each of the 13 intercostal nerves run on the posterior border of the rib, along the intercostal space with the artery and vein; they all supply intercostal muscles, pleura and thoracic skin and, depending on their location along the spine, also supply the pectoral muscles, transverse thoracic muscle, diaphragm, internal abdominal oblique muscle and rectus abdominal muscle.

A. Intercostal Block

The intercostal block provides effective analgesia and can be performed preemptively or post-operatively for lateral thoracotomies, and post-trauma of the lateral thorax, including fractured ribs. The analgesia associated with this block facilitates breathing and helps reduce the use of systemic analgesics. The block is more effective if several adjacent intercostal nerves are included, since there is common overlapping of nerve endings between adjacent individual intercostal nerves. Therefore, it is commonly recommended for thoracotomies to block the intercostal nerve where the incision occurred and the next 1–2 intercostal nerves immediately cranial and caudal to the incision.

The block is performed using a 22- or 23-gauge, 1–1.5 in needle or spinal needle, by palpating the desired intercostal space and introducing the needle as dorsal as possible to the rib's origin from the spine, directly on the caudal aspect of the shaft of the rib by making contact with it and walking the needle off to the medial aspect where the nerve is located with the artery and vein. Aspiration before injection is necessary to avoid intravascular injection and to assure that the needle is not in the thoracic cavity. A volume of 1.0 mL of local anesthetic per nerve is appropriate in a 20–30 kg dog (Figure 14.14).

Clipping: Yes
Surgical preparation: Yes
Sterile gloves: Yes

B. Interpleural Block

An alternative to the intercostal block is to deposit the anesthetic in the space between the parietal and visceral pleura in order to block the nerve endings from intercostal nerves at the parietal surface of the pleura. To allow for proper contact of the local anesthetic with the nerve endings at the pleura and the intercostal nerve emerging from the spinal cord, it is necessary to position the affected side down to facilitate the absorption of the anesthetic. In people, the supine position facilitates this process, and the same can be implemented in the heavily sedated or anesthetized patient. However, this is less practical in the conscious patient due to discomfort and pain. The mechanism of action of a local anesthetic injected between the parietal and visceral pleura involves reverse diffusion through the parietal pleura into the subpleural space. From there, the anesthetic can reach the intercostal nerve.

The block is performed using an over-the-needle catheter, the gauge selected according to the animal's size. A 20-gauge, 1.88 in is appropriate for dogs > 10 kg and can be introduced between the seventh and eighth rib, as per a thoracocentesis, at the middle or dorsal third of the affected side of the chest. The catheter is introduced in proximity to the cranial border of the rib to avoid the nerve on the caudal border, and then advanced slowly at a 45° angle through the parietal pleura into the pleural space. Some recommend attaching a syringe with saline and

Figure 14.14 Intercostal block in a dog that includes the intercostal nerve where the incision occurred (I) and the next 1–2 intercostal nerves immediately cranial and caudal to the incision.

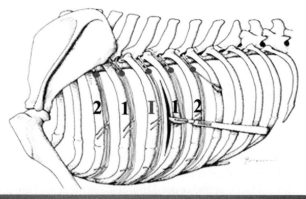

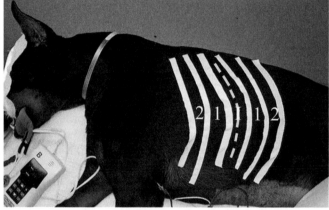

a bubble of air to the catheter during the insertion to recognize aspiration of the fluid and movement of the bubble from the syringe into the chest due to the negative intrapleural pressure; however, in patients with trauma and pneumothorax this may not be possible due to the lack of negative pressure or presence of fluid/blood in the cavity. The ease with which the catheter can be advanced away from the stylet, into the pleural space, is a good indicator of proper placement. Aspiration to verify negative pressure and absence of blood is completed before the injection of local anesthetic. Bupivacaine 0.25–0.5% is preferred over lidocaine due to a more prolonged duration of action (3–24 h) by this route, using a dose of 1.5 mg/kg (0.3 mL of 0.5% or 0.6 mL/kg of 0.25%) and injected slowly over 1 min. Lidocaine 1–2% can be administered using the same volumes described for bupivacaine. Once the volume is injected, the catheter is removed and the patient positioned to facilitate contact of the affected site with the local anesthetic. Contact time should be at least 5–10 min for lidocaine and 10–20 min for bupivacaine.

The block can be less effective if the pleural space contains blood and/or air, as often occurs after surgery, as these conditions predispose to pooling of local anesthetic and limited spread over the affected area.

For repeated injections or continuous administration, an indwelling catheter can be placed on the affected side using the same technique described above and securing the catheter to the skin of the thoracic wall. The volume held by the catheter has to be taken into account when calculating doses using this technique.

Although complications from interpleural injections are possible, proper technique minimizes most of them and the incidence is very low. Reported complications include pneumothorax, phrenic nerve paralysis, Horner's syndrome, infection and pleural effusion.

Clipping: Yes
Surgical preparation: Yes
Sterile gloves: Yes

C. Epidural Block

An epidural approach to the thoracic area is possible from a lumbosacral injection or from an intervertebral thoracic injection [10, 11]. The latter has been used only occasionally in dogs and involves the use of an epidural catheter that can be inserted between the last thoracic segments (T12–T13) through a paramedian approach and directed towards the desired thoracic segments. The lumbosacral injection is more commonly used and from this site an epidural catheter can also be directed to the desired thoracic segments. For either technique, the tip of the catheter is placed at the desired thoracic segment and the local anesthetic injected at a reduced dose to affect only those thoracic segments, usually 0.07–0.1 mL/kg versus 0.2 mL/kg injected directly at the lumbosacral space. The injection can affect both sides of the thorax, unless the patient is positioned with the affected side down, to emphasize the block on that side.

Epidural catheters are placed through a Tuohy needle, which has a curved bevel that facilitates direction of the threaded catheter through it into the epidural space. The needle is initially introduced perpendicular to the skin and the angle of insertion adjusted as required to facilitate the location of the intervertebral space until it pierces the *ligamentum flavum* and the needle is further introduced into the epidural space. To verify correct placement of the needle, several tests can be performed; a glass syringe that comes with the kit and offers minimal resistance upon injection of air or saline, due to the sub-atmospheric pressure of the epidural space. If this is the case, the catheter can be threaded through the needle and advanced slowly, especially from the lumbosacral space, due to the long distance to thoracic segments and the likelihood of encountering resistance from meningovertebral ligaments and the spinal cord along the path. Tuohy needles are 17-, 18- and 20-gauge, 2–3.5 in, and thread epidural catheters 19-, 20- and 24-gauge, respectively. The catheter is secured by suturing it or gluing it at the site of entry into the skin. The use of the filter that comes with the kit is recommended.

Complications from this approach include mechanical factors affecting the catheter itself, such as looping, kinking, knotting and dislodgment of the tip of the catheter outside of the vertebral canal. In addition, intrathecal and venous puncture and spinal cord damage are possible. In regards to volumes and dose, it is important to avoid overdosing and related complications, such as hypotension and Horner's syndrome from blocking sympathetic fibres along the sympathetic trunk, and respiratory impairment from blocking motor fibres that may affect diaphragm contractions.

Clipping: Yes
Surgical preparation: Yes
Sterile gloves: Yes

VI. Abdomen, Perineum and Pelvic Limb Blocks

The abdomen is innervated from nerves arising from the last thoracic (T10 to T13) and from the lumbar area (L1 to L6). The pelvis, pelvic limb and perineal area is innervated by the lumbosacral plexus, formed by ventral branches of spinal nerves L4 to S3, which exchange axons and give rise to individual nerves that contain axons from multiple segments.

The nerves to the pelvic limb include the obturator nerve (L4 to L6 nerve roots), which innervates the adductor muscles; the femoral nerve (L4 to L6 nerve roots), which innervates the cranial muscles of the thigh through its branch of the saphenous nerve; and the sciatic nerve (L6, L7 and S1, S2 nerve roots), which innervates the remaining muscles of the limb through the common peroneal nerve (cranial muscles) and tibial nerve (caudal muscles).

The sacral portion of the lumbosacral plexus is the origin of the pelvic nerve, for both afferent and efferent innervation of the pelvic viscera, and the pudendal nerve for both efferent and afferent innervation from pelvic structures, including the anus and penis/clitoris.

A. Epidural Block

An epidural injection that affects (1) abdomen, perineum or pelvic limbs can be performed at the **lumbosacral space** [11]. An epidural injection that affects (2) perineum and adjacent areas can be performed at the **sacrococcygeal space** [12].

1. Single Lumbosacral Epidural Block

Volumes of local anesthetic of at least 0.2 mL/kg injected in the lumbosacral space of dogs and cats have been shown to reach up to the T10 vertebrae and provide sufficient anesthesia for a laparotomy, the pelvis, perineal area and pelvic limbs. Lower volumes (0.1 mL/kg) limit the extent of the block to low lumbar segments and are sufficient for blocking sensory to the pelvis, perineal area and pelvic limbs. Opioids (Table 14.1) are almost always combined with the local anesthetic to achieve analgesia for a much longer duration than that achieved by local anesthetics used alone. Morphine is most commonly chosen because it has the longest duration of action among the opioids. When an opioid is used, the dose of the opioid is calculated, then the local anesthetic is added to the opioid for a total volume of 0.2 mL/kg of the mixture (e.g. the volume of 0.1% morphine dosed at 0.1 mg/kg for a 20 kg dog is 2 mL). As an example of a block for a 20 kg dog: 20 kg × 0.2 ml/kg = 4 mL, therefore, 2 mL of lidocaine is added to the 2 mL of morphine for the total of 4 mL.

Epidural injections can be performed in conscious, sedated or anesthetized animals with the patient in a lateral or sternal position. Proper aseptic preparation of the area is important for this technique. The lumbosacral space is located by palpation of the anterior aspect of both iliac crests with the thumb and middle finger of the operator's hand that is cranial to the patient's pelvis and tracing an imaginary line that crosses over the L6–7 space between both fingers. The operator then palpates the L6 spinous process caudal to the index finger of that same hand, so it can locate the space cranial to the finger (L6–7) to then continue advancing the finger over the spinous process of L7 to finally locate the lumbosacral space. Usually, the L6 spinous process is taller and more distinct than the L7 spinous process. In addition, caudal to L7, the spinous processes of the sacrum feel like a continuous ridge due to their fusion (Figure 14.15).

Table 14.1 Opioids used for epidural analgesia.

Opioid	Dose	Duration of action	Time of onset of action
Morphine	0.1 mg/kg	12–24 h	30–60 min
Oxymorphone	0.03–0.05 mg/kg	6 h	30 min
Hydromorphone	0.02–0.04 mg/kg	6–12 h	<30 min
Methadone	0.1–0.3 mg/kg	7 h	<20 min
Fentanyl	0.004 mg/kg	0.5 h	<10 min
Buprenorphine	0.005 mg/kg	10–15 h	30 min

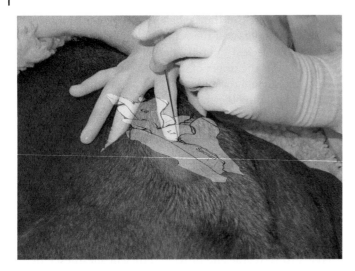

Figure 14.15 Lumbosacral epidural block. The lumbosacral space (L7–S1) is located by palpation of the anterior aspect of both iliac crests with the thumb and middle finger of the operator's hand that is cranial to the patient's pelvis and tracing an imaginary line that crosses over the L6–7 space between both fingers. The operator then palpates the L6 spinous process caudal to the index finger of that same hand, so it can locate the space cranial to the finger (L6–7) to then continue advancing the finger over the spinous process of L7 to finally locate the lumbosacral space.

The diameter of the L–S space is relatively small in dogs and cats and some authors recommend that the hind limbs are moved forward to enhance the L–S space. If the patient is in a sternal position with the legs extended caudally, the angle of insertion of the needle is perpendicular to the spine, but if the legs are flexed forward, the angle of insertion of the needle is perpendicular to the pelvis but not to the spine. The bevel of the needle is directed forward to facilitate the distribution of the injectate and adjustments to the angle of insertion are made as required to facilitate correct placement of the needle as it advances into deeper layers. Spinal needles, 20- or 22-gauge, 1.5–2.5 in, are recommended for medium and large dog breeds, whereas a 22-gauge, 1.5 in spinal needle is used in young and small dog breeds and cats.

For patients in sternal recumbency, the stylet of the needle can be removed once the needle is through the skin and saline or local anesthetic used to fill the hub of the needle; the needle is then slowly advanced deeper into the lumbosacral space. Occasionally, a "pop" can be felt when it pierces the *ligamentum flavum,* and at this time the fluid in the hub of the needle is aspirated into the epidural space because of the sub-atmospheric epidural pressure. This test is known as the "hanging drop technique". However, it only works for patients in sternal recumbency and can also have false-negatives due to clogging of the lumen of the needle with tissue as it is advanced or from the use of small spinal needles. Alternatively, a glass syringe, which offers low resistance, can be attached to the needle and air injected to test for resistance upon injection. This latter technique can be used with patients in lateral or sternal recumbency. For this latter technique in dogs, the spinal needle with or without a stylet can be advanced into the epidural space to the floor of the canal, the glass syringe attached at this time while the needle is steady in that location, and then the needle withdrawn 1–2 mm to test for resistance to a small volume of air injection (0.5–1 mL). If no resistance is encountered, then the glass syringe can be exchanged with the syringe containing the local anesthetic to be injected.

In cats, small dogs and young dogs, the spinal dura mater can extend slightly beyond the L7 vertebra, and the likelihood of piercing this membrane and obtaining cerebrospinal fluid (CSF) is high; therefore, it is preferable to not advance the needle to the floor, to avoid piercing the dura/arachnoid membranes and the risk of an intrathecal (subarachnoid) injection. It is not recommended to inject an epidural dose intrathecally, because of the risk of overdose; alternatively, the epidural dose can be adjusted to an intrathecal dose by decreasing it to 10% of the epidural dose. In these patients, flicking of the tail, movement of the hind limbs or twitching of the skin can be observed when the needle is in the epidural space and pricks, but does not necessarily pierce, the spinal cord or cauda equina, without adverse effects. At this time, the

Figure 14.16 Example of an epidural catheter placed at the lumbosacral space.

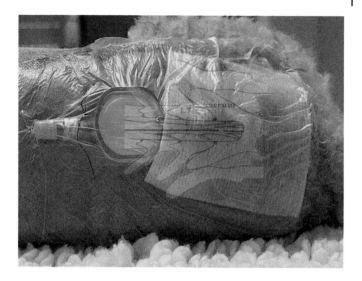

advancing of the needle is stopped and the air resistance test can be performed then, before injection. If CSF is obtained during epidural attempts, withdrawing the needle slowly may reposition the needle back into the epidural space and the epidural injection completed after verification of the air resistance test. The likelihood of anesthetic injected epidurally going intrathecally after the dura/arachnoid membrane has been pierced is very low due to the pressure gradient of CSF from the intrathecal to the epidural space.

Epidural catheters can also be placed through a Tuohy needle at the lumbosacral space, using the same general principles described above for thoracic epidural, except that the catheter is advanced only to lumbar segments, usually 5–10 cm into the spinal canal. The catheter is secured in place by suturing or gluing it at the site of entry into the skin. This facilitates continuous or repeated injections of local anesthetics and/or analgesics recommended for epidural use (Figure 14.16).

Regardless of the method used for epidural injection, the block is more effective if the affected side is lowermost, to facilitate the contact and absorption of the local anesthetic by the nerve tissue. For conditions requiring a block of both sides, sternal or dorsal recumbency is appropriate.

2. Repeated Drug Administration

For patients with severe pain that is difficult to manage, epidural drugs can be administered via an epidural catheter by intermittent or continuous infusion from the lumbosacral space, to allow for constant analgesic effects of the drugs. Continuous infusion is recommended for drugs with a short duration of action (e.g. lidocaine), in which the constant administration of the drug replaces the amount of drug taken away by systemic absorption and metabolism from the epidural space. Intermittent administration is recommended for drugs with a prolonged duration of action (bupivacaine).

i. Continuous Infusion

Lidocaine can be administered as a continuous infusion. A loading dose is used initially using a dose of 0.1–0.2 mL/kg (2–4 mg/kg), and then the specific expected duration of action (up to 1.5 h) of this dose is divided into hourly requirements and infused at that rate after the loading dose. Thorough monitoring is required to avoid overdosing and adverse effects (paralysis, excessive rostral spread, hypotension). Accurate administration is best via syringe pump, and aseptically through an epidural filter.

Table 14.2 Local anesthetics used for epidural anesthesia.

Local anesthetic agent	Dose	Duration of action	Time to onset of action
Lidocaine 2%	0.2 mL/kg	45–90 min	5 min
Mepivacaine 2%	0.2 mL/kg	60–90 min	5 min
Bupivacaine 0.5%	0.2 mL/kg	120–360 min	20 min
Ropivacaine 0.2%	0.5 mL/kg	90–420 min	15 min

ii. Intermittent Injection

For drugs with prolonged duration of action (>3 h), such as bupivacaine, intermittent injection is sufficient to maintain proper analgesic effects. Doses of 0.1–0.2 mg/kg (0.5–1 mg/kg) and timing of administration, subsequent to the first dose, should be adjusted according to the quality of analgesia and the observed duration of action, to avoid adverse effects from overdosing or insufficient analgesia from underdosing. Opioids are also given by intermittent injection (Table 14.1 and 14.2). However, for the very painful patient, q8h may be required.

Contraindications for epidural injections include patients that have coagulation disorders, deformity of the anatomy of the L–S area from traumatic injury or obesity that make the approach difficult or impossible and infection in the L–S area. A relative contraindication is unstable hemodynamic function that may be exacerbated by the possible vasodilatory effects of local anesthetics from blockade of the sympathetic trunk.

Clipping: Yes
Surgical preparation: Yes
Sterile gloves: Yes

3. Sacrococcygeal Epidural Block

This technique is recommended in cats with urethral obstruction to facilitate comfort of the patient and manipulation of the urethra [12]. Proper technique blocks the sacral portion of the lumbosacral plexus, including the pelvic, pudendal and caudal nerves, providing anesthesia of the perineum, penis, urethra, colon, anus and tail. The roots to nerves of the pelvic limb (obturator, femoral and sciatic) are not affected if the volume of injection of the local anesthetic does not exceed 0.1 mL/kg; therefore, motor function is not affected.

The advantage of this technique is that it is very specific to the perineum, and in cats it avoids the risk of intrathecal injections. Lidocaine is preferred for its rapid onset and can result in anesthesia within 5 min after injection and last up to 60 min.

After proper aseptic preparation of the area, the sacrococcygeal space is located, with the patient in sternal recumbency, by palpating the caudal portion of the sacrum (S3 vertebra) and the first coccygeal vertebra (Co1) by elevating and lowering the tail while palpating the area and identifying the space at which the tail hinges. Alternatively, the first intercoccygeal space (Co1–Co2) can also be used for the injection. A 25-gauge, 1 in needle can be used in cats, whereas 22- or 23-gauge, 1.5 in needles can be used in dogs. The angle of insertion of the needle is at 30–45° to the spine with the bevel of the needle directed forwards to facilitate the distribution of the injectate. The needle is advanced slowly towards the sacrococcygeal space and adjustments made as required until it pierces the *ligamentum flavum*, which may be associated with an occasional "pop". The hanging drop technique is not very effective at this location due to the smaller space and smaller gauge needles used. The injection of air is also not recommended because it can interfere with the distribution of the injectate and result in a patchy block. Therefore, ease of injection is the best indicator. This test is known as the hanging drop technique; however, it only works for patients in sternal recumbency and can also have false-negatives due to clogging of the lumen of the needle with tissue as it is advanced or from the use of small spinal needles. A volume of 0.1–0.2 mL/kg is recommended. The lower the volume, the less likely motor function of the pelvic limb is affected.

A video of the procedure can be accessed online. For example, on the website YouTube, search using "Wright sacrococcygeal block".

Clipping: Yes
Surgical preparation: Yes
Sterile gloves: Yes

B. Femoral and Saphenous Block

The femoral nerve is both motor and sensory; it descends on the medial aspect of the limb and soon becomes the saphenous nerve as it accompanies the femoral artery. The femoral nerve is in front of the femoral artery in the upper third of the thigh, before it travels downwards and cranial towards the quadriceps muscle between the vastus medialis and rectus femoris. The saphenous nerve is strictly sensory and is also present in the upper third of the thigh as it branches out of the femoral nerve. Both nerves supply the sensory innervation to the medial and cranial aspect of the thigh and stifle, and the medial aspect of the metatarsus (Figure 14.17A).

To block the femoral nerve, the approach is high in the inguinal area, in the triangle formed by the iliopsoas muscle at the base of the inguinal area, the sartorius muscle running downwards and cranial to the nerve, and the pectineus muscle running downwards and caudal to the nerve. The patient is positioned in lateral recumbency with the limb to be blocked uppermost; this limb is abducted 90° to visualize the inguinal area and extended to delineate the femoral triangle. Palpation of the femoral artery at the base of the inguinal area within the triangle of muscles will indicate that the femoral nerve is in front of it. The injection can be performed with a 22- or 23-gauge, 1–1.5 in needle, inserted at a 20–30° angle to the skin towards the base of the triangle, avoiding the femoral artery and the risk of hematoma [6, 8]. Alternatively, electrostimulation with a peripheral nerve stimulator using special needles with insulation can be used setting the initial current at 0.8–1 mA to stimulate the nerve and elicit quadriceps muscle contractions with extension of the knee joint; the current is then decreased to 0.4 mA to pinpoint that the muscle contraction is due to specific nerve stimulation; at this point, the injection is performed and the muscle will stop contracting. A volume of 0.1 mL/kg of local anesthetic is injected after verification of negative blood aspiration. Bupivacaine is preferred over lidocaine due to its longer duration of action.

A proper block of the femoral nerve also includes the saphenous nerve before the latter separates from the femoral nerve.

Clipping: Yes
Surgical preparation: Yes
Sterile gloves: Yes

C. Saphenous Block

The saphenous nerve travels downwards in front of the femoral artery up to the middle third of the thigh, between the sartorius muscle cranially and the gracilis muscle caudally. Then medial to the saphenous artery on the lower third, where it anastomoses with branches of the superficial peroneal nerve from the sciatic nerve. The saphenous nerve is sensory to the medial aspect of the limb between the knee and ankle.

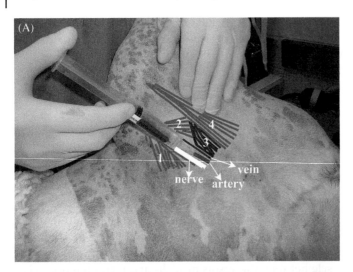

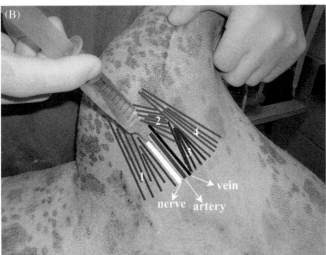

Figure 14.17 Femoral and saphenous block in a dog. Relevant anatomical structures include the femoral triangle, formed by the base of the inguinal area, the sartorius muscle (1) running downwards and cranial, and the pectineus muscle (3) running downwards and caudally. (A) To block the femoral nerve and the saphenous nerve at the femoral triangle, the pulsating femoral artery is palpated in the triangle and the femoral nerve is cranial to the artery at this location; therefore, the needle is inserted cranial to the artery. (B) To block only the saphenous nerve, the needle is inserted into the middle third of the thigh, in front of the adductor muscle (2) and gracilis muscle (4), and caudal to the sartorius muscle (1), by palpating the pulsating femoral artery, and the saphenous nerve is cranial to the artery at this location.

The injection site for the saphenous nerve is in the middle third of the thigh, between the femoral triangle and the medial epicondyle of the femoro-tibial joint (Figure 14.17B) [6, 8, 13, 14]. The limb to be blocked can be place uppermost or lowermost, as access to the middle third of the thigh is possible with both positions. If the limb is lowermost, the opposite limb is positioned caudally or abducted 90°; if the limb is uppermost, the limb is abducted 90° and for either approach, a 22- or 23-gauge, 1–1.5 in needle is inserted at a 20–30° angle towards the inguinal area, in front of the pulsating femoral artery and gracilis muscle and caudal to the sartorius muscle. A volume of 0.05–0.1 mL/kg of local anesthetic is injected. The nerve can also be identified by electrostimulation with a peripheral nerve stimulator and special needle, similar to the femoral nerve technique (see Section VI.B); however, stimulation of the nerve only results in sensory discomfort that can be quickly blocked by injection of local anesthetic. This approach is feasible in conscious people, but less useful in animals, whether conscious, sedated or anesthetized.

Clipping: Yes
Surgical preparation: Yes
Sterile gloves: Yes

D.   Sciatic, Common Peroneal and Tibial Block

The sciatic nerve emerges from the greater sciatic foramen and passes downwards and backwards on the lower part of the sacro-sciatic ligament to pass between the major trochanter of the femur and the ischiatic tuberosity of the pelvis. From here, it descends on the lateral and caudal part of the femur between the biceps femoris muscle laterally and the adductor, semimembranosus, and semitendinosus muscles medially as both the common peroneal and tibial nerve; they separate above the origin of the gastrocnemius (above the condyles of the femur), caudal to the femoro-tibial joint.

   Several techniques have been described to complete a sciatic nerve block [6, 8, 13, 14]. The easiest method is to position the patient in lateral recumbency with the affected limb uppermost and to insert a 20- or 22-gauge, 1.5 in needle, standing from the back of the patient, with a 45° angle between the major trochanter of the femur and the ischiatic tuberosity, closer to the former since the sciatic nerve descends over the pelvis to the femur at this location (Figure 14.18A). A volume of 0.05–0.1 mL/kg of local anesthetic is injected. The nerve can also be identified by electrostimulation with a peripheral nerve stimulator and special needle, similar to the femoral nerve technique (see Section VI.B), by observing dorsiflexion of the foot from the actions of the peroneal component of the sciatic nerve. Therefore, blocking of the sciatic nerve at this level also includes the innervation of the peroneal and tibial nerve. The peroneal nerve specifically innervates the caudolateral femoro-tibial joint capsule, the lateral meniscus, the flexors of the tarsus, the extensors of the digits, the skin of the dorsal aspect of the tarsus/metatarsus and the digits. The tibial nerve specifically innervates the caudal femoro-tibial joint capsule, the extensors of the tarsus, the flexors of the digits and the plantar aspect of the tarsus and digits.

   If the femoral nerve is also blocked, then there is complete block of the limb, except for the obturator nerve, which is sensory to the skin of the middle part of the medial thigh.

Clipping: Yes
Surgical preparation: Yes
Sterile gloves: Yes

E.   Peroneal and Tibial Block

The common peroneal and tibial nerves run as one, downward and deep along the thigh on the caudolateral aspect of the femur, as a continuation of the sciatic nerve, underneath the hamstring muscles (biceps femoris, semitendinosus and semimembranosus). The two nerves eventually divide caudal to the femoro-tibial joint, from where the common peroneal runs downwards and forwards across the lateral head of the gastrocnemius muscle, passes between the deep flexor of the digit and the peroneus longus and divides into superficial and deep branches that provide innervation to all digits on the dorsal aspect. The tibial nerve is the direct continuation of the sciatic nerve, runs on the medial aspect of the gastrocnemius muscle, along the tibia and divides into medial and lateral plantar branches at the tarsus to provide innervation to all digits on the plantar aspect.

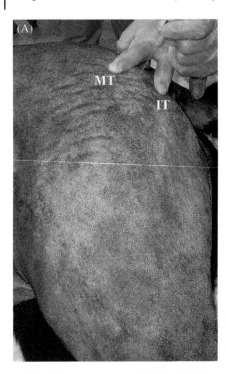 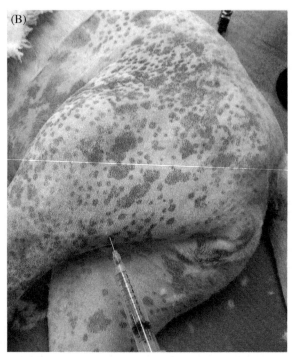

Figure 14.18 Sciatic, common peroneal and tibial nerve block in a dog. (A) To block all three nerves, a needle is inserted with a 45° angle between the major trochanter (MT) of the femur and the ischiatic tuberosity (IT), closer to the former since the sciatic nerve descends over the pelvis to the femur at this location. (B) To block the common peroneal and tibial nerve, a long needle is advanced in a caudal-to-cranial direction in the middle third of the thigh in the space between the biceps femoris muscle laterally and the semitendinosus muscle medially until it reaches the caudal surface of the femur and is slightly withdrawn for the injection at that location.

The block to include both peroneal and tibial nerves can be performed in the middle third of the thigh with the dog in lateral recumbency and the affected limb uppermost [6, 8, 14]. One hand palpates with the thumb in a caudal-to-cranial direction the space between the biceps femoris muscle laterally and the semitendinosus muscle medially until it reaches the caudal surface of the femur and a 20- or 22-gauge, 1.5–3.5 in spinal needle is directed perpendicular in the same fashion as the thumb until it contacts the bone and is then withdrawn a few millimetres, the stylet removed and the local anesthetic injected using a volume of 0.1–0.2 mL/kg of local anesthetic (Figure 14.18B). The nerve can also be identified by electrostimulation with a peripheral nerve stimulator and special needle, similar to the femoral nerve technique, by observing dorsiflexion of the foot.

Clipping: Yes
Surgical preparation: Yes
Sterile gloves: Yes

VII. Intra-Articular Block

Intra-articular blocks can be performed in any joint. However, they are most commonly used for the femoro-tibial joint before (preemptive) or after surgical intervention. A 22- or 23-gauge, 1–1.5 in needle can be inserted into any joint and correct placement verified by aspiration of joint fluid, before injection of local anesthetic (Figure 14.19). Bupivacaine is the most

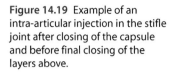
Figure 14.19 Example of an intra-articular injection in the stifle joint after closing of the capsule and before final closing of the layers above.

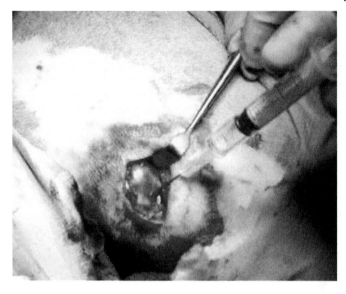

commonly used anesthetic because it provides a duration of action of 2–4 h. The volume varies with the size of the joint, usually 0.1–0.5 mL/kg.

Clipping: Yes
Surgical preparation: Yes
Sterile gloves: Yes

VIII. Intravenous Regional Anesthesia (IVRA) or Bier Block

This method provides complete anesthesia of the distal limb and consists of the injection of local anesthetic into a superficial vein on the thoracic or pelvic limb after proximal application of a tourniquet to occlude arterial blood flow. Sedation or general anesthesia is recommended for IVRA to decrease the discomfort of the tourniquet.

The tourniquet consists of a pneumatic cuff or a rubber style tourniquet, placed proximal to the region to be desensitized and pressurized or firmly wrapped to interrupt arterial blood flow and removal of the local anesthetic from the surgical area. A 22-gauge, 1 in catheter is placed in a vein of the limb, distal to the tourniquet, and close to the surgical site, for the injection of the local anesthetic. A volume of 0.1–0.2 mL/kg of lidocaine (2–4 mg/kg) can be injected. Bupivacaine should not be used IV due to toxicity to the central nervous and cardiovascular systems. After injection of the local anesthetic, the catheter can be removed and a bandage applied to prevent a hematoma.

The lidocaine injected diffuses into the vascular and eventually spills out of the vasculature and into the small veins surrounding the nerves, from where it can diffuse into the capillary plexi of the endoneurium and the vas nervorum capillary plexi that extends intraneurally, thereby blocking conduction. The onset of anesthesia is quick (5–10 min), and the tourniquet should be left in place for the duration of the procedure, which should not exceed 90 min. If the procedure is short, it is not recommended to remove the tourniquet earlier than 10 min after injection, to minimize adverse effects from systemic lidocaine.

Clipping: Yes
Surgical preparation: Yes
Sterile gloves: Yes

IX. Wound Management Block

Wounds resulting from soft tissue and orthopedic procedures can be managed by infusion of local anesthetics through direct injection or placement of special catheters into the surgical wound.

A. Direct Injection Block

This technique is used more commonly for soft tissue surgery that involves the abdomen and consists of injecting local anesthetic into the subcutaneous tissue of the wound edge, on both sides of the incision, from inside the wound, with the needle oriented parallel to the long axis of the wound. Lidocaine (2–4 mg/kg; 0.1–0.2 mL/kg) or bupivacaine (0.5–1 mg/kg; 0.1–0.2 mL/kg) can be used.

Clipping: Yes
Surgical preparation: Yes
Sterile gloves: Yes

B. Wound Infusion Catheter Block [15]

These catheters are known as "wound infusion catheters" or "soaker catheters" (PainBuster Soaker® catheter, dj Orthopedics, Inc. Vista California, or a Diffusion Catheter/Wound Catheter, Mila International), which allow for repeated or continuous administration of the local anesthetic for periods of up to 5 days. The catheter is small gauge with a sealed tip and multiple side fenestrations of very small diameter (170–750 μm) and high resistance to flow, which allows for uniform flow and passage of the local anesthetic through each and all the fenestrations along the entire diffusion length of the catheter when the local anesthetic is delivered as a bolus.

The surgeon primes the entire catheter system with the local anesthetic, at the concentration planned for future dosing, filling the dead space without regard for the amount that it takes, before inserting it into the wound. The catheter is positioned within the wound subcutaneously at the desired position with the working surface situated so that the tissues comprising the deepest aspect of the surgical wound are brought into close apposition to the catheter (e.g. sarcoma removal in cats). In addition to anesthetizing the actual wound, where nerves are observed, the catheter can be placed alongside the nerve with the primary consideration that the nerve should serve the wounded area. An example of a dual block is a wound catheter placed following a thoracic limb amputation that is positioned to also block the severed nerves of the brachial plexus. The catheter is then brought out through a separate skin stab incision close to the surgical incision and anchored securely to the skin by stay sutures. After skin closure, the patient's local anesthetic dose, lidocaine (1–2 mg/kg) or bupivacaine (0.25–0.5 mg/kg), is delivered through the catheter, which is then capped for subsequent injections. Subsequent injections can be administered every 2–3 h for lidocaine or every 4–6 h for bupivacaine. A continuous rate infusion of 1 mg/kg/h of lidocaine or 0.25 mg/kg/h of bupivacaine, through an infusion pump, is an alternative; however, the lower pressure frequently results in a patchy block. For a mobile patient, disconnecting the infusion pump to allow for walks can result in potential for contamination/infection of the lines and ports.

Regardless of the system used, all injections should be done without consideration of the catheter dead space. When using the intermittent injections, it is essential, for each dosing, to inject only 0.2–0.3 mL of the anesthetic initially under pressure, then wait 15 min to allow desensitization of the tissue immediately adjacent to the site and then complete the injection. This will prevent stinging of the bupivacaine upon injection. The catheter is never flushed with saline between treatments. The injected local anesthetic displaces the same volume of the local anesthetic from the catheter into the patient, so the volume in the tubing system remains unchanged.

Clipping: Yes
Surgical preparation: Yes
Sterile gloves: Yes

C. Prolonged-Release Bupivacaine

A prolonged-release formulation of bupivacaine consisting of multivesicular liposomes encapsulating aqueous bupivacaine has recently been approved for single dose administration in dogs (Nocita®, Aratana Therapeutics, Inc., Leawood, KS, USA) at a dose of 5.3 mg/kg (0.4 mL/kg). This technology has been used with good analgesic effects in human patients. In dogs, it is applied to the surgical site to provide post-surgical analgesia, and the slow release of the bupivacaine may provide up to 72 h of pain control [16].

Clipping: Yes
Surgical preparation: Yes
Sterile gloves: Yes

X. Local Anesthetics for Pediatric Patients

A. General Considerations

Local anesthetics are recommended wherever possible, but careful dosing based on accurate body weight is imperative. Infiltration of lidocaine is extremely painful even with 27- to 30-gauge needles, especially in the neonate or pediatric patient. To reduce pain, buffering, warming (37–42 °C) and slow administration are recommended. Buffering can be accomplished by mixing 1% lidocaine with sodium bicarbonate at a 10:1 ratio (1 mL 1% lidocaine with 0.1 mEq (0.1 mL of 1 mEq/mL) sodium bicarbonate). As most veterinary practices have a 2% solution, this can be diluted 1:1 with 0.9% sodium chloride (1% = 10 mg/mL), then mixed with sodium bicarbonate in a 10:1 ratio (1 mL 1% lidocaine: 0.1 mEq sodium bicarbonate) prior to administration. It may be advisable to use a maximum dose of lidocaine in **kittens** of 3 mg/kg in the neonate to 6 mg/kg to the older pediatric, and 5 mg/kg in the neonatal **pup** to 8 mg/kg in the older pediatric. Mepivacaine does not induce pain on injection; a maximum dose is half the adult dose for both kittens and puppies up to 10 days of age. The lower dose is required because of the immaturity of peripheral nerves and not because the younger animals are at any greater risk of toxic side effects. This dose should be diluted in 0.9% saline for accurate dosing, ease of administration and distribution over the site. Bupivacaine may also be used with a 2 mg/kg maximum dose in the older kitten and puppy, with half of this dose advised for the neonate and weanling. Buffering of a 0.5% bupivacaine solution (5 mg/mL) requires a 20:1 mixture with 1 mEq/mL sodium bicarbonate (~0.5 mL bupivacaine and 0.025 mL sodium bicarbonate) and warmed, as described for lidocaine.

B. Topical Local Anesthetic Creams

EMLA® (eutectic mixture of local anesthetic) cream is a prescription-only mixture of lidocaine 2.5% and prilocaine 2.5% combined with thickening agents to form an emulsion (EMLA cream, AstraZeneca LP, Wilmington, DE, USA). This product is not sterile and should be used only in intact skin to provide anesthesia for IV catheter placement, blood collection, lumbar puncture and other minor superficial procedures. EMLA cream should be covered with an occlusive dressing for at least 30 min and preferably longer. In children, the peak effect is at 2 h; however, our experience in animals is that 30 min facilitates such procedures as jugular catheter placement using the Seldinger technique; however, a longer dwell time may be necessary in the more active animal. Sterile prep is performed just prior to the procedure. In one veterinary study, there was no systemic uptake of the components of EMLA cream and its use appeared effective in preventing signs of discomfort during jugular catheter placement.

ELA-Max®, LMX™ (Ferndale Laboratories, Ferndale, MI, USA) is an over-the-counter liposome-encapsulated formulation of 4% lidocaine. Transdermal absorption did occur after application of 15 mg/kg of this product, but plasma concentrations remained significantly below toxic values. The area where it has been applied needs to be covered to prevent licking with subsequent absorption through the oral mucous membrane and concerns for lidocaine toxicity.

Maxiline® 4 (Ferndale Laboratories, Ferndale, MI, USA) is a product containing 4% lidocaine and may be preferred to EMLA cream, as the local anesthetic effect occurs faster. This product is only used on intact skin.

Lidocaine 2% is also available in a sterile gel, in a cartridge and is useful for sterile local desensitization (e.g. desensitization of the vaginal vault prior to urinary catheter placement in female cats and dogs) and may also be applied to the penis prior to urinary catheter placement.

References

1 Gwaltney-Brant, S. and Meadows, I. (2012) Use of intravenous lipid emulsions for treating certain poisoning cases in small animals. *Vet Clin North Am Small Anim Pract*, 42: 251–262.
2 Liu, P. L., Feldman, H. S., Giasi, R., *et al.* (1983) Comparative CNS toxicity of lidocaine, etidocaine, bupivacaine, and tetracaine in awake dogs following rapid intravenous administration. *Anesth Analg*, 62: 375–379.
3 Liu, P. L., Feldman, H. S., Giasi, R., *et al.* (1982) Acute cardiovascular toxicity of intravenous amide local anesthetics in anesthetized ventilated dogs. *Anesth Analg*, 61: 317–322.
4 Esteves, A., Ribeiro, C. F., Damaso, C. S., *et al.* (2009) Anatomical description of the trigeminal nerve [V] and its branching in mongrel dogs. *Braz J Morphol Sci*, 26: 187–192.
5 Viscasillas, J., Seymour, C. J. and Brodbelt, D. C. (2013) A cadaver study comparing two approaches for performing maxillary nerve block in dogs. *Vet Anaesth Analg*, 40: 212–219.
6 Campoy, L., Read, M. and Peralta, S. (2015) Canine and feline local anesthetic and analgesic techniques. In: Grimm, K. A., Lamont, L. L., Tranquilli, W. J., *et al.* (eds), *Veterinary Anesthesia and Analgesia: The fifth edition of Lumb and Jones*. Wiley-Blackwell, Ames, IA: 827–856.
7 Allam, M. W., Lee, D. G., Nulsen, F. E. and Fortune, E. A. (1952) The anatomy of the brachial plexus of the dog. *Anat Rec*, 114: 173–179.
8 Campoy, L., Bezuidenhout, A. J., Gleed, R. D., *et al.* (2010) Ultrasound-guided approach for axillary brachial plexus, femoral nerve and sciatic nerve blocks in dogs. *Vet Anesth Analg*, 37: 144–153.
9 Skelding, A., Valverde, A., Sinclair, M., *et al.* (2016) Anatomical characterization of the brachial plexus in dogs and comparison of the traditional block technique to 2 novel approaches. (Abstract) Annual Conference of the American College of Veterinary Anesthesiologists and Analgesia, and 22nd International Veterinary Emergency and Critical Care Symposium. Grapevine, Texas, September 2016.
10 Franci, P., Leece, E. A. and Corletto, F. (2012) Thoracic epidural catheter placement using a paramedian approach with cephalad angulation in three dogs. *Vet Surg*, 41: 884–889.

11 Valverde, A. (2008) Epidural analgesia and anesthesia in dogs and cats. *Vet Clin North Am Small Anim Pract*, 38: 1205–1230.

12 O'Hearn, A. K. and Wright, B. D. (2011) Coccygeal epidural with local anesthetic for catheterization and pain management in the treatment of feline urethral obstruction. *J Vet Emerg Crit Care*, 21: 50–52.

13 Costa-Farré, C., Blanch, X. S., Cruz, J. I. and Franch, J. (2011) Ultrasound guidance for the performance of sciatic and saphenous nerve blocks in dogs. *Vet J*, 187: 221–224.

14 Rasmussen, L. M., Lipowitz, A. J. and Graham, L. F. (2006) Development and verification of saphenous, tibial and common peroneal nerve block techniques for analgesia below the thigh in the nonchondrodystrophoid dog. *Vet Anaesth Analg*, 33: 36–48.

15 Hansen, B., Lascelles, D. X., Thomson, A. and DePuy, V. (2013) Variability of performance of wound infusion catheters. *Vet Anaesth Analg*, 40: 308–315.

16 Lascelles, B. D. X., Rausch-Derra, L. C., Wofford, J. A. and Huebner, M. (2016) Pilot, randomized, placebo-controlled clinical field study to evaluate the effectiveness of bupivacaine liposome injectable suspension for the provision of post-surgical analgesia in dogs undergoing stifle surgery. *BMC Vet Res*, 12: 168.

Further Reading

Search the website for the World Small Animal Veterinary Association for local anesthetic techniques: www.wsava.org or use the following direct link: http://www.wsava.org/sites/default/files/Local%20anesthetic%20educational%20videos_0pdf

15

Integrative Techniques for Pain Management

Cornelia Mosley and Shauna Cantwell

Integrative pain therapy is the philosophy that combines traditional and non-traditional approaches to pain management. The philosophy behind integrating traditional with non-traditional approaches to pain management is aiming to reduce the presenting pain and prevent the development of hypersensitivity or chronic maladaptive pain. This facilitates a reduction in pharmacologic management of pain, resulting in a reduction in the potential, or actual, side effects of conventional drugs. The functional ability of the patient will be supported with the additional benefit of keeping the patient engaged and, therefore, improving motivation and positive mentation. In particular, for the organ-compromised, unstable or geriatric patients, the benefits are multiple. As some classes of analgesics are contraindicated in these patients, the resultant "physical modifying effects" of traditional modalities have been shown to speed recovery, and improve well-being of the patient [1].

These therapies frequently require a more holistic and balanced approach to patient assessment and treatment, and an open mind may be necessary to incorporate some of these into the treatment plans. Physical therapy, massage therapy, laser therapy, diet (including food therapy) and traditional Chinese veterinary medicine (TCVM), including acupuncture and herbal medicine, to name a few, are commonly used. Most modalities are more commonly used for the treatment of chronic pain but can play an important role in the acute pain phase, if used correctly. It is sometimes missed that the patient with acute pain may also have some ongoing chronic pain which, if treated in addition to treating the acute pain, may speed recovery. This is often true for older patients in particular.

Modalities that are most commonly utilized in human and veterinary medicine for the acute recovery phase immediately after surgery are physiotherapy, manual therapies, thermal therapy, laser therapy and traditional Chinese veterinary medicine (including acupuncture, herbal medicine and food therapy). **The goals for such integrative therapy are**:

- to reduce the presenting pain;
- to prevent development of hypersensitivity or chronic maladaptive pain;
- to support the functional ability of the patient;
- to reduce some side effects from pharmaceutical drugs (e.g. chemotherapy, nausea, loss of appetite; corticosteroids, PU/PD; and opioids, maintain gastrointestinal (GI) motility);
- to increase activity and mobility of the patient and therefore hasten recovery;
- to keep the patient engaged, which may improve motivation and positive mentation.

It is important to recognize that most of the above-mentioned modalities require specific training for the full understanding, and application, of the principles behind these therapy

Analgesia and Anesthesia for the Ill or Injured Dog and Cat, First Edition. Karol A. Mathews, Melissa Sinclair, Andrea M. Steele and Tamara Grubb.
© 2018 John Wiley & Sons, Inc. Published 2018 by John Wiley & Sons, Inc.

modalities in order to successfully, and appropriately, use the techniques. Therefore, only qualified personnel should conduct physical therapy, acupuncture and massages.

The recovery from major surgery is, in general, divided into three phases [2]:

1. an immediate or post-anaesthetic phase;
2. an intermediate phase, encompassing the hospitalization period;
3. a convalescent phase, including the recovery/rehabilitation phase.

Phases 1 and 2 focus on:

- maintenance of homeostasis;
- treatment of pain;
- prevention and early detection of complications.

To improve phases 2 and 3, and returning the animals to normal function faster, complementary modalities can be added to the conventional methods.

There are many different ancillary methods to pain management with a broad variety of documentation, validation or understanding. Some are extrapolated from human medicine or compiled from clinically used techniques in veterinary medicine. Due to the tailored individualized therapy approach, generalizations are difficult to make. Evidence-based studies are often limited by the methodology, but scientific research and recent medical history and experiences have added to the rapidly growing understanding of different aspects of complementary pain management methods.

I.   Traditional Chinese Veterinary Medicine

TCVM has a long and rich history that dates back over 3000 years. Acupuncture is the most known modality of TCVM, but it is only one modality of the four main pillars of TCVM. The other three entail Tui na (a specific medical and meridian-based massage technique), herbal medicine and food therapy. The philosophy of TCVM is to find the underlying cause for pain. It is also known as the "root-and-branch treatment", which aims at finding and treating the root cause for the problem to effectively treat the symptoms. TCVM is based on the balance of energy (Qi) and its undisrupted flow through the body and aims to resolve any imbalances and stagnations (blockage), thereby promoting health and preventing disease. It is a useful tool for painful conditions, but most importantly it is also frequently able to solve the underlying cause leading to the painful problem [3–7].

A.   Acupuncture

Acupuncture is the stimulation of a specific point (acupuncture point) on the body that elicits a therapeutic homeostatic response. These points are located along, or around, specific pathways, called "meridians". Commonly, these points are located in an area with a high density of free nerve endings, mast cells, small arterioles and lymphatic vessels. The stimulation of the points releases beta-endorphins, serotonin and other neurotransmitters and provides some pain relief [3]. The actions of acupuncture are broad and multifactorial; besides pain relief, acupuncture stimulation also induces physiological effects such as regulation of GI motility, anti-inflammation and immuno-regulation, hormone-regulation, antipyretic effects and promotion of microcirculation [5]. All these effects can be important in the immediate post-operative phase. Acupuncture and trigger point therapy can have profound effects on the sympathetic nervous system [5, 6]. To be specific, the effects of acupuncture cannot be explained by one single mechanism of action. Research on neural-based mechanisms clarifies the neuro-humoral actions and immune-modulatory effects of acupuncture from a "Western point of view" [5]. Endorphins and monoamines play an important role locally, but also at the level of segmental and supra-segmental areas [5]. The needling itself stimulates the A-beta sensory fibres, which causes multiple reflex reactions to the motor-neuron tone, the vasculature and ligaments at the segmental level. Via the "gate-theory", the stimulation of the A-beta afferent fibres will facilitate the local inhibition of nociception. When C and A-delta nociceptive fibres are stimulated, the transmission may be blocked due to the inhibition by endogenous opioids, inhibitory interneurons and descending norepinephrine and serotonergic pathways. **Electro-acupuncture** is the stimulation of 2 acupuncture points with electric current for a stronger effect on the acupuncture point and to connect the current between the 2 needles. This form of acupuncture induces the release of endomorphins (µ-opioid agonist), dynorphins (k-opioid agonist), enkephalins and ß-endorphins (mixed µ- and k-opioid agonist) release with subsequent pain relief [8]. Endorphin release is one component occurring during acupuncture but other, equally important, complex interactions of other neurotransmitters, also contribute to local and central nociceptive effects [8, 9]. The anti-inflammatory effects of acupuncture can be explained with cytokine changes and leukocyte migration as well as with the influence of the cholinergic anti-inflammatory pathway [10–12]. Other studies have shown a significant effect on the autonomic nervous system [13, 14].

Various mechanisms have been researched and help us understand the effects of acupuncture from a Western point of view [1, 7, 9]. The principle of the mechanism of acupuncture from an Eastern point of view is based on Qi, the vital energy that flows throughout the body. This energy, and its undisturbed flow through specific pathways (called meridians), is important for health and protection from disease and pain. The health of an animal is influenced by the quality, quantity and balance of Qi. There are 14 meridians inside every body, each connecting specific organs and glands. When the flow of Qi on these meridians is obstructed, it will cause pain and illness. Under normal circumstances, the body can bounce back from a blockage or imbalance, but when the disruption is prolonged or excessive, treatment with acupuncture, by stimulating specific points on the meridian, can help unblock the obstruction to help the body recover.

Acupuncture can be useful for any painful condition in the post-operative recovery state, for example after intervertebral disk disease/surgery, fracture repair, ligament procedures and wound healing, to name a few [15–17]. Patients with polyarthritis and other causes of inflammatory pain will benefit from the pain relief, anti-inflammatory and fever-reducing effects of acupuncture. Patients with GI disease (post-surgical or primary) show significant improvement in appetite, and peristalsis when GI motility is decreased, after acupuncture treatment (Figure 15.1). Patients with diarrhoea and vomiting can also benefit. Dogs that show signs of

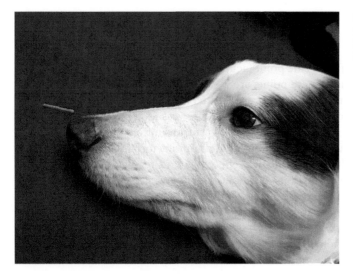

Figure 15.1 The stimulation of this acupuncture point (*Shan Gen*) helps stimulate appetite and can be useful in patients with anorexia.

vertigo and dizziness or patients that are admitted with vestibular disease can be helped with acupuncture by decreasing the severity of the symptoms [18].

B.   Herbal Pain Medication

Chinese herbs have been used for many years in both human and veterinary medicine for pain management. The anti-inflammatory properties of some Chinese herbs have been popular worldwide for humans and are also used for animals. Some have properties similar to the ancient natural remedies that Western culture is currently re-discovering (e.g. cranberry or currants to decrease inflammation, chamomile to sooth the stomach, lavender to calm). A variety of pain-relieving herbal combinations is commercially available and can be used in addition to conventional drugs or as an alternative for dogs and cats. This integrative approach will likely improve overall pain management and can help decrease dosing of drugs like non-steroidal anti-inflammatory analgesics (NSAIAs) or tramadol, and therefore reduce potential side effects. When using other pharmacologic agents with herbal medication, it is essential to ensure there are no adverse effects with these combinations (i.e. NSAIAs in combination with gingko, garlic, ginger, ginseng, meadowsweet and willow bark may inhibit platelet function [19]).

II.   Manual Therapy Techniques

Manual therapy techniques include massage, joint mobilization, stretching and range of motion exercises. These will advance tissue healing, in particular after surgery or an injury, as they increase circulation and help reduce swelling. Benefits include reduced muscle pain and overall aching, loosening muscle tension and spasms and increased muscle flexibility. The risk of adhesions, scar tissue formation and muscle contracture can be decreased with this modality, thereby preventing/reducing ongoing chronic pain. This technique is probably one of the more important ones for improving healing in post-operative care during the recovery phase, but knowledge and training are advised to not cause pain. Even though massage therapy is poorly regulated in veterinary medicine, its impact, when done correctly, is profound, while massage performed poorly can create backwards flow of lymph/blood/toxins that can lead to increased pain. Comprehensive courses with qualified instructors are offered and recommended to perform specific massage therapies adequately. Basic techniques can be explained by qualified instructors, but overall more specific techniques are the ones that improve healing and it is important to use this effective modality in the correct manner.

Animals in shock and/or with fever are not ideal candidates for massage. It is further contraindicated to massage directly over a fresh injury, wound, tumour or area with skin infection. Other contraindications of massage include, but are not limited to, lymphatic disease, liver or kidney disease or bowel obstruction. Some basic considerations are necessary, including the acceptance of the animal for the treatment. An intuitive personality helps to assess the benefits of the treatment for the animal, in particular to decide on duration and intensity of the massage. The animal, in general, will give subtle feedback for the therapist to adjust or end the treatment, which is important to notice and respect.

Some techniques that can be performed on a hospitalized animal:

- **A specific "swelling massage technique"** of the Swedish massage principle helps decrease swelling. The wound itself is not to be massaged, but on the outside edges of where the swelling of the tissue begins. Gentle circling and outward stroking massage techniques may reduce the swelling faster.
- **Effleurage strokes:** long relaxing, continuous gliding strokes with the whole flat palm along the length of the muscles. This increases blood circulation and lymph drainage as well as relaxes and stretches the muscles. It has an overall calming effect on a stressed animal and

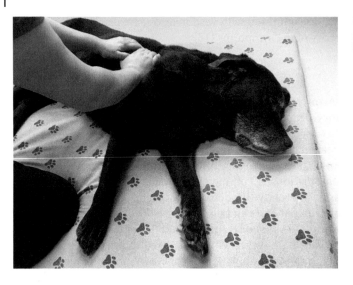

Figure 15.2 Massages can help in mobilizing specific muscles or bones.

can give the person an indication of tight spots, painful areas and swelling when used over the whole body (from head to tail, down the limbs).

- **Trigger point release:** trigger points are tight muscle knots that are tender and sensitive. A gentle application of light pressure with the thumb can help release the tension. After the gentle release with the thumb, gentle outward strokes with the palm of the hand will maintain the release of the tight knot (Figure 15.2).
- **Lymph drainage massage technique** can be a valuable method to assist lymph drainage for post-surgical cases.
- **Foot massage** is an easy technique to apply for all patients. It can be applied by gently stroking the carpus with the fingertips down to the digits. The lateral and medial side of the base of the nails can be gently squeezed between the thumb and the fingers. These are specific acupuncture points called "Ting points" (beginning and ending of the different meridians). Around the pads and toes, circular or pulling/stretching/bending techniques can be used.
- **Stretches:** once the muscles are warmed up and relaxed the different parts of the leg can be stretched in a gentle and slow manner, never past the point of resistance. Both joints on either side of the muscle/bone are supported with the hands. Warming up muscles can be done through massage, warm packs or exercise (when possible) (Figure 15.3).

Osteopathy is another specialized manual therapy modality that evaluates the tissue quality, tissue position and imbalances in motility via palpation to identify problems that may cause pain. The principle of osteopathic manual therapy is to maintain, improve or restore the normal physiological function of interrelated body structures and systems. It uses various manual assessment and treatment techniques/modalities to help animals with acute or chronic pain by reducing swelling, improving tissue mobility and promoting efficient healing. Specific training is required to use this modality effectively.

III. Animal Physical Rehabilitation

A. Overview

Clinical applications for physical therapy include restoration, maintenance and promotion of optimal physical function, and is increasingly used for the recovery phase of surgical, orthopedic and neurologic injuries and diseases. Physical therapy can be tailored to the specific problem

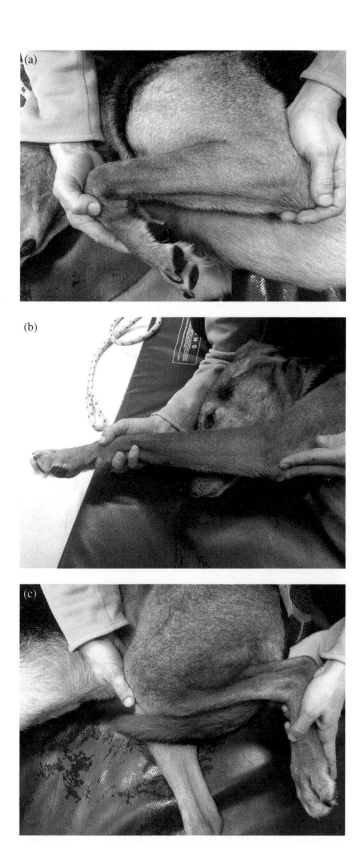

Figure 15.3(a–c) A gentle passive range of motion can be performed post-operatively to prevent joints from freezing and keep muscles flexible. Two hands are necessary to move a joint in a controlled and safe manner. The dog should be relaxed and slow movements are used in the early phase to avoiding causing discomfort.

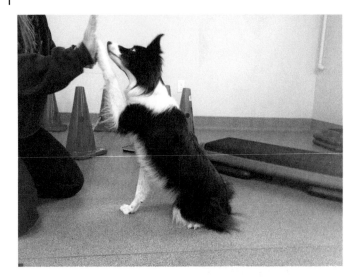

Figure 15.4 In physical therapy specific exercises are used for specific muscles and joint uses as well as weight distribution. Notice the mental engagement of the dog getting this exercise.

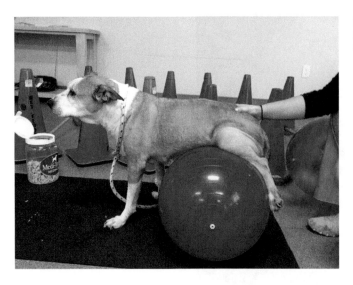

Figure 15.5 In physical therapy specific exercises can help stretch and flex specific parts of the body.

and may entail integumentary physical therapy, neurologic physical therapy and orthopedic physical therapy. Advanced training is mandatory for beneficial treatment. Immediate post-operative physical therapy involves primarily passive range of motion techniques (see Figure 15.3) and warm/cold therapies (Figure 15.4). This in particular is useful for post-fracture surgeries, lacerations, tibial-plateau-levelling osteotomy (TPLOs), etc. Other physical therapy techniques are mostly used in the later phases of recovery/rehabilitation physical therapy, the convalescent phase (Figure 15.5 and Figure 15.6) [20–24].

B. Cryotherapy

Cryotherapy uses "cold" temperature on the site of injury to decrease pain and inflammation in the immediate post-injury or post-surgical period. The principle thought is that a decreased tissue temperature will suppress the metabolic rate of the traumatized tissue and, by reducing swelling induced by vasoconstriction and decreased nerve conduction, decrease pain development. Analgesia is also enhanced due to the reduction in inflammatory mediators, in particular

Figure 15.6 An ice-filled Dixie cup is used to ice specific muscles or joints. The Dixie cup is rotated on the area to prevent freezing of the skin.

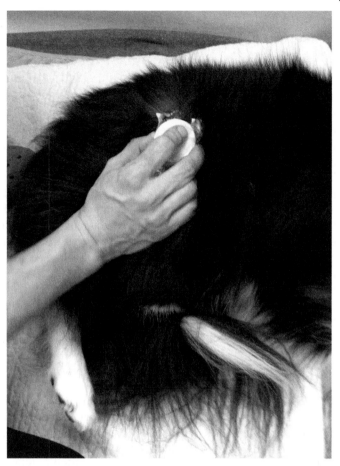

tumour necrosis factor and nitric oxide [25–32]. Ice packs are commonly covered in towels and directly placed on the inflamed area for a limited time (5–20 min range). Figure 15.6 shows icing of a specific muscle with the help of a paper Dixie cup filled with frozen water. The smaller surface area can target specific joints or muscles. The open part with the ice is rotated on the skin, while the paper part of the cup makes it easy to handle. Caution is required to avoid freezing injury when placed directly on skin. Intermittent pneumatic compressions (a form of controlled cryotherapy, or CCT) may be added to the cryotherapy to reduce swelling even further. Cryotherapy is commonly used for the first 24–48 h after acute injury.

C. Warm Therapy

Heat application results in vasodilation and increased blood flow in the injured area. The vasodilation of the blood and lymphatic vessels results in improved flow decreasing bruising and swelling [31, 32]. Warm therapy is commonly applied following the cryotherapy phase at 48–72 h. The warm packs should not be too hot (less than 40 °C, the temperature can be tested on the palmar side of one's own wrist). Any temperature at risk of burning skin is too high. The temperature should be maintained consistently over time. The warm packs are applied on the muscle and kept there for 20–30 min. This can be done multiple times during the day. Heat is contraindicated in an area with lack of sensation, poor perfusion, open ulcers or wounds. Neoplastic areas are contraindicated for warm therapy as local heat may promote blood flow and enhance the growth of neoplasm.

Alternating therapies (contrast therapy) has also been suggested for sport injury (1 min warm followed by 2–4 min cold therapy).

D. Phototherapy (Laser Therapy)

The acronym "laser" stands for "light amplification by stimulated emission of radiation" and follows the concept that light can be used for therapeutic purposes (Figure 15.7). In physical therapy "cold" or "low-level" lasers are most commonly used and have low power properties which allow penetration through the surface of the skin without any heating or skin-damaging effects. Laser is used to target a small area of the body at a specific wavelength. The purpose of laser therapy is wound healing, accelerated tissue repair and pain relief, with the main effects resulting from photobiomodulation of the tissues, including stimulation of cellular metabolism and growth. Angiogenesis may be accelerated from laser light in damaged tissues, which is thought to improve the rate of wound healing. Further, laser light therapy shows vasodilatory effects and improves lymphatic drainage, which can result in reducing edema and swelling caused by bruising or inflammation. Wound healing, bone, ligament and cartilage healing, nerve and spinal healing all show promising effects after laser treatment, although the literature is not cohesive on the effectiveness on some of the goals [33, 34]. An understanding of the principles of laser therapy will optimize the benefits of treatment, especially in the immediate post-operative phase. No certifying training is required, but high-quality courses are offered and recommended to make the treatment meaningful and beneficial for the patient.

E. Transcutaneous Electrical Nerve Stimulation (TENS)

The TENS device produces electrical current and uses it for therapeutic purposes, in particular to treat pain. It is used to stimulate the sensory nerves for inhibiting pain fibre input and to provide pain relief. It has traditionally been used for chronic pain; however, evidence also supports the effective and valid use of TENS for acute pain relief. The device connects to the skin with electrodes connected to adhesive patches with the ability to adjust pulse width (duration),

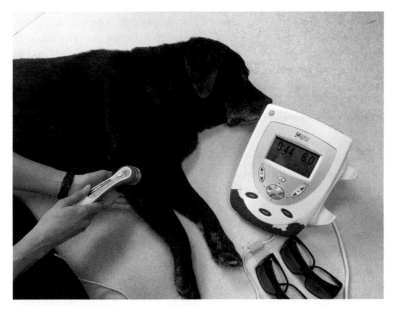

Figure 15.7 Laser therapy performed on an elbow.

frequency and intensity. Two modes of frequencies are clinically used, either low frequency (<10 Hz, believed to stimulate A-delta fibres) or high frequency (>50 Hz, believed to stimulate A-beta fibres). The intensity needs to be sufficient enough to depolarize the sensory nerves (low intensity). Higher-intensity or neuromuscular electrical stimulation (NMES) is used when motor contractions are generated aiming at muscle activity, which is commonly used during physical therapy sessions. The electrode patches can be positioned across painful joints, over muscles or in the general area of discomfort, and can be quite useful in the post-operative period. In particular, in human medicine, it is commonly used with various studies showing conflicting, but overall promising, results. The analgesic mechanism of action is not fully understood. The gate control theory of stimulating the A-beta nerve fibres is thought to be one of the mechanisms of action, but other mechanisms of central modulation may also play a role. For example, the release of neurotransmitters and activation of opiate, serotonergic and muscarinic receptors are activated through the use of TENS. The TENS system can be used on any post-surgical patient [33].

F. Pulsed Electromagnetic Field (PEMF) Therapy and MBST® Nuclear Magnetic Resonance Therapy

The principle of the pulsed electromagnetic field therapy is the penetration of this dynamic natural electromagnetic field (low frequency) through the body, creating a cascade of effects within the body due to stimulating ions in the tissue. The PEMF has shown promising results for a variety of pathologies and conditions but is most commonly used for bone healing, wound healing, decreased inflammation and pain relief. The mechanism of action is considered to be on a cellular level by restoring and maintaining optimal cellular function. This is based on the magnetic spin of specific ions, protons and electrons, but in particular the ions. Ferrum ions (iron), for example, are part of hemoglobin and show that magnetic momentum and exposure to a magnetic field will affect blood flow and microcirculation. Further $Ca2^+$ ions and $Ca2^+$ channels play an important role in many physiological processes, and seem to be sensitive to the magnetic field and show activation resulting in increased movement of $Ca2^+$ ions across membranes. Proteins play another role when affected by the magnetic field. It is FDA approved for post-operative edema and pain. It also shows promising effects on chronic wound healing, osteogenesis and anti-inflammation. Electric and electromagnetic fields may be applied through the use of skin patches, or magnetic devices, that can be placed in collars or on bandages or wraps [35].

The MBST nuclear magnetic resonance therapy stimulates mainly the hydrogen protons similar to an MRI, but on a much lower energy level, treating osteoarthritic pain, back pain and other conditions [36]. The MBST therapy stimulates the hydrogen protons by using radio waves and, therefore, increases the energy state of the protons. This energy is then released, absorbed and used by the tissue. This principle of recharging the cells is used by this modality. Specific veterinary products like MBST's nuclear magnetic resonance therapy are on the market, particularly in Europe, and its use has been increasing significantly for chronic and acute inflammatory pain conditions. No certifying training is required for both modalities, but high-quality courses are offered and recommended to make the treatment meaningful and beneficial for the patient.

IV. Emotional Component to Pain Management

It is not new to the scientific literature that pain is closely linked to emotional factors. In human pain management strategies, cognitive behaviour changes and mindfulness are regular treatment components. In veterinary medicine, this is also recognized. Anxious dogs are often treated with trazodone, acepromazine or dexmedetomidine post-operatively until they leave the clinic. An anxiety-reducing drug certainly can help significantly in improving the recovery phase, but other options for engaging an anxious/fearful/depressed dog can be applied. Some of the above-mentioned modalities, in particular the manual therapies, are very useful in engaging a patient. Downtime spent sitting next to an animal providing calm time with or without gentle strokes and talking can further put a patient at ease, which will improve appetite and improve quality of sleep and therefore speed recovery. Consistent interaction with a patient will make pain assessments significantly easier and more accurate.

Acknowledgements

Thank you to Brenna L. Cairncross, BA, REMT, for her input to the manual therapies and Wendy Davies, BA, CVT, CCRA for proofreading. Special thanks to Hank, Rue, Texas, Jade and Moka for being excellent models for the pictures.

References

1 Cantwell, S. L. (2007) Pain management: III: Ancillary therapies. In: Seymor, C. and Duk, D. (eds), *BSAVA Manual of Canine and Feline Anaesthesia and Analgesia*, 2$_{nd}$ edn. BSAVA, Cheltenham.

2 Doherty, G. M. (2010) Postoperative care. In: G. M. Doherty (ed.), *Current Diagnosis and Treatment: Surgery*, 13th edn. McGraw-Hill, New York: 24–32.

3 Xie, H. and Preast, V. (2013) *TCVM Fundamental Principles*, 2nd edn. Chi Institute Press, Reddick, FL.

4 Fratkin, J. P. (1996) Root and branch: Clinical applications of Japanese meridian therapy. *North American Journal of Oriental Medicine*, 3(7), http://drjakefratkin.com/articles/root-and-branch-clinical-applications-of-japanese-meridian-therapy.

5 Cantwell, S. L. (2014) Mechanism of acupuncture analgesia. In: C. M. Eggers, L. Love and T. Doherty (eds), *Pain Management in Veterinary Practice*, 1st edn. John Wiley & Sons, Ltd, Chichester: 177–182.

6 Cantwell, S. L. (2010) Traditional Chinese veterinary medicine: The mechanism and management of acupuncture for chronic pain. *Top Companion Anim Med*, 25(1): 53–58.

7 Schoen, A. M. (2010) *Veterinary Acupuncture: Ancient art to modern medicine*, 2nd edn. Mosby, London.

8 Lin, J. G. and Chen, W. L. (2008) Acupuncture analgesia: A review of its mechanisms of actions. *American Journal Chinese Medicine*, 36(4): 635–645.

9 Zhang, R., Lao, L., Ren, K. and Berman, B. M. (2014) Mechanisms of acupuncture-electroacupuncture on persistent pain. *Anesthesiology*, 120(2): 482–503.

10 Lee, H. G., Lee, B., Choi, S. H., *et al.* (2004) Electroacupuncture reduces stress-induced expression of c-fos in the brain of the rat. *American Journal Chinese Medicine*, 32: 597–606.

11 Yim, Y. K., Lee, H., Hong, K. E., *et al.* (2007) Electroacupuncture at acupoint ST36 reduces inflammation and regulates immune activity in collagen-induced arthritic mice. *Evidence Based Complementary Alternative Medicine*, 4: 51–57.

12 Kavoussi, B. and Ross, B. E. (2007) Neuroimmune basis of anti-inflammatory acupuncture. *Integrative Cancer Therapy*: 6(3): 251–257.

13 Kimura, Y. and Hara, S. (2008) The effect of electro-acupuncture stimulation on rhythm of autonomic nervous system in dogs. *Journal Veterinary Medical Science*, 70(4): 349–352.

14 Fabrin, S., Soares, N., Yoshimura, D. P., *et al.* (2016) Effects of acupuncture at the Yintang and the Chengjiang Acupoints on cardiac arrhythmias and neurocardiogenic syncope in emergency first aid. *J Acupunct Meridian Stud*, 9(1): 26–30.

15 Laim, A., Jaggy, A., Forterre, F., *et al.* (2009) Effects of adjunct electroacupuncture on severity of postoperative pain in dogs undergoing hemilaminectomy because of acute thoracolumbar intervertebral disk disease. *Journal American Veterinary Medical Association*, 234(9): 1141–1146.

16 Joachim, J. G. F., Luna, S. P. L., Brondani, J. T., *et al.* (2010) Comparison of decompressive surgery, electroacupuncture, and decompressive surgery followed by electroacupuncture for the treatment of dogs with intervertebral disk disease with long-standing severe neurological deficits. *JAVMA*, 236(11): 1225–1229.

17 Liu, C. M., Holyoak, G. R. and Lin, C. T. (2016) Acupuncture combined with Chinese herbs for the treatment in hemivertebral French bulldogs with emergent paraparesis. *Journal of Traditional and Complimentary Medicine*, 6: 409–412.

18 Chiu, C.-W., Lee, T.-C., Hsu, P.-C., *et al.* (2015) Efficacy and safety of acupuncture for dizziness and vertigo in emergency department: A pilot cohort study. *BMC Complementary and Alternative Medicine*, 15: 173.

19 Trepanier, L. A. (2005) Potential interactions between NSAIDs and other drugs. *J Vet Emerg Crit Care*, 15(4): 248–253.

20 Monk, M. L., Preston, C. A. and McGowan, C. M. (2006) Effects of early intensive postoperative physiotherapy on limb function after tibial plateau leveling osteotomy in dogs with deficiency of the cranial cruciate ligament. *American Journal of Veterinary Research*, 67(3): 529–536.

21 Sharp, B. (2012) Feline physiotherapy and rehabilitation. *Journal of Feline Medicine and Surgery*, 14(9): 622–632.

22 Sharp, B. (2008) Physiotherapy in small animal practice. *In Practice*, 30(4): 190.

23 Darryl, L., Millis, D. F. and Adamson, C. (2005) Emerging modalities in veterinary rehabilitation. *Vet Clin North Am Small Anim Pract*, 35(6): 1335–1355.

24 Levine, D., Millis, D. L. and Marcellin-Little, D. J. (2005) Introduction to veterinary physical rehabilitation. *Vet Clin North Am Small Anim Pract*, 35(6): 1247–1254.

25 Drygas, K. A., McClure, S. R. and Goring R. L. (2011) Effect of cold compression therapy on postoperative pain, swelling, range of motion, and lameness after TPLO in dogs. *JAVMA*, 238(10): 1284–1291.

26 Caldwell, F. (2013) Postoperative cryotherapy: It's more than just cold. *Veterinary Nursing Journal*, 28(0): 316–318.

27 Ohkoshi, Y., Ohkoshi, M., Nagasaki, S., *et al.* (1999) The effects of cryo- therapy on intra-articular temperature and postoperative care after anterior cruciate ligament reconstruction. *Am J Sports Med*, 27: 357–362.

28 Ho, S. S., Coel, M. N., Kagawa, R., *et al.* (1994) The effects of ice on blood flow and bone metabolism in knees. *Am J Sports Med*, 22: 537–540.

29 Martin, S. S., Spindler, K. P., Tarter, J. W., *et al.* (2001) Cryotherapy: An effective modality for decreasing intra-articular temperature after knee arthroscopy. *Am J Sports Med*, 29: 288–291.

30 Yenari, M. A. and Han, H. S. (2006) Influence of hypothermia on post-ischemic inflammation: Role of nuclear factor kappa B (NfkappaB). *Neu rochem Int*, 2: 164–169.

31 Lehmann, J. F., Warren, C. G. and Scham, S. M. (1974) Therapeutic heat and cold. *Clin Orthop Relat Res*, 99: 207–245.

32 Nadler, S. F., Weingand, K. and Kruse, R. J. (2004) The physiological basis and clinical applications of cryotherapy and thermotherapy for the pain practitioner. *Pain Physician*, 7(3): 395–399.

33 Millis, D. L., Francis, D. and Adamson, C. (2005) Emerging modalities and veterinary rehabilitation. *Vet Clin North Am Small Anim Pract*, 35(6): 1335–1355.

34 Kurach, L. M., Stanley, B. J., Gazzola, K. M., *et al.* (2015) The effect of low-level laser therapy on the healing of open wounds in dogs. *Veterinary Surgery*, 44: 988–996.

35 Strauch, B., Herman, C., Dabb, R., *et al.* (2009) Evidence-based use of pulsed electromagnetic field therapy in clinical plastic surgery. *Anesthetic Surgery Journal*, 29(2): 135–143.

36 Kullich, W., Schwann, H., Walcher, J. and Machreich, K. (2006) The effect of MBST with complex 3-dimensional electromagnetic nuclear resonance fields on patients with low back pain. *Journal of Back and Musculoskeletal Rehabilitation*, 19: 79–87.

16

The Veterinary Technician/Nurse's Role in Pain Management

Andrea Steele

The veterinary technician or nurse (VT/N) has a vital role in the management of their patient's pain that should never be minimized. The VT/N is the primary caregiver for each patient. Over the course of a shift, or days, the VT/N begins to understand their patient; they recognize when the patient is comfortable, when they are beginning to experience discomfort and quickly notice signs of pain in each patient. As always, pain is better avoided than treated. Treating at the earliest sign of discomfort will ensure the patient does not experience significant pain.

I. Analgesic Orders

While the use of bolus dosing versus continuous rate infusion (CRI), and the dosing for each, are discussed elsewhere in this book (refer to Chapter 18), it is important to discuss the orders for analgesics that will be provided to the VT/Ns so that they may best optimize their patients' care.

Every practice uses VT/Ns in different ways, and pain management can be modified to provide the very best possible outcome. Regardless of the type of patient observation in use, ensuring that VT/Ns are part of the pain plan, and encouraging active participation in pain management, will result in not only more comfortable patients but also happier team members. There is no need for pain management to be solely the responsibility of the veterinarian.

In a busy practice, with VT/Ns who are conscientious about pain management, and dedicated to patient observation and care in an ICU type environment, the veterinarian will usually find that standing orders for analgesia using dose ranges or PRN (as needed) bolus dosing will provide the most effective analgesia. Allowing the VT/N to intervene when they feel the patient is beginning to show signs of pain, or allowing them to modify the dose as needed, ensures flexibility and individualization of dosing. The other benefit is that the veterinarian does not need to be interrupted from their other duties to assess the patient each time a dose change is required. If the patient's needs seem excessive, or appear to require dosing outside of the range provided, the veterinarian should always be consulted.

In practices where continuous observation is impossible, as VT/Ns are required to perform other duties, using standardized dosing at regular intervals will likely be the best choice. It remains important to titrate opioids to effect when provided intravenously, to avoid dysphoria and other negative effects. Patients should still be observed as frequently as possible, and the response to the analgesic noted at each opportunity.

Analgesia and Anesthesia for the Ill or Injured Dog and Cat, First Edition. Karol A. Mathews, Melissa Sinclair, Andrea M. Steele and Tamara Grubb.

II. The Patient Advocate

Both human and veterinary nurses have long been referred to as "patient advocates". In veterinary medicine, this is a particular challenge with non-verbal patients. VT/Ns are required to identify often subtle cues that a patient is more, or less, painful. VT/Ns should always feel comfortable discussing these findings with the case veterinarian, as a patient's condition can rapidly change, causing a patient to be suddenly over- or underdosed with analgesic. Having open dialogue between the veterinarians and technicians, discussing patient goals (i.e. pain expectations or "the go home" plan) ensures that everyone is aware of the plan for the patient each day.

A. Ask for Analgesic Orders

When presented with a serious emergency patient, the veterinarian's focus is often on fluid therapy, containing hemorrhage or performing life-saving procedures, and often management of pain is easy to overlook in the heat of the moment. Once a catheter is placed, and fluid and oxygen therapy initiated, VT/Ns are often able to step back slightly and inquire about pain management, and they should be encouraged to do so. As discussed in Chapters 7 and 8, there are rarely situations where an analgesic is not appropriate, whether it be a local block or systemic opioid. This should not be looked upon as a failure on the part of the veterinarian. It is simply a vital aspect of the "team approach to pain management" and indicates the different focus of the two veterinary professionals.

Similarly, there are often patients in the veterinary hospital that are not thought to be painful upon admission. It is important that pain assessment of **all** patients take place on a frequent basis, as often the patient's condition may change. For example, a patient with dietary indiscretion may develop pancreatitis and a painful abdomen. Pain may develop at any point, and the VT/N should bring their findings to the veterinarian and ask for analgesic orders.

B. Ask for Changes to Analgesics

Oftentimes, a patient may be on a specific opioid, as a bolus or CRI, but it becomes obvious that the medication isn't right for that particular patient. The patient may have an opioid sensitivity, resulting in excessive sedation, or develop ileus, nausea or rapid dysphoria. Sometimes trying something different will have a better effect. Adding an adjunct analgesic may provide more complete analgesia, while allowing the reduction of the opioid causing the problem. Often, the VT/N will notice these issues, and should bring them to the attention of the veterinarian. Offering a suggestion, "Can we try buprenorphine instead?" or "Can we add a ketamine CRI?", and a reason for the suggestion, can help the veterinarian provide orders that may work better for that individual.

In every practice, VT/Ns should be encouraged to speak up about analgesia and be part of the pain plan for each patient. Suggestions should be welcomed, but the VT/N should not expect every suggestion to be taken by the veterinarian. When there is disagreement, it should be discussed as a team, as open dialogue encourages further learning and participation.

17

Optimal Nursing Care for the Management of Pain

Andrea Steele

It is known that stress heightens the sensation of pain. In addition, stress is known to inhibit healing, increase serum glucose concentrations and affect cortisol levels [1]. The ambient noise and 24 h lighting of a hospital is stressful to all patients in addition to their physical discomfort. Stress reduction is essential in the overall pain management plan of the ill or injured patient in pain. There are numerous non-pharmacological methods available to ensure that a painful patient is provided with the most comfort possible, in addition to judicious use of analgesics. Veterinary technicians/nurses (VT/Ns) can institute these techniques as part of their nursing care plan, which should be part of the team discussion and management of the case. Integrative techniques should also be considered (refer to Chapter 15).

I. The Nursing Care Plan

VT/Ns should always prepare an ongoing nursing care plan for every patient in their care. The nursing care plan is an individualized plan that has several benefits for the patient:

- **Continuity of care:** Provides communication within the VT/N team, providing a framework for rounds between shifts. The nursing plan should be continually updated, including milestones reached (patient eating well, patient able to ambulate, etc.) or, alternatively, appearing more painful and less responsive to prescribed analgesics/dosages. Both of these situations require changes in medication dosages/frequency/additions (reduction or increases).
- **Documentation in the medical record:** Accurate and timely recordings ensure that the nursing aspects of the case, such as those mentioned above, are in the medical record, and so are available for the continuity of care by nursing staff and veterinarians and the well-being of the patient. VT/Ns who are encouraged to think critically, troubleshoot and communicate within the veterinary team will have increased job satisfaction and retention. In addition, the VT/N, using these skills, will ensure that concerns are brought to the attention of the veterinarian much sooner, expediting intervention and improving patient outcome.

Analgesia and Anesthesia for the Ill or Injured Dog and Cat, First Edition. Karol A. Mathews, Melissa Sinclair, Andrea M. Steele and Tamara Grubb.

A. Formulating the Nursing Care Plan for the Painful Patient

The process of developing a nursing care plan arises from a procedure termed the "nursing process". This is a five-step procedure that assists the VT/N in establishing goals (shift goals or therapeutic goals, as prescribed), and include:

- **The nursing assessment:** The information collection stage. Both objective and subjective data is collected and analysed before moving to the next step. Objective data includes hard numbers associated with temperature, pulse and respiration, urine output, SpO_2, etc. Subjective data, in human nursing, includes things that the patient tells the nurse, for example: "I feel pain here", "I would rank it as 7 on a scale of 1–10" or "I feel anxious". Veterinary patients cannot communicate with the VT/N in this way. Subjective data for the VT/N may include discussion with the owner to find out how the pet normally reacts to hospitalization, for example: "He never eats while in hospital", "He will not urinate on a leash" or "He gets very anxious when away from home". All of this data can be of value while formulating the plan. The data must be assessed, determining whether the objective values are normal or abnormal or meet the parameters provided by the veterinarian.
- **The nursing concerns:** In human medicine, a complete list of approved nursing "concerns" (diagnoses) are provided and frequently updated for nurses by NANDA International (formerly the North American Nursing Diagnosis Association) [2]. The **nursing** concerns take the information gathered in the nursing assessment, as well as the medical diagnosis, to determine what nursing interventions may help the patient's outcome and prevent possible complications. For example:
    - The recumbent patient may be at risk of decubital ulcers or urine scalding (Figure 17.1).
    - The painful patient may have fluctuations in pain level.

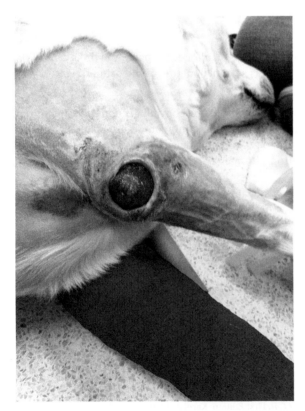

Figure 17.1 A patient referred to manage a severe decubital ulcer following one week of lateral recumbency. Ulcers can form rapidly and the skin must be observed closely for any irritation.

- **Planning:** In this phase, the VT/N takes the information gathered in the first two phases to develop short and long-term goals, ultimately creating an individualized plan for the patient. For example:
  - The patient's position should be changed q4h, and the skin assessed for early signs of redness.
  - Each hour, the patient should have a complete pain score completed to ensure adequate, but not excessive, analgesia. Analgesia should be adjusted within the dosing limits, or discussed with the veterinarian if adjustments outside of the dosing limits are recommended.
- **Implementing:** In this phase, everything identified for the individual patient is put into action.
  - The patient's position is adjusted every 4h, and the VT/N notices some redness at the stifle.
  - The pain score is completed hourly and the analgesia adjusted accordingly.
- **Evaluation:** Finally, the VT/N must assess the outcome of the plan that they have put into place. This may take place at the end of the shift before handing over the patient to the next shift, or it may take place many times during the shift, for example a patient receiving a fluid or analgesic bolus should be evaluated for response when complete. For example:
  - Redness was noted, and additional padding was provided to the area of concern, also ensuring the area was kept clean and dry.
  - The patient maintained an adequate level of analgesia; however, it was noted that the patient required an additional bolus of fentanyl prior to changing sides or trolleying outdoors.

In addition to the nursing care plan being an important communication tool to use between the VT/Ns over the course of the patient's hospitalization, the plan is also important to share with the case veterinarian as it may be useful in determining adjustments to treatments. It should be continually updated and modified to include both improvements in the patient's condition (requires less analgesia, eating or drinking) and backwards steps (develops aspiration pneumonia, prolonged anorexia) over time.

Some suggested plans that would be useful for the veterinary technician to prepare for the painful patient include different techniques for non-pharmacological comfort. Many have already been alluded to above, but are discussed in more detail below.

B. Non-Pharmacological Nursing Interventions for Patient Comfort

- **Reducing hospital stress:** There are several aspects of being in hospital that are very stressful for most pets. Some have never been away from home before or been housed in a cage. This in itself can be very stressful. Barking dogs, loud machines such as oxygen cages or alarming equipment all contribute to noise-related stress. Foam earplugs or cotton balls in the ears of recumbent patients may reduce their sensitivity to noise.

Cats in particular should be housed away from barking dogs. This may be difficult in a typical ICU environment, but providing cats with cages in an enclosed glass room or glass-fronted cages may help to reduce noise, while allowing them to be observed closely. Consider strategies such as boxes in the cage for the cat to hide within, with an opening large enough for observation.

Barking can have a cumulative effect in the ICU, with one barker getting several dogs going at once. This can be very stressful for all the patients, as well as the veterinary team. Occasionally, providing some light sedation for the vocal instigator will have the benefit of calming the followers. The VT/N should discuss the use of an appropriate sedative with the veterinarian. In many cases, the veterinarian will provide an "as needed" (PRN) order for a dosage of sedative

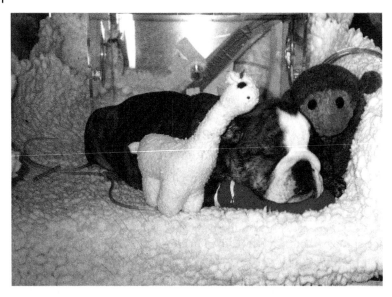

Figure 17.2 A toy from home and comfortable environment reduces stress and, therefore, pain.

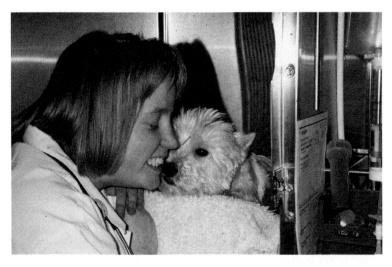

Figure 17.3 A little TLC.

on the patient's flowsheet for these instances. Removing patients that are feeling better, and are disruptive, to a step-down unit, general wards or home as soon as possible is recommended.

Providing bedding, toys (Figure 17.2), food dishes, or owners' clothing from home can be soothing for the pet that is having trouble adjusting to the hospital environment.

TLC and extra attention for the patient that is anxious or stressed will be comforting (Figure 17.3).

- **Ensuring adequate sleep:** While poorly documented in veterinary medicine, the importance of sleep for hospitalized human patients has been well researched. In humans, sleep disturbances in the ICU environment include fragmented sleep cycles, often 15–20 min in length, many times a day and night, resulting in many cycles of light broken sleep and lack of deep restorative sleep [3]. Sleep disruption has been attributed to noise, light, patient–nurse interactions, etc. Physical consequences of sleep deprivation include hormonal and metabolic, ventilatory, cardiovascular and immunologic disruption.

Presumably, veterinary patients experience similar issues with sleep deprivation in the ICU environment. A recent study showed that dogs have diurnal sleep–wake cycles similar to humans, and total locomotor activity varied with the presence of the owner in the home [4]. Cats in the same study exhibited no rhythmicity to total locomotor activity with owner's presence and had nocturnal restlessness. This suggests that dogs especially may benefit from maintaining a diurnal environment in the ICU, with reduced lighting and noise, minimal nursing interventions and disturbances at night, to encourage sleep during the night-time hours.

- **Reducing other sources of pain:** The ICU environment is rife with invasive devices such as intravenous, arterial, nasal and urinary catheters, as well as other tubes such as esophagostomy/gastrostomy tubes, thoracic drains and abdominal drains. All of these various tubes add to the pain and discomfort of the patient. Overall nursing care must include awareness of the pain associated with managing these devices, for example aspirating thoracic drains and nasogastric tubes with minimal negative pressure, and monitoring for phlebitis. Managing the pain these devices incur should be included in the overall pain plan, and considering whether to add additional analgesia prior to manipulating the device, removing the device if no longer necessary or replacing the device. Monitoring for tightness of bandages and associated swelling must also be included in the plan.
- **Positional comfort:** Patients can become very uncomfortable when left in the same position for extended periods of time. This will be exacerbated in geriatric patients, which have less muscle and fat reserves, and in those with arthritis. Providing ample padding between the limbs will reduce stress on joints by keeping limbs in a natural position, with subsequent reduction in discomfort (Figure 17.4).

Many patients choose not to move around in their cage for many reasons – pain or discomfort, fear or anxiety being very common. Assisting these patients with changes in position will help to reduce this discomfort. A common example is the dog recovering from surgical repair

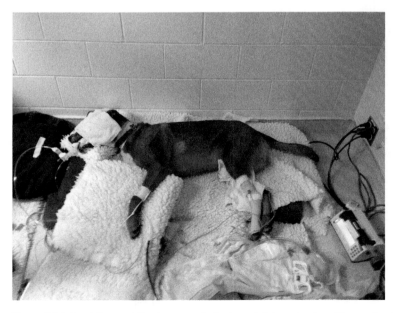

Figure 17.4 Providing padding between limbs to maintain natural position and reduce strain on joints and pressure points.

of intervertebral disk herniation. Frequently, these dogs sit upright on the tail with hind limbs extended and with fairly rigid forelimbs (Figure 17.5). These dogs frequently have difficulty lying down, and need assistance to move into the down position. Often, they will immediately go to sleep once placed in lateral recumbency.

There are more complex situations where careful observation with respect to discomfort and pain is needed. This is especially so for patients that cannot move themselves due to their disease (paralysis, shock) or because they are sedated or anesthetized (status epilepticus or ventilator patients). These patients require changes in position to minimize discomfort and the risk of decubital ulcer formation (Figure 17.1). This is especially important in a ventilator patient that is lightly anesthetized. Discomfort is frequently manifested by an increase in heart rate and blood pressure under a light plane of anesthesia or restlessness, such as movement of the limbs (if not paralysed) or head, threatening to dislodge the endotracheal tube. Changing the position of these patients, even from lateral to sternal, will often allow the patient to relax without increasing anesthetic/analgesic doses.

- **Addressing need to urinate or defecate:** Many patients become anxious when they need to urinate or defecate, the stress of which may increase the sensation of pain. The need to urinate is assessed by bladder palpation or cage-side bladder ultrasound. The bladder can be gently expressed in recumbent patients if placement of a urinary catheter is contraindicated.

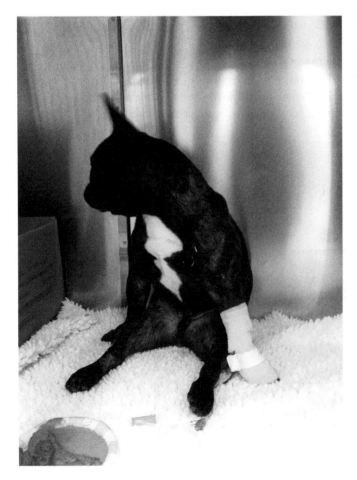

Figure 17.5 Typical posture of a patient with intervertebral disc disease (IVDD). Gently assisting the patient into a recumbent position will often help them to sleep.

Placing a temporary or indwelling urinary catheter may be beneficial to relieve the anxiety of needing to urinate, and also to prevent urine scalding.

In general, veterinary patients do not defecate as frequently when hospitalized as when at home. Some patients may find the posture, or straining, to defecate very uncomfortable and is thus avoided. Observe for signs that they need to defecate (feces on the thermometer, flatulence or prolonged time between bowel movements). Ideally, the patient that is eating and has normal stool should produce a bowel movement daily. Occasionally, the act of taking a temperature will stimulate a bowel movement, so having a diaper pad handy is advisable. Enemas may be prescribed in the recumbent patient to empty the rectum should constipation be diagnosed.

For patients that are mobile, allowing more time to urinate or defecate outdoors, by capping and flushing IV lines so they can roam in a safe space for a few extra minutes, may encourage elimination. Asking the owners for commands associated with urination or defecation may be of benefit.

Using assist devices such as slings or harnesses may allow the patient to assume an elimination posture more easily without risk of a fall.

- **Temperature/humidity of the environment:** The environmental temperature can greatly impact the comfort of a patient. Consider a large, heavy fur-coated dog that is panting in a cage: the temperature and humidity in the space is going to increase and hinder their ability to lose heat. Providing a fan, placing the dog in a run or having wall tie-downs that allow patients to be left on the floor can help prevent this problem. New gel pads are available that offer cooling effect by dissipating heat.

Conversely, patients may struggle with hypothermia when critically ill. Providing supplemental heat should be part of the nursing plan. It is important to provide for both warm and normal room temperature areas within the cage, so that the animal can move away from the heat if they feel too warm. Using safe heat sources such as oat bags, microwaveable heating discs or warming devices such as a warm-water-circulating blanket, Hot Dog Warmer® or Bair Hugger® can provide warm zones in the cage.

- **Addressing thirst:** Many patients may not be able to move towards a water bowl, or lift their head to drink, but may benefit from small amounts of water syringed into the mouth. Many patients will give subtle cues that they are ready for a little more water by lip smacking or nudging their heads towards the bowl. Using a small syringe (6–12 mL), cautiously drip water into the mouth and allow the patient to swallow. Placing the patient's head and thorax on a 30° incline may assist with swallowing and minimize risk of aspiration. Aspiration is indeed a concern and only small amounts of water should be administered at one time (Figure 17.6). Excessive thirst suggests inadequate fluid administration requiring re-assessment of fluid therapy.
- **Addressing hunger:** Hunger can be another factor leading to distress in the hospitalized patient. While many painful patients will not be willing to eat, well-managed patients may enjoy food. Make a nutritional plan based on the patient's underlying disease, and offer nutritious choices at intervals that are comfortable for the patient. Some patients may prefer their daily requirement split into q2–4h feedings, and others may suffice with twice daily feedings. To begin eating, some patients may need coaxing with extra fragrant "sauces" added to their meals, such as chicken or beef baby food, juice from a can of tuna or sardines, gravy or other flavour enhancers. Minimize the use of these treats to only enough to encourage eating the nutritious food, which should be the mainstay of their diet. Some patients have preference for dry food, whereas others may prefer canned – trying both options may lead to success.

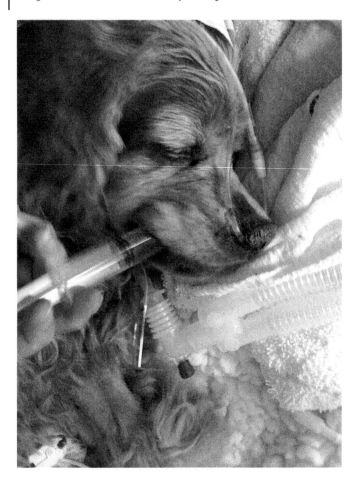

Figure 17.6 Recumbent patients are unable to reach a water bowl and appreciate water being offered by syringe.

II. Formulating the Pain Plan: The Team Approach [5]

After addressing all the potential situations (noted above) to rule out non-medical or surgical causes of potential contributors to the painful experience, a pain plan should be created for every patient that is hospitalized and requiring analgesia. The initial, or default, dosages and medications chosen will be based on several factors:

- What is the expected pain level for the procedure, disease or trauma?
- Are there any individual, breed or species considerations?
- Are there any pre-existing pain conditions, such as chronic pain?
- Are there any drug contraindications or drug sensitivities in this patient?

The pain plan should be formulated between the veterinarian and VT/N. The veterinarian will be familiar with the pre-existing conditions, sensitivities and contraindications, while the VT/N will have a good grasp of the individual behaviour and idiosyncrasies of the patient. Ideally, a dose range and PRN orders will be provided for bolus analgesics, allowing the VT/N to titrate analgesia to the desired effect, and also give flexibility for the time of dosing. For patients requiring continuous rate infusion (CRI) analgesics, an acceptable dose range provided by the veterinarian will allow for flexibility in dosing. If the VT/N reaches the limits of the dose range, and feels that the patient needs higher or lower doses of the CRI, they should discuss this with the veterinarian.

After the initial doses of analgesics are given by bolus ± CRI, a pain assessment should be completed within 15–30 min. Observing and recording the response to the analgesic is critical, and part of the nursing plan.

Observations should include details and a subsequent plan should be formulated, such as:

- The initial response to a bolus dose of an opioid, for example:
  - The VT/N noted the patient vomited and panted for 15 min after a 0.05 mg/kg bolus of hydromorphone, before lying down and going to sleep.
    - The plan should be to titrate the opioid and note the dose given before the patient appears slightly nauseated (drooling, lip smacking) or begins to pant. This approach identifies when the effective dose has been reached (refer to Chapter 8). The dose required will also give an indirect assessment of the level of pain the patient is experiencing.
    - This effective dose can be used to plan the CRI.
  - The pain score changed from x to y.
    - The plan will be to lower the current analgesic dose.
- The duration of effect of the analgesic:
  - It is important to note whether the analgesic effect lasted longer or shorter than the expected duration of action for the medication (utilizing pain scoring techniques).
  - If longer, this may indicate the patient has a lower pain level, and is ready for reduction of dosage, or transitioning to other analgesics.
  - If shorter, this may indicate the patient has a higher level of pain, and may need a higher dosage, alterations to method of delivery or addition of adjunct analgesics.
- Transition to oral analgesics: Depending on the illness or injury, transitioning to oral medication can be difficult (it's definitely the "fussy" stage). Some tips to enhance the experience:
  - Where less than 100 mg of gabapentin is required, ask the compounding pharmacy to suspend gabapentin 200 mg/mL in a chicken-flavour oil base. Dogs really like chicken flavour, as do cats. With this high concentration, the dose volume is very small (Robin Downing, personal communication)
  - Hickory smoke flavour Canine Pill Pockets® are enjoyed by both dogs and cats. These pills do not crumble like the other flavours and are moist enough to pinch off a little to wrap around the medication. They are very cost-effective. There is no concern for patients with pancreatitis (Robin Downing, personal communication).
  - Reward all medication episodes with appropriate treats or canned food. As an example, when this technique is used by cat owners when administering insulin, the cat gets the "high sign" and sits for its insulin injection (Margie Scherk, personal communication).
  - For small dogs and cats that are prescribed amitriptyline, prepare in size 4 gel capsules (Margie Scherk, personal communication).

III. Anesthetic Recovery

The anesthetic recovery period requires increased vigilance and observation of the patient.

Recovery is a critical phase of anesthesia and begins when the anesthetic agents are discontinued, continues **after** the patient is extubated and is complete when the patient returns to its normal physiological and behavioural state. Most anesthetic-associated deaths occur during the first 3 h of the post-operative period once the anesthetic agent is turned off. Forty-seven per cent of canine anesthesia mortalities and 60% of feline anesthesia mortalities are reported to occur within this post-anesthetic period [6]. Hence, monitoring should be performed by those trained in the recognition of anesthetic complications.

Generally, the patient is only moved to its cage once swallowing, conscious and extubated. Until that time, a team member should be at the patient's side assessing adequate ventilation, return to consciousness and readiness to extubate to prevent an endotracheal accident with aspiration of the tube. Following extubation, the patient should continue to be observed closely for adequate respiration, oxygen saturation as well as signs of pain or delirium. A quiet separate recovery area from the anesthetic induction and surgical preparatory area is ideal for the patient. However, this requires adequate staffing and transfer of information to the VT/N team if different from the anesthesia team. Pertinent details of the patient's anesthesia and surgery should be fully communicated by the anesthetist. This case transfer information should include any peri-operative complications that may have occurred, medications used, last systemic analgesic doses, details of nerve blocks, epidural or other analgesic modalities with intraoperative efficacy, recent blood gas/laboratory values and temperature, pulse, respiration (TPR) at time of extubation.

Upon entry to the recovery area, the TPR, and depending on the patient and surgery, a blood pressure and SpO2 should be repeated. Continuous ECG or blood pressure monitoring may be required, and initiated as soon as possible. Oxygen support may be indicated. Supplemental heat and/or blankets should be applied until return to low normal temperature. The patient's respiration rate should be continuously monitored throughout the recovery period. Pulse and temperature should be obtained every 15–30 min, until they return to normal values. A pulse oximeter while the patient is sedated is useful for monitoring adequate respirations and heart rate.

Analgesic delivery during the recovery period may involve bolus, or CRI, drug delivery. As with any pain management regimen, the ideal is for the VT/N to have dose ranges and frequency orders from the veterinarian; however, frequency should be flexible and based on the patient's needs, sooner or later depending on pain assessment. Where PRN orders are given, to facilitate flexibility, it is essential that the VT/N be experienced in pain assessment (refer to Chapter 8) to avoid the painful experience. The veterinarian should assess the analgesic requirements based on the original problem, tissue trauma and manipulation during surgery, and provide initial analgesic dose ranges based on this information. The recovery period often leads to the most variability in dosing, and frequency if bolus doses are prescribed, due to individual patient variability, the effectiveness of local analgesia, the use of analgesics during the procedure and the surgical procedure. It may take some time to find the ideal analgesic level. Orders for low-dose sedation may be useful to combat delirium and anxiety in the recovery period. It is important that the VT/N be proactive and discuss potential analgesic requirements with the veterinarian, and request orders for additional analgesics.

Pain assessment (refer to Chapter 8) should be performed with the initial intake examination, and at frequent intervals during the recovery period. Extra care should be taken with the sedated patient, to ensure that they are not painful. A patient lying quietly in the cage should not be assumed to be pain-free; a pain assessment may reveal the patient has splinting or guarding of the incision site upon gentle palpation, reluctance to move, as well as elevated heart rate and blood pressure.

Ideally, during the recovery period, the patient's pain level would be expected to decrease. Obviously, the timeframe will differ based on the individual and surgery performed, but the post-operative period should reflect decreasing analgesic needs over time as the patient's condition improves. Sudden increases in analgesic needs during the immediate post-operative period should be considered suspect, and immediately brought to the veterinarian's attention. Nerve entrapment or impingement, for example, will acutely increase a patient's pain level, and will need to be evaluated and treated immediately. During the remaining 24–48 h of the recovery period, an increase in analgesic needs should be suspect and underlying surgical or medical complications be assessed.

References

1 Stanford, G. (1994) The stress response to trauma and critical illness. *Crit Care Nurs Clin N Am*, 6: 693–702.

2 Kamdar, B. B., Needham, D. M. and Collop, N. A. (2012) Sleep deprivation in critical illness: Its role in physical and psychological recovery. *J Intensive Care Med*, 27(2): 97–111.

3 NANDA International (2012) *Nursing Diagnoses: Definitions and classifications: 2012-2014*. Wiley-Blackwell, Ames, IA.

4 Piccione, G., Marafioti, S., Giannetto, C., *et al.* (2012) Comparison of daily rest/activity in companion cats and dogs. *Biol Rhythms Res*, 45(4): 615–623.

5 Shaffran, N. (2008) Pain management: The veterinary technician's perspective. *Vet Clin North Am Small Anim Pract*, 38: 1415–1428.

6 Brodbelt, D. C., Blissit, K. J., Hammond, R. A., *et al.* (2008) The risk of death: The confidential enquiry into perioperative small animal fatalities. *Vet Anaesth Analg*, 35(5): 365–373.

18

Preparation and Delivery of Analgesics

Andrea Steele

Analgesics can be delivered orally (PO), subcutaneously (SC), intramuscularly (IM) and intravenously (IV). It is important to assure that each injectable formulation is licensed for the route being considered, as some medications may have specific routes of administration. In general, analgesics are administered IV to ill or injured patients and may be delivered as a bolus or continuous infusion following the bolus.

I. Bolus Dosing

Bolus dosing is the simplest method of administering analgesics; however, when not performed cautiously, it can lead to complications. When administering opioids, it is only in the rare, excruciatingly painful patient that a bolus dose of pure mu-opioid should be administered as a fast push of the prescribed dose. In these patients, the use of fentanyl as the first-line opioid may be the most gentle and effective, as it is least likely to produce unwanted side effects such as vomiting, panting and dysphoria. If only morphine, hydromorphone or oxymorphone are available, be prepared for side effects with rapid administration of an empirical dose, although with a severely painful patient the benefit of rapid analgesia may outweigh the potential negative side effects. A painful patient will also be less likely to exhibit negative side effects, when compared with a patient that is mild–moderately painful. As a warning, morphine should not be delivered as a rapid bolus IV, as this will trigger histamine release, resulting in marked hypotension.

In general, when a mu-opioid is indicated to control pain, titrating the drug in small aliquots of the dose (often in 1/8–1/4 of the dose) over several minutes will allow for careful monitoring and prevention of any negative side effects. The maximal effective dose of the medication – the point at which maximal analgesia and minimal side effects are noted – will be a guide as to the severity of pain and repeat dosing requirements.

Other considerations to remember when titrating an opioid include:

- **Speed of fluid administration if delivering through the IV line.** If administering at the time of a fluid bolus, the fluids are running at a very fast rate, and therefore the drug will be administered at a very fast rate. Consider making the aliquots of drug smaller (1/10–1/8 of the total expected dose). If administering an analgesic bolus through a line with the fluid running very slowly, be sure to administer the medication close to the patient, and either flush the medication in or leave sufficient time for the medication to reach the patient before adding more.

Analgesia and Anesthesia for the Ill or Injured Dog and Cat, First Edition. Karol A. Mathews, Melissa Sinclair, Andrea M. Steele and Tamara Grubb.
© 2018 John Wiley & Sons, Inc. Published 2018 by John Wiley & Sons, Inc.

- **Nausea or vomiting may not be the endpoint of analgesic requirement.** In some cases, the rapidity of the opioid administration may trigger the chemoreceptor trigger zone for emesis, causing signs of nausea (lip smacking, drooling, excessive swallowing) or vomiting, which rapidly subsides. Consider that the rapidity of administration alone may have caused this reaction, and that the maximal effective dose may not yet be reached. Pause, until the adverse effects subside. Don't make the assumption that the patient is not painful without a full pain assessment. If the patient still appears painful, administer the analgesic at a much slower rate until the patient is pain-free, or consider adding a different class of analgesic (e.g. non-steroidal anti-inflammatory analgesic, ketamine).

Intermittent bolus dosing of opioids has some drawbacks. The most important of which is that the patient will exhibit some level of pain prior to administration of the next timed dose. Generally, the doses are timed based on the expected half-life of each drug. For example, hydromorphone is typically prescribed for q4–6h. While this may be in the treatment plan, it is recommended that the veterinarian technician/nurse (VT/N) or veterinarian assess the patient, using pain assessment techniques, prior to the 4 or 6h mark and titrate the opioid as needed, which will provide analgesia before the patient is exhibiting significant pain. On the other hand, should the patient's condition be improved, delaying a 4h treatment will reduce the potential for adverse effects of a continuing set dose given at a set interval.

As with opioids, bolus dosing of adjunct analgesics such as ketamine, dexmedetomidine and lidocaine are commonly used to rapidly raise serum levels prior to beginning a continuous rate infusion (CRI). A bolus may also be used to assess the efficacy of the drug for the individual patient, prior to a CRI; if relief is apparent, a CRI will be started. In general, these analgesics are best used as a CRI for long-term pain relief, rather than as bolus doses. Boluses of dexmedetomidine or ketamine may provide sedation in the patient experiencing delirium post- anesthesia.

II. Continuous Rate Infusion

CRI allows for continuous analgesia, with constant or variable dosing, without the "peaks and valleys" of bolus dosing; the patient does not need to be exhibiting pain before receiving the next dose – the dose is being trickled in at a continuous rate, approximately the same rate as it is being metabolized. The benefit is continuous analgesia, and the hope that the patient will remain at a continuous level of analgesia, thus avoiding breakthrough or cyclic pain.

Experience has shown that the initial dosing of a CRI is estimated from the maximal effective dose of the opioid identified during the initial bolus dose. For example, a patient that required a very high initial bolus will begin a CRI at the high end of the dose range, while a patient that required a low dose may have the CRI started at the low to mid-range of the dose. On average, the duration of analgesia of hydromorphone, methadone and morphine is 4–6h; therefore, the effective bolus dose is used to maintain a steady-state analgesia, as a CRI, over 4h (1/4 the bolus dose/h). Whereas the duration of fentanyl is approximately 1h, the effective bolus dose is administered as an hourly infusion. This also applies to ketamine and lidocaine.

CRIs can be delivered in several formats, depending on what equipment is available at the veterinary clinic. The authors prefer doses that are individualized to the patient, often delivered in the fluid bag, burette, elastomeric pump or via syringe pump into the hourly fluids. Many clinics prefer to create a standard stock solution in an appropriately sized fluid bag to provide easy dosing such as 1 mL/kg/h through a fluid pump. This method may require a second line, bag and pump in order to meet the patient's hourly fluid requirement. The authors do not recommend sharing leftover stock solution between patients, but rather discard according to local or provincial/state-controlled drug legislation.

A. How to Prepare Drug Solutions for Infusions

There is considerable room for error when making admixtures, and it is vitally important to ensure the proper technique is used. Use the following tips to reduce errors:

- Use the closest syringe size for the volume of initial drug concentration (whether full-strength or previously diluted) you need for the admixture.
- Ensure you have chosen a compatible carrier fluid; use the product monograph or a drug compatibility chart.
- Never flush the syringe/needle by repeatedly pulling back fluid and re-injecting the volume into the syringe.

B. Fluid Bag Delivery

Delivery of one or more analgesics added to the maintenance fluid bag is a very effective method of delivering a CRI. There are some drawbacks that should be mentioned, however.

- **Less flexibility in dosing:** If the CRI is running with the maintenance fluids, there is less flexibility in dosing without exceeding, or reducing, the amount of fluid the patient is receiving. This method may be more appropriate for drugs such as lidocaine, ketamine or dexmedetomidine, as they are not necessarily as variable as opioids in their dosing; likely, they can remain at the same level for a longer period of time.
- **More wastage:** The bag method is best for patients that will use the entire bag in a 24h period, such as large dogs, or patients with higher fluid rates. Using smaller fluid bags – such as 100, 250 or 500 mL bags – may help alleviate the wastage, but these bags are typically more expensive/mL than their 1 L counterparts.
- **Overfilling of fluid bags leads to inaccuracies:** Fluid bags are overfilled ~10% by the manufacturer. When stored for long periods, bags lose volume due to evaporative losses and may contain less than stated on the label. This will cause the concentration of the bag to be different than expected. Likely, this will not cause a concern. However, it is important to be aware of this source of error. Because of overfill and evaporative losses, human compounding pharmacies will not provide CRI medication in an IV bag, as the concentration cannot be guaranteed (the exception being if the drug and the fluid in measured quantities are added to an empty, sterile bag). Prefilled IV bags are only used for drug admixtures when they are providing a set number of milligrams, by using the entire contents of the bag in a short period of time (e.g. diluting 500 mg of ampicillin in 50 mL of saline, and giving over half an hour). The final concentration is not as important as knowing the number of milligrams being administered. For this reason, CRI delivery in a fluid bag should be considered the least desirable method of administering analgesic drugs.

The method for preparing a CRI in a fluid bag or burette is discussed in Section III. The method for both deliveries are similar. However, there are additional considerations for fluid bags alone that must be taken into account when preparing the CRI.

- **The 10% rule:** This is a rule that hospital pharmacies use to ensure consistency in the final admixture product. If the drug to be added to the bag is 10% or more of the volume in the bag then that volume should be removed from the bag prior to addition of the drug. For example, to make a 5% dextrose solution using 50% dextrose, in a 1 L bag of fluid, 100 mL of dextrose must be added to the container; 100 mL of fluid should be removed from the bag before the addition. In the case of 2.5% dextrose solution, 50 mL must be added to 1 L. As this is < 10% of the volume in the fluid bag, there is no need to remove 50 mL prior to addition. By ensuring that all parties are following the 10% rule in your practice, you can be assured that if the solution is made up correctly the final concentration should be similar from person to person.

- **Mixing:** After addition of an admixture drug, it is important to invert the bag several times to ensure adequate mixing.
- **Adjust based on patient response:** Knowing that the final concentration of a drug in a fluid bag can never be precise due to the overfill of the bag, it is important the veterinarian and VT/N are aware that the delivered dose per hour may vary slightly. This highlights the importance of assessing the patient for response to therapy and adjusting the fluid rate/dosing accordingly.

III. Drug Infusions Using a Burette

A burette is an inexpensive tool for IV fluid therapy. It is an inline, graduated volume cylinder that allows for accurate portioning of IV fluids into a smaller volume. Adjustments to drug dose rate are easily made by adding more fluid (decrease concentration), or more drug (increase concentration), or emptying the burette and adding a fresh solution. The 150 mL burette is frequently used: it has an IV spike at the top that is inserted into the IV fluid bag and a roller clamp below the spike facilitates controlled fluid entry into the burette. The proximal end of a standard IV delivery solution set is spiked into the bottom of the burette and the distal end is attached to the patient's IV catheter. Drug infusions in a burette should be administered using an IV fluid pump for accuracy. Where an IV pump is not available, frequent monitoring within the hour is essential.

There is an injection port at the top of the burette for addition of medication. Some models (usually needleless port types) have a volume of dead space within the injection port; therefore, following addition of a medication, instil ~1 mL of a sterile fluid (0.9% NaCl or fluid drawn aseptically from the fluid bag, into a syringe) to flush the port to ensure that the entire dose of medication is delivered into the burette.

Avoid squeezing the burette. Squeezing the burette ultimately causes a pressure change within the chamber and will actually impede flow by gravity into the chamber. This will worsen each time the burette is squeezed, air will collect in the bag above and eventually it will be impossible to fully fill the burette. Fill the burette approximately halfway by gravity from the fluid bag, add the calculated drug volume through the injection port and then continue to fill with fluid to the final volume. When adding a volume of medication greater than ~1 mL, withdraw the same amount of air from the burette using the syringe. This will minimize pressure change affecting the fill of the burette by gravity. Swirl the burette to mix the drug thoroughly, and avoid inverting it, as this would damage the air inlet at the top of the burette.

A. Preparation of Drug Infusions for Bag/Burette

To prepare medications for infusion in a fluid bag or burette, the following information is required:

- the dose to be provided per hour
- the initial concentration of the drug
- the weight of the patient
- the volume of the fluid bag **or** the actual or desired volume of the burette
- the prescribed fluid rate/h.

Using the provided dose, calculate the number of mL/h of drug that is required. For example: hydromorphone CRI, at 0.01 mg/kg/h for a 20 kg dog.

- $0.01\,\text{mg/kg/h} \times 20\,\text{kg} = 0.2\,\text{mg/h}$

Using the 2 mg/mL concentration of hydromorphone:

- 0.2 mg/h / 2 mg/mL = 0.1 mL/h

Next, determine how many hours of fluid will fit in the burette, if the hourly rate is 35 mL/h and the burette holds 150 mL

- 150 mL/35 mL/h = 4.3 h

Finally, how many mL of hydromorphone are needed for 4.3 h?

- 4.3 × 0.1 mL/h = 0.43 mL

The same calculation is performed for a fluid bag.

- Using a 500 mL 0.9% NaCl bag, calculate how much fentanyl should be added to deliver 3 µg/kg/h to a 30 kg dog receiving 75 mL/h.

Calculate the number of mL/h of fentanyl that is required:

- 3 µg/kg/h × 30 kg = 90 µg/h

Fentanyl concentration of 50 µg/mL:

- 90 µg/h/50 µg/mL = 1.8 mL/h

Next, calculate the number of hours, assuming an approximate volume of 500 mL:

- 500 mL/75 mL/h = 6.67 h

Finally, how much fentanyl do we need for 6.67 h?

- 6.67 h × 1.8 mL/h = 12.0 mL

Since 12.0 mL is < 10% of the volume of the bag, add it to the bag, and invert to mix.

B. Labelling the Drug Infusion

It is very important to appropriately label the drug infusion, not only to accurately identify the contents but also to ensure consistency, or in some cases to identify an error in the previous drug calculation. The admixture should be recalculated as a verification each time a new solution is made.

A simple label can be made for you at the local print shop, or on the clinic printer (Figure 18.1).

A bright label readily identifies there is a drug in the bag or burette, to avoid inadvertent changes in the fluid rate. The final line "# mls drug in ____ mls" refers to the number of mL of drug in a final volume of × mL. For example, the label for the hydromorphone example above would read:

Drug: Hydromorphone
Dose: 0.01 mg/kg/h
Fluid Rate: 35 mL/h
0.43 mL drug in 150 mL

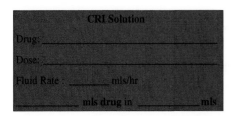

Figure 18.1 Label to be applied to drug infusions.

CRI Solution

Drug: _____

Dose: _____

Fluid Rate : _____ mls/hr

_____ mls drug in _____ mls

IV. Standardized Concentration Infusions

As mentioned above, some clinics prefer to use standardized concentrations of analgesics, delivered on a sliding scale based on patient weight.

A. Benefits

- **Less likely to have calculation errors:** The same amount of drug is added to the same size bag each time it is made up, reducing the chance of a calculation error.
- **Less likely to have administration errors:** Likewise, there is less chance of an administration error, when the dose is standardized. If prescribed at 1 mL/kg/h, this is simply the body weight of the patient entered into the pump.
- **Recipes can be used to make multidrug bags:** Fairly advanced CRIs can be created using a standard recipe. This delivers each drug at a set rate. Commonly morphine–lidocaine–ketamine infusions are prepared in this manner.
- **Flexibility in dosing:** While the standard recipe may be delivered at 1 mL/kg/h, increasing, or decreasing, the hourly rate will allow titration. For multidrug bags, the infusion of each medication is increased or decreased.

B. Drawbacks

- **Additional fluid line and pump required:** Often the mL/h supplied with the standardized concentration method is not sufficient to meet the patient's hourly fluid requirements; therefore, an additional line and bag with maintenance crystalloid may be required. If only one fluid pump were available, the pump could be used for the analgesic bag, and gravity used for the maintenance fluids for medium- to large-sized dogs. Pumps offer a safety feature for smaller dogs and cats.
- **Wastage:** Wastage can be significant with this method, as the patient may not use the entire bag of medication. Consider recipes for 100/250/500/1000 mL bags to adjust for patient size.
- **Lack of individualization:** Especially with multidrug bags, this method allows increasing or decreasing the dosage of all drugs, but not each drug individually. Frequently, finding the right level of each drug for the patient is a challenge, and this type of system makes it more difficult.

All things considered, the standardized infusion bag is an acceptable method of providing a CRI, and may be preferable in veterinary clinics with a limited number of fluid pumps available.

Preparing a standardized infusion bag is similar to following a recipe. Several organizations offer "recipes" online and CRI calculators, which makes set up simple. To produce your own customized recipe, the following information is needed:

- volume of fluid bag
- concentration of each drug
- desired dose for each drug.

For example, ketamine has a dose range as a CRI of 0.1–2.0 mg/kg/h. Most commonly, it is delivered in the 0.1–1.0 mg/kg/h range, for moderate pain. Note: a patient in severe pain would require the higher-concentration bag, to reduce the fluid rate. The following example is using the moderate range of ketamine CRI.

Starting at a mid-range dose for the standardized bag to deliver 1 mL/kg/h of fluid will allow for some flexibility. The dose can be decreased or increased by changing the fluid rate (i.e. 0.5 mL/kg/h will reduce the dose to 0.25 mg/kg/h). Doubling the fluid rate to 2 mL/kg/h will deliver ketamine at 1 mg/kg/h.

Therefore, calculate based on 0.5 mg/kg/h:

- Initial concentration of ketamine is 100 mg/mL.
- Desired dose of 0.5 mg/kg/h ketamine delivered in 1 mL/kg/h gives a final concentration of 0.5 mg/mL ketamine (0.5 mg/kg/h per 1 mL/kg/h = 0.5 mg/mL).
- For a 1 L bag of fluid: 0.5 mg/mL × 1000 mL = 500 mg of ketamine.
- 500 mg/100 mg/ml = 5 mL of ketamine to add to the bag.
- For alternate bag sizes: 2.5 mL/500 mL, 1.25 mL/250 mL, 0.5 mL/100 mL.

If fentanyl at 3 μg/kg/h is added to the same bag to be delivered at 1 mL/kg/h rate:

- 3 μg/kg delivered in 1 mL/kg/h of fluids = 3 μg/mL of final solution.
- 1000 mL bag, need 3000 μg.

Fentanyl is 50 μg/mL, therefore:

- 3000 μg/50 μg/mL = 60 mL of fentanyl to a 1000 mL bag.

For alternate bag sizes:

- 6 mL/100 mL
- 15 mL/250 mL
- 30 mL/500 mL.

Keep in mind that, due to overfill/evaporative losses, the actual concentration may vary by ±10%.

V. Drug Infusion Using an Elastomeric Pump

Elastomeric pumps are another option for infusion delivery of a CRI to a patient. An elastomeric pump is also known as a "balloon pump", and uses a balloon made from a material that rebounds at a set rate, thus pushing the infusion into the patient at a set rate. It is designed to be a single-use device, which delivers a set volume over a period of time. Different manufacturers make different sizes, and flow rates, but generally they will infuse 0.5–2 mL/h over a period of 24 h to seven days depending on the capacity. It is accurate to ±10–12%, which can be affected by changes in temperature or outside pressure.

Drug preparation for an elastomeric pump will differ from a bag or burette, as the hourly volume of analgesic must be in the hourly delivery volume of the device. For example, the hydromorphone example above requiring 0.1 mL/h of hydromorphone would require that 0.1 mL of hydromorphone and 1.9 mL of 0.9% NaCl be delivered per hour for a 2 mL/h device.

A two-day, or 48 h, infuser holds 100 mL and delivers 2 mL/h. For our patient above, we would calculate the volumes required:

- 100 mL total volume/2 mL/h = 50 h.
- 50 h × 0.1 mL/h of hydromorphone = 5 mL of 2 mg/mL hydromorphone.

To calculate 0.9% NaCl needed to make a final volume:

- 100 mL − 5 mL = 95 mL.
- Final pump volume contains 5 mL hydromorphone and 95 mL of saline, 2.5 mL is residual in the device at the end of delivery and therefore the pump will run for 47.5 h at 2 mL/h.

VI. Drug Infusions Using a Syringe Pump

Syringe pumps are becoming more popular in the practice setting as they are very easy to use and generally very reliable and accurate. One distinct advantage is the ability to readily adjust drug dose rate. The drug can be prepared full-strength. However, if very small hourly volumes are required, some syringe pumps may not be able to deliver with accuracy, requiring dilution of the drug. Please see information below on proper dilution of drugs for administration. Many syringe pumps offer on-board programmes that allow the manager to create drug libraries, and set the concentration, dose range, dosing limits for the drug (min/max) and programme boluses. Some basic syringe pumps will be programmed simply with mL/h, and in some cases pumps are programmed using a chart that converts mL/h for each possible syringe size and manufacturer to mm/h. These latter pumps are very inexpensive devices, but care must be taken to ensure training is appropriate to avoid errors.

A. How to Dilute Stock Analgesic Drugs

Diluting drugs for ease of handling in syringe pumps, or for adding to solutions, is one of several steps in preparing drugs for infusion where errors may occur.

- To make a drug dilution, the full-strength drug, a diluent (usually D5W or 0.9% NaCl) and the desired final concentration is required. The diluent volume will be the **desired final volume** of diluted drug, less the calculated full-strength drug volume (i.e. a 1:10 dilution is 1 part of full-strength drug diluted in 9 parts of diluent to make a total of 10 parts). A common 1:10 drug dilution is dexmedetomidine, 500 μg/mL diluted to 50 μg/mL. To make 10 mL of diluted drug, take 1 mL of full-strength dexmedetomidine and add to 9 mL of 0.9% NaCl. A 1:100 dilution of dexmedetomidine 500 μg/mL would be a 5 μg/mL final solution, or 1 part drug in 99 parts diluent.
- Draw up the drug to be diluted and the diluent in **separate syringes**. The needle, the hub of the needle and the hub of the syringe have dead space, which can total 0.1–0.2 mL depending on the size of the needle and the type of syringe. This dead space reflects the volume that is left behind following an injection, or remains in the hub/needle when a drug is drawn up. Figure 18.2 illustrates the measured volume of drug and the syringe hub, needle hub and needle dead space that will contain residual drug. The dead space volume is unmeasured and unaccounted for when drawing up a specific dose of drug, and therefore, drawing diluent into the same syringe as the drug will cause the dead space volume of concentrated drug to be added to the syringe. This will result in a significant increase in the final concentration of drug in the syringe, especially where small volumes of total drug are required. Drawing concentrated drug directly into a syringe of diluent will cause a similar error.

Consider the example of a 1:10 dilution of dexmedetomidine. If you draw up 1.0 mL of dexmedetomidine in a 10 mL syringe with a 20-gauge × 1 in needle, the approximate needle and hub dead space is 0.15 mL. If 9 mL of 0.9% NaCl is drawn up using the same syringe and needle, an additional 0.15 mL of dexmedetomidine is added to the syringe. This results in a final concentration of 57.5 μg/mL, rather than the desired 50 μg/mL, the equivalent of a +15% error.

Consider a 1:100 dilution of dexmedetomidine, where 0.1 mL of dexmedetomidine is diluted into 10 mL of diluent. Using the same needle and syringe to draw up dexmedetomidine, followed by diluent, would result in 0.25 mL (0.1 + 0.15 in hub) being added to 10 mL, not 0.1 mL. This gives a final concentration of 12.5 μg/mL, instead of the desired 5 μg/mL, a 250% stronger concentration than desired! Fortunately, this is unlikely to happen, because 0.1 mL cannot be accurately measured in a 10 mL syringe.

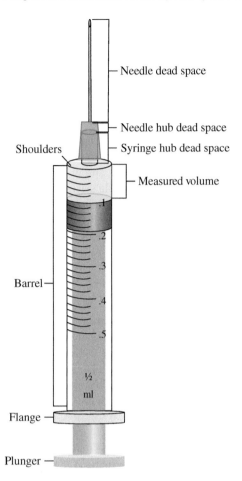

Figure 18.2 "Anatomy" of a syringe and needle.

B. How Should a Dilution Be Prepared?

The steps are illustrated in Figure 18.3. Draw up the drug and the diluent separately in two appropriately sized syringes (A). A 1 mL syringe is advised for volumes < 1.0 mL. When the diluents has been collected to the desired volume (i.e. 9 mL in the 10 mL syringe), leave the needle in place on the diluent syringe, draw air until the diluent is no longer in the hub of the syringe and needle but sits at the shoulders of the syringe (base of the syringe hub) (B). The air will aid in assessing the dead space volume. Read the volume at the base of the syringe (i.e. 9.0 mL of diluent now reads 9.2 mL, indicating there is 0.2 mL of hub dead space). Push the plunger forward and expel the measured hub volume of air (C). What remains in the diluent syringe, hub and needle is the required 9.0 mL. Draw back on the plunger once again to give some room in the syringe for the drug to be added and remove the capped needle. Insert the needle of the concentrated drug syringe into the hub and barrel of the diluent syringe and inject the drug (D), allowing residual drug to remain in the hub/needle. As the measured volume of drug has been added to the measured diluent (E), this is now the desired concentration of drug. Discard the drug syringe and needle, place the capped needle on the diluent syringe, expel the air and mix the contents by inverting several times.

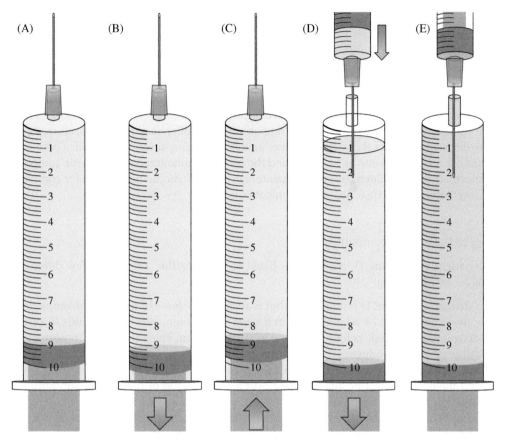

Figure 18.3 The drug dilution method.

VII. Drug Compatibility

As most ill or injured dogs and cats may receive more than one analgesic, and some will also be receiving medication unrelated to analgesia, being aware of compatibility data of all drugs being administered is essential. The compatibility refers to the reaction of two, or more, drugs within the IV tubing, not within the patient. Drug interactions within the patient should be known before prescribing a drug. Drugs contacting each other within the IV tubing can result in a number of reactions that may be physical, chemical or therapeutic in nature, and can alter pharmacokinetics and efficacy. It is, therefore, essential that the compatibility of each drug is known prior to mixing. This also applies to compatibility with fluids (i.e. the pH of fluids may influence drug activity).

Physical incompatibilities often result in a precipitate or hazy appearance, immediately or over a period of time. However, this may not be readily visible with smaller volumes of a drug but may still be occurring. The individual particulates formed may settle out within the IV tubing – furosemide and diazepam readily precipitate. Particulates may be a risk for microvascular pulmonary emboli.

Other physical incompatibilities include colour change or gas formation in the IV line. With any observed physical incompatibility, the infusion must be immediately stopped and the lines must be changed. The patient should be observed closely for negative reaction.

Chemical incompatibilities are those that result in a loss of potency of greater than 10% over a period of time in which they were tested (e.g. Plasma-Lyte A has pH 7.4, which may reduce the activity of lidocaine requiring a pH < 6. Unfortunately, these incompatibilities are not as obvious as physical incompatibilities but may be noted as a lack of response to a medication. Both physical and chemical incompatibilities are often related to the pH of the carrier solution or other admixtures.

Therapeutic incompatibilities are those in which the drug combination results in unexpected synergistic or antagonistic effects of one or all drugs.

There are comprehensive guides to drug compatibility that offer easy-to-use charts covering all IV medications. Each of these offers pocket guides and online resources as well. There are numerous other online resources available, and the product monographs also provide compatibility information. The diluent (often the maintenance fluids) should be checked for compatibility as well. If in doubt, treat drugs as incompatible.

A.   How to Deal with Incompatible Drugs

When a patient is receiving IV medications listed as incompatible, there are a few different methods for administering.

- **Bolus drugs:** If a patient is not on a CRI but is receiving boluses of multiple, incompatible drugs, the drugs should be administered in a staggered fashion, allowing IV fluids to carry each drug into the patient before giving the next medication. Flush the injection port with 0.9% saline prior to introducing the next drug.
- **CRI and incompatible bolus or slow push drugs:** Often, a CRI of one drug is running, and a second medication must be administered over a short period of time (often antibiotics). This situation is managed by:
  - Turning off the CRI during administration of the bolus/slow push drug. This is easiest when using a syringe pump for the CRI, as the syringe pump can be put in standby mode, while the IV fluids are allowed to continue flowing to clear the line, and carry in the bolus or slow push drug; **or**
  - If the CRI is within a burette or IV fluid bag, the pump should be turned off and the line cleared of the CRI drug with a bolus of a few mL of 0.9% saline at the port closest to the patient. The bolus drug can now be administered via this port, followed by a flush with 0.9% saline. The fluids and CRI are then restarted.
  - For slow push drugs (administered over 10 min or more) that need to be given in the same line with a CRI in a bag or burette, the same procedure can be followed as above; clear the line with a small bolus of saline, followed by a small volume of the drug and another small bolus of saline. Repeat this procedure every 2–5 min until the dose is complete. For small volume drugs, consider diluting the drug further into a larger volume prior to administering.
- **Multiple incompatible CRI drugs:** ICU patients may be receiving multiple CRIs at the same time, requiring specialized delivery of the medications:
  - Place a multi-lumen central lines to split the CRI drugs.
  - Place an additional peripheral IV line to split the CRI drugs.
  - Use "double-T" extension sets for incompatible drugs. These extensions divide the line close to the catheter, allowing for a reduced contact time. Note, some drugs will react instantly, and this method may cause the reaction to be unobserved as it may happen in the hub of the catheter. **This is the least desirable option.**

Providing accurate CRI delivery is dependent on many factors. Errors can occur at many phases of preparing a CRI of a drug, including: calculations, dilution errors/inaccurate concentration and improper technique in admixture preparation. It is important to be aware of the potential for error and where best practices can be used to ensure a predictable concentration. While it is unlikely to ever achieve a perfect concentration, guidelines suggest that the final concentration should be within 10% of the expected concentration.

B. Common Drug Incompatibilities

For the purposes of this text, incompatibilities of common analgesics used as a CRI, with other common medications used IV, are listed for your reference. This list is not exhaustive, but focuses only on the most common medications and interactions.

Dexmedetomidine

Compatible	Incompatible
Ampicillin	Diazepam
Butorphanol	Pantoprazole
Cefoxitin	
Fentanyl	
Famotidine	
Hydromorphone	
Lidocaine	
Metoclopramide	
Propofol	
Magnesium sulfate	

Fentanyl

Compatible	Incompatible
Dexmedetomidine	Ampicillin
Famotidine	Enrofloxacin
Furosemide	Pantoprazole
Lidocaine	
Ketamine	
Metoclopramide	
Midazolam	
Ondansetron	
Potassium chloride	
Propofol	

Hydromorphone

Compatible	Incompatible
Ampicillin	Heparin
Cefazolin	Diazepam
Cefoxitin	Pantoprazole
Famotidine	Sodium bicarbonate
Furosemide	

Compatible	Incompatible
Ketamine	
Magnesium sulfate	
Propofol	

Ketamine

Compatible	Incompatible
Cefazolin	Ampicillin
Famotidine	Cefoxitin
Fentanyl	Diazepam
Midazolam	Furosemide
Morphine	Pantoprazole
Propofol	

Lidocaine

Compatible	Incompatible
Dexmedetomidine	Pantoprazole
Famotidine	Propofol
Fentanyl	

Methadone

Compatible	Incompatible
Diazepam	Furosemide
Metoclopramide	
Midazolam	
Pantoprazole Dopamine, Dobutamine Ketamine* Dexmedetomidine* Medetomidine* Lidocaine*	*no compatibility studies; however, these drugs are frequently combined in a CRI in veterinary practice

Morphine

Compatible	Incompatible
Ampicillin	Furosemide
Cefazolin	Pantoprazole
Cefoxitin	
Famotidine	
Ketamine	
Lidocaine	
Midazolam	

Further Reading

Adapa, R. M., Mani, V., Murray, L. J., *et al.* (2012) Errors during the preparation of drug infusions: A randomized controlled trial. *British Journal of Anaesthesia*, 109(5): 729–734.

American Society of Health-System Pharmacists (2014) *Handbook on Injectable Drugs*, 18th edn. American Society of Health-System Pharmacists, Bethesda, MD.

Institute for Safe Medication Practices (2013) *Understanding and Managing IV Container Overfill.* ISMP Medication Safety Alert, http://www.ismp.org/newsletters/acutecare/showarticle. aspx?id=63, accessed 31st July 2017.

King Guide to Parenteral Admixtures (2017) Internet, print, and wall chart editions. Available at https://www.kingguide.com/.

19

Cardiovascular Disease as a Co-Morbidity for Anesthesia and Analgesia of Non-Related Emergencies

Tamara Grubb

The cardiovascular system comprises the heart, the vasculature and the blood/plasma. Dysfunction of any or all of these components can occur in patients with cardiovascular disease or disease that secondarily affects the cardiovascular system (e.g. hyperthyroidism, sepsis, anemia). Unfortunately, anesthetic drugs (e.g. inhalants), perioperative manipulations (e.g. recumbency, positive pressure ventilation) and surgical complications (e.g. uncontrolled pain, hemorrhage) can exacerbate this dysfunction – and can even cause cardiovascular changes that mimic cardiovascular disease. Thus, a fair number of anesthetized patients may need cardiovascular support, even in the absence of cardiovascular disease. Because of the vast number of diseases/conditions that affect the cardiovascular system, one anesthetic protocol may not be appropriate for all patients in this category, but an understanding of cardiovascular physiology and the cardiovascular effects of the anesthetic drugs will promote appropriate anesthetic/analgesic protocol selection. In addition to appropriate dose/drug selection, diligent patient monitoring and support are crucial.

I.   Analgesic Considerations and Drug Choices

Pain causes sympathetic nervous system stimulation that can result in tachycardia, and increased peripheral resistance, arterial blood pressure, cardiac work and cardiac oxygen consumption. These changes are generally well tolerated in patients with a healthy cardiovascular system but are extremely dangerous in a patient with cardiovascular disease, possibly resulting in decompensation and cardiac failure. Therefore, pain must be controlled in patients with cardiovascular disease.

- **Opioid** agonists (e.g. fentanyl, hydromorphone, morphine, methadone), agonist-antagonists (e.g. butorphanol) and partial agonists (buprenorphine) are the analgesics of choice in patients with cardiac disease because they have minimal impact on the cardiovascular system [1], they can be titrated to effect and their effects are reversible in the event that adverse effects occur. A mild vagally mediated bradycardia can occur after the administration of most opioids [2], but the opioids do not tend to cause other arrhythmias [1]. Opioids do not contribute to myocardial depression and are, in fact, considered cardioprotective, meaning that they allow a reduction in the dose of drugs that may cause adverse cardiac effects (e.g. inhalant drugs). Opioids appear to induce pharmacologic preconditioning of the myocardium [1] and tend to decrease afterload. Large dosages of morphine, but not most other

Analgesia and Anesthesia for the Ill or Injured Dog and Cat, First Edition. Karol A. Mathews, Melissa Sinclair, Andrea M. Steele and Tamara Grubb.
© 2018 John Wiley & Sons, Inc. Published 2018 by John Wiley & Sons, Inc.

opioids, delivered by rapid intravenous (IV) bolus can cause histamine release and subsequent hypotension. However, the histamine release is minimal to non-existent when morphine is administered intramuscularly (IM), or very slowly IV using clinically relevant continuous rate infusion (CRI) dosages [3]. Opioid effects can be reversed with naloxone or partially reversed with butorphanol. Rapid reversal of opioid effects will also antagonize analgesia. In humans, rapid IV administration of naloxone has been associated with development of cardiac dysrhythmias and even sudden death [4].Thus, for preservation of analgesia and safety, slowly titrated reversal drug is preferred **if** reversal is necessary. Suggested reversal is naloxone 0.4 mg/mL, 0.1 mL diluted in 5 mL saline for cats and small dogs, 0.25 mL diluted in 10 mL saline for medium and large breed dogs. Titrate at 0.5 mL/min (small animals)-1 mL/min until adverse effects are gone and the patient appears comfortable. This may have to be repeated. If the patient is not comfortable after reversal, add an alternate class of analgesic. The choice of opioid and route of delivery (e.g. bolus, infusion, regional block) should be based primarily on the level of analgesia required but also on the patient's health status and the site/extent of the painful condition or lesion. Frequent assessment of the patient's pain state or intraoperative depth and responses will aid in the determination of the appropriate administration interval. Refer to Chapter 10 for information on dosing, duration of action and selection of opioids.

- **Local/regional anesthetic blockade** can provide fairly profound analgesia with little to no systemic effects and allow a dose reduction of systemically administered analgesic drugs. Local/regional anesthetic blockade should be considered in patients with cardiovascular disease that have lesions that can be desensitized, even if surgery is not imminent. Administration of an opioid, potentially combined with a benzodiazepine, may be required to accomplish the block. In addition, the local anesthetic should be buffered with bicarbonate. **For initial placement in the awake patient** prepare a mixture of 0.5% (5 mg/mL) bupivacaine (0.2 mL/kg = 1 mg/kg) based on ideal body weight in the obese patient, and sodium bicarbonate (1 mEq/mL). Buffering of a 0.5% bupivacaine solution (5 mg/mL) requires a 20:0.1 mixture with sodium bicarbonate 1 mEq/mL (~0.2 mL bupivacaine and 0.001 mL sodium bicarbonate). Warm to body temperature. Overdosage of local anesthetic drugs can cause profound hypotension and even cardiac arrest so, as is always advised, dosages should be calculated carefully and good technique (i.e. aspirate prior to injection of the drug) should be utilized.

- **Ketamine** infusions have not been specifically studied in patients with cardiovascular disease. However, infusions at a dose slightly higher than that used for analgesia did not produce negative cardiovascular effects in healthy human patients [5]. In addition, ketamine infusions have been utilized in human medicine in patients that may have cardiovascular compromise, similar to veterinary patients presented on an emergency basis [6]. Ketamine caused minimal, clinically insignificant hemodynamic changes in sedated, mechanically ventilated children with pulmonary hypertension [7]. However, a low incidence of tachyarrhythmia [8] and both hypotension and hypertension [9] have been reported in human patients receiving ketamine infusions. In veterinary medicine, ketamine infusions administered to endotoxemic dogs did not change cardiovascular status [10]. With appropriate monitoring, the author commonly uses low-dose ketamine infusions for analgesia in dogs and cats with cardiovascular disease.

- **Lidocaine** infusions are commonly used in dogs for analgesia [11] and are used in both cats and dogs for treatment of select arrhythmias, e.g. ventricular tachycardia (VT) [12]. Because of the chance of adverse effects in patients with cardiovascular disease, analgesia provided by opioid and/or ketamine infusions may be preferred for most patients. However, in conscious human patients with "significant myocardial disease", lidocaine doses of a 1.5 mg/kg bolus followed by a CRI infusion of 50 µg/kg/min (3 mg/kg/h) caused no adverse hemodynamic effects [13].

- **Non-steroidal anti-inflammatory analgesics (NSAIAs)** do not negatively impact cardiovascular function and are commonly used in patients with cardiovascular disease. In human medicine, the highly selective cyclooxygenase-2 (COX-2) inhibiting NSAIDs (cox-ibs), especially rofecoxib and valdecoxib were shown to contribute to myocardial infarction (MI) by causing both vasoconstriction and platelet aggregation [14]. This does not appear to be a concern in veterinary medicine, likely due to the fact that MI is uncommon or even non-existent in veterinary species. However, NSAIDs can reduce the efficacy of some medications administered for the control of cardiac disease (e.g. diuretics, ACE inhibitors, beta-blockers) [15]. NSAIDs can cause renal damage, especially in low-flow states [14, 15]. Thus, NSAIDs should not be administered to patients that are hypovolemic or hypotensive. Because some NSAIDs (primarily aspirin) can cause platelet dysfunction and prolonged bleeding times, these select should not be used in patients with bleeding tendencies [15]. However, the anti-clotting effects of aspirin may be used therapeutically in some diseases [16]. Refer to Chapter 11 for further contraindications and drug interactions.
- **Gabapentin** has no known cardiac effects, but dose reduction may be necessary if decreased cardiac output has caused secondary renal or hepatic insufficiency as the drug depends on both organs for elimination, at least in dogs [17, 18]. In other species that have been studied (humans, primates, rats), elimination is primarily via the urine [17, 18]. Although there are no studies in veterinary medicine, gabapentin did not cause or exacerbate cardiovascular adverse events in human patients with cardiovascular disease [19, 20]. In fact, perioperative use of gabapentin has been shown to improve cardiovascular stability in human patients [21, 22] and those with some co-morbidities that impact cardiovascular function, like diabetic peripheral neuropathy [23].
- **Other drugs** may be appropriate but most have not been evaluated in patients with cardiovascular disease.

II. Anesthetic Considerations

The ultimate goal of the cardiovascular system is to work in concert with the respiratory system to provide adequate oxygen delivery to the working cells. On the cardiovascular side, the support of oxygen delivery is dependent on adequate cardiac output. Unfortunately, both cardiac disease and anesthetic drugs can negatively impact cardiac output so the goals of the anesthetist include both alleviation of the impact of the disease (if possible) and careful selection of anesthetic drugs/drug dosages.

A. Patient Preparation

1. Pre-Operative Examination and Laboratory Testing
Of course, a thorough physical exam and history are extremely important, as are a complete blood count (CBC) and serum chemistry analysis, since cardiac disease can cause impairment of other organ systems through decreased perfusion and oxygen delivery. An ECG should be performed in all patients prior to anesthesia, and a thoracic radiograph may be useful in certain diseases. A more thorough cardiac workup including advanced techniques such as cardiac ultrasonographic examination may be necessary in some patients.

2. Stabilization
The **first goal** of the anesthetist is stabilization. Stabilization of **any** patient, especially one with cardiovascular disease, is crucial and can drastically decrease the likelihood of morbidity or mortality during anesthesia. Stabilization can mean immediate stabilization (e.g. pre-operative

judicious administration of IV fluids to maintain appropriate circulating blood volume) or more long-term stabilization (e.g. support of myocardial function through administration of beta- or calcium channel-blockers for days to weeks prior to anesthesia). The goal of stabilization is to return cardiovascular function to as close to normal as possible in order to support oxygen delivery and should include:

- **Normalization of heart rate:** Abnormal heart rate may be due to the disease itself but is often due to underlying causes (pain, hypoxemia, anemia, etc.) so those causes must be identified and treated.
- **Alleviation of arrhythmias:** At best, arrhythmias can contribute to decreased cardiac output and, at worst, they can be fatal.
- **Support of cardiac contractility:** The patient may need inotropic drugs either long-term (e.g. pimobendan) or immediately prior to and/or during anesthesia (e.g. dopamine or dobutamine).
- **Provision of adequate, but not excessive, circulating blood volume through judicious use of crystalloids and/or colloids:** In other words, administer at fluid volume adequate to rehydrate the patient and to replace ongoing losses (e.g. urine production) but not large enough to overload the heart and lungs.
- **Provision of adequate blood volume for oxygen delivery:** Blood transfusions may be more important in patients with cardiovascular disease than in other patients. Decreased cardiac output combined with decreased arterial blood oxygen content (due to a decreased number of red blood cells) can lead to a substantial decrease in tissue oxygen delivery. Transfusions should be considered in dogs with PCV (packed cell volume) < 25% and cats with PCV < 20%, although a PCV of down to 18% in both species may be tolerated if the anemia is chronic.

3. Pre-Medication/Pre-Anesthesia Support

- In order to support oxygen delivery during induction when mild/moderate drug-induced respiratory depression may occur, oxygen should be administered by facemask or flow-by for 3–5 min prior to administering induction drugs ("pre-oxygenate").
- Excitement, struggling and fear cause tachycardia and increased peripheral resistance, arterial blood pressure, cardiac work and cardiac oxygen consumption. These changes are extremely dangerous in a patient with cardiovascular disease, possibly resulting in decompensation and cardiac failure. Pain causes the same sympathetic response as excitement, struggling and fear. Therefore, all of these stressors must be avoided in patients with cardiovascular disease and calm handling, along with the administration of a low dose of a tranquilizer and preemptive analgesic drugs, is crucial.

B. Anesthetic Drugs and Dosing

In addition to the cardiovascular dysfunction caused by the disease itself, most anesthetic drugs cause some degree of cardiovascular dysfunction. The **second goal** of the anesthetist is to choose anesthetic drugs that will have minimal impact on the patient's injury or illness. Furthermore, the cardiovascular effects caused by anesthetic drugs are generally **dose dependent**, and selection of the appropriate dose is even more important than selection of the appropriate drug.

Circulation becomes "centralized" in patients with moderate to severe cardiac disease, resulting in greater delivery of blood, and drugs carried by the blood, to highly perfused tissues, including the brain. However, cardiac output may be decreased in these patients, resulting in **slower** drug delivery to the brain. Thus, the dosage of anesthetic drugs administered to patients with cardiac disease should be decreased and drugs that are administered IV should be administered slowly and with ample time between doses for delivery to the brain.

1. Pre-Medicant Drugs

- As stated in Section I, opioids cause minimal to no adverse cardiovascular effects and allow a decrease in the dose of drugs that do cause adverse cardiovascular effects, such as the inhalant anesthetic drugs. Thus, opioids should be included in all anesthetic protocols for patients with cardiovascular disease, even if pain is not expected. Opioids used alone may not provide adequate sedation in young, healthy patients but are often sufficient for compromised patients, such as those with moderate to severe cardiovascular disease. The choice of opioid should be based on the level of analgesia required, the overall health of the patient and the reason for anesthesia (e.g. non-invasive diagnostics versus surgical procedures).
- If an opioid alone will not/does not provide adequate sedation, midazolam or diazepam should be added to the protocol. Midazolam may be preferred as it can be administered either IV or IM (so less struggling if no catheter in place) and does not cause a sting upon injection. Sedation with a benzodiazepine alone is not recommended since paradoxical excitement can occur, although this is less likely in patients with moderate to severe systemic disease. The benzodiazepines produce minimal cardiovascular effects, although both diazepam and midazolam can cause a small, generally clinically insignificant decrease in systemic blood pressure. Because this effect is primarily mediated by a slight drop in systemic vascular resistance, especially with midazolam, it may actually be beneficial in improving cardiac output [24]. Drug effects can be reversed with the benzodiazepine antagonist flumazenil.
- Acepromazine decreases afterload secondary to alpha-adrenergic blockade with subsequent vasodilation. This may result in increased cardiac output following a low dose (0.01 mg/kg) of acepromazine but could result in hypotension following a higher dose or following any dose in patients already suffering from hypotension. A low dose of acepromazine with an opioid is often an appropriate tranquilizer choice in a patient with increased afterload and/ or hypertrophic cardiomyopathy. Acepromazine can protect against arrhythmias by causing an increase in the dose of epinephrine required to induce ventricular arrhythmias, possibly due to alpha$_1$ blockade [25].
- The alpha$_2$-adrenoceptor agonists (e.g. medetomidine and dexmedetomidine) cause profound vasoconstriction and an increase in cardiac work and are thus not appropriate for patients with cardiovascular disease. There is evidence that administration of medetomidine to cats with dynamic left ventricular outflow obstruction may improve output [26], but this is the exception rather than the rule for using alpha$_2$ agonists in patients with most types of cardiac disease.
- Other pre-medicant drugs: Anticholinergics (e.g. atropine, glycopyrrolate) could be considered for the treatment of bradycardia that adversely impacts cardiac output but **should not be routinely administered**. Anticholinergics increase myocardial oxygen consumption, heart rate and the possibility of certain cardiac arrhythmias while decreasing the threshold for ventricular fibrillation. Patients with cardiovascular disease may not tolerate the increased heart rate and myocardial oxygen consumption, and may be prone to disease-induced arrhythmias.

2. Induction Technique and Drugs

Induction should occur smoothly with rapid intubation and immediate initiation of supplemental oxygen delivery. As previously stated, the circulation becomes centralized, and so lower induction drug dosages should be administered and more time should be allowed for the drug to reach the brain before re-dosing (e.g. propofol should take effect within 10 s in patients with normal cardiac function but can take up to 30 s in patients with decreased myocardial contractility).

Induction Drugs/considerations include:

- Etomidate causes minimal to no change in myocardial contractility, heart rate, stroke volume or cardiac output, making it the drug of choice for most patients with moderate to severe cardiac disease [27]. Etomidate causes adrenocortical suppression, but the clinical relevance of this is controversial and unlikely to have an impact in most patients following an induction bolus of the drug. Etomidate should never be used without adequate pre-anesthetic sedation as it commonly causes muscle rigidity, muscle twitching and vocalization in unsedated patients.

- Ketamine and tiletamine increase heart rate, afterload, cardiac output and arterial blood pressure through stimulation of the sympathetic nervous system [28]. In patients with no sympathetic reserve, as may occur in end-stage cardiac disease, ketamine and tiletamine cause direct myocardial depression [28]. In patients with more moderate disease, the cardiac effects can be detrimental or beneficial, depending on the disease. The effects may be detrimental in patients with hypertrophic disease, hypertension or tachycardia but could be beneficial in patients with decreased cardiac contractility (e.g. dilated cardiomyopathy), hypotension or bradycardia. The increase in heart rate and contractility could increase myocardial oxygen consumption and could precipitate myocardial ischemia [28]. However, both the positive and negative effects of ketamine and tiletamine are attenuated by the concurrent or prior administration of tranquilizers (e.g. benzodiazepines, acepromazine) [29]. Tiletamine is commercially available only in combination with a benzodiazepine (zolazepam) but the long duration of action of this combination can cause delayed recovery, which may not be ideal in compromised patients that require intensive support.

- Propofol causes dose-dependent myocardial depression and hypotension but the effect is brief and is attenuated by the concurrent or prior administration of benzodiazepines [30]. Propofol can be dosed "to effect", thereby decreasing the likelihood of overdosing. Propofol is rapidly cleared from the body, which minimizes the duration of anesthesia-induced physiological depression.

- Alfaxalone has not been studied extensively in patients with cardiovascular disease, but current evidence suggests that the cardiovascular depressive effects are similar to those caused by propofol [31].

- The barbiturates cause moderate to profound dose-dependent cardiovascular depression, making them a poor choice for patients with cardiovascular disease.

- High dosages of inhalant gases should be avoided in patients with cardiovascular disease since the gases cause a moderate to profound dose-dependent decrease in arterial blood pressure that is primarily caused by systemic vasodilation with contribution from decreased cardiac contractility [28]. Induction to anesthesia by mask or chamber is often accompanied by stress and struggling with subsequent tachycardia and increased oxygen consumption. The use of inhalant gases alone to induce and maintain anesthesia increases the risk of anesthesia-related mortality [32]. These factors make mask or chamber induction with inhalant gases inappropriate for patients with cardiovascular disease.

3. Anesthetic Maintenance Drugs and Techniques

- **Inhalant anesthetic gases,** as part of a balanced anesthetic protocol with appropriate sedatives and induction drugs, are the drugs of choice for maintenance of anesthesia. Analgesic drugs should be used in order to allow low dosages of inhalants. In humans, sevoflurane may be less likely than isoflurane or desflurane to cause tachycardia and may be preferable in patients prone to myocardial ischemia [28].

- **Monitoring:** Diligent monitoring and patient support are imperative for successful anesthetic outcome. Excessive anesthetic depth is one of the main contributors to cardiovascular dysfunction. Thus, the patient should be constantly evaluated for appropriate anesthetic depth and anesthetic drugs should be delivered to effect. Blood pressure **must be monitored** along with ECG, SPO$_2$ and ETCO$_2$. Pulse oximetery (SpO$_2$) can create a false sense of security in anemic patients as oxygen delivery can be inadequate even with a normal SpO$_2$ since fewer red blood cells are available to carry oxygen. An abnormally low ETCO$_2$ can be due to poor perfusion and a sudden decrease in ETCO$_2$ can be predictive of cardiac arrest.

- **Support:** In order to maximize oxygen delivery, support of the anesthetized patient includes support of both the cardiovascular **and** respiratory systems.
- **Blood pressure** should be maintained with a mean arterial blood pressure (MAP) > 60 mmHg and a systolic arterial pressure (SAP) > 90 mmHg.
  - ○ A judicious dose of IV crystalloids (2–5 mL/kg/h for the first hour; half that dose for every hour after the first hour – unless the patient is experiencing major fluid loss, in which case the fluid rate will need to be increased) should be administered to correct any dehydration and to replace ongoing fluid losses (e.g. urine production, evaporation from the airway). However, excessive fluid administration must be avoided as fluid overload can exacerbate cardiovascular dysfunction. Furthermore, IV fluids delivered to treat hypotension will not resolve the hypotension if cardiac contractility (as opposed to hypovolemia) is the problem.
  - ○ If hypotension persists after an initial crystalloid fluid bolus, a bolus of colloids (1–2 mL/kg) can be considered, but colloids can also cause volume overload so must be used carefully. Colloid use is controversial with co-existent renal dysfunction in the septic patient.
  - ○ Correction of hypotension will likely require the use of positive inotropic drugs like dopamine or dobutamine. In fact, if impaired cardiac contractility is known or presumed, start delivery of the positive inotropic drug as soon as hypotension is identified. As stated in the introduction, some patients that are presumably cardiovascularly healthy prior to anesthesia may require positive inotropic drugs for support of normal blood pressure, likely due to the negative inotropic effects of the inhalant anesthetic drugs. If decreasing the inhalant anesthetic dose and administering a bolus of crystalloids and/or colloids does not improve blood pressure, assume contractility is the problem and start an infusion of dopamine (1–15 μg/kg/min) or dobutamine (1–10 μg/kg/min).
  - ○ The last step in treatment of hypotension is the use of vasopressors, e.g. norepinephrine (0.1–0.5 μg/kg/min) or vasopressin (0.8 units/kg, once). This is a tricky step since vasoconstriction increases cardiac work so the need for improved blood pressure must be carefully weighed against the negative impact on myocardial function. Fortunately, this step is not often necessary except in select patients (e.g. patients with extreme vasodilation, such as those in shock).
- **Support of the respiratory system** should include provision of supplemental oxygen in all patients anesthetized or moderately/deeply sedated. Support of adequate gas exchange through maintenance of adequate respiratory rate and/or tidal volume using assisted ventilation may be necessary.
- Finally, **the patient should be kept warm** as hypothermia can further contribute to cardiac dysfunction and can cause VT and coagulation abnormalities [33]. Shivering can increase oxygen consumption by up to 200%.

4. Recovery from Anesthesia

Patient observation, support and monitoring **must** continue well into the recovery period. Oxygen and fluids may be necessary, active warming should be included and all appropriate drugs should be continued (e.g. dopamine, anti-arrhythmic drugs) Analgesia should be re-addressed. If the patient experiences excitement or fear, a low dose of a sedative drug should be administered.

Box 19.1 Example anesthetic plan for dogs and cats with cardiovascular disease

Patient with Mild to Moderate Cardiovascular Disease

Patient Preparation
- Stabilize to the greatest extent possible.
- Place monitors (ECG and blood pressure) on patient prior to induction.
- Pre-oxygenate using mask or flow-by oxygen.

Pre-Medication: Drugs and Dosages
- **Pre-medication** with an opioid plus a sedative for most patients. Drug dosages are at the low end or slightly lower than those used for healthy patients.
- Choose an **opioid**. The pure μ-agonist drugs are preferred vs. butorphanol or buprenorphine for surgical procedures but the latter two drugs may be appropriate for procedures that cause only mild pain (some diagnostics) and/or for augmentation of sedation. These drugs can be administered IV or IM. In general, use the low end of the dose for IV administration.
  - o **Methadone** 0.3–0.5 mg/kg, **or**
  - o **Oxymorphone** 0.05–0.1 mg/kg, **or**
  - o **Hydromorphone** 0.1 mg/kg, **or**
  - o **Fentanyl IV** 2–5 µg/kg.
- Add a **sedative** if necessary – likely necessary in patients that are fairly healthy. Weigh the expected adverse effects of the sedative with the fact that the sedative will allow a decrease in induction and maintenance drug dosages. Adverse effects of anesthetic drugs (as with most drugs) are largely dose-dependent.
  - o Midazolam (can be administered IM or IV), diazepam (**IV only**).
    - ▪ May cause paradoxical excitement in healthy patients.
  - o Acepromazine (**in select patients**) 0.01 mg/kg IM or IV.
  - o Alfaxalone can be administered IM to cats or really small dogs at 0.5 mg/kg IM. Higher dosages = induction. Remember that alfaxalone does cause some cardiovascular depression.

Induction
- Any of the induction drugs are acceptable. Start at the low end of the dose and titrate carefully to effect. If the patient isn't adequately sedated, 0.1–0.2 mg/kg midazolam or diazepam can be administered immediately prior to, or concurrent with, the induction drug.
- Etomidate: 1–3 mg/kg.
  - o Ideal for patients with severe cardiovascular disease but not required for those with mild to moderate disease.
- Propofol: Initial bolus 1–3 mg/kg, IV then to effect.
  - o Although brief cardiovascular effects may occur, these are minimized by pre-medications and by titrating to effect.
- Alfaxalone: Initial bolus 1–2 mg/kg, IV, then to effect.
  - o Although brief cardiovascular effects may occur, these are minimized by pre-medications and by titrating to effect.
- Ketamine: 3–5 mg/kg, IV.
  - o Not ideal for patients with tachyarrhythmias.
- **Do not mask induce:** The inhalant dose for induction is higher than that for maintenance and will cause hypotension.

(Continued)

Box 19.1 (Continued)

Maintenance
- Isoflurane, sevoflurane or desflurane.
  - ○ **Carefully titrate the dose to effect**; expect to use the low end of the dose range.
  - ○ Add analgesia to support low dosing of inhalant. Opioid boluses or infusions and local anesthetic blocks are ideal.
- Monitor and support.

Recovery
- Keep patient pain-free, warm and quiet.
- Continue monitoring and support as needed.

Patient with Severe Cardiovascular Disease

- Patient preparation
  - ○ **Stabilize.** Unstable patients with severe cardiovascular disease should not be anesthetized unless anesthesia is required to save the patient's life (e.g. a patient with profound intra-abdominal hemorrhage).
  - ○ Place monitors (ECG and blood pressure) on patient prior to induction and ensure that physiologic parameters are as close to normal as possible prior to induction.
  - ○ Pre-oxygenate using a mask or flow-by oxygen.
- Pre-medication: Drugs and dosages
  - ○ An opioid alone is generally sufficient pre-medication for patients with severe cardiovascular disease.
  - ○ The patient should have an IV catheter in place and the opioid can be administered IV a few (2–5) minutes prior to administration of the induction drug.
  - ○ Drug dosages are at the low end or slightly lower than those used for healthy patients. One recommendation is to **start with half of the dose** for a healthy patient.
  - ○ The pure μ-agonist drugs are preferred vs. butorphanol or buprenorphine for surgical procedures, but the latter two drugs may be appropriate for procedures that cause only mild pain (some diagnostics) and/or for augmentation of sedation. These drugs can be administered IV or IM. In general, use the low end of the dose for IV administration.
    - ▪ **Methadone** 0.1–0.3 mg/kg, **or**
    - ▪ **Oxymorphone** 0.05–0.1 mg/kg, **or**
    - ▪ **Hydromorphone** 0.05–0.1 mg/kg, **or**
    - ▪ **Fentanyl IV** 1–2 (up to 5 if titrated carefully) μg/kg.
- Induction
  - ○ Administer **low** end of the dose and at a **slow** rate. Cardiac output is decreased, so drug delivery to the brain is slowed.
  - ○ Etomidate 0.5–1.0 (up to 3.0 but titrate carefully) mg/kg.
    - ▪ Ideal for patients with severe cardiovascular disease.
    - ▪ If patient is not sedate from the opioid, administer 0.1–0.2 mg/kg midazolam immediately prior to administering the etomidate.
  - ○ **Low-dose** propofol and alfaxalone can also be used (i.e. half the dose listed for patients with mild to moderate disease).

- o **Do not mask induce:** The inhalant dose for induction is higher than that for maintenance and will cause hypotension.
- Maintenance
  - o Isoflurane, sevoflurane or desflurane.
    - **Carefully titrate the dose to effect**; expect to use the low end of the dose range.
    - Administer a fentanyl or other opioid CRI in order to keep inhalant dosages as low as possible.
    - Add other analgesia as needed. Local anesthetic blocks are ideal.
  - o Monitor and support.
- Recovery
  - o Keep patient pain-free, warm and quiet.
  - o Continue support and monitoring.

References

1 Bovill, J. G. (2006) Intravenous anesthesia for the patient with left ventricular dysfunction. *Semin Cardiothorac Vasc Anesth*, 10(1): 43–48.

2 Gutstein, H. B. and Akil, H. (2001) Opioid analgesics. In: Hardman, J. G. and Limbird, L. E. (eds), *Goodman & Gilman's The Pharmacologic Basis of Therapeutics*, 10th edn. McGraw-Hill, New York: 569–620.

3 Guedes, A. G., Rudé, E. P. and Rider, M. A. (2006) Evaluation of histamine release during constant rate infusion of morphine in dogs. *Vet Anaesth Analg*, 33(1): 28–35.

4 Pallasch, T. J. and Gill, C. J. (1981) Naloxone-associated morbidity and mortality. *Oral Surg Oral Med Oral Pathol*, 52(6): 602–603.

5 Miller, A. C., Jamin, C T. and Elamin, E. M. (2011) Continuous intravenous infusion of ketamine for maintenance sedation. *Minerva Anestesiol*, 77(8): 812–820.

6 Ahern, T. L., Herring, A. A., Miller, S., *et al.* (2015) Low-dose ketamine infusion for emergency department patients with severe pain. *Pain Med*, 16(7): 1402–1409.

7 Friesen, R. H., Twite, M. D., Nichols, C. S., *et al.* (2016) Hemodynamic response to ketamine in children with pulmonary hypertension. *Paediatr Anaesth*, 26(1): 102–108.

8 Umunna, B. P., Tekwani, K., Barounis, D., *et al.* (2015) Ketamine for continuous sedation of mechanically ventilated patients. *J Emerg Trauma Shock*, 8(1): 11–15.

9 Kator, S., Correll, D. J., Ou, J. Y., *et al.* (2016) Assessment of low-dose IV ketamine infusions for adjunctive analgesia. *Am J Health Syst Pharm*, 73(5 suppl. 1): S22–S29.

10 DeClue, A. E., Cohn, L. A., Lechner, E. S., *et al.* (2008) Effects of subanesthetic doses of ketamine on hemodynamic and immunologic variables in dogs with experimentally induced endotoxemia. *Am J Vet Res*, 69(2): 228–232.

11 Ortega, M. and Cruz, I. (2011) Evaluation of a constant rate infusion of lidocaine for balanced anesthesia in dogs undergoing surgery. *Can Vet J*, 52(8): 856–860.

12 DeFrancesco, T. C. (2013) Management of cardiac emergencies in small animals. *Vet Clin North Am Small Anim Pract*, 43(4): 817–842.

13 Grossman, J. I., Cooper, J. A. and Frieden, J. (1969) Cardiovascular effects of infusion of lidocaine on patients with heart disease. *Am J Cardiol*, 24(2): 191–197.

14 Papich, M. G. (2008) An update on nonsteroidal anti-inflammatory drugs (NSAIDs) in small animals. *Vet Clin North Am Small Anim Pract*, 38(6): 1243–1266.

15 Gwaltney-Brant, S. M. and Talcott, P. A. (2013) Nonsteroidal antiinflammatories. In: Peterson, M. E. and Talcott, P. A. (eds), *Small Animal Toxicology*, 3rd edn. Saunders/Elsevier, Philadelphia: 687–708.

16 Smith, S. A. (2012) Antithrombotic therapy. *Top Companion Anim Med*, 27(2): 88–94.

17 Radulovic, L. L., Türck, D., von Hodenberg, A., *et al.* (1995) Disposition of gabapentin (neurontin) in mice, rats, dogs, and monkeys. *Drug Metab Dispos*, 23(4): 441–448.

18 Vollmer, K. O., von Hodenberg, A. and Kölle, E. U. (1986) Pharmacokinetics and metabolism of gabapentin in rat, dog and man. *Arzneimittelforschung*, 36(5): 830–839.

19 Ucak, A., Onan, B. and Sen, H. (2011) The effects of gabapentin on acute and chronic postoperative pain after coronary artery bypass graft surgery. *J Cardiothorac Vasc Anesth*, 25(5): 824–829.

20 Menda, F., Köner, O., Sayın, M., *et al.* (2010) Effects of single-dose gabapentin on postoperative pain and morphine consumption after cardiac surgery. *J Cardiothorac Vasc Anesth*, 24(5): 808–813.

21 Neogi, M., Basak, S., Ghosh, D., *et al.* (2012) A randomized double-blind placebo-controlled clinical study on the effects of gabapentin premedication on hemodynamic stability during laparoscopic cholecystectomy. *J Anaesthesiol Clin Pharmacol*, 28(4): 456–459.

22 Misra, S., Koshy, T., Unnikrishnan, K. P., *et al.* (2011) Gabapentin premedication decreases the hemodynamic response to skull pin insertion in patients undergoing craniotomy. *J Neurosurg Anesthesiol*, 23(2): 110–117.

23 Ermis, N., Gullu, H., Caliskan, M., *et al.* (2010) Gabapentin therapy improves heart rate variability in diabetic patients with peripheral neuropathy. *J Diabetes Complications*, 24(4): 229–233.

24 Stoelting, R. K. (2006) Benzodiazepines. In: Stoelting, R. K. (ed.), *Pharmacology and Physiology in Anesthetic Practice*, 4th edn. Williams & Wilkins, Philadelphia: 140–154.

25 Lemke, K. A. (2007) Anticholinergics and sedatives. In: Tranquilli, W. J., Thurmon, J. C. and Grimm, K. A. (eds), *Lumb & Jones Veterinary Anesthesia and Analgesia*, 4th edn. Blackwell Publishing, Ames, IA: 203–239.

26 Lamont, L. A., Bulmer, B. J., Sisson, D. D., *et al.* (2002) Doppler echocardiographic effects of medetomidine on dynamic left ventricular outflow tract obstruction in cats. *J Am Vet Med Assoc*, 221(9): 1276–1281.

27 Darrouj, J., Karma, L. and Arora, R. (2009) Cardiovascular manifestations of sedatives and analgesics in the critical care unit. *Am J Ther*, 16(4): 339–353.

28 Evers, A. S. and Crowder, C. M. (2001) General anesthetics. In: Hardman, J. G. and Limbird, L. E. (eds), *Goodman & Gilman's The Pharmacologic Basis of Therapeutics*, 10th edn. McGraw-Hill, New York: 337–366.

29 Jacobson, J. D. and Hartsfield, S. M. (1993) Cardiorespiratory effects of intravenous bolus administration and infusion of ketamine-midazolam in dogs. *Am J Vet Res*, 54(10): 1710–1714.

30 Short, C. E. and Bufalari, A. (1999) Propofol anesthesia. *Vet Clin North Am Small Anim Pract*, 29(3): 747–778.

31 Chiu, K. W., Robson, S., Devi, J. L., *et al.* (2016) The cardiopulmonary effects and quality of anesthesia after induction with alfaxalone in 2-hydroxypropyl-β-cyclodextrin in dogs and cats: A systematic review. *J Vet Pharmacol Ther*, 39(6): 525–538.

32 Brodbelt, D. C., Blissitt, K. J., Hammond, R. A., *et al.* (2008) The risk of death: The confidential enquiry into perioperative small animal fatalities. *Vet Anaesth Analg*, 35(5): 365–373.

33 Leslie, K. and Sessler, D. I. (2003) Perioperative hypothermia in the high-risk surgical patient. *Best Pract Res Clin Anaesthesiol*, 17(4): 485–498.

20

Kidney Disease as a Co-Morbidity for Anesthesia and Analgesia of Non-Related Emergencies

Melissa Sinclair

Mild, moderate to very significant renal disease may exist in a patient requiring anesthesia and analgesia for surgery of a traumatic injury or medical management of a critical disease. The kidneys play an important role in fluid, electrolyte, acid-base regulation, solute waste removal, hormone secretion and clearance of drugs.

The severity of kidney disease may range from asymptomatic, in a seemingly normal patient, to a severely critical and debilitated animal. In cats and dogs, chronic kidney disease (CKD) is commonly diagnosed and is likely present in many patients requiring anesthetic and analgesic management. In cats, CKD is approximately two to three times more prevalent than in dogs, especially in the geriatric feline population. Older reviews have estimated CKD to be prevalent in 15–20% of geriatric dogs and cats [1]. Considering this prevalence, veterinary awareness of the main renal physiological considerations and common abnormalities with optimal anesthetic and analgesic protocols are important to prevent further renal failure and minimize the impact during anesthesia.

Patients with renal disease require pre-operative assessment and stabilization prior to anesthetic management in non-emergency situations. In emergency anesthetic situations, time should be taken to stabilize the condition of the patient as much as possible. In animals with renal disease special attention, and assessment, of the following is critical: low-circulating volume, blood pressure, hyperkalemia or hypokalemia, metabolic acidosis, anemia and the impact of various analgesics and anesthetics on kidney function as well as the effect of renal disease on the pharmacokinetic handling of drugs. Regardless, renal insufficiency suggests a reduced functional renal mass, renal blood flow (RBF) and glomerular filtration rate (GFR). The early stage of renal disease likely goes underdiagnosed as elevations in blood urea nitrogen (BUN) and creatinine only occur when renal function is reduced by 50–70%. Once BUN and creatinine are increased, significant renal damage is already present. Using guidelines from the International Renal Interest Society (IRIS), and correlations with symmetrical dimethylarginine (SDMA) testing, an earlier indication and staging of renal insufficiency or CKD can be made, which will aid in selecting the analgesic and anesthetic protocols wisely. A balanced anesthetic and analgesic approach is imperative to minimize cardiovascular depression and to ensure optimal circulation, blood flow and oxygen delivery are maintained to the kidney to limit further nephron damage.

This chapter gives a general outline of the specific findings in cats and dogs with kidney co-morbidities and their impact on anesthetic and analgesic administration. Anesthetic and analgesic considerations for the urinary bladder and urethra are detailed in Chapter 30.

Analgesia and Anesthesia for the Ill or Injured Dog and Cat, First Edition. Karol A. Mathews, Melissa Sinclair, Andrea M. Steele and Tamara Grubb.
© 2018 John Wiley & Sons, Inc. Published 2018 by John Wiley & Sons, Inc.

I. Analgesia Considerations for Patients with Kidney Disease

- **Opioids** are the analgesics of choice for patients with kidney disease because they can be titrated to effect, are cardiovascularly sparing, do not rely on renal function for metabolism and are reversible. Upon initial presentation, a μ-agonist opioid should be administered to a patient with an injury, whilst determining the patient's overall cardiovascular and volume status. The choice of opioid should be based on the patient's health status and level of analgesia required. The initial dose of an opioid does not necessarily need to be reduced if kidney disease is present. The appropriate analgesic dose can be determined by titration to effect; however, the duration between single dose administration may need to be increased in severely debilitated patients suffering from other co-morbidities, i.e. liver or cranial diseases/injury. Frequent assessment of the patient's pain state, or intraoperative depth and responses, will aid in the determination of the appropriate administration interval. Morphine given as a bolus intravenously (IV) may precipitate plasma histamine release, resulting in a decreased arterial blood pressure and potentially reduced renal blood flow if dramatic, and compounded by the presence of a hypovolemic or hypotensive state. However, slow IV administration with monitoring does not preclude its use in these patients if it is the only opioid available. Meperidine should not be administered IV. Refer to Chapter 10 for further information on dosing, duration of action and selection of opioid.

- **Alpha₂ adrenoceptor agonists** are excellent analgesics but also have profound cardiovascular effects that may impact renal perfusion and natriuresis. Renal vascular resistance in dogs is increased by both alpha$_1$ and alpha$_2$ adrenoceptor subtype agonists but alpha$_1$ agonists are more potent [2]. Hence, both new alpha$_2$ agonists such as dexmedetomidine (alpha$_2$ adrenoceptor subtype selective) and older alpha$_2$ agonists such as xylazine (alpha$_1$ adrenoceptor subtype selective) may both reduce renal blood flow in dogs. Comparative studies are not available in cats.

  Activation of alpha$_2$ adrenoceptors on pancreatic beta cells inhibits the release of insulin with subsequent increase in serum glucose and urine production, with a decrease in urine-specific gravity [3, 4]. Alpha$_2$ adrenoceptor agonists also reduce the release of vasopressin (antidiuretic hormone) and its actions, which decreases medullary interstitial osmolality and reduces passive Na^+ reabsorption, which increases the production of dilute urine.

  Administration of IV medetomidine (20 or 40 μg/kg) versus IM (80 μg/kg) resulted in an increase in mean arterial blood pressure after IV administration for 5–15 min, but not intramuscular (IM), administration, which was followed by a decrease in blood pressure in both groups from baseline for approximately 90–120 min. This was more profound after IM injection. Renal blood flow (RBF) and GFR increased after IV injection and decreased after IM injection [4], and although the route of administration may be responsible for these differences, the difference in dose has to be considered, especially in a sick patient.

  Dexmedetomidine undergoes almost complete biotransformation through direct glucuronidation and cytochrome P450 metabolism and very little excretion of unchanged molecules in the urine or feces, but metabolites are almost completely (95%) excreted in the urine, although they probably do not possess any intrinsic activity. In patients with renal related diseases, the alpha$_2$ agonists may be administered; however, they should be avoided in hypovolemic patients and patients with urinary tract obstruction, due to the diuretic effect, with further volume loss and increased bladder size, respectively.

- **Ketamine** can be used at subanesthetic doses to provide analgesia. In dogs, 62% of ketamine is biotransformed [5] via N-demethylation or hydroxylation and glucuronidation via cytochrome P450 metabolism to metabolites (norketamine) that have reduced activity (<20%) and inactive metabolites, all excreted in the urine in dogs [6], whereas in cats only norketamine results from biotransformation [7]. In cases of CKD, the effects of ketamine may be more prolonged through delayed renal excretion of active metabolites or unchanged drug. This effect can be more pronounced in the cat due to greater reliance on renal clearance of the active drug norketamine.

- **Lidocaine** IV 1–2 mg/kg followed by this as an hourly continuous rate infusion (CRI; ~25–30 μg/kg/min) in an awake patient – **dogs only**; can be added to a multi-modal regimen utilizing the above analgesics where pain scores are > 7 (refer to Chapter 8) or a reduction in opioid dosing is required. Under general inhalant anesthesia, higher doses, 3–7 mg/kg/h CRI (~50–120 μg /kg/min) may be used in dogs to allow for minimum alveolar concentration (MAC) sparing properties and a balanced analgesic approach to reduce inhalant levels and thus cardiovascular depression. Refer to Chapter 12 for lidocaine administration in cats.

- **Non-steroidal anti-inflammatory analgesics (NSAIAs)** should be avoided in patients with acute or chronic kidney disease/injury. Suppression of leukotrienes and prostaglandins, which control renal blood flow autoregulation, with any NSAIA, will exacerbate kidney injury through reduced renal blood flow.

- **Gabapentin** has a high renal elimination with up to 65% being eliminated unchanged in the urine. This can result in higher than expected plasma concentrations in patients with acute kidney injury (AKI) and CKD. Dose reductions are recommended to avoid toxicity [8].

- **Amantadine** has minimal hepatic elimination and is excreted largely unchanged in the urine. This potentially increases the likelihood for toxicity in patients with kidney disease due to decreased elimination and drug accumulation [9].

- **Amitriptyline** undergoes extensive hepatic metabolism and is biotransformed to its active metabolite nortriptyline. Patients with CKD have decreased concentrations of amitriptyline, nortriptyline and their unconjugated hydroxymetabolites, all of which are active metabolites, compared to patients with normal kidney function. This reduction may decrease the clinical effectiveness of the drug [10]. However, the reasoning for this and clinical significance is unclear. Amitriptyline is not renally excreted and can be used at recommended doses in patients with kidney disease.

II. Anesthetic Considerations for Patients with Kidney Disease/Injury

Patients requiring anesthesia with mild to moderate kidney disease are commonly anesthetized by the veterinary practitioner. In most cases, patients are not presenting with acute kidney injury/failure (AKI/F) but with various degrees of CKD. Clinical signs of AKI/F are severe and non-specific such as lethargy, depression, anorexia, vomiting, diarrhea and dehydration, with more specific renal clues of enlarged or swollen kidneys, hemoconcentration, metabolic acidosis, normal body condition and urinary casts or sediment. Animals with CKD may have a similar level of azotemia as the patient with AKI/F but may be more likely to be anemic, dehydrated, polyuric/polydipsic (PU/PD), have smaller than normal kidneys and in poor body condition. More commonly, anesthesia is required for animals with CKD due to a traumatic injury or surgery than in animals with AKI/F. Heavy sedation or anesthesia for the patient with AKI/F may be necessary to obtain renal biopsies, radiographs, diagnostic imaging or renal angiography, versus emergency surgery.

With either CKD or AKI/F, the anesthetic goals are to prevent further kidney damage and progression of the disease by preventing hypotension and ensuring adequate oxygen delivery and renal blood flow. Ideally, only anesthetics that do not rely on the kidney for metabolism or excretion of active metabolites, and are not nephrotoxic, should be used. A specific anesthetic or analgesic "recipe" for use in cats and dogs with CKD or AKI/F does not exist, as concurrent co-morbidities – such as electrolyte disturbances, cardiac or endocrine abnormalities – are frequently present in this patient population. High doses of a sole anesthetic agent, or combinations that result in hypotension and dramatic decreases in cardiac output, should be avoided. A balanced anesthetic approach to provide analgesia, prevent sympatho-adrenal responses and maintain normal blood pressure and cardiac output intraoperatively, thereby supporting renal blood flow, is imperative.

Key aspects of pre-operative and anesthetic management are outlined below. A full review of renal function testing is beyond the scope of this chapter; however, specific parameters are highlighted. For specific details of management and renal function testing in patients with AKI/F or CKD, additional reading is suggested [11].

A. Pre-Operative Examination and Laboratory Testing prior to Anesthesia

A thorough history, physical examination with attention to hydration status, pre-operative fluid therapy, laboratory evaluation (complete blood count, serum biochemistry and urinalysis) with attention to renal values, acid-base status and electrolytes are important. A baseline arterial blood pressure should be obtained prior to anesthesia and considered in light of the overall pain state, additional co-morbidities and hydration status of the patient.

- CKD and AKI patients are azotemic with elevations in serum creatinine. Based on the CKD staging, they may, or may not, have normal renal concentrating ability or proteinuria prior to anesthesia. Every effort should be made with fluid therapy to correct dehydration and improve the azotemia and potentially hyperkalemia, which can cause bradyarrhythmia and increase myocardial sensitivity to anesthetics.

  Staging CKD involves BUN, creatinine and SDMA evaluation. In a non-azotemic animal, a persistent increase in SDMA of > 14 μg/dL suggests a reduced renal function in a dog with creatinine values of < 124 mmol/L (1.4 mg/dL) or a cat 144 mmol/L (1.6 mg/dL) and is considered IRIS CKD stage 1. In these patients, attention to anesthetic management and monitoring is also critical to prevent the progression to CKD stage 2–4.
- As renal function deteriorates, there is a reduction in the ability of the kidney to secrete hydrogen ions and reabsorb bicarbonate ions resulting in a metabolic acidosis. This metabolic acidosis exacerbates muscle wasting, and azotemia. With muscle wasting, the patient is likely to require ventilatory support, especially with prolonged procedures. The acidemia will also decrease the plasma protein binding of drugs, resulting in an increase in free active drug concentrations. Titration of anesthetics to effect will be important to prevent relative overdosages and minimize the clinical impact of protein binding.
- Patients with CKD may have a non-regenerative anemia, as the kidney is the source of erythropoietin. The exact optimal value of the packed cell volume (PCV) in these patients will depend on the chronicity of the anemia, hydration status, procedure or surgery planned with duration, as well as other co-morbidities of the animal. A **general guideline** is that packed red cell transfusions are indicated for surgical procedures or prolonged anesthesia when the PCV is < 25%.

B. Specific Anesthetic Considerations

1. Hydration, Fluid Therapy and Pre-Operative Fasting

Hypovolemia and dehydration should be corrected prior to general anesthesia. The presence and level of anemia may necessitate blood product administration. Cats and dogs can be fasted for 6–8 h. However, water should be available for the patient up until pre-medication. Fluid rates of 5–10 mL/kg/h of lactated Ringer's solution or Plasma-Lyte fluids are appropriate. Rates should be adjusted if the patient is anuric, as fluid overload is common.

2.   Renal Blood Flow with Anesthesia and Surgery

The kidney receives 25% of the total cardiac output. This level of cardiac output is required to support the high metabolic oxygen demands and functions of the kidney and to maintain renal blood flow. The kidneys are susceptible to the effects of a reduced renal blood flow under general anesthesia and can be trended by measuring blood pressure. Treatment of hypotension (MAP < 60–80 mmHg) to prevent a reduced blood flow or ischemia to the kidney is important.

Anesthetic agents can reduce renal blood flow and GFR in a dose-related fashion with the largest decrease in GFR associated with inhalant use. No anesthetic is safer than the other. A reduction in anesthetic time is always important, but it is especially critical in patients with significant renal insufficiency.

3.   Sedative and Anesthetic Considerations

- **Opioid** (see Box 20.1) pre-medication on its own is likely sufficient for sedation and preemptive analgesia in this patient population with evidence of CKD or AKI. The choice of opioid should be based on the patient's status, level of analgesia required and planned duration of surgery. The main advantages of opioids in patients with kidney disease are that they have minimal to no negative cardiovascular effects; confer sedation, analgesia and MAC reduction; do not rely on the kidney for metabolism; and are reversible with naloxone. If warranted, an anticholinergic such as atropine (0.02–0.04 mg/kg, SC or IM) or glycopyrrolate (0.005–0.01 mg/kg, SC or IM) may be used to prevent opioid-induced bradycardia.
- The decision to administer **acepromazine** in these patients should be made on a case-by-case basis related to their personality, pre-operative status and stage of CKD. With significant CKD, and AKI, high doses of acepromazine (>0.05 mg/kg) could additively reduce arterial blood pressure with the induction agents and inhalants. Acepromazine will reduce arterial blood pressure with alpha$_1$ antagonism, and these vasodilatory effects may be beneficial in patients with renal disease because, despite a lower arterial blood pressure, it does not affect GFR [12]. In a research study, acepromazine 0.03 mg/kg administered to dogs did not prevent the low-dose dopamine-mediated receptor effects of vasodilation [13]. The anxiolysis and sedation from acepromazine at doses of 0.01–0.03 mg/kg may be beneficial for sympatholysis pre-operatively in cases not sedated sufficiently from the opioid alone. In critical patients with CKD/AKI and other significant co-morbidities, small doses (<0.02 mg/kg, IV or IM) should be reserved for potential administration post-operatively, in the recovery or ICU setting, for further sedation or relief of dysphoria if required
- **Benzodiazepines** are typically recommended for ill or injured patients, including patients with CKD. They have the advantage of minimal negative cardiovascular effects when used as a sedative agent for pre-medication, and can be used during induction for co-induction. The main disadvantages of benzodiazepines are that they may not provide effective sedation in anxious patients and they are not analgesic. Benzodiazepines should be avoided where liver disease is a co-morbidity and the reversal agent flumazenil is not available.
- **Alpha$_2$ adrenoceptor agonist** use, like dexmedetomidine, in animals with CKD/AKI should be considered carefully based on the individual animal's condition, personality and procedure. Their dose-related sedative and negative cardiovascular effects should be kept in mind to determine whether their use is justified, as the reduction in cardiac output, and hence renal blood flow, usually negate their use.

Box 20.1   Example anesthetic plan for an animal with CKD

Pre-Medication

- **Fentanyl** 2–5 µg/kg, **or**
- **Methadone:** 0.1–0.5 mg/kg, **or**
- **Oxymorphone** or **hydromorphone:** 0.02–0.05 mg/kg, **or**
- **Morphine:** 0.1–0.5 mg/kg, IM preferred. Only IV in compromised patients if none of the opioids above is available and monitoring of blood pressure and heart rate is available.
- **Acepromazine:** 0.01–0.03 mg/kg can be considered pre-operatively in stable cats and dogs with mild CKD. Doses of < 0.02 mg/kg may be used post-operatively for anxiolysis.
- **Benzodiazepines**
  - **Diazepam:** 0.1–0.4 mg/kg, IV
  - **Midazolam:** 0.1–0.5 mg/kg, IM or IV
- **Propofol:** Initial bolus dose of 2–2.5 mg/kg, IV. Incremental additional boluses every 6–12 s of 0.5 or 0.75 mg/kg can be given until endotracheal intubation is achieved. In compromised patients (ASA 3–4), an initial bolus of 1 mg/kg of propofol should be used.
- **Alfaxalone:** Initial bolus dose of 1–1.5 mg/kg, IV. Incremental additional boluses every 6–12 s of 0.3–0.4 mg/kg can be given until endotracheal intubation is achieved. In compromised patients (ASA 3–4); then an initial bolus of 0.5 mg/kg of alfaxalone should be used.
- **Ketamine:** A single induction bolus of ketamine and diazepam or midazolam 1:1 volume given as 0.1–0.2 mL/kg in cases of mild CKD with limited options. (This volume mixture results in doses of ketamine of 5–7 mg/kg and diazepam or midazolam doses of 0.25–0.3 mg/kg.)
- **Ketamine co-induction dose:** 0.5–1 mg/kg, IV after the initial lower bolus dose of propofol (1 mg/kg) or alfaxalone (0.5 mg/kg) to lower the dose and negative cardiovascular effects of propofol or alfaxalone in an unstable or compromised patient may be used.
- **Isoflurane or sevoflurane maintenance**

Adjunct Medications during Anesthesia of Patients with Renal Disease

Dopamine
Dopamine is commonly recommended for patients with renal disease due to its potential effects of renal arterial vasodilation and an increase in renal blood flow in healthy animals and humans. These effects are associated with low infusion rates (<2 µg/kg/min). Unfortunately, in patients with renal disease, other factors, such as hypovolemia, hypoxemia and concurrent disease, prevent dopamine from exerting its renal beneficial effects. Retrospective and prospective studies in human patients with renal disease have not demonstrated better outcomes with dopamine use, and in fact dopamine can have negative effects that include an increase in renal vascular resistance and an increase in oxygen demand in the proximal tubule through the diuretic effect of increasing Na^+ delivery to tubular cells [17, 18]. Norepinephrine (0.4 µg/kg/min) has been shown to be a better renal vasodilator than dopamine in animal models [19], although clinical evidence is not available.

Mannitol
Mannitol has been considered a renal protective agent. Mannitol is a small particle that filters freely at the glomerulus and is not reabsorbed by the tubules, which increases urine output. Conditions of hypotension and hypovolemia are damaging to the kidneys, especially the renal medulla, because of its reduced blood flow (5–10%), compared to the renal cortex (90–95%), despite the more active role of the medulla. Hypoperfusion can result in acute tubular necrosis and worsening of kidney function. Mannitol can be useful in these circumstances in preventing

acute tubular necrosis by filtering into the tubules and inducing osmotic diuresis that helps remove necrotic cell debris and casts, but it is ineffective if there is already complete occlusion [20]. Mannitol can also increase renal blood flow and decrease renal vascular resistance [21].

However, mannitol can also induce acute renal tubular injury if serum osmolarity exceeds 320 mOsm/L [22], and this detrimental effect can be exacerbated by concomitant administration of other nephrotoxic drugs and agents, volume depletion and pre-existing renal disease [23].

Fenoldopam
Fenoldopam mesylate is a potent dopamine-1 receptor agonist that increases blood flow to the renal cortex and outer medulla and can be beneficial in patients with acute renal injury by reducing the need for renal replacement therapy, and mortality [24]. Unlike dopamine, which has agonistic actions on dopamine$_1$, dopamine$_2$, and alpha$_1$ receptors, fenoldopam can produce selective renal vasodilation through its dopamine-1 actions and has been shown to improve renal function when infused at a dose of 0.1 µg/kg/min, compared with renal dose dopamine (2 µg/kg/min) in human patients with acute early renal dysfunction [25].

- **Induction** agents will have an impact on arterial blood pressure and thus renal blood flow and perfusion. The specific choice of propofol or alfaxalone is less critical and should always be tailored to the individual needs of the patient with attention to other co-morbidities. Propofol has been shown to have minimal effects on renal blood flow. However, correction of fluid deficits prior to induction, with titration to effect to minimize the potential for acute hypotension, is important to maintain renal blood flow. Minimal information exists for alfaxalone for cats and dogs with CKD/AKI. However, the same considerations stated for propofol likely apply. Clinical studies evaluating etomidate for anesthetic induction in cases with CKD/AKI in veterinary medicine are not available.

  Ketamine benzodiazepine combinations for induction should be avoided in cats and dogs with significant CKD/AKI. In cases with mild or early evidence of CKD, this induction drug combination (ketamine 5–7 mg/kg and diazepam or midazolam 0.3 mg/kg) may be acceptable for a single, or carefully titrated, induction dose if propofol or alfaxalone is not available. In cats with CKD/AKI, minimizing the total dose of ketamine is recommended by using it with propofol or alfaxalone. (See Box 20.1.)
- **Inhalant anesthetics** will reduce renal blood flow. Isoflurane and sevoflurane will maintain renal blood flow better than that previously described with halothane. A balanced anesthetic approach with optimal analgesia to enable the lowest possible inhalant level is always recommended to prevent the reduction in glomerular filtration that occurs with high inhalant doses. It is important to note that urine production can be greatly decreased under inhalant anesthesia due to an increase in vasopressin secretion [14–16]; therefore, assessing urine production in anesthetized patients is unreliable.

References

1 Burkholder, W. J. (2010) Dietary considerations for dogs and cats with renal disease. *JAVMA*, 216: 1730–1734.
2 Strandhoy, J. W. (1985) Role of alpha-2 receptors in the regulation of renal function. *J Cardiovasc Pharmacol*, 7(suppl. 8): S28–S33.
3 Burton, S., Lemke, K. A., Ihle, S. L. and Mackenzie, A. L. (1998) Effects of medetomidine on serum osmolality, urine volume, osmolality and pH, free water clearance, and fractional clearance of sodium, chloride, potassium, and glucose in dogs. *Am J Vet Res*, 59: 756–761.

4 Saleh, N., Aoki, M., Shimada, T., *et al.* (2005) Renal effects of medetomidine in isoflurane-anesthetized dogs with special reference to its diuretic action. *J Vet Med Sci*, 67: 461–465.

5 Kaka, J. S. and Hayton, W. L. (1980) Pharmacokinetics of ketamine and two metabolites in the dog. *J Pharmacokinet Biopharm*, 8: 193–202.

6 Capponi, L., Schmitz, A., Thormann, W., *et al.* (2009) In vitro evaluation of differences in phase 1 metabolism of ketamine and other analgesics among humans, horses, and dogs. *Am J Vet Res*, 70: 777–786.

7 Hanna, R. M., Borchard, R. E. and Schmidt, S. L. (1988) Pharmacokinetics of ketamine HCl and metabolite I in the cat: A comparison of I.V., I.M., and rectal administration. *J Vet Pharmacol Ther*, 11: 84–93.

8 Zand, L., McKian, K. P. and Qian, Q. (2010) Gabapentin toxicity in patients with chronic kidney disease: A preventable cause of morbidity. *Am J Med*, 123: 367–373.

9 Ing, T. S., Daugirdas, J. T., Sound, L. S., *et al.* (1979) Toxic effects of amantadine in patients with renal failure. *Can Med Assoc J*, 120: 695–698.

10 Sandoz, M., Vandel, S., Vandel, B., *et al.* (1984) Metabolism of amitriptyline in patients with chronic renal failure. *Eur J Clin Pharmacol*, 26: 227–32.

11 Langston, C. E. (2009) Acute renal failure. In: Silverstein, D. C. and Hopper, K. (eds), *Small Animal Critical Care Medicine*. Elsevier, St Louis, MO.

12 Boström, I., Nyman, G., Kampa, N., *et al.* (2003) Effects of acepromazine on renal function in anesthetized dogs. *Am J Vet Res*, 64: 590–598.

13 Monteiro, E. R., Teixeira, F. J., Castro, V. B. and Campagnol, D. (2007) Effects of acepromazine on the cardiovascular actions of dopamine in anesthetized dogs. *Vet Anaesth Analg*, 34: 312–321.

14 Adams, H. A., Schmitz, C. S. and Baltes-Gotz, B. (1994) Endocrine stress reaction, hemodynamics and recovery in total intravenous and inhalation anesthesia: Propofol versus isoflurane. *Anaesthetist*, 43: 730–737.

15 Hauptman, J. G., Richter, M. A., Wood, S. L. and Nachreiner, R F. (2000) Effects of anesthesia, surgery, and intravenous administration of fluids on plasma antidiuretic hormone concentrations in healthy dogs. *Am J Vet Res*, 61: 1273–1276.

16 Connolly, C. M., Kramer, G. C., Hahn, R. G., *et al.* (2003) Isoflurane but not mechanical ventilation promotes extravascular fluid accumulation during crystalloid volume loading. *Anesthesiology*, 98: 670–681.

17 Jones, D. and Bellomo, R. (2005) Renal-dose dopamine: From hypothesis to paradigm to dogma to myth and, finally, superstition? *J Intensive Care Med*, 20: 199–211.

18 Lauschke, A., Teichgräber, U. K., Frei, U. and Eckardt, K. U. (2006) Low-dose dopamine worsens renal perfusion in patients with acute renal failure. *Kidney Int*, 69: 1669–1674.

19 Di Giantomasso, D., Morimatsu, H., May, C. N. and Bellomo, R. (2004) Increasing renal blood flow: Low-dose dopamine or medium-dose norepinephrine. *Chest*, 125: 2260–2267.

20 Shawkat, H., Westwood, M. M. and Mortimer, A. (2012) Mannitol: A review of its clinical uses. *Contin Educ Anaesth Crit Care Pain*, doi: 10.1093/bjaceaccp/mkr063.

21 Bragadottir, G., Redfors, B. and Ricksten, S. E. (2012) Mannitol increases renal blood flow and maintains filtration fraction and oxygenation in postoperative acute kidney injury: A prospective interventional study. *Critical Care*, 16: R159.

22 Zhou, T. B. and Zong-Pei, J. (2014) Systematic review of the role of mannitol in renal diseases. *Am J Med Stud*, 2: 31–33.

23 Visweswaran, P., Massin, E. K. and Dubose, T. D. Jr (1997) Mannitol-induced acute renal failure. *J Am Soc Nephrol*, 8: 1028–1033.

24 Landoni, G., Biondi-Zoccai, G. G., Tumlin, J. A., *et al.* (2007) Beneficial impact of fenoldopam in critically ill patients with or at risk for acute renal failure: A meta-analysis of randomized clinical trials. *Am J Kidney Dis*, 49: 56–68.

25 Brienza, N., Malcangi, V., Dalfino, L., *et al.* (2006) A comparison between fenoldopam and low-dose dopamine in early renal dysfunction of critically ill patients. *Crit Care Med*, 34: 707–714.

21

Liver Disease as a Co-Morbidity for Anesthesia and Analgesia of Non-Related Emergencies

Melissa Sinclair

Mild, moderate to very significant liver disease may exist in a patient requiring anesthesia and analgesia for diagnosis and surgery of a traumatic injury or medical management of a critical illness. A detailed history from the owner is necessary to identify or highlight the existence or the progression of liver disease. The liver plays an important role in drug metabolism and excretion of all anesthetic and analgesic agents. It is essential to obtain baseline laboratory evaluation to assess hepatic function prior to administration of anesthetic or analgesic agents, and for trending after the emergency event. This is especially important when selecting analgesics and anesthetics that are not reversible. The following gives a general outline of the specific findings in cats and dogs with liver disease and their impact on anesthetic and analgesic administration.

The liver has several major functions, which include the production of albumin, coagulation factors and peptides. It is also responsible for glycogen storage, nutrient metabolism, detoxification and exclusion of many endogenous and exogenous substances, including almost all anesthetic and analgesic agents. The liver has a major reserve capacity to perform all of these functions. The clinical appearance of hypoglycemia, icterus, bleeding tendencies, hepatic encephalopathy (HE) or ascites indicates significant liver dysfunction and loss of reserve. It is in these patients where the administration of anesthetics and analgesics must be tailored specifically to the liver disease, as outlined below. In other cases, signs of early liver disease may be non-specific (polyuric/polydipsic, lethargy, vomiting, anorexia) and the patient will not have exhausted liver function capabilities; however, specific liver disease considerations and appropriate anesthetic and analgesic management will still be necessary.

I. Analgesia Considerations for Patients with Liver Disease

- **Opioids** are the analgesics of choice in patients with liver disease because they can be titrated to effect, and are reversible with naloxone. Initially, a mu-agonist opioid should be administered and titrated to effect whilst determining the patient's cardiovascular and volume status. The choice of opioid should be based on the patient's status and level of analgesia required. The opioid effects may last longer in patients with hepatic dysfunction and administering the shortest-acting opioid available for a given pain state is generally recommended [1]. The initial dose of opioid does not necessarily need to be reduced if liver disease is present [2]. The appropriate analgesic dose can be determined by titration to effect; however, the duration between single dose administrations may need to be increased. Where a continuous rate infusion is established, a lower hourly dose than that generally recommended is required;

Analgesia and Anesthesia for the Ill or Injured Dog and Cat, First Edition. Karol A. Mathews, Melissa Sinclair, Andrea M. Steele and Tamara Grubb.
© 2018 John Wiley & Sons, Inc. Published 2018 by John Wiley & Sons, Inc.

however, to determine this, frequent assessment is required. Similarly, frequent assessment of the patient's pain state, or intraoperative depth and responses, will aid in the determination of the appropriate administration interval or infusion dose. Morphine given as a bolus intravenously (IV) may precipitate plasma histamine release, resulting in decreased arterial blood pressure and reduced hepatic blood flow. However, slow IV administration with monitoring does not preclude its use in these patients if it is the only opioid available. Meperidine should not be administered IV. Refer to Chapter 10 for information on dosing, duration of action and selection of opioids.

- **Lidocaine** IV, 1–2 mg/kg followed by this at an hourly rate (~25–30 µg/kg/min), **dogs** only; can be added to the above regimen where pain scores are ≥ 8/10 in patients with liver disease or for reduction in opioid dosages. With significant liver disease, reductions in the initial dose and infusion rate are required due to lower liver extraction rates and flow and the potential for accumulation. Prolonged infusions > 3–4 h may be acceptable at reduced doses of ≤ 1–1.5 mg/kg (25 µg/kg/min) infusion rates in extremely painful cases. Attention to dose reduction is necessary to prevent cumulative effects if maintained for prolonged periods. Nausea and vomiting tend to occur with accumulation. Refer to Chapter 12 for lidocaine administration to cats.
- **Non-steroidal anti-inflammatory analgesics (NSAIAs)** are commonly used for pain control in veterinary medicine; however, their use in patients with liver disease should be avoided due to NSAIAs' potential to cause liver injury either intrinsically or idiosyncratically. In addition, NSAIAs have the potential to impact platelet aggregation and clot formation, which, in this patient population, is of concern. As there are no prospective clinical studies evaluating the use of NSAIAs in veterinary patients with liver dysfunction, their use cannot be recommended.
- **Gabapentin** undergoes some biotransformation in the liver in dogs into N-methyl-gabapentin, but most of the gabapentin (up to 65%) is eliminated unchanged in urine. The relative half-life (3.3 h) and low biotransformation contribute to its low to nil rate of hepatotoxicity in dogs. In humans, signs of liver disease have been rarely associated with gabapentin, and complete recovery is expected; therefore, it is considered safe to use in patients with hepatic disease. No specific information is available related to use in cats with liver disease; however long-term continuous use for up to 3–5 months followed by intermittent use for an additional 2–12 months in three separate feline cases with musculoskeletal trauma did not result in any hepatic side effects, despite a reduced ability of hepatic glucuronidation in this species [3].
- **Amitriptyline** can induce liver enzyme elevation (serum aminotransferase) in 10–12% of human patients, which may reflect hepatocellular to cholestatic alterations. Amitriptyline undergoes extensive hepatic metabolism and is biotransformed to its active metabolite nortriptyline, an active metabolite. Liver injury may be associated with the production of a toxic intermediate of metabolism, hence dose reductions, or avoidance in patients with significant liver dysfunction, should be considered [4].
- **Amantadine** undergoes minimal hepatic metabolism and is excreted largely unchanged in the urine. These factors make it an unlikely drug to induce hepatotoxicity but increase its likelihood for toxicity in patients with kidney disease due to decreased elimination and a potential for drug accumulation [5].

II.   Anesthetic Considerations for Patients with Liver Disease

Patients with liver disease requiring anesthesia impose a unique challenge. The anesthetic goals are to prevent further liver damage, ensure maximal oxygen delivery to the liver, use anesthetics that are short acting or do not rely on the liver for metabolism and/or to use reversible anesthetics.

Human patients with liver disease requiring anesthesia are categorized as those with: (1) mild liver disease or injury and (2) clinically apparent liver dysfunction. For the second category, human patients have a mortality rate of 11.6% and morbidity of 30% when undergoing anesthesia for procedures unrelated to the liver [6]. The main pre-anesthetic risk factors in these patients are ascites, a higher ASA classification score (which is a component of many confounding factors), high creatinine and pre-operative bleeding. In veterinary medicine, there are no studies specifically related to the incidence of anesthetic mortality in cats or dogs with liver disease undergoing anesthesia. A retrospective study of dogs with liver carcinoma undergoing hepatic resection found a poorer prognosis to discharge in dogs with a high ALT (alanine aminotransferase), AST (aspartate aminotransferase), a coagulopathy or a large percentage of the liver excised during surgery [7]; however, the results were not related to the anesthesia itself.

Most cats and dogs that have mild liver disease, represented by an increase in liver enzymes, may require sedation ± anesthesia for further diagnosis of liver disease (ultrasonography and biopsy). Others may require general anesthesia for surgical procedures either related to (e.g. liver resection) or unrelated to their liver disease. The underlying liver disease will compound the anesthetic risk in patients with an additional injury or illness. As anesthetics mainly rely on cytochrome P450 enzyme liver systems for hepatic biotransformation to active or inactive compounds, liver injury or dysfunction raises the concern of the ability of the liver to metabolize anesthetics. Liver injury or disease may increase the side effects, or result in a prolonged recovery, from use of analgesics, sedatives and general anesthetics.

Considering this, key aspects of pre-anesthetic assessment and anesthetic goals should be addressed in this patient population, as outlined below, to prevent further morbidities. A full review of all biochemistry, carbohydrate metabolism and coagulation testing is beyond the scope of this chapter; however, specific parameters will be highlighted. The reader is referred to [8].

A. Pre-Operative Examination and Laboratory Testing prior to Anesthesia

- These patients require a biochemical profile, coagulation panel and, potentially, pre- and post-prandial bile acids. Elevations in ALT, AST, GGT (gamma-glutamyl transferase) and ALP (alkaline phosphatase) are sensitive for hepatobiliary injury but are not specific for cause. Although the increase usually reflects the increase in hepatobiliary injury, it does not predict the remaining functional capacity, prognosis or ability to metabolize anesthetics. An elevation in liver enzymes refers to hepatocellular damage and not necessarily hepatic dysfunction.
- With significant liver dysfunction, normoglycemia cannot be maintained during fasting. Over 70% of liver function must be lost prior to the development of hypoglycemia. Glucose monitoring is important during anesthesia, and supplementation is required when glucose is < 3.5 mmol/L.
- Albumin is synthesized in the liver, and normally the liver only functions at 33% of its synthesis capacity. The half-life of albumin is 8–9 days. Considering these two factors, hypoalbuminemia is typically associated with significant liver disease and loss of reserve if other causes have been ruled out (protein losing enteropathy, nephropathy, acute blood loss, etc.). For anesthesia, the importance of hypoalbuminemia is related to its major contribution to providing plasma oncotic pressure and maintaining intravascular volume. With hypoalbuminemia, the development of hypotension is typical with general anesthetics. In addition, there is a reduction in the bound fraction of highly protein-bound drugs, including many anesthetics, such as propofol, and benzodiazepines, which will increase the portion of free active drug and plasma concentration. This alters the plasma concentration and volume of

distribution of the anesthetics, making slow IV titration, to effect, very important with highly protein-bound drugs to prevent increases in drug effects for a given dose.

- If surgery is required with evidence of an abnormal coagulation profile, blood typing and cross-matching are warranted. Coagulation factors have a relatively short half-life, so alterations in coagulation can be seen with more acute liver injury. Patients should be stabilized as much as possible with fluid therapy and blood products, where appropriate, prior to anesthesia and surgery.

III. Specific Anesthetic Considerations

A. Hepatic Blood Flow with Anesthesia and Surgery

The liver receives 25% of the total cardiac output and serves as a blood reserve for the body. It receives its blood flow and oxygenation from a dual supply with approximately 75% flow from the portal vein, which provides 50–55% of the oxygenation, and 25% flow from the hepatic artery, which provides 45–50% of the oxygenation. Increases in oxygen demand are solved with an increase in oxygen extraction and not a further increase in hepatic blood flow. Systemic hypotension or reductions in cardiac output are mainly accompanied by a reduction in portal venous flow and offset by hepatic arterial autoregulation and increases in hepatic arterial flow. The hepatic arterial vasculature, rich in alpha$_1$ adrenergic receptors, will constrict with sympathetic stimulation, resulting in a decrease in hepatic arterial flow. Increases in central venous pressure will increase portal venous pressures and reduce arterial blood flow.

The physiology above is important to consider in relationship to anesthesia, analgesia and surgery to enable maintenance of hepatic flow and oxygenation, especially in patients with signs of liver injury. Hepatic arterial autoregulation is not maintained with high inhalant or IV anesthetic concentrations. A balanced anesthetic approach to enable use of lowered doses of inhalant or IV anesthetics is always advised.

In addition, abdominal surgery will reduce hepatic blood flow via direct compression from surgical manipulation as well as sympathetic stimulation intraoperatively. A balanced anesthetic approach with appropriate analgesia is important to reduce the sympathetic stimulation to alpha$_1$ adrenergic receptors in the hepatic artery and resultant deceases in blood flow. High peak inspiratory pressures (PIPs) during manual or mechanical ventilation, or positive end-expiratory pressures, will increase portal vein pressures and reduce hepatic blood flow. Minimizing PIP as much as possible to an ideal maximum of 10–12 cmH$_2$O should be attempted while monitoring of PaO$_2$, PaCO$_2$ and SPO$_2$ to meet the individual patient's needs when significant liver disease exists. Dramatic elevations in PaCO$_2$ under general anesthesia can also reduce hepatic blood flow via sympathetic stimulation.

B. Biotransformation and Drug Elimination

The liver has a primary function of drug metabolism. It is responsible for the conversion of lipid-soluble drugs into water-soluble components, which will be excreted in the urine or bile. The cytochrome P450 hepatic microsomal enzyme located in the endoplasmic reticulum is important in this regard and liver dysfunction will impair this system. There are differences in type of cytochrome systems in, and within, species and location in hepatocyte zones of the liver, hence extrapolation across species for drug metabolism is difficult. However, with significant liver impairment, the result is consistently prolonged anesthetic effects.

C. Sedative and Anesthetic Considerations

- **Opioid** pre-medication on its own is frequently sufficient for sedation and preemptive analgesia in this patient population. The choice of opioid should be based on the patient's status and level of analgesia required. Frequent assessment of the patient's pain state or intraoperative depth and responses will aid in the determination of the appropriate administration interval.

  Earlier reports suggest that in people morphine causes constriction of the sphincter of Oddi, leading to spasm of the common bile duct [9]. This has led to the recommendation of avoiding morphine in cases with hepatobiliary disease; however, there is no clear evidence in veterinary patients of this occurrence. In general, with cholecystitis, it is advisable to avoid morphine; however, in cases without hepatobiliary disease, morphine may be used if it is the only opioid available for analgesia.

- The decision to administer **acepromazine** in these patients should be made on a case-by-case basis related to their personality, pre-operative status and degree of liver dysfunction present. With significant liver dysfunction signs, e.g. coagulopathy, ascites, hypoglycemia and hypoalbuminemia, clinical doses of acepromazine pre-operatively are not recommended. Acepromazine will reduce arterial blood pressure with $alpha_1$ antagonism. The impact of acepromazine on hepatic arterial blood flow is unknown; however, the cumulative effect with hypovolemia and other necessary anesthetics makes its use less ideal. Small doses (<0.02 mg/kg, IV or intramuscularly (IM)) may be possible in the recovery or ICU setting for further sedation, or relief of dysphoria if required; however, titration with naloxone for treating dysphoria is recommended. In patients with significant liver dysfunction and other co-morbidities, acepromazine is not recommended.

- **Benzodiazepines** are typically recommended in sick patients as they have the advantage of causing minimal negative cardiovascular effects; however, in patients with liver disease, the use of benzodiazepines is controversial. Benzodiazepines should not be administered to patients with HE. For patients without HE, having flumazenil available for benzodiazepine reversal is necessary as the sedative effects of the benzodiazepines are likely to be prolonged from hepatic enzyme reduction and slowed biotransformation. The pathogenesis of HE is complex and most commonly noted in portosystemic shunt (PSS) patients. The signs of HE are due to accumulation of neurotoxins from the gastrointestinal track that the liver cannot efficiently metabolize, resulting in central nervous system (CNS) effects and is indicative of greater than 70% of liver function being lost. Ammonia and other blood compounds (tryptophan, glutamine, GABA and endogenous benzodiazepines) in excess due to liver dysfunction result in excitatory as well as inhibitory CNS effects. In people with HE, flumazenil is used to lessen the clinical signs of HE. While clear clinical research is not available in veterinary medicine, benzodiazepines are generally avoided in veterinary patients with HE.

- The **alpha$_2$ adrenoceptor agonist** most commonly used is dexmedetomidine. Despite the dramatic (up to 50%) reduction in cardiac output with clinical dosages, 10 µg/kg did not reduce hepatic blood flow in dogs [10]. The overall sedative and cardiovascular effects should be considered to determine whether their use is justified for each individual patient. If used, lowered doses should be selected. However, when using this class of drug in patients with liver disease, their ability to provide analgesia and significantly reduce the amount of IV injectable and inhalant levels, with reversibility, may offer some advantages.

- **Induction** agents will have an impact on hepatic blood flow. Both propofol and thiopental maintain hepatic blood flow during induction via arterial vasodilation. Propofol clearance is higher than hepatic arterial blood flow, and also undergoes extra-hepatic metabolism, making it a good, and commonly reported, option in feline hepatic lipidosis [11] and for induction of anesthesia in PSS cases. Alfaxalone is another potential anesthetic induction option in veterinary patients with liver disease; however, clinical trials evaluating alfaxalone are not available. Alfaxalone has a large clearance and is primarily metabolized in the liver; however, the gastrointestinal tract, lungs and kidney also have a role in clearance [12, 13]. Titration to effect for a single IV anesthetic dose, or short-term maintenance, is a viable option in cats and dogs with liver dysfunction.

The barbiturates rely on hepatic metabolism and are not recommended for use in patients with liver dysfunction. Ketamine modestly reduces hepatic blood flow in comparison to thiopental and etomidate [14]. Ketamine relies on hepatocytes for metabolism in dogs and somewhat in cats. The main factor to consider is that ketamine is most commonly administered with a benzodiazepine and the benzodiazepine may require reversal in recovery. The metabolites of ketamine are highly dependent on renal excretion. In cats, the liver does function to metabolize ketamine to norketamine, a first step active metabolite, but this active metabolite is not metabolized further, which is different in dogs, requiring renal elimination [15]. Hence, in both cats and dogs with significant liver disease, use of high doses of ketamine or intermittent dosing for anesthetic maintenance could result in prolonged or rougher recoveries. However, a single clinical bolus of ketamine for anesthetic induction is not completely contraindicated in patients with mild liver disease if alternative options do not exist [16]. Individual patient considerations are important to assess the best option if limited options exist.

In human anesthesia, etomidate is seen as a good option for anesthetic induction due to minimal negative cardiovascular effects causing only minor alterations in hepatic blood flow. However, it should be noted that it has a 50% hepatic extraction ratio and requires hepatic metabolism. Clinical studies evaluating etomidate for anesthetic induction in veterinary medicine are not available.

- **Inhalant anesthetics** have differing effects on hepatic blood flow, oxygen consumption and autoregulation. Isoflurane, sevoflurane and desflurane have been shown to maintain hepatic blood flow and oxygen delivery compared to halothane or enflurane. However, the key aspect with inhalant anesthesia is that there is a dose-dependent decrease in flow and oxygenation to the liver irrespective of the inhalant anesthetic. That is, what is more important is how the inhalant is administered rather than which one. Despite the fact that inhalants are eliminated

---

Box 21.1 Example anesthetic plan for an animal with significant liver disease

- **Pre-medication:**
  - **Opioid alone:** pure μ-agonist preferred vs. butorphanol or buprenorphine for surgical procedures
    - **Fentanyl** 2–5 μg/kg, **or**
    - **Methadone** 0.1–0.5 mg/kg, **or**
    - **Oxymorphone or hydromorphone** 0.02–0.05 mg/kg
  - **Anticholinergic** should be considered on a case-by-case basis
    - Atropine 0.02–0.04 mg/kg, SC or IM, **or** glycopyrrolate 0.005–0.01 mg/kg, SC or IM
- **Pre-oxygenation** or flow by oxygen recommended after sedation
- **Induction:**
  - Propofol preferred: initial bolus 2 mg/kg, IV then to effect
  - Alfaxalone: initial bolus 1–2 mg/kg, IV, then to effect
  - Midazolam or diazepam co-induction (0.2–0.4 mg/kg, IV) possible in cases without HE, but flumazenil should be available for reversal
- **Maintenance:** isoflurane or sevoflurane.

primarily through alveolar ventilation and do not rely on the liver, mask induction and/or use of inhalants as a sole method of anesthesia will require higher levels of inhalant which will have a greater negative impact on hepatic blood flow and autoregulation. A balanced anesthetic approach with optimal analgesia to enable the lowest possible inhalant level is always recommended.

References

1 Tegeder, I., Lotsch, J. and Geisslinger, G. (1999) Pharmacokinetics of opioids in liver disease. *Clinical Pharmacokinetic*, 37: 17–40.

2 Bower, S., Sear, J. W., Roy, R. C. and Carter, R. F. (1992) Effects of different hepatic pathologies on disposition of alfentanil in anesthetized patients. *Br J Anaesth*, 68: 462–465.

3 Lorenz, N., Comerford, E. and Iff, I. (2015) Long-term use of gabapentin for musculoskeletal disease and trauma in three cats. *J Fel Med Surg*, 15: 507–512.

4 Sandoz, M., Vandel, S., Vandel, B., *et al.* (1984) Metabolism of amitriptyline in patients with chronic renal failure. *Eur J Clin Pharmacol*, 26: 227–32.

5 Ing, T. S., Daugirdas, J. T., Sound, L. S., *et al.* (1979) Toxic effects of amantadine in patients with renal failure. *Can Med Assoc J*, 120: 695–698.

6 Brovida, C. and Rothuizen, J. (2010) World Small Animal Veterinary Association (WSAVA) Guidelines. In: Ettinger, S. E. and Feldman, E. C. (eds), *Veterinary Internal Medicine*, 7th edn. Saunders, Elsevier, St Louis, MO: 1609–1611.

7 Liptak, J. L., Dernell, W. S., Monnet, E., *et al.* (2004) Massive hepatocellular carcinoma in dogs: 48 cases (1992–2002). *JAVMA*, 225(8), 1225–1230.

8 Webster, C. R. L. (2010) History, Clinical signs and physical findings in hepatobiliary disease. In: Ettinger, S. E. and Feldman, E. C. (eds), *Veterinary Internal Medicine*, 7th edn. Saunders, Elsevier, St Louis, MO: 1612–1625.

9 Flancbaum, L., Alden, S. M. and Trooskin, S. Z. (1989) Use of cholescintigraphy with morphine in critically ill patients with suspected cholecystitis. *Surgery*, 106: 668–673.

10 Flacke, W. E., Flacke, J. W., Bloor, B. C., *et al.* (1993) Effects of dexmedetomidine on systemic and coronary hemodynamics in the anesthetized dog. *J Cardiothoracic Vasc Anesth*, 7: 41–49.

11 Posner, L. P., Asakawa, M. and Erb, H. N. (2008) Use of propofol for anesthesia in cats with primary hepatic lipidosis: 44 cases (1995–2004). *J Am Vet Med Assoc*, 232: 1841–1843.

12 Warne, L. N., Beths, T., Whittem, T., *et al.* (2015) A review of the pharmacology and clinical application of alfaxalone in cats. *The Vet Journal*, 203: 141–148.

13 Whittem, T., Pasloske, K. S., Heit, M. C., *et al.* (2008) The pharmacokinetics and pharmacodynamics of alfaxalone in cats after single and multiple intravenous administration of Alfaxan at clinical and supraclinical doses. *Journal of Vet Pharm and Therap*, 31: 571–579.

14 Thomson, I. A., Fitch, W., Hughes, R. I., *et al.* (1986) Effects of certain IV anesthetics on liver blood flow and hepatic oxygen consumption in the greyhound. *Br J Anaesth*, 58: 69–80.

15 Baggott, J. D. and Blake, J. W. (1976) Disposition kinetics of ketamine in the domestic cat. *Arch Int Pharmacodyn Ther*, 220: 115–124.

16 Kaka, J. S. and Hayton, W. I. (1980) Pharmacokinetics of ketamine and two metabolites in the dog. *J Pharmacokinetics Biopharm*, 8: 193–202.

22

Managing the Aggressive Patient

Andrea Steele and Tamara Grubb

Handling an aggressive animal with force is never a good choice, and more likely to cause additional stress to the animal and/or injury to the staff. The veterinary staff must also ensure that the owner is safe, especially with a traumatized patient. Even the friendliest patient may bite when experiencing extreme pain. At no time should an owner restrain their own pet.

Whenever possible, gentle handling techniques and the use of appropriate analgesia or sedatives is important, and will produce the best results.

I. General Handling Strategies

The goal in dealing with an aggressive patient that is in need of intravenous (IV) catheterization, stabilization, pain management, etc., is to minimize the initial handling stress, and keep the handlers safe.

A. Aggressive Dogs

Dogs can be aggressive for many reasons: pain, fear, anxiety, protection of self or protection of the owner, being the most common. When a dog is hospitalized for surgery, or in an ICU environment, the owners have usually left the patient behind. In some cases, this makes the dog much more manageable, having removed the protection/guarding instinct. Fear and anxiety, however, are often exaggerated in hospitalized patients. It is important to remember that many dogs have been trained not to growl, resulting in a dog that bites without obvious warning. A growl should always be considered a warning, and appropriate precautions taken.

B. Handling Strategies for Dogs

A dog that is showing signs of aggression for any reason should not be handled alone. There should be two persons present at all times to prevent injury or call for help if needed. At all times, protection of self is the most important, and staff should not be putting themselves at risk.

The nervous/fearful/aggressive dog should be sedated (see Section II) prior to placing in a cage when they first arrive. This will be safer for staff, and also make it easier to retrieve the patient after the sedative has taken effect. Sedatives will often have a better effect if the patient is placed in a quiet area, as the patient will relax. Make placement of an IV catheter and attaching IV fluids a priority once the patient is sedate, to allow for repeated sedation from a safe distance.

Analgesia and Anesthesia for the Ill or Injured Dog and Cat, First Edition. Karol A. Mathews, Melissa Sinclair, Andrea M. Steele and Tamara Grubb.
© 2018 John Wiley & Sons, Inc. Published 2018 by John Wiley & Sons, Inc.

Ideally, the dog will be removed from the cage to avoid cage aggression, and provide the staff with a safer opportunity to restrain the patient. Large mobile dogs should be coaxed out of the cage with food, or asking if they want to go for a walk, and a loop type leash applied. A nervous dog that will not come out through the door of the run or cage should be approached very slowly and sideways, while avoiding eye contact. Allow the dog to relax in your presence prior to trying to apply the leash. A dog that is very aggressive and lunging will be difficult to retrieve from a cage, and a capture pole may be the safest tool to prevent injury.

A thick blanket or towel placed over the head and body of the aggressive small dog may allow the patient to be lifted out of the cage, and will also afford a brief window to provide sedation or analgesia via an intramuscular (IM) injection. Often the handler can place the patient on the table, under the towel, and simply push the patient down on the neck/shoulders and backend gently, while the injection takes place. Restraint of the head and neck is often easier with the towel over the head to buffer bites. Thick protective leather gloves can be used, but these often reduce the handler's dexterity, making a patient difficult to subdue. Once the sedation ± analgesic is injected, place the patient back into the cage to allow it time to work.

Muzzles may be difficult to place in the aggressive dog that has been muzzled previously and is not comfortable with them. Leather muzzles, maintain their shape and may be easier to place than cloth muzzles. Muzzles should not be used in patients that are dyspneic, vomiting or have head trauma.

A large rolled towel wrapped around a dog's neck and held high under the jaw may offer some protection from a patient that is trying to bite those behind him by preventing the dog from swinging around. This may allow time to sedate with an injection in the hind end, or even access the saphenous vein for an injection or catheter. This works particularly well for recumbent, but alert, patients who are aggressive.

Placing and maintaining an Elizabethan collar on an aggressive dog may make hospitalization and patient handling much easier by protecting the handler from bites. Caution must always be used in the patient that begins struggling, as they may also manage to remove the collar and be a danger. Often, the lack of peripheral vision afforded by the collar will calm the patient, and moving slowly and gently may allow a minimum examination/treatment.

C. Aggressive Cats

Cats rarely guard their owners; however, they frequently exhibit fear, anxiety and self-protective behaviours. Pain can make a normally docile cat very aggressive. An aggressive cat may be very difficult to calm, and a mildly aggressive cat will escalate rapidly into a very aggressive animal.

Leather cat muzzles are often effective as they also remove visual stimuli by covering the eyes. Muzzles, however, must be avoided with dyspnea, vomiting or head trauma.

In general, cats respond very well to "less is more". They become highly fearful when forced into a position and will retaliate. Begin with the least restraint possible, and increase only as needed. Less cooperative cats can be wrapped in large towels or a cat bag to contain sharp claws and allow for an injection for chemical restraint. In recent years various initiatives such as "Fear Free"™ and "Cat Healthy"™ have stressed the importance of gentle handling techniques for cats. Techniques such as avoiding scruffing, using pheromone products, having cat only waiting areas and examination areas can help to reduce the stress experienced by cats, and thus, their aggression in hospital.

Once sedate, prioritize an IV catheter so that further analgesics, sedation and/or anesthesia can be given IV, from a distance. Ensure the catheter is well secured and bandaged in place. Take a moment to trim the claws of the patient while sedate, to minimize future risk of injury. Each time the patient is sedated, examine the catheter and leg for any potential issues (kinking, phlebitis, leaking around site, etc.) and change the bandage. Replace the IV at the first sign of an issue to reduce the risk of losing the catheter.

II. Sedation/Anesthesia for the Aggressive/Fractious Patient

A. Start Treatment at Home

This is generally not an option for patients presented as an emergency but can be used for recheck and repeat visits since, ideally, treatment of the fractious/aggressive patient should start at home before the patient leaves its house or yard. Having a calmer patient to anesthetize not only is extremely beneficial for the patients but also makes our jobs easier and safer. The dose of drugs needed to sedate/anesthetize patients escalates as fractiousness/aggression escalates and, since the adverse effects of most sedative/anesthetic drugs are dose-dependent, this can lead to a dangerous potential for drug overdose. Depending on the reason for the aggressive/fractious behaviour, analgesic drugs, benzodiazepines, trazodone and gabapentin may be good choices for treatment at home.

B. At the Hospital

Once in the hospital, the patient should spend minimal (or no) time in noisy lobbies, should be placed in a quiet exam room and should be handled by veterinarians/technicians/staff with appropriate training and compassion for the behaviour status of the animal. The use of pheromones, music and other calming techniques may also benefit the patient.

When it is time to examine or treat the patient, gentle handling may be sufficient if the patient has mild fear/anxiety or pain or even moderate fear/anxiety or pain that has responded to therapy at home. **Don't be afraid to sedate the patient** and **don't wait until the situation has irrevocably escalated** if the patient is showing signs of fractiousness/aggression. This is dangerous for everyone, including the patient, and early use of sedatives/analgesics can prevent a bad situation. If the situation has already escalated beyond what can be controlled by sedation/analgesia, consider general anesthesia immediately (even if no examination has been done).

Drugs – and, more importantly, the drug dosages – for sedation/anesthesia/analgesia should be chosen based on the patient's degree of fear/anxiety or aggression, level of anticipated pain and sedation/anesthesia risk level (Table 22.1), if possible. Often when sedating a very aggressive patient, a full physical examination is impossible and selection of drugs may be made based on the patient's presenting history and a few vital parameters.

There is no "one size fits all" in these situations. "Appropriate drugs" and "appropriate dosages" will be very patient- and situation-dependent and the protocols presented here are guidelines, but each veterinarian should choose individualized protocols using their clinical experience.

Remember: response to drugs can be quite varied in patients with fear/anxiety, fractiousness/aggression and/or pain. Expect an unpredictable response – especially in unpredictable patients – and be ready to escalate your protocol

Table 22.1 American Society of Anesthesiologists (ASA) risk factor for anesthesia- adverse events.

ASA status	Risk
I	Low: free from disease or conditions that may impact anesthetic drug/management choices
II	Low but with mild disease or conditions that may impact anesthetic drug/management choices
III	Moderate: has disease or condition that may moderately impact anesthetic drug/management
IV	Severe: disease or condition that may profoundly impact anesthetic choices; patient may die
V	Profound: patient has life-threatening disease and may die with or without anesthetic intervention

C. Sample Protocols Based on Patient ASA, Fear/Aggression and Pain Levels

Dosages for drugs listed in the protocols are listed in Table 22.2. Unless indicated otherwise, drugs are generally administered IM to decrease stress from restraint for IV injection. In aggressive patients, IV injection should not be attempted. The subcutaneous route of administration is not recommended because the absorption is too slow and results in low circulating concentrations of the drug. Some analgesics/sedatives will be absorbed via the oral mucosa. Ketamine, buprenorphine and dexmedetomidine have all been used via a spray into the mouth.

1. Low Fear/Anxiety, Mild Pain, ASA I–II (Low Risk)
- Dexmedetomidine low dose
  - ○ Low-end range (Table 22.2): large cats and dogs, older patients
  - ○ High-end range: smaller patients, younger patients, if used solo (without opioid).
- And/or dose of **acepromazine**
  - ○ Not an anxiolytic so may add a benzodiazepine to the protocol if not using alpha$_2$ agonist
  - ○ **Add** if long duration sedation is necessary
  - ○ **Not reversible; no analgesia.**
- ± the **opioid** of your choice
  - ○ Match the opioid to the degree of pain; butorphanol and/or buprenorphine may be appropriate for mild pain.

2. Low Fear/Anxiety, Mild Pain, ASA III–IV (Moderate to High Risk)
- Midazolam or alfaxalone.
- **Plus** opioid appropriate for level of pain. **Do not administer benzodiazepines alone** – may cause paradoxical excitement.
- If the patient becomes extremely fractious, consider low dose of dexmedetomidine:
  - ○ This level of fear/anxiety/aggression is likely more detrimental than a low dose of a reversible drug
  - ○ Staff safety must be considered along with health status of the pet.

3. Moderate Fear/Anxiety or Pain, ASA I–II
- Start calming therapy pre-visit for rechecks and subsequent visits if possible.

For the initial emergency visit, use the drug protocol:

- Dexmedetomidine higher dose:
  - ○ Dosing caveats same as for ASA I–II.
- ± acepromazine or midazolam.
  - ○ Comments are the same as for ASA I–II.

Table 22.2 Sedative, analgesic and anesthetic drugs.

Drug and dosage (mg/kg)	Advantages	Disadvantages/ concerns	Notes
Drugs to administer at home			
Acepromazine **Dog** and **Cat:** 0.025–0.05 oral transmucosal	Inexpensive	Effects are not consistent with oral administration	Effects are highly variable
Benzodiazepines	True anxiolytics	May take days – weeks for full effect	Variety used for anxiolysis
Clonidine **Dog** and **Cat:** 0.01–0.05 mg/kg PO	Oral alpha$_2$ agonist	Bradycardia	Little to no information for using in this context
Dexmedetomidine gel (see label for dose)	Effective for mild calming	Unlikely to be potent enough for aggressive patients	FDA-approved for noise phobia, but can be used for fractiousness and aggression
Diphenhydramine	–	–	Effects are highly variable
Gabapentin **Dog:** 10–20 PO **Cat:** 50–100/cat PO	Safe	No major concerns	Effective for calming, mild to moderate sedation
Trazodone **Dog:** 5–7 (up to 15) PO **Cat:** 50 mg/cat PO	Safe	No major concerns	Effective for calming, mild to moderate sedation
Sedative/analgesic drugs for in-hospital use			
Acepromazine **Dog:** 0.01–0.03 IV or IM **Cat:** 0.03–0.05 IV or IM	Mild to moderate sedation for several hours Can be given orally or transmucosally but higher doses will be required and onset of effects are slow	Not anxiolytic, analgesic or reversible Duration may be longer than desired	If anxiolysis rather than sedation is required, a benzodiazepine should be added to the protocol No absolute contraindications but use with caution in patients with hepatic disease, clotting dysfunction or hypotension. Recent evidence proves that it does **not** cause seizures. Can be used alone but best used in combination with opioids and/or other sedatives
Alfaxalone 0.5–1.0 IM	Mild to moderate sedation for 20–40 min	Mild cardiovascular and respiratory depression	Alfaxalone is an anesthetic induction drug that can be used IM for sedation It is best used with opioids and in cats and small dogs since the injectate volume can be very large for medium to large patients

Drug and dosage (mg/kg)	Advantages	Disadvantages/ concerns	Notes
Alpha₂ agonists *Dexmedetomidine* **For light to moderate sedation:** **Dog:** 0.001–0.003 IV or 0.003–0.01 IM **Cat:** 0.001–0.005 IV or 0.005–0.015 IM **For deeper sedation: Dog:** 0.008–0.03 IV or 0.01–0.04 IM **Cat:** 0.02–0.04 IM or IV Use low end of dosing range if used in conjunction with opioids or other sedatives, for older patients and patients with low level of fear/anxiety Use high end of range if used alone, for younger patients and patients with higher level of fear/anxiety or aggression *Medetomidine* Dosages are roughly double the mg/kg of dexmedetomidine dosages	Provide analgesia and sedation Effects are reversible Rapid onset Titratable sedation from mild to profound Decreased stress as evidenced by decreased cortisol release	Cardiovascular effects including hypertension and increased cardiac work due to vasoconstriction Sudden, brief arousal can occur with painful stimulus – alleviated by concurrent opioid administration	Generally the best drugs for patients exhibiting moderate to profound fear/anxiety and/or fractiousness/aggression Most predictable effects when used in combination with opioids Dosages in this handout are based on, but not exactly the same as, the FDA-approved label dosages See the product insert for more information on dosing Can reverse drug effects once procedure is complete and patient is in a calm, quiet area where restraint is possible if necessary Contraindication: do not use in patients with most types of cardiovascular disease An oral dexmedetomidine paste is available for treatment of noise phobia that may also be effective for mild calming in some patients
Benzodiazepines *Midazolam* **Dog or Cat:** 0.1–0.2 IM or IV *Diazepam* **Dog or Cat:** 0.1–0.2 IV only	Minimal to no adverse physiologic effects Enhance calming when used in combination with true sedatives Midazolam can be administered IM	True sedation is minimal May not be effective if patient is already exhibiting fear/anxiety/aggression Paradoxical excitement can occur if used alone	Never use alone Use in combination with an opioid and/or true sedative for those exhibiting fear/anxiety/aggression and/or aggression Be cautious with reversal as it may cause sudden arousal Generally no need to reverse effects

(Continued)

Table 22.2 (Continued)

Drug and dosage (mg/kg)	Advantages	Disadvantages/ concerns	Notes
Opioids: Low pain *Butorphanol* **Dog** and **Cat:** 0.2–0.4 IM or IV *Buprenorphine* **Dog** and **Cat:** 0.02–0.03 IM or IV; 0.03–0.05 oral transmucosal (slow onset)	Opioids provide mild to potent analgesia depending on the drug and have a wide safety margin Fast onset except buprenorphine (10–30 min) Reversible	May cause vomiting, slow gastrointestinal (GI) motility and some respiratory depression if used with other respiratory-depressing drugs (e.g. inhalants) More potent opioids may cause excitement and/or hyperthermia in cats	Combine with a sedative to avoid excitement in cats With mild pain can use butorphanol or buprenorphine With moderate to severe pain use hydromorphone, methadone, morphine or oxymorphone No absolute contraindications but use with caution in patients in which vomiting or slowed GI motility would be detrimental
Opioids: High pain *Hydromorphone* **Dog:** 0.1–0.2 IM or IV **Cat:** 0.1 IM or IV *Methadone* **Dog:** 0.3–0.5 IM or IV **Cat:** 0.3–0.5 IM or IV *Morphine* **Dog:** 0.3–1.0 IM **Cat:** 0.1–0.3 IM	Many to choose from Variety of routes of administration; synergistic with sedatives		

Anesthetic drugs
Any of the anesthetic drugs can be used if IV access is available. Listed here are the anesthetics used IM

Drug and dosage (mg/kg)	Advantages	Disadvantages/ concerns	Notes
Ketamine **Dog** and **Cat:** 1.0–2.0 IM when used in combination with a sedative may provide dissociation without anesthesia while the same dose IV will provide light anesthesia 5.0–10.0 mg/kg IM for true anesthesia IM is a good for route for cats but the volume at this dose may be too high for medium-large dogs **Tiletamine-zolazepam** **Dog** and **Cat:** 1.0–2.0 IM or IV can be added to sedatives/opioids for light to moderate sedation For anesthesia **with pre-meds:** **Dog:** 5–6 IM; 2–3 IV **Cat:** 6–8 IM; 2–3 IV	Decrease central nervous system response to circulating neurotransmitters in those already exhibiting fear/anxiety and/or aggression Decrease incidence of sudden arousal to stimulus Ketamine (and maybe tiletamine) can contribute to pain relief	Duration and/or depth may be longer and/or more profound than desired Ketamine and tiletamine are not reversible Ketamine is painful on injection Prolonged, rough recoveries are possible with tiletamine-zolazepam, especially in dogs	**This is anesthesia so patients should be monitored** There are no absolute contraindications, but use with caution in patients with sympathetically driven cardiac arrhythmias or seizures and those with clinically significant hepatic or renal disease since these drugs are cleared by the liver and kidneys

Note: Not all of the drugs in these charts are FDA-approved for use in dogs and cats. Drugs like the alpha$_2$ agonists and acepromazine are often used at lower than the FDA-approved dose as profound sedation is not always necessary. However, all of the dosages in this chart are commonly used and are referenced in the veterinary literature. A variety of drugs/protocols are available. Choices should be made based on the veterinarian's experience. Drugs are presented in alphabetical order in each category.
Source: Adapted from FearFreeTM In-hospital sedation module Grubb TG author.

- Midazolam is an excellent addition as a true anxiolytic (but not likely to need **both** ace and midazolam).
- ± the opioid of your choice.
  - Match the opioid to the degree of pain.
- Moderate–high pain: morphine, hydromorphone, methadone, oxymorphone.
- If the procedure is painful, use other analgesics as appropriate for the procedure:
  - E.g. local anesthetic blockade, continuous rate infusion.

4. Moderate Fear/Anxiety/Fractiousness or Pain, ASA III–IV
- Start calming/sedating therapy pre-visit for rechecks and subsequent visits if possible.

For the initial emergency visit, use the drug protocol:

- Midazolam or alfaxalone.
- **Plus** opioid (standard doses – low end of range) appropriate for degree of pain.
- If painful procedure, use other analgesics as appropriate for the procedure.

5. Severe Fractiousness/Aggression, Any ASA
- **Start calming/sedating treatment pre-visit** for rechecks and subsequent visits.

For the initial emergency visit, use the drug protocol:

- **Do not** put personnel in danger or stress the patient any further.
- Go straight to deep sedation/anesthesia.

Protocol 1
- High dose dexmedetomidine (can use **label dose**).
- Plus an opioid appropriate for the level of pain.
- Will get calmer patient in about 20 min – but may still need IV or IM anesthetic drugs (Protocol 2).

Protocol 2
- Next step if previous protocol not effective **or** first step if patient is dangerous.
- Add IM ketamine to protocol above:
  - 1–2 mg/kg may provide dissociation without anesthesia; often called "ketamine stun"
  - 5–10 mg/kg added for true anesthesia – often used in cats but volume too high for most dogs.
- Or add telazol to protocol above.
- Combine all drugs in same syringe and administer together IM by quick hand injection, pole syringe or dart.

Further Reading

Cohen, A. E. and Bennett, S. L. (2015) Oral transmucosal administration of dexmedetomidine for sedation in 4 dogs. *Can Vet J*, 56(11): 1144–1148.

Gilbert-Gregory, S. E., Stull, J. W., Rice, M. R. and Herron, M. E. (2016) Effects of trazodone on behavioral signs of stress in hospitalized dogs. *J Am Vet Med Assoc*, 249(11): 1281–1291.

Gruen, M. E., Roe, S. C., Griffith, E., *et al.* (2014) Use of trazodone to facilitate postsurgical confinement in dogs. *J Am Vet Med Assoc*, 245(3): 296–301.

Gruen, M. E. and Sherman, B. L. (2008) Use of trazodone as an adjunctive agent in the treatment of canine anxiety disorders: 56 cases (1995–2007). *J Am Vet Med Assoc*, 15, 233(12): 1902–1907.

Hammerle, M., Horst, C., Levine, E., *et al.* (2015) 2015 AAHA Canine and Feline Behavior Management Guidelines. *J Am Anim Hosp Assoc*, 51(4): 205–221.

Overall, K. L. (2013) *Manual of Clinical Behavioral Medicine for Dogs and Cats*, http://www.dvm360.com/sites/default/files/u11/Medications_fearful-dogs_cats.pdf, accessed 1st August 2017.

Rodan, I., Sundahl, E., Carney, H., *et al.* (2011) AAFP and ISFM feline-friendly handling guidelines: American Animal Hospital Association. *J Feline Med Surg*, 13(5): 364–375.

Sheldon, C. C., Sonsthagen, T. and Topel, J. (2006) *Animal Restraint for Veterinary Professionals*. Mosby, St Louis, MO.

Yin, S. (2007) Simple handling techniques for dogs. *Compend Contin Educ Vet*, 29(6): 352–358.

23

Analgesia and Anesthesia for Pregnant Cats and Dogs

Karol Mathews and Melissa Sinclair

Where anesthesia and/or analgesia are required during pregnancy, drugs and protocols require careful consideration for both mother and fetus. Anesthesia and /or analgesia may be indicated in pregnant animals for an injury, a painful medical illness, an unrelated surgical procedure or cesarean section itself. Unfortunately, there are no clinical studies investigating the safety of any analgesics in the pregnant dog or cat. Although many analgesic and anesthetic regimens have been recommended and used clinically for cesarean sections with no apparent ill effects, the long-term effects of analgesics in pregnant dogs and cats have not been studied. Only a few reports have investigated injectable anesthetics in small animals, and most information is extrapolated from the human literature.

The information currently available in veterinary medicine for analgesia in pregnant dogs and cats is extrapolated from information published from research in laboratory animals and humans. As a consequence, veterinarians may withhold or restrict analgesic use in pregnant animals because the effects of these drugs on the developing fetus are not known, leading to inadequate analgesia in the pregnant cat and dog. For pregnant women, the Food and Drug Administration (FDA) classifies five categories of various drugs, including anesthetic and analgesic agents, used in pregnancy based on teratogenicity research: categories A, B, C, D and X. Category A is considered the safest category and category X is absolutely contraindicated in women who are, or may become, pregnant [1]. This provides therapeutic guidance for the care of women and should be considered in animals undergoing non-cesarean anesthetic events.

The following information is a general guideline of the anesthetic and analgesic literature to provide anesthesia safely in the dam/queen to ensure viable neonates, and to provide analgesia safely to avoid suffering of the dam/queen.

I. Physiological Changes in the Pregnant Cat and Dog Affecting Analgesic Selection and Dosing [2]

Drug pharmacodynamics, pharmacokinetics and distribution to the fetus are altered due to the physiological changes associated with the maternal–placental–fetal unit regardless of the route of administration. Reduced plasma levels of a drug may occur as an increase in total body fat, which may occur during pregnancy, and results in a larger volume of distribution for lipid-soluble drugs with less plasma availability. Low plasma levels may also occur with orally administered medication as decreased gastrointestinal (GI) motility, esophageal reflux and vomiting may alter drug absorption. Transdermally administered drugs may have enhanced absorption due

Analgesia and Anesthesia for the Ill or Injured Dog and Cat, First Edition. Karol A. Mathews, Melissa Sinclair, Andrea M. Steele and Tamara Grubb.
© 2018 John Wiley & Sons, Inc. Published 2018 by John Wiley & Sons, Inc.

to the maternal increase in cutaneous blood flow in the late stage of pregnancy. However, as the volume for distribution of drugs is also increased due to an increase in total body water, and with distribution throughout the maternal tissues, amniotic fluid, placenta and fetus, this may not be a problem. Other factors that may alter the response of pregnant animals to analgesic drugs include altered hepatic enzymatic activity, increased renal function (with an associated increased elimination of water-soluble drugs and metabolites) and reduced serum albumin relative to intravascular volume. It is hypothesized that reduced serum albumin could result in more free, normally protein-bound, drug which would then be available for action on maternal receptor sites and transport across the placenta to the fetus. In dogs and cats, however, laboratory-measured albumin levels may drop to low normal values, but this is felt to be secondary to the increased plasma volume and, therefore, associated dilution and is not attributable to reduced albumin load in the normal pregnancy. As the total albumin volume is unchanged, this should not affect the availability of a drug.

As the placental barrier is considered a lipoprotein, lipophilic compounds diffuse passively along a concentration gradient to the fetus [3]. Many pharmacologic compounds have a molecular size smaller than 600 Da, which also readily cross the placenta. As the concentration increases within the fetus, equilibrium with the maternal plasma concentration is reached, limiting further transport. The placenta is an enzymatically active organ in all species, but with variable activity amongst species. Cytochrome P450 enzymes, N-acetyltransferase, glutathione transferase and sulfating enzymes can alter the activity of drugs into their active or inactive forms with variable activity in the fetus. While drugs with high lipid solubility are permeable, drugs that are water soluble, protein-bound, polar or ionized are less likely to cross the placenta into the fetus [3]. Blood flow also determines the rate of drug entering the placenta, and increased or decreased placental flow influences delivery of drugs to the fetus [3]. Placental thickness decreases as the placenta ages, facilitating further diffusion into the fetus. Cotyledons in the human placenta are a potential site for drug storage and ongoing release making direct extrapolation from humans to cats and dogs difficult for specific drugs, such as morphine. Because dogs and cats do not have placental cotyledons, the site of potential placental storage of analgesics will differ from humans.

The stage of gestation of the fetus influences the effects of the various analgesics; drugs administered in the early stage have a different effect than when administered during the later stages [1, 2]; however, there are species differences. As an example, the human fetal liver can perform many enzymatic and metabolic activities as it matures; however, it cannot perform glucuronidation, which is important for the metabolism of many lipophilic drugs, such as some opioids [1]. This feature may be of value when extrapolating information of placental transfer of opioids from humans to dogs. Unlike the human fetus, the liver of the canine fetus has no drug-metabolizing capabilities; therefore, elimination of drugs from the canine fetal circulation is by means of immature fetal renal mechanisms or diffusion back through the placenta to the mother [4, 5]. There is no information available for the potential of feline fetal liver metabolic function, hence it cannot be considered. Fetal body water and albumin increase, and body fat decreases, during development, all of which influences the plasma concentrations of various analgesics.

There are no specific dosages given for the various analgesics administered during pregnancy; however, the recommendation for human patients is a reduction of 20% or more. This is due to an increase in progesterone and progesterone metabolites, which are potent positive allosteric modulators of GABAA nociceptors and increased hormonal prevention of pain transmission activated by estrogen and progesterone during pregnancy. However, analgesics should be administered to effect; therefore, a reduction in dosage may be variable, or not at all. Epidural vessels are engorged, resulting in a reduction of the epidural space by 30–50% and is, therefore, essential to reduce the epidural volume of drug (e.g., morphine ± lidocaine or bupivacaine) administered by this route.

Acid-base status is also important as fetal acidosis results in "ion-trapping" of some opioids, preventing diffusion back into the maternal circulation. This results in an increase in fetal opioid and/or local anesthetic accumulation in tissues and plasma, especially with repeated administration.

II. Which Analgesics Can Be Administered to Pregnant Patients?

While the concerns for analgesic administration are focused on the fetus and potential interference with breeding, painful animals must be managed appropriately and the owner notified of potential fetal loss or unsuccessful breeding.

A. Opioids

This class of analgesics is used in pregnant dogs and cats. Methadone, morphine and hydromorphone are used during pregnancy in humans as they are less lipid-soluble when compared to other compounds, which may reach higher concentrations in the fetus (e.g. meperidine > sufentanil > butorphanol, buprenorphine and nalbuphine >> fentanyl > methadone > hydromorphone > oxymorphone > morphine). Based on the human literature, short-term opioid analgesic administration does not seem to be a problem and this is likely so in veterinary patients. With prolonged non-methadone opioid use (several weeks) during pregnancy in human mothers, the reported adverse effects on the fetus are a low birth weight and behavioral deficits. Similar findings have been reported in laboratory animals [6]. The behavioural problems incurred with chronic use may be a result of reduced nervous system plasticity secondary to the opioid action on the development of normal synaptic connections, neurotransmitter production and metabolism [7]. Chronic use during pregnancy would be extremely rare in veterinary patients; however, the benefit to the mother must be considered. In veterinary medicine, opioids are frequently used pre-operatively for cesarean section, and most puppies and kittens are successfully delivered and are vigorous.

Methadone appears to be safe for the treatment of pain during pregnancy in humans and is the recommended opioid for the addicted patient. Methadone is a very good analgesic, unfortunately only the parenteral route can be used in dogs because this opioid is not absorbed via the oral route in this species, limiting its use for short-term analgesia. Both parenteral and oral transmucosal (OTM) routes have been reported in the cat [8].

Fentanyl's high lipid solubility facilitates rapid crossing into the placenta and into the fetal brain. Fentanyl was present in the fetal brain of first and early second trimester aborted human fetuses after clearance from the maternal blood. A study investigating human fetal and maternal plasma opioid concentrations after epidural fentanyl-bupivacaine mixture administered for analgesia during labour and delivery, noted that fentanyl administration was associated with lower neurobehavioral test scores when compared to sufentanil-bupivacaine at 24h of life, although none of the neonates had clinically significant depression [9]. Several forms of fentanyl, including the patch, have been available to manage chronic pain in humans, for many years without reports of serious adverse effects. However, there are only two case reports in the literature describing chronic use in pregnancy. One woman required a 125 μg/h fentanyl patch throughout pregnancy, and the newborn infant manifested mild withdrawal symptoms at 24–72h after birth with subsequent normal behaviour [10]. In the other, a much lower dose (25 μg/h) of fentanyl patch was used throughout pregnancy with no apparent adverse effects in the infant [11].

Sufentanil's placental transfer is greater than that of fentanyl; however, there is significant reuptake of sufentanil to the maternal circulation, which reduces neonatal opioid exposure considerably. This was noted when epidural sufentanil–bupivacaine mixture was administered during labour in the above study. In this study, the investigators concluded that both drugs are acceptable for use with epidural bupivacaine during labour but that reduced neonatal opioid exposure with sufentanil suggests that it may have some advantages over fentanyl [9].

Morphine therapeutic use has not been linked to any major congenital defects [1]; however, maternal addiction to morphine during pregnancy, with subsequent neonatal withdrawal syndrome, is well documented. Morphine was widely used during labour in women until the 1940s, when it was replaced by meperidine. The clinical impression was that less respiratory depression was noted with meperidine when compared to that when morphine was used [1]. This appears counterintuitive based on the lipid solubility of meperidine; however, the dosage and duration of action differences between the two drugs are likely accountable. For postoperative analgesia in women; however, morphine, and not meperidine, is recommended.

Hydromorphone is frequently administered to veterinary patients but there are no reports on its use during pregnancy. As a pregnant cat and dog may acquire a painful medical condition, the safest class of analgesic to consider is an opioid. As an example of potential medical pain, a case report of a woman at 34 weeks gestation presented with acute biliary pancreatitis. She was managed with intravenous (IV) fluids, parenteral nutrition and hydromorphone for seven days. At this time fetal heart rate increased and cesarean section was performed. There were no adverse effects noted in the neonate upon delivery [12].

Buprenorphine is deposited into the intervillous space, where it acts as a depot resulting in low transplacental transfer to the fetal circuit. The direct effect of buprenorphine on the fetus depends on its concentration in the fetal circulation. Less than 10% of placental buprenorphine, which is slowly released from the placenta, reaches the fetal circulation. With repeated administration, however, an increased depot of the drug would result in continuous release into the fetal circulation, which may contribute to neonatal withdrawal in a small number of neonates [13, 14].

Butorphanol rapidly crosses the placenta and neonatal serum concentrations are 0.4–1.4 times maternal concentrations. The mean neonatal serum concentration of butorphanol was not different from the mean maternal serum concentration of butorphanol, following a 1 or 2 mg intramuscular dose [15].

When opioid analgesia is required, as in any other painful situation, one should dose to effect and treat the underlying problem. It is also important to ensure that there are no other stresses and the patient has an environment that is comfortable, clean and at normal ambient temperature.

B. Opioid Antagonism

When "overdose" or adverse effects of an opioid are noted after any surgical procedure required during pregnancy, reversal by titration with naloxone is effective. For cautious administration, combine naloxone (0.4 mg/mL) 0.1 mL or 0.25 mL (for larger animals) with 10 mL saline and titrate at 1 mL/min only until unwanted affects are eliminated; with this technique, the analgesia still persists. Do not administer by bolus injection, as this may precipitate hyperalgesia. The opioid adverse effects may outlast the naloxone, and re-dosing in the same manner may be required. Naloxone does not alter the transfer or clearance of morphine across the placenta; its effects are likely antagonistic by direct actions on fetal mu-receptors [16].

C. Non-Steroidal Anti-Inflammatory Analgesics (NSAIAs)

A study in women taking aspirin, other NSAIAs or acetaminophen for seven days or longer, during the first 20 weeks of gestation, showed an 80% miscarriage rate in those administered aspirin, or other NSAIAs, but not in those administered acetaminophen. Because acetaminophen has a different mechanism of action than other NSAIAs, this may be why miscarriage did not occur [17]. The 20 weeks of gestation in human beings may equate to approximately 4–5 weeks in dogs and cats. In addition, this class of analgesics should not be administered to pregnant animals, as several studies have demonstrated teratogenicity and development-interfering effects such as orofacial clefts, with NSAIA administration, especially during the first trimester, at which time much fetal organogenesis occurs. A renal embryopathy syndrome, which developed in babies when mothers were administered indomethacin for more than 48 h, has been recognized [18]. Other complications include transient renal insufficiency, which can decrease fetal urinary output and lead to oligohydramnios. Placental transfer of the NSAIAs may cause arrest of nephrogenesis in the fetus as cyclooxygenase -2 (COX-2) is essential for maturation of the embryologic kidney [18]. Fetal abnormalities in hemostasis that extend into the post-birth period predisposes the neonate to conditions such as intraventricular hemorrhage, and reduction in mesenteric blood flow predisposing to necrotizing enterocolitis. The NSAIAs block prostaglandin activity, which may result in cessation of labour and disruption of fetal circulation, and failure of closure of the ductus arteriosus (PDA), should they be administered during labour. However, even short-term use of NSAIAs in late pregnancy is associated with a substantial increase in the risk of premature ductal closure [19].

There are no studies specifically examining the safety or potential adverse effects of the more recently approved NSAIAs in veterinary medicine (e.g. meloxicam, carprofen, deracoxib, firocoxib, tolfenamic acid, ketoprofen, robenacoxib, grapiprant) to pregnant cats or dogs; however, the same effects are expected. "After pregnancy", following cesarean section, carprofen may be considered based on measured drug levels in cows' milk and a canine study investigating the presence of carprofen in breastmilk when administered at 2 mg/kg subcutaneously to Labrador retrievers immediately post-cesarean and continuing with 2 mg/kg PO q12h for six days [20]. A follow-up random retrospective study was carried out on 50 offspring of various canine breeds, delivered by cesarean section, suckling from dams given carprofen in the above protocol. The ages of these dogs ranged from five to 106 months with a median age of 33.4 months and an average age of 41.9 months. Serum creatinine on all subjects was within normal reference ranges [21]. No other veterinary NSAIA has been studied in this setting and all others have withdrawal times in dairy cattle; carprofen has no withdrawal time as none within analyzer range enters the milk. Refer to Chapter 24 for further information.

As COX-2 induction is necessary for ovulation and subsequent implantation of the embryo, should any breeding animal be experiencing a painful condition requiring an NSAIA, the owners should be instructed to spare breeding at this time and focus on managing the pain of the dog or cat.

Ketamine rapidly crosses the placenta to the fetus in animals and human beings [1]; however, no adverse effects have been observed during organogenesis and near term in rats, mice, rabbits and dogs [22]. Of concern, however, is that ketamine increases uterine tone and can potentially result in abortion [22], but this appears to be dose-dependent. Ketamine, an N-methyl-D-aspartate (NMDA) receptor antagonist, has become a useful adjunctive analgesic for severe pain in hospitalized patients. In this setting, it is necessary to administer ketamine as a continuous rate infusion (CRI) because of its short duration of action. There are no reports in the veterinary or human literature examining the effects on the mother or fetus at doses used in this setting (0.2–1.0 mg/kg/h). Based on ketamine's effect on uterine contractions and tone, the potential for maternal discomfort and miscarriage may be a concern with higher dosages. When administered at anesthetic dosages, no teratogenic or other adverse fetal effects have been observed in reproduction studies during organogenesis and near delivery with rats, mice, rabbits and dogs [1]. Doses of 2 mg/kg administered to mothers before delivery resulted in profound respiratory depression and increased muscle tone of the infant at birth. When lower dosages (>0.25–1.0 mg/kg) were used, these complications did not occur; however, the mother's uterine contractions increased. Dosages of 0.25 mg/kg are used in women without evidence of uterine contractions. Dosages of 2.2 mg/kg administered IV, resulted in a marked increase in uterine tone [1]. The effect of ketamine on intrauterine pressure varies depending on the stage of pregnancy. A 2 mg/kg intravenous dose of ketamine, given to women before termination of an 8-to 19-week pregnancy, greatly increased intrauterine pressure, intensity and frequency of contractions when compared to those prior to delivery, which are painful. This effect in companion animals is unknown. The higher doses resulted in increased maternal systolic and diastolic pressure, and the low doses had no effect on fetal blood pressure [1]. Neurobehavioural tests demonstrate that human infants are depressed for up to two days after high-dose ketamine administration peri-delivery. This same effect would be expected in companion animals and follows neonatal viability reported in puppies [23, 24]. During pregnancy, where multimodal analgesia including ketamine is required, dosages of up to and including 0.25 mg/kg appear to be safe. Ideal body weight is suggested; however, the weight details are not given in the various studies.

Alpha₂ adrenoceptor agonists: There are no published studies reporting on the use of medetomidine or dexmedetomidine clinically in dogs and cats during pregnancy and, therefore, they should not be administered.

Gabapentin is being prescribed more frequently for chronic and neuropathic pain conditions in veterinary patients. It is also used as part of a post-operative multi-modal analgesic regimen. The safety of prolonged gabapentin administration has not been reported in cats and dogs. In humans, the information pertains to women receiving gabapentin for seizure control and cluster headaches. Of the few reported studies, most report an incident of teratogenic change; however, gabapentin was not used alone; therefore, it is difficult to assess the absolute culprit. One study showed that the rates of maternal complication – cesarean section, miscarriage, low birth weight and malformation – were less than, or similar to, those seen in the general population or among women with epilepsy. Conclusions were that gabapentin exposure during pregnancy did not lead to an increased risk for adverse maternal and fetal events; because of the small number of patients examined in this study, additional data from more pregnancies and outcomes is needed [25]. However, for short-term analgesia, gabapentin appears safe. A case reported of a 24-year-old 732 kg (1,610 lb) pregnant Belgian draft horse mare developing neuropathy and signs of intractable pain following colic surgery. Following recovery, the mare had signs of femoral neuropathy involving the left hind limb. Within 36 h after recovery, the mare developed signs of severe pain that were unresponsive to conventional treatment. No GI tract or muscular abnormalities were found, and the discomfort was attributed to neuropathic pain. The mare was treated with gabapentin 2.5 mg/kg (1.1 mg/lb) PO q12h. Shortly after this treatment was initiated, the mare appeared comfortable and no longer had signs of pain. Treatment was continued for six days, during which the dosage was slowly decreased, and the mare was discharged. The mare subsequently delivered a healthy foal [26]. From this report, gabapentin appears to be a safe, effective and economical treatment for neuropathic pain in the horse and may also be in the cat and dog. The suggested starting of gabapentin in dogs and cats is 10 mg/kg q8h; however, as with other analgesics, an increase or decrease may be required based on the patient's response and the underlying problem being treated.

Pregabalin has been associated with an increased risk of major birth defects after first trimester exposure in women [27].

Amantadine is not recommended during pregnancy in women and should, therefore, be avoided in pregnant cats and dogs.

Local anesthetics are considered safe and non-teratogenic, and are highly recommended where appropriate. **Lidocaine** is able to cross the placenta, but it does not seem to have any adverse effect on pregnancy outcome. In prospective studies of more than 1200 pregnant women, there was no increase in major or minor anomalies [28]. Lidocaine is also used for epidural analgesia in labour to alleviate pain without affecting uterine contractions. It is also used to treat arrhythmias in pregnant women [29]. Although epidural anesthesia has been associated with rare abnormalities of neurobehavioural testing in the neonate in some studies, more recent studies have shown that such abnormalities are rare and, if occurring, they are mild or transient. None has been reported in veterinary patients. Should systemic lidocaine be considered in a multi-modal regimen to manage severe pain in dogs (not to be used in cats), the patient should be observed closely. Based on reports in human medicine where numbness of the tongue and oral cavity have been reported, and personal observation of nausea at ~24h, it is advised to restrict the infusion to a few hours to avoid vomiting. Where epidural lidocaine is planned, the dose should be reduced as the spread and depth of the local anesthetic is greater in pregnant patients. See Section V.E.1.

D. Amitriptyline [1, 30]

Amitriptyline is recommended as an adjunct, or alone, for neuropathic pain in veterinary patients. It is listed in the US FDA pregnancy risk category C. Nortriptyline, is **pregnancy** category D, which is confusing because nortriptyline is the active metabolite of amitriptyline. This is based on animal reproduction studies showing an adverse effect on the fetus at high dosages. There are no adequate and well-controlled studies in humans, but there is no evidence of human fetal risk. The information from the National Teratology Information Service states that epidemiological studies have shown no evidence that therapeutic doses of tricyclic antidepressants are associated with an increased incidence of birth defects. Chronic use, or the use of high doses near term, has been associated with neonatal withdrawal symptoms in some cases. If amitriptyline is required throughout pregnancy, it is recommended that the dose be tapered 3–4 weeks prior to delivery to reduce the likelihood of neonatal withdrawal symptoms. Cardiac problems, irritability, respiratory distress, muscle spasms, seizures and urinary retention have been reported in infants whose mothers received tricyclic antidepressants immediately prior to delivery. Limb deformities and developmental delay have been reported in infants whose mothers had taken this drug during pregnancy. In humans, amitriptyline and imipramine are the recommended drugs of choice for the treatment of depression during pregnancy, based on the length of time that they have been in use and the cumulative data on their lack of fetotoxicity.

Amitriptyline would be the drug of choice for neuropathic pain. Based on the lack of adverse effects in general, compared with imipramine in humans, amitriptyline is the drug of choice in veterinary patients. Refer to Chapter 12 for more information.

E. Herbal Analgesic Medications

Due to a lack of information of the use of this class in dogs and cats, and potential concerns for some, herbal analgesic medications should be avoided.

F. Non-Pharmacologic Methods

Where dystocia resulted in injury, or episiotomy was performed, to reduce swelling apply cold compresses to the area following delivery, and for the next 2–3 days.

G. Conclusion

Other than the NSAIAs and pregabalin, analgesics used in therapeutic doses for acute and chronic pain in humans appear to be relatively safe during pregnancy. Unfortunately, similar studies have not been performed in cats and dogs.

III.   Anesthesia during Pregnancy

A.   General Considerations

In most instances, anesthesia will be undertaken only for an emergency situation in a pregnant dog or cat, including a cesarean section. Hence, prompt anesthetic drug decisions will have to be made by the veterinarian in addition to detail and management of specific anesthetic considerations associated with the pregnancy. Owners should be made aware that there is the potential for a spontaneous abortion when anesthesia is required for a non-obstetrical procedure. In women, the incidence of spontaneous abortion is increased when anesthesia is required during the first trimester of pregnancy. However, there is no increased risk of congenital abnormalities [30]. The main finding in humans is a lower birth weight. Comparable studies are not available in dogs and cats. In pregnant mares with colic, an increased rate of abortion of up to 50% was found when mares were treated medically and 20% abortion rate in those with surgery [31]. In mares undergoing surgical management of the colic, hypotension increased the risk of abortion. Hence, it is likely that the incidence of hypotension, hypoxemia and the disease itself has a greater impact on the loss of the fetus than the specific anesthetic agents themselves in these cases. The overall anesthetic management and monitoring are key to fetal viability.

B.   Specific Anesthetic Considerations with Pregnancy

1.   MAC Requirements

Elevated progesterone levels associated with pregnancy have been shown to reduce the MAC (minimum alveolar concentration) of inhalants by up to 40% [32]. The depth of anesthesia should be adjusted accordingly to each individual animal for the required procedure with attention to an appropriate depth. Ventilation may require assistance to deliver the inhalant to the dam and maintain an adequate anesthetic depth from the enlarged uterus and reduced functional residual capacity in the lungs. Without assisted ventilation, the MAC reduction of pregnancy may not be realized on the vaporizer setting alone.

2.   Anesthetic Effects on the Cardio-Respiratory Systems

Attention to anesthetic depth and maintenance of optimal cardio-respiratory variables are especially important in the pregnant dog and cat. When an animal is anesthetized, a reduction in cardiovascular function such as cardiac output, myocardial contractility, bradycardia and hypotension is possible, especially with excessive anesthetic depth. These negative effects can alter blood flow and oxygen delivery to all organs, including the uterus. Excessive depth and negative cardio-respiratory effects of the dam will also impact the fetus.

Adequate blood flow and oxygenation to organs is also impacted by the weight of the gravid uterus itself. This is very important in small animals as cats and dogs have a higher weight of the uterus in proportion to the dam's weight (13–16%, respectively), compared to women (5%). With anesthesia and positioning in lateral or especially dorsal recumbency, the weight impact of the uterus on the diaphragm and vena cava significantly reduces the efficiency of both the respiratory and cardiovascular functions. Assistance to ventilation is always required with mid- to late-term pregnancies because of this weight. Higher inspiratory pressures (of even up to 15–20 cmH$_2$O) will be required to expand the lungs during each breath, especially in dorsal recumbency. Venous return to the right side of the heart will also be negatively impacted by the weight of the uterus on the vascular structures in lateral or dorsal recumbency. These higher inspiratory pressures required in pregnancy will also hinder venous return to the heart. The veterinarian needs to be aware of these cardio-respiratory effects and monitor effectively with the ability to intervene as required.

3. Teratogenicity

When anesthesia is required in the pregnant animal, avoidance of teratogenic anesthetic drugs is necessary. The two main reportedly teratogenic anesthetic agents in humans are nitrous oxide and repeated use of benzodiazepines (midazolam and diazepam). Nitrous oxide is listed as an X for classification and should not be used during pregnancy. Both diazepam and midazolam are listed as level D for risk, with reports of neural tube and cardiac defects, and a higher incidence of cleft palate formation with chronic prolonged usage or high dosages during pregnancy. Anesthesia itself of women during pregnancy is not reported to increase the chance of congenital defects in infants [30]. Comparable teratogenic reports are not available in companion animals. The teratogenic effects of single doses of either midazolam or diazepam (0.2–0.3 mg/kg) as sedation or with the primary induction agent are unknown for final organ development in the to-term puppy or kitten.

4. Placental Blood Barrier

Large quaternary ammonium drugs do not cross the placenta. For anesthetic management, these drugs are the anticholinergic glycopyrrolate, the depolarizing muscle relaxant succinyl-choline and a non-depolarizing muscle relaxant class of drugs: atracurium/cisatracurium. All other sedatives and anesthetic agents, including inhalant anesthetics, cross the placenta. Glycopyrrolate administration during anesthetic management would not cause fetal tachyar-rhythmia, but would also not treat fetal bradycardia.

IV. Anesthesia Protocols

A. Non-Obstetrical Procedures

In these anesthetic situations, the dam will be responsible for metabolizing the anesthetic drugs. The focus of the anesthetic management is related to the needs of the individual patient, surgical requirements and duration, as well as maintaining normal cardio-respiratory function of the dam. The balance of normal cardio-respiratory function will be imperative to maintain uterine perfusion, fetal viability and prevent an abortion. If anesthesia is required for an emergency situation then stability of the dam prior to the anesthetic event is imperative. As with all other emergency situations, an assessment of hydration status, blood loss and analgesic requirements must be made, as well as baseline laboratory tests to evaluate organ function, acid-base and electrolyte status.

B. Sedation and Pre-Medication for Non-Cesarean Procedures (Refer to Chapter 9, 10 and 13)

Opioids are the main class of pre-medicants used for pregnant cats and dogs undergoing non-cesarean anesthetic events. The opioid should be based on the duration and type of surgical procedure being initiated (see Anesthesia sections in the relevant scenario chapters).

Acepromazine can be used for sedation in a stable animal that is pregnant; however, lower doses should be used (0.01–0.03 mg/kg). Higher doses may lower blood pressure in the dam when combined with inhalant anesthetics, promoting hypotension and a reduction in uterine blood flow. Hypotension would likely be most prevalent in a sick unstable pregnant patient, hence acepromazine should be withheld or reserved for mild sedation post-operatively upon recovery in a very anxious patient versus pre-medication.

Alpha$_2$ adrenoceptor agonist use during pregnancy, specifically dexmedetomidine, is controversial in pregnant cats and dogs. Use of xylazine in cattle in late-term pregnancy has been reported to cause abortion, presumably due to alteration in uterine blood flow and xylazine-induced oxytocin like effects and increase in myometrial contractility [33]. Fetal death is likely due to hypoxia from prolonged constriction of blood vessels in the myometrium and placenta from the alpha$_2$-induced intrauterine hypertensive effects. Detomidine has not been reported to have the same uterine effects in cattle [34]. In addition, the administration of small doses of detomidine in pregnant cows [32] and clinical doses of medetomidine in pregnant dogs [35] leads to a decrease in myometrial contractility without abortions. Therefore, the uterine effect of drugs stimulating the α-adrenoceptors depends to a high degree on the level of steroid hormones. That is, an increased level of estrogen increases the sensitivity of the alpha adrenoceptors while a high level of progesterone during pregnancy stimulates the sensitivity of beta adrenoceptors and actually decreases the contractility of the uterus [36]. No studies have been reported related to the effects of alpha$_2$ agonists on the feline uterus. Due to the lack of supporting evidence for use, medetomidine and dexmedetomidine are not recommended for use in breeding or pregnant dogs and cats. The pharmaceutical company also has pregnancy as a contraindication for dexmedetomidine use. This may largely be due to the unknown potential for abortion and the alterations in cardiovascular function, which may impact uterine blood flow.

C. Anesthetic Induction for Non-Cesarean Procedures

Induction options are as follows:

- **Propofol:** 2–4 mg/kg, IV to effect. The initial bolus amount may be reduced to 1 mg/kg when used with co-induction agents or in a depressed, sick patient.
- **Alfaxalone:** 1–3 mg/kg, IV to effect. The initial bolus amount may be reduced to 0.5 mg/kg when used with co-induction agents or in a depressed, sick patient.

Ketamine benzodiazepine combinations can be used if no other alternative is available. However, midazolam and diazepam are seen as teratogenic risk D level, or high (see above). Information for companion animals is unknown and, based on the human literature, a single use is not contraindicated. As stated above, ketamine at doses of 2.2 mg/kg induced intrauterine contractions, which were uncomfortable in women. The dose for induction of ketamine in cats and dogs is 5–10 mg/kg with the mL/kg mixtures of ketamine benzodiazepines when combined as equal parts (1:1) titrated to effect. Similar effects in veterinary medicine are unknown. However, it is assumed that this would occur, especially at induction dosages. Propofol or alfaxalone are preferred for non-obstetrical anesthesia based on the above concerns.

Mask induction with inhalant anesthetics is not recommended by this author when other alternatives are available. Disadvantages of mask induction are related to the stress/excitement phase, increased potential for vomiting with pregnancy, and reduced respiratory reserve in the dam with the increasing uterine size.

V. Anesthesia for Cesarean Section

The dam will be responsible for metabolism of some of the anesthetic and sedative drugs administered; however, some will cross the placenta. Once the puppies or kittens are removed, any anesthetic drugs remaining will require metabolism and exhalation in the newborn or the appropriate reversal agent to improve their viability and survival. With this in mind, the anesthetics used for cesarean section should be of (1) short duration, (2) reversible and (3) without any negative cardio-respiratory side effects. The last is not possible with anesthetic agents when administered at surgical maintenance levels; however, the veterinarian should be familiar with proper dosing and the expected negative cardio-respiratory effects and be prepared for appropriate supportive management of the dam and neonate.

A. Sedation and Pre-Medication for Cesarean Section

Pre-medication to reduce the dam's stress and anxiety associated with IV catheterization, pre-anesthetic examination and pre-oxygenation is warranted. In addition, effective pre-medication will reduce the injectable induction agent as well as the inhalant anesthetic for a balanced anesthetic approach and potentially improved neonatal viability. Opioids, especially the mu-agonists, will provide preemptive analgesia and also assist in lowering the induction and inhalant anesthetic dose. However, the pure mu-agonists with a longer duration of action (4h) will also have a prolonged sedative effect in the neonate after delivery, approximately double that of the dam, which will require monitoring and reversal for hours afterwards. Beyond the immediate sedative effects, the administration of opioids prior to delivery has not been shown to adversely affect the outcome of puppies [23]. If opioids have been administered to the dam and the offspring are bradycardic or appear sedate, naloxone (one drop) can be administered sublingually or via the umbilical vein.

The dam should be considered to have a full stomach resulting from overall decreased GI motility, physical displacement of the stomach from the enlarged uterus and the effects of progesterone delaying gastric emptying and lower esophageal sphincter pressure. For this reason, if opioids are given pre-operatively, those that are least likely to induce vomiting (e.g. fentanyl, methadone and meperidine) may be warranted if available. Hydromorphone may induce vomiting. However, it can still be used if most readily available. Buprenorphine and butorphanol will not induce vomiting; however, they do not provide an ideal level of analgesia for cesarean section in this author's opinion. The class of the opioid should always be considered related to the necessary analgesia. Where buprenorphine or butorphanol are used, a higher than recommended dose of a pure mu-agonist may be required to manage post-operative pain in the dam, and reversal of buprenorphine and butorphanol in puppies or kittens upon delivery will require higher repeated dosing of naloxone.

Acepromazine is generally not necessary for sedation unless the dam is very anxious. It is not reversible and, due to its alpha$_1$ antagonism, it will promote hypotension in combination with the inhalants, dorsal recumbency and impact of the uterine weight on venous return. Lowered doses of acepromazine (see below) may be acceptable in very anxious dams. Older drugs such as xylazine and methoxyflurane are associated with an increase in maternal and/or neonatal mortality [23]. Comparable information of dexmedetomidine and medetomidine are not available. Considering the negative cardiovascular side effects of medetomidine or dexmedetomidine, both should be avoided in cesarean sections.

B. Pre-Medication Options for Cesarean Sections

- **Meperidine** is a mu-agonist of short duration and does not cause vomiting. It also has a reduced incidence of panting. Although some reports suggest meperidine could be given IV slowly, it does induce a greater histamine release after IV injection than morphine and is not recommend IV use. Duration of action, cat and dog: 0.5–2h.
  - Dog: 5–10 mg/kg, IM
  - Cat: 3–5 mg/kg, IM, SC.
- **Fentanyl.** Duration of action 0.5–1h depending on the dose and route.
  - Cat and dog: 2–10 μg/kg, IV
  - An initial bolus of 2–5 μg/kg should be given IV; this dose could be repeated
  - 5–15 μg/kg, IM, SC.
- **Methadone** is a mu-agonist and has beneficial NMDA-antagonist properties. It has the advantage of not causing vomiting. Duration of action, cat and dog: 3–4h.
  - Dog: 0.3–0.5 mg/kg, IM or IV
  - Cat: 0.3–0.5 mg/kg, IM, IV.

- **Hydromorphone**. Duration of action: 3–4h.
  - Cat and dog: 0.02–0.05 mg/kg, IM, SC or IV.

1. Anesthetic Induction

Prior to induction, pre-oxygenation is always recommended in the dam. The physiologic effects of pregnancy make pregnant cats and dogs more likely to develop hypoxemia during the induction process due to their higher oxygen requirement and reduction in the functional residual capacity of the lungs. Pregnant animals require a rapid sequence of induction to allow control of the airway and prevent aspiration of contents from a full stomach. Endotracheal intubation is always warranted to protect the dam's airway from aspiration, deliver oxygen with the inhalant and assist ventilation.

2. Neonatal Vitality

In one study [24] respiratory rate (RR) and neurologic reflexes of puppies were compared after the dam received ketamine/midazolam, thiopentone, propofol induction agents or an epidural local anesthetic. The RR was higher after epidural anesthesia, and neurologic reflexes were best after epidural, followed by propofol, thiopentone and ketamine/midazolam. Moon also reports that although ketamine did not increase puppy mortality it decreased the vigour of newborn puppies; therefore, resuscitation efforts should be anticipated if ketamine is used [23]. There was no difference in survival between puppies whose dams received propofol or alfaxalone [37]. However, this one report demonstrates puppy vitality to be better with alfaxalone compared to propofol. No data is available to assess and compare the anesthetic drugs related to vigour in kittens following cesarean sections.

C. Anesthetic Induction for Cesarean Sections

Induction options
- **Propofol:** 2–4 mg/kg, IV to effect. The initial bolus amount may be reduced to 1 mg/kg in a depressed, sick patient.
- **Alfaxalone:** 1–3 mg/kg, IV to effect. The initial bolus amount may be reduced to 0.5 mg/kg in a depressed, sick patient.

Co-induction with midazolam or diazepam before or after the propofol or alfaxalone is not recommended for cesarean sections unless flumazenil is available as the benzodiazepines will add to sedation of the neonate and increased muscle relaxation. If neither propofol nor alfaxalone is available, ketamine–benzodiazepine combinations could be considered. However, attention and support of the puppies and kittens after delivery is required due to the likelihood of decreased vigour. Ketamine is not reversible and will contribute significantly to the respiratory depression in the neonate. Flumazenil, if available, could be given to the puppies or kittens (one drop sublingually) if ketamine–benzodiazepine combinations were necessary.

D. Anesthetic Maintenance for Non-Obstetrical or Cesarean Sections

Maintenance of general anesthesia with an inhalant is preferred compared to total intravenous anesthesia (TIVA). Maintenance with propofol or alfaxalone TIVA is possible; however, a recent comparison of alfaxalone TIVA with isoflurane demonstrated that recovery was faster, and the vitality of the puppies was better, with isoflurane versus alfaxalone. There was no difference in the overall puppy survival [38].

Inhalant anesthesia with isoflurane or sevoflurane is appropriate and both have similar effects on the maternal/fetal unit in sheep [32]. Isoflurane requires less metabolism (0.2%) compared to sevoflurane (5%). However, sevoflurane with a lower blood gas partition co-efficient has a faster recovery in sheep, in both the dam and the neonate, offering advantages which would also be expected in companion animals. At delivery, once the neonate begins to breathe, the inhalant will be exhaled. It is important to note that the initial 5–10 min of resuscitation efforts required for the depressed neonate is for the large part a result of the inhalant and any pre-medication, if propofol or alfaxalone has been used.

Regardless of the maintenance agent, appropriate monitoring and maintenance of depth, to prevent extremes in depth, is essential to avoid significant fluctuations in uterine blood flow.

E.   Local Anesthetic Techniques

Incisional line blocks provide supplemental analgesia and are recommended for cesarean sections. This should be administered pre-incisional as well as post-operatively, depending on the duration of surgery. The local anesthetic, or combination, used will depend on the timing of administration and surgery.

- Local anesthetic dosages: General rule = 0.2 mL/kg with concentrations noted below.
- Total dose of lidocaine (2%): 2–4 mg/kg; onset 5–10 min; duration ≈ 1 h.
- Total dose of bupivacaine (0.5%): 1 mg/kg; onset 20–30 min; duration ≈ 4 h.

When local anesthetics are combined, each dose should be halved, as toxicity is additive.

1.   Epidural Analgesia

Epidural anesthesia (refer to Chapter 14) can be used to support the anesthetic protocol and reduce inhalant levels required as well as provide analgesia. The epidural should be performed efficiently, however, and not delay the cesarean section. Few to no canine patients will remain calm for a cesarean section in dorsal recumbency without general anesthesia and unconsciousness. However, epidural administration of morphine, 0.1 mg/kg, can be administered pre- or post-operatively to supplement systemically administered analgesia, and provide up to 18–20 h of analgesia for the dam. This volume of morphine can be mixed with sterile saline to achieve a final volume of 1 mL/7 kg to a maximum of 6 mL. The total volume administered epidurally to the pregnant animal is less due to venous engorgement of epidural vessels, a smaller space and a greater potential for anterior spread of the local. Once administered epidurally, onset of morphine action takes approximately 60 min; therefore, to minimize the sedative and respiratory depressant effects of the morphine in the neonate, it is ideal to complete the cesarean section prior to this. There is controversy related to administering a local anesthetic epidurally in the dam as hind end paralysis, or weakness, in recovery could distress the dam or cause harm to the neonates if she falls. Administration of lidocaine epidurally (1 mL/7 kg to a maximum of 6 mL) would be the preferred local anesthetic for a cesarean section due to shorter duration of action. Local anesthetics can be combined with morphine for epidural injection.

F.   Post-Cesarean Management

1.   Neonate

If the puppies or kittens are depressed after delivery and not responding to appropriate post-delivery care of rubbing and warming, a drop of naloxone placed sublingually should reverse these effects; however, repeat dosing may be required. Repeated dosing of naloxone is more likely to be required if the dam is sedated with butorphanol or buprenorphine. Naloxone will reverse butorphanol's K-agonist effects, but a higher dose may be required. In addition, repeated naloxone doses sublingually may be necessary to offset buprenorphine's partial mu-agonist receptor binding efficacy.

If continual re-narcotization in the newborn is a concern with discharge from the clinic, the owner should be given instructions on sublingual administration of a drop of naloxone dispensed in a tuberculin syringe. Other potential causes for perioperative depression must be considered if the cesarean section was not routine.

2. Dam

Controversy exists related to the administration of NSAIAs to the dam pre- or post-operatively in regards to neonatal renal maturation and potential negative effects of the NSAIA. Information exists related to the safety of carprofen 2 mg/kg PO q12h for six days in dogs post-cesarean without an impact on the neonatal renal maturation and uterine involution in the dam [20, 21]. Carprofen measured in breastmilk was below analyser range [20] (refer to Chapter 24 for details and supporting study). Currently, there is no information on NSAIA administration in cats.

Opioids are given post-operatively to the dam after a cesarean section. In most cases without complications, the opioid is switched to buprenorphine (0.02–0.04 mg/kg) from the pure mu-agonist initially chosen. Post-operative pain control requirements of the dam should be evaluated on a case-by-case basis.

References

1 Briggs, G. G., Freeman, R. K. and Yaffe, S. J. (2011) *Drugs in Pregnancy and Lactation*, 9th edn. Lippincott Williams and Wilkins, Philadelphia.

2 Wunsch, M. J., Stanard, V. and Schnoll, S. H. (2003) Treatment of pain in pregnancy. *Clin J Pain*, 19(3): 148–155.

3 Ward, R. (1989) Maternal-placental-fetal unit: Unique problems of pharmacologic study. *Pediatr Clin North Am*, 36: 1075–88.

4 Papich, M. G. and Davis, L. E. (1986) Drug therapy during pregnancy and in the neonate. *Vet Clin North Am Small Anim Pract*, 16(3): 525–538.

5 Johnston, S. D., Root Kustritz, M. V. and Olson, P. (1995) *Canine and Feline Theriogenology.* W B Saunders, Philadelphia.

6 Pascoe, P. J. (2000) Perioperative pain management. *Vet Clin North Am Small Anim Pract*, 30(4): 917–932.

7 Di Giulio, A. M., Tenconi, B., Malosio, M. L., *et al.* (1995) Perinatal morphine: I: Effects on synapsin and neurotransmitter systems in the brain. *J Neurosci Res*, 42: 479–485.

8 Ferreira, T. H., Rezende, M. L., Mama, K. R., *et al.* (2011) Plasma concentrations, behavioural and antinociceptive and physiological effects of methadone after intravenous and transmucosal administration in cats. *Am J Vet Res*, 72(6): 764–771.

9 Loftus, J. R., Hill, H. and Cohen, S. (1995) Placental transfer and neonatal effects of epidural sufentanil and fentanyl administered with bupivacaine during labor. *Anesthesiology*, 83: 300–308.

10 Regan, J., Chambers, F., Gorman, W. and MacSullivan, R. (2000) Neonatal abstinence syndrome due to prolonged administration of fentanyl in pregnancy. *BJOG*, 107(4): 570–572.

11 Einarson, A., Bozzo, P. and Taguchi, N. (2009) Use of a fentanyl patch throughout pregnancy. *J Obstet Gynaecol Can*, 31(1): 20.

12 Ko, C. (2006) Biliary sludge and acute pancreatitis during pregnancy. *Nature Clinical Practice: Gastroenterology & hepatology*, 3(1): 53–57.

13 Fischer, G., Rolley, J. E., Eder, H., *et al.* (2000) Treatment of opioid-dependent pregnant women with buprenorphine. *Addiction*, 95: 239–244.

14 Nanovskaya, T., Deshmukh, S., Brooks, M., *et al.* (2002) Transplacental transfer and metabolism of buprenorphine. *J Pharmacol Exp Ther*, 300(1): 26–33.

15 Pittman, K. A., Smyth, R. D., Losada, M., *et al.* (1980) Human perinatal distribution of butorphanol. *Am J Obstet Gynecol*, 138: 797–800.

16 Kopecky, E. A., Sione, C., Knie, B., *et al.* (1999) Transfer of morphine across the human placenta and its interaction with naloxone, *Life Sci*, 65(22): 2359–2371.

17 De-Kun, L. L. and Odouli, R. (2003) Exposure to non-steroidal anti-inflammatory drugs during pregnancy and risk of miscarriage: Population based cohort study. *BMJ*, 327: 368–373.

18 Drukker, A. (2002) The adverse renal effects of prostaglandin synthesis inhibition in the fetus and the newborn. *Paediatr Child Health*, 7(8): 538–543.

19 Koren, G., Florescu, A., Costei, A. M., *et al.* (2006) Nonsteroidal anti-inflammatory drugs during third trimester and the risk of premature closure of the ductus arteriosus: A meta-analysis. *Ann Pharmacother*, 40(5): 824–829.

20 Escobar, S. R. (2010) Carprofen exposure via lactation in canine neonates post caesarian section. SFT/ACT Annual Conference Track 2.

21 Escobar, S. R. (2016) *Carprofen exposure via lactation in canine neonates post-caesarian section: Follow-up.* Proceedings for the Society for Theriogenology, September, 8(3): 191.

22 Oats, J. N., Vasey, D. P. and Waldron, B. A. (1979) Effects of ketamine on the pregnant uterus. *Br J Anaesth*, 51: 11636.

23 Moon, P. F., Erb, H. N., Ludders, J. W., *et al.* (2000) Perioperative risk factors for puppies delivered by cesarean section in the United States and Canada. *J Am Anim Hosp Assoc.* 36(4): 359–368.

24 Luna, S. P., Cassu, R. N., Castro, G. B., *et al.* (2004) Effects of four anaesthetic protocols on the neurological and cardiorespiratory variables of puppies born by caesarean section. *Vet Rec*, 154(13): 387–389.

25 Montouris, G. (2003) Gabapentin exposure in human pregnancy: Results from the Gabapentin Pregnancy Registry. *Epilepsy and Behavior*, 4(3): 310–317.

26 Davis, J. L., Posner, L. P. and Elce, Y. (2007) Gabapentin for the treatment of neuropathic pain in a pregnant horse. *J Am Vet Med Assoc*, 231(5): 755–758.

27 Winterfeld, U., Merlob, P. and Baud, D. (2016) Pregnancy outcome following maternal exposure to pregabalin may call for concern. *Neurology*, 86(24): 2251–2257.

28 Jürgens, T. P., Schaefer, C. and May. A. (2009) Treatment of cluster headache in pregnancy and lactation. *Cephalalgia*, 29: 391–400.

29 Lalkhen, A. and Grady, K. (2008) Non-obstetric pain in pregnancy. *Reviews in Pain*, 1(2): 10–14.

30 Allaert, S. E., Carlier, S. P., Weyne, L. P., *et al.* (2007) First trimester anesthesia exposure and fetal outcome: A review. *Acta Anaesthesiol Belg*, 58(2): 119–123.

31 Chenier, T. S. and Whitehead, A. E. (2009) Foaling rates and risk factors for abortion in pregnant mares presented for medical or surgical treatment of colic, 153 cases (1993–2005). *Can Vet J*, 50: 481–485.

32 Okutomi, T., Whittington, R., Stein, D. and Hisayo, M. (2009) Comparison of the effects of sevoflurane and isoflurane anesthesia on the maternal-fetal unit in sheep. *J Anesth*, 23: 392–398.

33 Jedruch, J. and Gajewski, Z. (1986) The effect of detomidine hydrochloride on the electrical activity of the uterus in cows. *Acta Vet Scand*, 82 (suppl.): 198–192.

34 Jedruch, J., Gajewski, Z. and Ratajska-Michalczak, K. (1989) Uterine motor responses to an α_2-adrenergic agonist medetomidine hydrochloride in the bitches during the end of gestation and the post-partum period. *Acta Vet Scand*, 85: 129–134.

35 Leblanc, M. M., Hubbell, J. A. E. and Smith, H C. (1984) The effect of xylazine hydrochloride in intrauterine pressure in the cow and the mare. *Proceedings of the Ann Meeting Soc Theriogenol*, 148: 386.

36 Rexroad, C. E. and Barb, C. R. (1978) Contractile response of the uterus of the estrous ewe to adrenergic stimulation. *Biol Repro*, 19: 297–305.

37 Doebeli, A., Bettschart, M. E., Hartnak, R. and Reichler, I. M. (2013) Apgar score after induction of anesthesia for canine Cesarean section with alfaxalone versus propofol. *Theriogenology*, 80(8): 850–854.

38 CondeRuiz, C., Del Carro, A. P., Rosset, E., *et al.* (2016) Alfaxalone for total intravenous anesthesia in bitches undergoing elective caesarean section and its effects on puppies: A randomized clinical trial. *Vet Anaesth Analg*, 43(3): 281–290.

24

Analgesia and Anesthesia for Nursing Cats and Dogs
Karol Mathews, Tamara Grubb, Melissa Sinclair and Andrea Steele

Nursing cats and dogs will benefit from ongoing analgesia post-cesarean, or to manage post-surgical or traumatic pain or inflammatory illness. However, there are no veterinary clinical studies published on the use of commonly prescribed human and veterinary analgesics in this group of cats and dogs; therefore, it is difficult to make evidence-based recommendations. The concerns are related to the transfer of the administered analgesic through the milk to the puppy or kitten and potential negative effects on the offspring. The veterinary product monographs state that "no studies have been conducted to evaluate use in lactating cats and dogs". It is important for the clinician to realize that the information currently available, and presented here, is restricted to human and laboratory animal studies, and information obtained from drug levels in cows' milk with some extrapolation to cats and dogs. An unpublished study in dogs is discussed. Some of the information available is conflicting and based on acute, perinatal pain management. There is very little published on non-acute or non-perinatal pain management in breastfeeding human mothers, with most chronic use published in the addiction literature, and nothing in the veterinary literature. It is hoped that future studies investigating the commonly prescribed analgesics, including the secretion of analgesics in milk of lactating dogs and cats, will be undertaken to offer guidance in managing this group of animals.

In human medicine, it is generally accepted that, for drugs without significant toxicity in the infant, a relative infant dose (RID) of < 10% of the weight-adjusted therapeutic dose is unlikely to cause harm to a full-term infant [1, 2]. The RID is calculated by dividing the infant's dose, obtained from the milk, in mg/kg/day, by the mother's dose in mg/kg/day. Using this calculation, a weight-normalized dose is determined that the baby may receive, which has been determined to be more accurate than when the weight of the mother and the baby are not taken into account [1]. It is estimated that the neonate receives approximately 1–2% of the maternal dose of a drug that is approved for use during breastfeeding [2]. High lipid solubility, low molecular weight, low protein binding and the non-ionized state are characteristics of a drug which would facilitate secretion into milk [2]. However, other rare transporters may also influence drug passage against a "normal" gradient. The fat and protein content of dog and cat milk is higher than other species' milk, whereas human and cows' milk is similar [3]. Dogs' colostrum is similar to humans' in that the fat content is lower and protein content is higher than that of "mature" milk. The pH of milk is not known in dogs; however, in humans the pH approaches that of plasma [2]. Also, the volume of colostrum is lower than "mature" milk. With these characteristics, less analgesic will be partitioned into the colostrum, which is produced during the first few days after birth in humans [2] but may vary between 12 and 24 h in dogs; not known in cats. If colostrum's characteristics are true for cats and dogs, the presence of an opioid

Analgesia and Anesthesia for the Ill or Injured Dog and Cat, First Edition. Karol A. Mathews, Melissa Sinclair, Andrea M. Steele and Tamara Grubb.

required peri- and post-cesarean will be low in colostrum. Drug characteristics are given with each class of analgesics below and calculations for transfer into breastmilk for some of the opioids used in veterinary medicine can be found in [4].

I. Analgesics

For dosing and drug details, refer to Chapters 9, 10, 11 and 13.

A. Opioids

Opioids circulate through the mammary gland/milk, and the general circulation, resulting in peak and trough levels in the milk. Opioids are administered peri-cesarean [5], with potential for a minimal amount to enter the colostrum; however, concerns for this have not been reported in cats and dogs. See below for the individual opioid's transfer into milk. For the majority the levels are low, and oral absorption of opioids in dogs is extremely low or may not be absorbed at all. However, as this has not been researched in cats and dogs, allowing suckling to occur after peak levels of the drug have waned and immediately prior to repeat administration is advised. Rather than withhold opioid analgesic therapy due to a potential concern for the puppies and kittens, administer the opioid in this manner with very frequent observation of behaviour. Recommendations are based on this approach. Should lack of vigour or respiratory depression occur in puppies or kittens, attributed to opioid administration to the dam, one-drop of naloxone (0.4 mg/mL) under the tongue, with further titration to effect if required, will reverse adverse effects.

The lipid solubility of the opioid influences its appearance in the milk; meperidine > sufentanil > buprenorphine, butorphanol and nalbuphine > fentanyl > methadone > hydromorphone ≥ oxymorphone > morphine; therefore, a less hydrophilic opioid, such as hydromorphone or morphine, appears in a smaller amount than a more lipid-soluble opioid, such as meperidine. When a continuous rate analgesic infusion is required after cesarean section, fentanyl is frequently used.

- **Hydromorphone HCl** distributes rapidly from plasma to human breastmilk but partitions into fat; protein binding is minimal in milk and plasma [6]. The infant receives approximately 0.67% of the maternal dose, which is well below that used to treat human neonates and is unlikely to have a deleterious effect [6], and anecdotally appears clinically safe in dogs and cats.
- **Methadone** is prescribed for human mothers, predominantly reported in the addiction literature, as there is low transfer into breastmilk [7–9]. If it is distributed to the milk of nursing mothers, methadone is not absorbed orally in dogs [10]; therefore, there should not be a problem with absorption in puppies following oral or parenteral administration to the dam, especially when suckling occurs a few hours following injection. Methadone in cats may be administered at 0.6 mg/kg oral transmucosal (OTM) for home management [11]. Based on human data, with low levels in breastmilk, kittens should not be, or minimally, affected.
- **Fentanyl** transfer into milk is low with < 0.01% detected in human breastmilk following parenteral administration in one study and an average of 0.033% in two other studies with a RID of < 3%; therefore, it is considered safe [6]. However, neither sufentanil nor fentanyl was detected in human breastmilk after epidural administration [12]. Epidural analgesia with local anesthetic, to reduce the post-operative pain associated with cesarean or vaginal/perineal injury/surgery, is recommended. An alternative, or as post-operative analgesia a fentanyl, continuous rate infusion (CRI), with careful titration to a minimal effective dose, is

suggested for cats and dogs. While measured levels of fentanyl in human breastmilk after a single dose are low [13], careful monitoring for neonatal effects is essential as this information is not known for cats and dogs. However, as an example of potential safety, a case report of a human patient requiring a transdermal fentanyl patch (100 μg/h) for four weeks reported that the mother's milk fentanyl level was 6.4 ng/mL with no measurable blood levels in the infant [14]. While searching for home care medication, fentanyl patch may be a method to consider; however, based on inconsistent absorption and up to 72 h to reach effective plasma levels in some dogs, and as puppies or kittens will be able to access the patch on the dam, it cannot be recommended. Transdermal fentanyl solution (Recuvyra®) should not be administered based on the strong warning in the product monograph that children should not contact the animal; this would also apply to puppies and kittens. At the time of writing, this product has recently been discontinued; however, it is not known whether this may be re-evaluated in the future. Should opioid analgesia be instituted, the owner must be prepared to remove puppies and kittens should there be evidence of sedation or poor suckling. Pumping and discarding the milk, and bottle feeding with milk replacer, is recommended at this point.

- **Oxymorphone** has been administered to dogs by the authors for perioperative orthopedic or soft-tissue pain following recommendations to avoid feeding during peak levels in the dam. The mothers were attentive and the puppies playful; no abnormalities were noted with the mother or puppies (Figure 24.1).
- **Morphine** levels are low in human breastmilk and potentially so in cats and dogs [15]. Oral morphine is not absorbed in dogs; therefore, the small amount reaching mother's milk would be of little concern [10]. There are no oral absorption studies in cats.
- **Meperidine (pethidine)**, based on human studies, is not recommended due to the amount reaching mother's milk causing heavy sedation in the infant and inability to suckle [15, 16]. In addition, cyanosis, bradycardia and the risk of apnea have been noted with intrapartum administration in humans [17, 18].
- **Butorphanol** information is inconsistent. Butorphanol was detected in the milk of lactating women following oral and intramuscular administration. Serum and milk concentrations

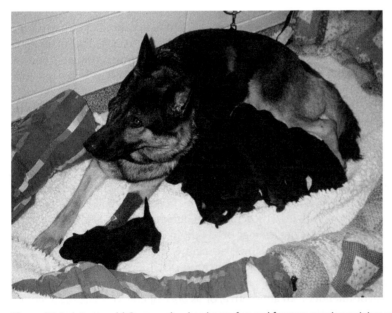

Figure 24.1 A 4-year-old German shepherd post-femoral fracture repair receiving oxymorphone analgesia.

appeared to be parallel with time. It was calculated that 4 μg would be the maximum amount of butorphanol, which would be expected to be present in the full daily milk output (1 L) following administration four times a day of 2 mg intramuscular or of 8 mg oral doses. An oral dose of 4 μg to an infant weighing 4 kg corresponds to the negligible oral dose of 0.7 mg to a 70 kg adult [19]. In another study, levels of butorphanol transferred into human milk were reported to be approximately 0.5% of the weight adjusted maternal dose. The conclusion of this study was that the minimal butorphanol content is probably of no concern to a breastfeeding neonate in the first week postpartum [15]. However, these recommendations are based on one study performed in humans where a single dose of butorphanol was used pre-delivery. There are no studies examining extended use in breastfeeding mothers. Based on information at hand, recommendations for humans are: "breast-feeding appears to be acceptable after a single maternal dose of butorphanol due to the low doses secreted in milk. No data exist on the possible effects on the infant after repeated administration, but as butorphanol is mainly excreted by the kidneys it cannot be excluded that detrimental effects may arise in the offspring after long term treatment" [20]. This would apply even more in dogs due to the delay in maturation of the kidney. Based on the current recommendations for single dose use in humans, transfer into breastmilk is assumed to be low in cats and dogs. While butorphanol is listed in some pre/post-operative protocols for cesarean section in veterinary patients [21] it is only effective for mild painful conditions. A veterinary case report using butorphanol as pre-medication in a Golden retriever prior to surgical repair of a peritoneopericardial diaphragmatic hernia, and again seven days later prior to cesarean section, found no adverse effects in the puppies at birth. Unfortunately, post-operative analgesia was not reported [22]. The use of butorphanol during labour in women has been reported to produce sinusoidal fetal heart rate patterns and irritability in newborns [15].

- **Buprenorphine** may be an appropriate choice for mild to moderate pain; however, information regarding milk production is inconsistent [23–25]. Buprenorphine enters the milk of human mothers in low levels and risk versus benefit is assessed with benefits outweighing risks. Previous reports in laboratory animals noted a reduction in, or lack of, milk production. This was not specifically mentioned in a later human study that notes suppressed breastfeeding in human infants with a significant decrease in milk fed and subsequent decrease in weight gain [23]. A more recent human report comparing bupivacaine and buprenorphine to bupivacaine alone also notes that the neonates consumed slightly less milk when compared to the control neonates [24]. There is no comment as to whether this was due to reduced production. The relative dose of buprenorphine per kg infant body weight was less than 1% of the body weight of the mother and no known adverse effects on infants has been reported; however, it is recommended that infants be monitored closely [24]. Of the case studies reported regarding buprenorphine and breastfeeding, all include small numbers of participants and contain conflicting data. All, however, concur that the amounts of buprenorphine in human milk are small and unlikely to have negative effects on the developing infant. A review of the human addiction literature concludes that a buprenorphine-maintained mother's breastmilk does not appear to place her infant at risk of experiencing adverse effects [25]. No known neonatal- or child-adverse consequences related to exposure to buprenorphine in breastmilk has been reported in the literature. Finally, the most recent guidelines recommend breastfeeding for mothers stabilized on either methadone or buprenorphine [25]. Based on extrapolation of this information from humans, and where OTM buprenorphine can be administered to cats, and potentially small dogs (<10 kg due to volume) at 0.02–0.04 q4–8h (refer to Chapter 10), this may be an option for managing ongoing pain. Feeding should occur at assumed trough levels, prior to each q6–8h administration to reduce kitten/puppy exposure. Buprenorphine injection SC (Simbadol®) at 240 μg/kg once per day may be an option in some situations. It is imperative that the owner be informed of the potential for reduction in suckling.

- **Nalbuphine** levels in human milk are quite low with an estimated weight adjusted RID of 0.59%. Nalbuphine is only effective for mild pain.
- **Tramadol**'s analgesic efficacy, when given orally to dogs, is questionable based on experimental and clinical studies where the anti-nociceptive effects were mild or did not differ from placebo [10]. Dogs, unlike cats and humans, cannot produce the active (desmethyl) metabolite which confers the opiate effects [26]. (Refer to Chapter 10 for details.) In addition, plasma levels in dogs tend to wane following continual oral administration, reducing any potential analgesic effects. A clinical interpretation of analgesia may be due to the behavioural changes and sedation produced by serotonin re-uptake inhibition [26]. Approximately 0.1% of an intravenous (IV) dose was measured in human breastmilk and it was concluded that there was low potential for adverse effects in breastfed infants exposed to short-term administration of tramadol [8]. The analgesic effects may be beneficial in cats; however, the dysphoria and bizarre behaviour that may occur require careful dosing to avoid these effects and potential lack of mothering. Anecdotal evidence of tramadol in lactating dogs varies from rare potential efficacy to extreme sedation and inability for the mother to care for the puppies.

Where opioids are selected for analgesia, mothers and offspring should be carefully observed and monitored for signs of potential opioid-adverse effects. Reports of rare genetic polymorphism and opioids in human patients indicate the opioid in breastmilk may adversely affect the infant.

B.   Non-Steroidal Anti-Inflammatory Analgesics (NSAIAs)

Most NSAIAs are not lipid-soluble, are highly protein bound to plasma proteins and may be present to a great degree in an ionized form in the plasma. Reports in human medicine indicate safety of some NSAIAs while breastfeeding, and the American Academy of Pediatrics considers ibuprofen, naproxen, indomethacin and acetaminophen safe for infants during breastfeeding; unfortunately, with the exception of acetaminophen for dogs, these NSAIAs are contraindicated for dogs and cats due to poor safety profiles in general for these species. From a coxib perspective, celecoxib (cyclooxygenase-2, COX-2, preferential) is found in human breastmilk at approximately 0.23% of the maternal dose, corrected for weight, and is substantially less than the national cut-off of 10% that is used to guide the use of wide therapeutic index drugs in mothers feeding healthy term infants [27]. Cimicoxib is approved for osteoarthritic pain in dogs in the European Union. A study investigating a single 2 mg/kg PO dose of cimicoxib administered to the dam on D0 and D28 post-cesarean noted high transfer into milk with a milk-to-plasma ratio of 1.7 to 1.9. Plasma samples obtained from the puppies on D28, at variable times after suckling the milk from the dams, had plasma cimicoxib concentrations below or very close to the limit of quantification (0.01 µg/mL). Plasma samples of the neonates were not obtained at D0−1. The conclusions of the study were, "the data obtained suggests that after administration of a single clinical dose of cimicoxib to nursing dams, suckling puppies should be minimally exposed to the drug through the dam's milk and no serious adverse effect should occur" [28]; however, as D0−1 plasma samples were not measured and follow-up kidney assessment was not included, awaiting this data is recommended prior to recommending safety in nursing mothers.

Veterinary-approved drug levels are measured in cows' milk and can be an indication of drug presence in breastmilk in general. As fat and protein content of dogs' and cats' breastmilk is higher than humans' and cows', it should not be assumed that all veterinary NSAIAs share the same milk pharmacokinetics; this should be confirmed with canine and feline studies. In Europe and Canada cows' milk withdrawal interval for meloxicam is five days [29] and four days, respectively. Meloxicam labelling states no studies have been conducted for breastfeeding mothers. Carprofen levels in healthy cows' milk is below detectable limits (<0.022 μg/mL) when examined for up to 24h after administration, resulting in no withdrawal time for milk for human consumption [29]. In experimentally induced mastitis, carprofen levels in cows' milk were 0.16 μg/mL at 12h and < 0.022 μg/mL (below analyser range) at 24h [30, 31]. A pilot study investigating the presence of carprofen 2 mg/kg administered subcutaneously to Labrador retrievers immediately post-cesarean and continuing with this dose PO q12h for 6 days included the mother's serum levels and validated milk assays. The blood levels measured in the mother were consistent with known PK-PD data for carprofen. Milk assays were performed daily at approximately 4h post-administration of the carprofen; all levels were below the low end limit of the analyser range of 0.001 μg/mL [32]. At this measurement, milk expression and puppy exposure would be in the picogram range at most and considered to be minimal exposure. The concern for neonatal puppies is based on immature renal function at birth and possible NSAIA exposure affecting the kidneys. To assess a potential affect on neonatal renal development, a random retrospective study was carried out on 50 offspring of various canine breeds, delivered by cesarean section, suckling from dams given carprofen in the above protocol. The ages of these dogs ranged from 5 months to 106 months with a median age of 33.4 months and an average age of 41.9 months. Serum creatinine on all subjects was within normal reference ranges of 44–140.8 μmol/L (0.5–1.6 mg/dL). Blood urea nitrogen was normal in all but two subjects (normal reference range 6–31 mg/dL). The two subjects out of range were 44 and 32 mg/dL. These dogs had a normal creatinine and no clinical signs of renal disease. The conclusion of this study was that the minimal expression of carprofen in milk does not adversely affect canine neonatal kidney function [33]. Based on measured drug levels in cows' and dogs' milk, and the follow-up canine renal function study, carprofen may be considered after cesarean section. A similar study in only one dog, where carprofen 2 mg/kg q12h was administered for five days, milk levels were measured on days 3, 5 and 10 with the highest measurement of 0.0036 μg/mL [34].

Where veterinary studies have not been performed, the concern is the potential continual presence of COX-2 preferential or COX-2 selective NSAIAs in milk as these have a high potential to inhibit maturation of the kidney in puppies [35]. The same concern exists for cats; however, the effect is not known. This is not a concern in humans. Complete maturation of the canine embryologic kidney does not occur until approximately three weeks after birth, and normal function does not occur until approximately 6–8 weeks of age [36]. This information is not known for cats. Where NSAIAs are essential to manage pain, carprofen appears to be the analgesic of choice based on known presence of levels in the milk. Uterine involution and placental expulsion occurs normally after carprofen administration (S. R. Escobar, personal communication). Hemorrhage is a potential concern following the administration of non-COX selective or COX-1 selective NSAIAs immediately after cesarean section, and potentially natural birth. If a client is apprehensive about carprofen use, but an NSAIA is considered essential for the mother for humane reasons, and to protect offspring from potential maternal aggression caused by pain, it can be suggested that the milk should be pumped and discarded during treatment, and for 12h after the last dose before allowing suckling. Puppies and kittens should be bottle-fed milk replacer during this time. Until studies similar to the carprofen study [32, 33] are performed to ascertain presence and levels of other veterinary-approved NSAIAs in milk of lactating cats and dogs, these should be administered with caution and as single doses only

Salicylates (e.g. aspirin) transfer into human breastmilk is 9–21% of the maternal dose and this has the potential to accumulate in human infants due to slow elimination [37]. This would likely apply to puppies and kittens also and, therefore, should not be administered to cats and dogs.

Acetaminophen (paracetamol) enters the milk poorly and is reported to be safe in low to moderate doses in human infants; however, long-term high doses should be avoided [38]. The estimated dose in the infant via breastfeeding is estimated at 6% of the maternal dose. Acetaminophen is listed as a drug of choice for breastfeeding mothers [1]. In general, acetaminophen is safe for use in dogs, but studies of use in lactating dogs have not been reported. Acetaminophen cannot be administered to cats.

II. Adjunctive Analgesics

A. Serotonin Re-Uptake Inhibitors

Based on overall adverse effects (e.g. serotonin toxicity) and emergency room visits reported in human patients taking imipramine, amitriptyline is the authors' choice in general for this class of drug for dogs and cats. Amitriptyline's safety profile, and some NMDA receptor antagonist properties, renders it a good adjunct analgesic.

B. Amitriptyline

Amitriptyline, after oral administration, showed low concentrations in human breastmilk based on large volume of distribution, extensive first pass metabolism and low plasma levels [8, 40]. Despite widely ranging milk-to-plasma ratios and variable infant serum levels of amitriptyline and nortriptyline (either as parent drug or as a metabolite of amitriptyline), there were no reports of adverse effects in the breast-fed infants. Similarly, pharmacokinetic studies in humans indicate that infants are exposed to 1% of the maternal dose of amitriptyline, and so it is recommended where indicated in breastfeeding mothers [39]. Recommended doses for amitriptyline in general, **dogs**: 1–2 mg/kg PO q12–24h; **cats**: 1–1.5 mg/kg LBW, PO q24h. However, in humans it is generally assumed that analgesic effects may take up to 2–3 weeks.

C. Gabapentin

Gabapentin is prescribed for cluster headaches in women. A study examining transfer into breastmilk demonstrated extensive passage into breastmilk 10–15h after dosing. It is assumed that levels may be higher prior to this sampling time. However, this resulted in low concentrations in the infant's serum, approximately 12% of the maternal values, and was not associated with adverse effects. Conclusions were that breastfeeding in most cases is safe to moderately safe; however, it is advisable to monitor nursed infants for potential adverse effects until more experience has been gained [40, 41]. Another study reported the absolute infant dose received was approximately 3% of the children's dose for gabapentin, and the infant plasma level of 0.4 mg/L was approximately 6% of the maternal plasma drug concentration [42]. No adverse effects attributable to gabapentin were noted in the infant. The conclusions were that in combination with previously published reports this limited data supports the prescription of gabapentin to a breastfeeding mother after a careful individual risk–benefit analysis [42]. Based on various studies, the RID is 1.3–6%. These reports indicate that where pain, especially where a neuropathic component, exists in the dam/queen, gabapentin could be considered, with careful assessment of the offspring. Dosing in cats and dogs is variable based on pharmacokinetic studies (refer to Chapter 12 for details) and anecdotal use based on individual patient efficacy. Based on human studies, if the lower dosages are used, the RID should be safe. Where compounding into a liquid is considered, human gabapentin formulations often contain xylitol. Discuss an alternative vehicle with the compounding pharmacist as xylitol is toxic to cats and dogs.

D. Amantadine

There is very little information on safety during lactation in humans but what exists recommends not using during breastfeeding.

III. Sedatives

A. Benzodiazepines

Information is conflicting [6, 43]. While diazepam may be of benefit for added sedation in some patients when combined with opioids in managing pain, diazepam and its metabolites have been reported to transfer at a high level into milk of human mothers [43]. A case report of a human mother receiving diazepam notes levels of the drug in the infant for up to 10 days after a single injection [43]. However, a study examining a combination of fentanyl, midazolam and propofol in human breastmilk for up to 24h after administration identified only 0.005% of the administered midazolam dose in the milk [13]. As midazolam transfer into milk is low, the conclusions, based on these levels with no untoward effects in the neonate, were that breastfeeding should not be interrupted [6]. Lorazepam resulted in a slight delay in establishing feeding after the mother received an oral dose, with an RID of 2.8% [6]. The RID for diazepam is calculated at 3–4.7% [6]. In babies, benzodiazepines can cause sedation, and poor feeding and extensive use is not recommended [44]. Based on this information, where a benzodiazepine is required, midazolam appears to be the safest choice. However, repeat administration to the dam/queen will result in accumulation in puppies and kittens as maturation of hepatic function, required for benzodiazepine metabolism, does not occur until approximately 4 weeks of age.

B. Acepromazine

Acepromazine has not been studied; however, chlorpromazine transfer into human breastmilk was low with levels that would not produce sedation in the neonate [44]. Chlorpromazine has also been used as a galactagogue [45]. In human case reports, a dose of 25 mg orally three times daily for one week has been used successfully to promote lactation. The mechanism is due to chlorpromazine being conformationally similar to the dopamine molecule which binds and blocks the dopamine receptor, resulting in increased prolactin levels [45].

IV. Local Anesthetics

A. Lidocaine

Lidocaine and its metabolites have low solubility and are secreted into human breastmilk. At therapeutic doses (e.g. dental procedures in humans), the quantities of lidocaine and its metabolites in breastmilk are small, and oral absorption of lidocaine is low; therefore, it is not expected to be a risk for the infant [46]. Where lidocaine is administered IV to nursing mothers, for treatment of a cardiac arrhythmia, only a limited amount passes into the mother's milk [46]. In women who received epidural anesthesia for a cesarean section and received, on average, 183 mg of lidocaine, the expected percentage of the weight-adjusted maternal daily dose transferred to a fully breastfed child in 24h (defined as relative dose) was no more than 1 to, at maximum, 4% of the active agent, which has a limited oral availability. No adverse effects were noted in the babies [46]. No risks have been reported in veterinary patients following line block for cesarean section using lidocaine and/or bupivacaine. In fact, these are highly recommended and confer excellent analgesia (refer to Chapter 14 and 23 for details).

B. Bupivacaine

Bupivacaine lipid solubility is greater than lidocaine (lidocaine 3.0 < ropivacaine 14.0 < L-bupivacaine and bupivacaine 30). Local anesthetics are poorly absorbed orally and are safe when administered to postpartum breastfeeding mothers [15]. Milk levels of bupivacaine and ropivacaine are exceedingly low [47]. A case report describing interpleural administration of bupivacaine after cholecystectomy in a breastfeeding human patient showed that the infant received at most 0.614 mg/day of bupivacaine. This corresponds to 0.1% of the maternal dose. The author concludes that interpleural analgesia by infusion of bupivacaine offers comfortable conditions for the breastfeeding mother and is apparently safe for the infant [48]. Evaluation of puppies and kittens suckling the dam receiving bupivacaine via diffusion catheters for continual analgesia for several hours following cesarean section are not reported. However, anecdotal reports state that the offspring "look fine", but the catheters are associated with technical problems. The veterinarian and owner must ensure protection from adverse events in both the offspring and dam.

V. NMDA-Receptor Antagonists

Ketamine: No studies investigating passage into breastmilk have been reported; however, it is expected to pass into breastmilk [15].

VI. Alpha₂ Adrenergic Agonists

Xylazine at 12 h and **detomidine** at 23 h, administered to horses and cows, were not detected in the milk. No studies examining transfer into breastmilk have been reported for dexmedetomidine in large or small animals, but proprietary information from the drug manufacturer states that dexmedetomidine is excreted into the milk of rats. The company states that lactating women "may consider" interrupting breastfeeding and discarding milk for 10 h (five half-lives) after drug administration [49]. Xylazine is detectable at very low levels in bovine milk for < 12 h [50], and detomidine is detectable in bovine and equine milk at very low levels for < 23 h [51]. However, the detomidine dose was twice the high end of the clinically recommended dose for horses and four times the high end of the clinically recommended dose for cattle. Alpha₂ agonists are commonly administered to cows and mares without apparent effect on the neonatal calf or foal, but the effects may be different in puppies and kittens. If alpha₂ agonists are needed in cats and dogs, the neonate can be monitored for sedation and the effects of the alpha₂ agonist can be reversed if necessary.

VII. Herbal Analgesic Medications

Due to a lack of information, these should be avoided.

VIII. Anesthetics

Refer to Chapter 13 for specific information.

A. Propofol

A study examining a combination of fentanyl, midazolam and propofol in human breastmilk for up to 24 h after administration identified 0.027% of the administered propofol dose in the milk. The conclusion on these levels is that breastfeeding should not be interrupted.

B. Etomidate

Etomidate has a very brief plasma distribution phase and should have minimal to no uptake in the milk [15], thus interruption of nursing is unlikely to be necessary.

C. Alfaxalone

There are no reports of alfaxalone use in nursing mothers of any species but the brief plasma distribution phase makes it unlikely that alfaxalone would accumulate in the milk and interruption of nursing is unlikely to be necessary.

D. Ketamine

As stated above, ketamine is likely to be excreted in breastmilk but the clinical impact is unknown. Although little information is available in any species, a small number of women anesthetized with ketamine for cesarean section breastfed their babies immediately after surgery with no reported adverse effects on the babies [52]. In a separate study, a low dose S-ketamine (an isomer of racemic ketamine) infusion delivered to the mother during cesarean section caused no adverse effects in breastfed babies [53]. However, ketamine concentrations in the milk were not measured in either of these studies.

E. Inhalants

The fairly insoluble inhalant anesthetic gases (i.e. isoflurane, sevoflurane and desflurane) undergo little to no tissue uptake, no tissue accumulation and a very brief plasma distribution phase so it is unlikely that inhalants would be found in the milk [15].

IX. General Anesthesia

Anesthesia and analgesia protocols should be designed based on the health status of the dam/queen, the procedural need (sedation versus general anesthesia) and the expected pain level. **In general, drug protocols/dosages appropriate for specific patients and procedures, as presented in other chapters, can be applied to the nursing mother.** More specifically, drugs with low secretion in the milk and/or reversible drugs are preferred but, as previously stated, milk can be discarded and the puppies/kittens fed with milk replacer if other drugs are more appropriate for the health of the dam/queen. For all drugs, in order to avoid excessive plasma concentrations that may increase the incidence of uptake of the drug in the milk, dosages should be kept low by using balanced anesthesia and multi-modal analgesia.

A. Pre-Medication

As stated above, opioids are an excellent choice for pre-medication for nursing mothers. There is minimal secretion in breastmilk for most opioids and any rare adverse event that may occur in the neonate can be reversed with naloxone. Sedation and decreased nursing activity are the most likely adverse effects and are easily remedied with reversal. Choose the opioid most appropriate for the expected pain level of the mother.

If an opioid alone is not sufficient for pre-medication, either an alpha$_2$ receptor agonist or acepromazine could be added. Alpha$_2$ receptor agonists are reversible in the neonate (if necessary), whereas acepromazine must be metabolized. However, as stated above, acepromazine is unlikely to be secreted in breastmilk and may promote lactation.

B. Induction

Drugs that are rapidly cleared from the plasma with little chance for accumulation in the milk are preferred. Propofol and etomidate have little secretion in breastmilk of humans and it is expected that alfaxalone would be the same.

C. Intraoperative

Anesthesia, even for short procedures, is best maintained by the inhalant anesthetic gases isoflurane, sevoflurane or desflurane because of their almost non-existent accumulation in plasma, and thus none in milk. Maintain the dam/queen on the lowest effective dose in order to promote a quick recovery and return to puppies/kittens. Addition of analgesic drugs will allow reduction of the inhalant dose.

As previously stated, the use of local anesthetics as an incisional block, or in the epidural space, result in little to no uptake into breastmilk. Morphine delivered in the epidural space provides long-duration analgesia (18–24 h) with negligible drug in the maternal serum, resulting in no, to negligible, morphine in milk. Thus, local incisional blocks and morphine epidurals are strongly recommended in all patients undergoing procedures in which these blocks are appropriate. The intraoperative use of local/regional anesthesia will not only provide intraoperative analgesia but also decrease the pain level and, therefore, analgesic requirements in the recovery period.

As previously stated, lidocaine and opioid infusions, titrated to the lowest effective dose, are unlikely to result in secretion of either drug in the milk. Based on the data on infusions of a ketamine isomer [53], this may also be true of ketamine. However, without further data, lidocaine and opioid infusions should be the first choices with the addition of ketamine reserved for dams/queens that have a specific need for that drug (i.e. high pain scores, neuropathic pain, pain from central sensitization).

D. Recovery

Pain should be re-addressed. Boluses of opioids are appropriate and carprofen (dogs only), as described earlier in this chapter, should be considered. Patients in the dysphoric phase of anesthesia can have unpredictable responses and could inadvertently injure the neonates. Where indicated, add any of the above analgesics recommended for nursing mothers. Ensure that the dam/queen is fully conscious before returning her to the pups/kittens.

X. Discharge Home

Select the appropriate analgesic(s) from those listed above.

References

1 Ito, S. (2000) Drug therapy for breastfeeding women. *NEJM*, 343(2): 118–126.
2 Britt, R. and Pasero, C. (1999) Pain control using analgesics during breastfeeding. *Am J Nurs*, 99(9): 20.
3 Lopate, C. (ed.) (2012) *Management of Pregnant and Neonatal Dogs, Cats and Exotic Pets.* Wiley-Blackwell, Ames, IA.
4 Sachs, H. C. (2013) The transfer of drugs and therapeutics into human breast milk: An update on selected topics. *Am Academy of Pediatrics*, 132(3): e796–e809.

5 Pascoe, P. J. and Moon, P. F. (2001) Periparturient and neonatal anesthesia. *Vet Clin North Am Small Anim Pract*, 31(2): 315–341.

6 Ostrea, E. M., Mantaring, III J.B., and Silvestre, M. A. (2004) Drugs that affect the fetus and newborn infant via the placenta or breast milk. *Pediatr Clin N Am*, 51: 539– 579.

7 Jansson, L. M. and The Academy of Breastfeeding Medicine Protocol Committee (2009) ABM Clinical Protocol #21: Guidelines for Breastfeeding and the Drug-Dependent Woman. *Breastfeed Med*, 4(4): 225–228.

8 Coluzzi, F., Valensisi, H. and Sacco, M. (2014) Chronic pain management in pregnancy and lactation. *Review Minerva Anestesiologica*, 80(2): 211, 224.

9 Briggs, G. G., Freeman, R. K. and Yaffe, S. J. (2011) *Drugs in Pregnancy and Lactation*, 9th edn. Lippincott Williams and Wilkins, Philadelphia.

10 KuKanich, B. (2013) Outpatient oral analgesics in dogs and cats beyond nonsteroidal antiinflammatory drugs: An evidence-based approach. *Vet Clin North Am Small Anim Pract*, 43: 1109–1125.

11 Ferreira, T. H., Rezende, M. L., Mama, K. R., *et al.* (2011) Plasma concentrations, behavioural and antinociceptive and physiological effects of methadone after intravenous and transmucosal administration in cats. *Am J Vet Res*, 72(6): 764–771.

12 Madej, T. H. and Strunin, L. (1987) Comparison of epidural fentanyl with sufentanil: Analgesia and side effects after a single bolus dose during elective caesarean section. *Anesthesia*, 42(11): 1156–1161.

13 Nitsun, M., Szokol, J. W. and Saleh, H. J. (2006) Pharmacokinetics of midazolam, propofol, and fentanyl transfer to human breast milk. *Clin Pharmacol Ther*, 79(6): 549–557.

14 Cohen, R. S. (2009) Fentanyl transdermal analgesia during pregnancy and lactation. *J Hum Lact*, 25(3): 359–361.

15 Montgomery, A., Hale, T. and The Academy of Breastfeeding Medicine (2012) ABM Clinical Protocol #15: Analgesia and anesthesia for the breastfeeding mother: Revised 2012. *Breastfeed Med*, 7(6): 547–5653.

16 Wittels, C., Scott, D. T. and Sinatra, R. S. (1990) Exogenous opioids in human breast milk and acute neonatal neurobehavior: A preliminary study. *Anesthesiology*, 73: 864–869.

17 Hamza, J., Benlabed, M., Orhant, E., *et al.* (1992) Neonatal pattern of breathing during active and quiet sleep after maternal administration of meperidine. *Pediatr Res*, 3: 412–416.

18 Hodgkinson, R., Bhatt, M., Grewal, G., *et al.* (1978) Neonatal neurobehavior in the first 48 hours of life: Effect of the administration of meperidine with and without naloxone in the mother. *Pediatrics*, 62: 294–298.

19 Pittman, K. A., Smythe, R. D., Losada, M., *et al.* (1980) Human perinatal distribution of butorphanol. *Am J. Obstet Gynaecol*, 138: 797–800.

20 Spigset, O. and Hagg, S. (2000) Analgesics and breast-feeding: Safety considerations. *Paediatr Drugs*, 2(3): 223–38.

21 Traas, A. M. (2008) Surgical management of canine and feline dystocia. *Theriogenology*, 70(3): 337–342.

22 Statz, G., Moore, K. E. and Murtaugh, R. J. (2007) Surgical repair of a peritoneopericardial diaphragmatic hernia in a pregnant dog. *J Vet Emerg Crit Care*, 17(1): 77–85.

23 Hirose, M. and Hosokawa, T. (1997) Extradural buprenorphine suppresses breast feeding after caesarean section. *Br J Anesthesia*, 79: 120–121.

24 Lindemalm, S., Nydert, P., Svensson, J.-O., *et al.* (2009) Transfer of buprenorphine into breast milk and calculation of infant drug dose. *J Hum Lact*, 25(2): 199–205.

25 Jones, H. E., Heil, S. H., Baewert, A., *et al.* (2012) Buprenorphine treatment for opioid-dependent pregnant women: A comprehensive review. *Addiction*, 107(1): 5–27.

26 Kukanich, B. and Papich, M. G. (2011) Pharmacokinetics and antinociceptive effects of oral tramadol hydrochloride administration in Greyhounds. *Am J Vet Res*, 72: 256–262.

27 Gardiner, S. J., Doogue, M. P., Zhang, M., *et al.* (2006) Quantification of infant exposure to celecoxib through breast milk. *British Journal of Clinical Pharmacology*, 61(1): 101–104.

28 Schneider, M., Kuchta, A, Dron, F., *et al.* (2015) Disposition of cimicoxib in plasma and milk of whelping bitches and in their puppies. *BMC Veterinary Research*, 11: 178.

29 Smith, G. W., Davis, J. L., Tell, L. A., *et al.* (2008) Extralabel use of nonsteroidal anti-inflammatory drugs in cattle. *JAVMA*, 232(5): 697–701.

30 Lohuis, J. A., van Werven, T., Brand, A., *et al.* (1991) Pharmacodynamics and pharmacokinetics of carprofen, a nonsteroidal anti-inflammatory drug, in healthy cows and cows with *Escherichia coli* endotoxin-induced mastitis. *J Vet Pharmacol Ther*, 14: 219–229.

31 Raffe, M. R. (2015) Anesthetic considerations during pregnancy and for the newborn. In: Grimm, K. A., Lamont, L. L., Tranquilli, W. J., *et al.* (eds), *Veterinary Anesthesia and Analgesia: The fifth edition of Lumb and Jones*. Wiley-Blackwell, Ames, IA: 708–722.

32 Escobar, S. R. (2010) Carprofen exposure via lactation in canine neonates post caesarian section. SFT/ACT Annual Conference Track 2.

33 Escobar, S. R. (2016) *Carprofen exposure via lactation in canine neonates post-caesarian section: Follow-up.* Proceedings for the Society for Theriogenology, September, 8(3): 191.

34 Persson, A. (2012) Carprofen som postoperative esmartlingdrin vid kejsnarsitt par hund. Doctoral thesis. Sverigens Lantbruksanuniversitet, Uppsala, Sweden.

35 Horster, M. and Valtin, H. (1971) Postnatal development of renal function: Micropuncture and clearance studies in the dog. *J Clin Invest*, 50: 779–795.

36 Kleinman, L. I. and Lubbe, R. J. (1972) Factors affecting the maturation of glomerular filtration rate and renal plasma flow in the newborn dog. *J Physiol*, 223: 395–409.

37 Bloor, M. and Paech, M. (2013) Nonsteroidal anti-inflammatory drugs during pregnancy and the initiation of lactation. *Anesth Analg*, 116(5): 1063–1075.

38 Baka, N. E. (2002) Paracetamol (acetaminophen) and methadone levels in breast milk do not justify interruption of nursing. *Anesth Analg*, 94: 184–187.

39 Breyer-Pfaff, U., Nill, K., Entenmann, A. and Gaertner, H. J. (1995) Secretion of amitriptyline and metabolites into breast milk. *Am J Psychiatry*, 152: 812–813.

40 Öhman, I. and Vitols, S. (2001) Committee on Drugs, American Academy of Pediatrics: The transfer of drugs and other chemicals into human milk. *Pediatrics*, 108: 776–789.

41 Öhman, I. and Vitols, S. Tomson, T. (2005) Pharmacokinetics of gabapentin during delivery, in the neonatal period, and lactation: Does a fetal accumulation occur during pregnancy? *Epilepsia*, 46(10): 1621–1624.

42 Kristensen, J. H., Ilett, K. F. and Hackett, L. P. (2006) Gabapentin and Breastfeeding: A case report. *J Hum Lact*, 22(4): 426–428.

43 Rathmell, J. P., Viscomi, C. M. and Ashburn, M. A. (1997) Management of non-obstetric pain during pregnancy and lactation. *Anesth Analg*, 85: 1074–1087.

44 Weichert, C. E. (1980) Prolactin cycling and the management of breast-feeding failure. *Adv Pediatr*, 27: 391–407.

45 Gabay, M. (2002) Galactogogues: Medications that induce lactation. *J Hum Lact*, 18(3): 274–279.

46 Jürgens, T. P., Schaefer, C. and May, A. (2009) Treatment of cluster headache in pregnancy and lactation. *Cephalalgia*, 29, 391–400.

47 Matsota, P. K., Markantonis, S. L., Fousteri, M. Z., *et al.* (2009) Excretion of ropivacaine in breast milk during patient-controlled epidural analgesia after cesarean delivery. *Reg Anesth Pain Med*, 34: 126–129.

48 Baker, P. A. and Schroeder, D. (1989) Interpleural bupivacaine for postoperative pain during lactation. *Anesth Analg*, 69: 40–42.

49 Mylan Institutional LLC. (2017). *Dexmedetomidine Hydrochloride – Dexmedetomidine Hydrochloride Injection, Solution, Concentrate.* https://dailymed.nlm.nih.gov/dailymed/drugInfo.cfm?setid=ebdfe2e8-30ca-4f18-935a-41bcbbce4937 (accessed 19 December 2017).

50 Delehant, T. M., Denhart, J. W., Lloyd, W. E. and Powell, J. D. (2003) Pharmacokinetics of xylazine, 2,6-dimethylaniline, and tolazoline in tissues from yearling cattle and milk from mature dairy cows after sedation with xylazine hydrochloride and reversal with tolazoline hydrochloride. *Vet Ther*, 4(2): 128–134.

51 Salonen, J. S., Vähä-Vahe, T., Vainio, O. and Vakkuri, O. (1989) Single-dose pharmacokinetics of detomidine in the horse and cow. *J Vet Pharmacol Ther*, 12(1): 65–72.

52 Ortega, D., Viviand, X., Lorec, A. M., *et al.* (1999) Excretion of lidocaine and bupivacaine in breast milk following epidural anesthesia for cesarean delivery. *Acta Anaesthesiol Scand*, 43: 394–397.

53 Suppa, E., Valente, A., Catarci, S., *et al.* (2012) A study of low-dose S-ketamine infusion as "preventive" pain treatment for cesarean section with spinal anesthesia: Benefits and side effects. *Minerva Anestesiol*, 78(7): 774–781.

Further Reading

Drukker, A. (2002) The adverse renal effects of prostaglandin synthesis inhibition in the fetus and the newborn: A review. *Paediatr Child Health*, 7(8): 538–543.

25

Physiologic and Pharmacologic Application of Analgesia and Anesthesia for the Pediatric Patient

Karol Mathews, Tamara Grubb and Andrea Steele

Normal physiological parameters of this group are presented as changes from normal can occur with analgesic administration and can also be affected by pain and associated illness or injury. The term "pediatric" generally refers to the first six months of life. Due to important physiologic changes which occur during this timeframe, a further demarcation will be defined for this review: neonatal (0–2 weeks), infant (2–6 weeks), weanling, (6–12 weeks) and juvenile (3–6 months). This distinction is made to make the reader aware of the metabolic changes that are occurring during these periods of maturation [1].

I. Physiologic Importance of Preventing Pain [2, 3]

While most of the information in this group of patients is obtained from human and laboratory animal studies, it is assumed that similar physiological events occur in kittens and puppies. The nerve pathways essential for the transmission and perception of pain (refer to Chapter 2) are present and functioning by 24 weeks of gestation in humans [4], and at a similar stage in laboratory animals. A lower threshold to a noxious stimulus, increased pain sensitivity, appears to be more pronounced in the newborn compared to adults due to increased number of pain receptors and neuronal reorganization in the neonate. The initial noxious stimulus produces transduced electrical signals that are transmitted by afferent sensory neurons to projection neurons in the spinal cord, each of which has receptors that are under developmental control, contributing to neuronal plasticity. These peripheral sensory neurons are overproduced during embryonic development and normally approximately 50% undergo programmed cell death in the adult. During this postnatal developmental period, the perception of pain and its inhibition undergo a waxing and waning physiological change making interpretation of behaviour/pain for a given stimulus difficult from one day to the next. In addition, the inhibitory pathway is not fully developed at birth, leaving the neonate, and potentially the infant, susceptible to increased pain sensation for a given stimulus. It has been demonstrated that sensory nerve cells in the infant spinal cord are more excitable than those of the adult, with a greater, and more prolonged, response and a larger receptive field [5]. Pain transmission occurs primarily along C fibres in neonates, rather than the A-delta fibres as occurs in adults prior to C fibre transmission. Reflex response can be triggered from a wider body area, and there is less precise localization than in adults [5]. These physiological events emphasize the high level of pain potentially experienced by young animals and is demonstrated so in human babies when responses to a given stimulus are greater when compared to the adult response.

Analgesia and Anesthesia for the Ill or Injured Dog and Cat, First Edition. Karol A. Mathews, Melissa Sinclair, Andrea M. Steele and Tamara Grubb.
© 2018 John Wiley & Sons, Inc. Published 2018 by John Wiley & Sons, Inc.

Because the central nervous system (CNS) is extremely plastic during development and an unmanaged painful experience may have a permanent negative impact on the animal, adequate analgesia is essential for any procedure no matter how minor it may seem. Where any traumatic or surgical injury or painful (inflammatory) illness is experienced without adequate analgesia, in the young animal (and human), a neural reorganization occurs and is permanent. This results in hyperalgesia, potential allodynia and behavioural abnormalities – the characteristics of central neuronal sensitization. Early adverse events of these physiologic systems and the ability to adapt can be altered, and this seems to increase the animal's susceptibility to the negative effects of stress in later life. Early life events can permanently influence the development of central corticotropin-releasing hormone (CRH) systems, which, in turn, mediate the expression of behavioural/emotional, autonomic and endocrine responses to stress. Studies in neonates and infants show that when anesthesia or analgesia was withheld altered pain sensitivity and increased anxiety occurred with subsequent painful experiences, when compared to children receiving analgesia [6]. This suggests that infants retain a "memory" of a painful experience with subsequent altered response to a painful stimulus. This has also been shown in laboratory animals [7] and there is no reason to believe this to be any different in cats and dogs. This is a very important reason to stop **all** cosmetic surgeries in young puppies. We **must** negotiate with the Kennel Clubs that "designer dogs" are not in the best interests of the dog. Historical reasons for tail docking are many but, as an example, in England was a proof of owning a dog for tax rebate. Note that the wealthy didn't need to do this (hounds keep their tails: a symbol of wealth). This ended in 1796! Consider behavioural problems in some dogs of docked breeds, this is likely neuropathic pain stemming from chronic nerve injury or potential neuroma formation – case experience. We have the Veterinarian's Oath to support us when insisting that the procedure be made **illegal**. This is so in some Canadian provinces, Europe, Australia and New Zealand. Many pet owners would like non-docked puppies but many breeders won't comply. Why must North America remain as the outlier, with the implication of cruelty made by our colleagues in other countries?

II. Physiologic Aspects to Consider When Managing Pain [2, 3]

As total body water (TBW) is important to consider when assessing heart rate (cardiac output) and analgesic selection, assessment of hydration status and intravascular volume is essential. Neonatal, infant and weanling puppies and kittens have a greater TBW volume (~80% when extrapolated from human babies) when compared to the adult, with approximately one-half being extracellular. During the following months of growth, a gradual reduction to 60% TBW occurs. Due to the high surface-area-to-body-water ratio facilitating greater heat loss and evaporation, this, along with a smaller reserve of intracellular water and a higher relative fluid and energy requirement, requires careful attention to fluid intake when healthy and constant assessment during illness and fever. Assessment of hydration is important and essential when considering anesthesia. Dehydration in kittens and puppies occurs rapidly, and is difficult to detect by skin turgor when younger than 6 weeks of age. With more advanced dehydration, the skin will lose turgor and remain tented or spontaneously wrinkle; however, this is best examined on the ventral abdomen. Urine colour can be a good indicator of dehydration. As puppies less than 3 weeks of age cannot metabolize bilirubin, their urine is normally colourless; where even slight colour is noted, dehydration is present. However, kittens can metabolize bilirubin, so there may be some colour to the urine. Should the colour diminish with fluid therapy, the patient was dehydrated. Constipation may be another sign of dehydration. Determination of degree of dehydration is difficult, but objective assessments can be made through the recent history of intake and losses (vomiting, diarrhea, polyuria), heart rate, mucous membrane moistness, colour and capillary refill time, eyes sunken within the orbit, heart rate and peripheral pulse character.

Blood pressure, peripheral vascular resistance and stroke volumes in puppies and kittens are lower than for adults; however, plasma volume, heart rate and central venous pressure are higher. Heart sounds can be difficult to auscultate; therefore, a pediatric stethoscope chest piece (2 cm bell, 3 cm diaphragm) should be used at the left fifth to sixth intercostal space. Rate and rhythm, presence or absence of a heart murmur, location if present, must be determined. Normal heart rate ~200/min. Hearts of puppies and kittens generate less force (stroke volume) than the adults', relying on heart rate primarily for cardiac output. At approximately 6 weeks of age, mean arterial pressure gradually increases reaching normal adult values when several months of age. The parasympathetic innervation to the pediatric heart is dominant; therefore, these patients are more vulnerable to bradycardia and hypotension.

Body temperature for < 2 weeks of age is 35.5–36 °C (96–97 °F), for > 4 weeks is 37.7 °C (100 °F) with gradual increase to 38.5 °C during the juvenile phase. Puppies and kittens also have a higher surface-area-to-body-weight ratio than adults, facilitating greater heat loss and subsequent evaporation. Due to the large surface-area-to-body-weight ratio, puppies and kittens have increased evaporative heat loss and poor thermoregulation, resulting in hypothermia given the right conditions. At a young age they cannot shiver, another factor contributing to hypothermia. The potential for hypothermia must always be considered when using any "liquid" and antiseptic; therefore, these should be warmed to a temperature equal to that of the palmar surface of the human wrist. Also, heat loss is enhanced when placed on cool surfaces. Hypothermia causes bradycardia (resulting in low cardiac output and hypotension), which may be potentiated with opioid administration. Therefore, re-warming the puppy or kitten is a priority, along with administration of fluids as appropriate. Body temperature may also influence glomerular filtration rate.

III. Pain Assessment

Evaluating the degree of pain experienced by puppies and kittens is very difficult; however, one can assume that the illness or injury acquired will be as painful as, or potentially more than, the adult humans and animals.

Prior to examining the patient, observe attitude (alert, depressed, distressed, etc.) and respiratory pattern (rate, rhythm, character); normal respiratory rate 15–35/min, followed by heart rate and rhythm assessment. A confounding problem is interpreting crying when no obvious injury is present. The neonate and infant, puppy and kitten cries when in pain, hungry (failure to nurse), cold or when they lose contact with the mother. Usually, the duration of crying when not ill or painful (behavioural) can last ~20 min, but where injury or illness is present, crying can be constant. The owner will have noticed a change in behaviour. Depression (facial expression) is difficult to ascertain at this age; however, a change in behaviour, not eating, a change in sleeping patterns and movement away from a painful area, a limp and poorly responsive animal, is an indication of illness or injury and pain may, or may not, be a component of the illness. The weanling and juvenile tend to be more demonstrative with respect to pain. Careful physical examination of the whole patient will localize an area of pain. There will be some degree of increase in heart and respiratory rates and blood pressure.

IV. Analgesics

Animals between 3 and 6 months of age appear to require adult dosing regimens to confer analgesia. There tends to be apprehension in administering analgesic drugs, especially opioids, to young animals due to the often-cited "decreased drug metabolism and high risk of overdose". While this may be a potential concern in the neonate, it is not necessarily so through all stages of maturation. Based on the human literature, the analgesic requirement may be higher at a certain stage of development, especially in the pediatric human patient, than the adult. Children of 2–6 years of age have greater weight-normalized clearance than adults for many drugs. Higher rates of drug metabolism by cytochrome P450 in children compared with adults have been attributed to a larger liver mass per kilogram of body weight, rather than to age-related changes in intrinsic enzyme catalytic rates [8]. More rapid clearance in children may require more frequent dosing [8]. While there are no reports in the veterinary literature suggesting increased dosing should be considered in the young cat or dog, personal experience with intensive monitoring of young (4- to 6-month-old) very painful animals, revealed no adverse effects; on the contrary, these animals appeared very comfortable. This is not to suggest that the opioid dose should automatically be increased but emphasizes that administering the analgesic to effect, rather than a pre-determined dose, is the most important method by which to manage pain (Table 25.1). As the effects of the opioid occur quite rapidly after administration, it is wise to monitor for potential adverse effects, and reverse with naloxone should these occur, rather than not treat because of fear of a "potential" problem, which may not happen. Opioids can be reversed by careful titration of naloxone (Table 25.1) should there be clinical evidence of CNS depression with associated respiratory depression, hypotension and bradycardia. In the authors' experience, naloxone administered carefully until adverse effects are eliminated should not reverse analgesia. Most animals that are comfortable and sleeping have lower heart rates than when awake, especially the larger breeds; this does not warrant concern unless respiratory depression and hypotension are noted. However, if bradycardia (heart rate < 150 bpm, a slightly lower rate with the older pediatric patient) is noted, and is associated with poor perfusion only, glycopyrrolate may be administered rather than reversing the opioid. Glycopyrrolate takes longer to exert its effect than atropine, but lasts longer (2–3 h) and is less likely to cause tachycardia. Increasing the heart rate to normal in this setting will increase cardiac output. Maintaining a normal heart rate to ensure appropriate cardiac output is important in pediatric patients.

Neonates, and potentially infants, need to be considered separately from the weanling or juvenile patient when considering analgesics [9]. Due to the potential delay in development of the descending inhibitory mechanism and enhancement of peripheral sensory neurons, which increases the perception of pain in neonates, the nociceptive threshold is lower than in the adult. Due to the slower development of some neurotransmitters or receptors, certain drugs may not be effective at this stage of development. The neonate also has reduced clearance of many drugs as compared with infants, children and adults largely because of the (1) greater water composition of their body weight, (2) a larger fraction of body mass that consists of highly perfused tissues, (3) a lower plasma concentration of proteins that bind drugs and (4) incomplete maturation of the hepatic system. Combined, these may result in reduced metabolism and excretion, which may require alterations in dosing and dosing intervals [1]. The hepato-renal system continues to develop until 3 to 6 weeks of age.

For all young animals, the presence of milk in the stomach may inhibit the absorption of some orally administered drugs, potentially resulting in lower blood levels.

Table 25.1 Opioid analgesic dosages for pediatric patients. (Suggestions only. Higher dosages may be required.)

Drug	Species	Dose mg/kg (1/4 to 1/2 dosages less than 4 weeks of age)	Route of Administration (SC suggested for less than 4 weeks of age but uptake from IM or IV is more predictable and preferred in older patients)	Interval (hours)
Mild to moderate pain				
*Opioid agonists: Titrate IV to effect where possible				
*Methadone	Dog and Cat	0.1–0.5	IV, IM, SC (PO cat) CRI	1–4 /4 h
*Hydromorphone	Dog Cat	0.05+ 0.05 to <0.1	IV, IM, SC CRI	2–4 (6) h /4 h
*Fentanyl	Dog and Cat	0.002–0.005 0.001–0.005	IV loading to effect IV/ 20–60 min or CRI	0.5–1 h /1 h
*Morphine (above opioids preferred)	Dog	0.1–0.5 0.05+ 0.25+	IM, SC, IV, v slowly to effect IV, CRI	1–4 h /4 h
	Cat	0.05–0.1 0.025+ 0.25+	IM, SC IV, v slowly to effect IV, CRI	1–4 h /4 h
*Meperidine for >6 weeks of age	Dog and Cat	1–2	IM	0.5–1 h
Opioid agonist-antagonists				
Butorphanol	Dog and Cat	0.2–0.4	IM, SC	1–4 h
	Dog and Cat	0.02–0.05 (or to effect)	IV	1–4 h
	Dog and Cat	0.05–0.01+	IV, CRI	/h

Opioid partial agonists				
Buprenorphine	Dog and Cat	0.005–0.02 0.03–0.06*	IV, IM, OTM – cats and dogs < 10 kg	~6 h

Moderate to severe pain

*Opioid agonists: Titrate IV to effect where possible

*Methadone	Dog and Cat	0.5–1+	IM, SC, IV (PO cat) IV CRI	1–4 h /4 h
*Hydromorphone	Dog	0.05–0.1+	IV, IM, SC IV CRI	2–4 (6) h /4 h
	Cat	0.05 to <0.1	IV, IM, SC IV CRI	2–4 (6) h /4 h
*Fentanyl	Dog and Cat	0.005–0.010+ 0.001–0.005	IV loading IV CRI	0.5–1 h /1 h
*Morphine (above opioids preferred)	Dog	0.05–0.1 0.05+	IM, SC IV v slowly to effect IV CRI	1–4 h /4 h 1–4 h
	Cat	0.05–0.1 0.025+	IV v slowly to effect CRI	/4 h

Naloxone (an opioid antagonist) should always be available when opioids are used. The dose depends on the administered opioid, dose and duration. When adverse effects are experienced, I start by slowly titrating naloxone IV. Mix 0.1 mL (cats, small dogs) or 0.25 mL of naloxone (0.4 mg/mL) with 5–10 mL saline. To avoid adverse effects, titrate this at 1 mL/ min until the side effects of opioids have subsided; using this technique analgesic effects will be maintained. May have to re-dose at varying intervals, as duration of opioid action is longer than naloxone. Single or non-titrated doses may result in hyperalgesia, hyperexcitability, cardiac arrhythmias and aggression

*Adult dose but may be required for the older pediatric patient. As pain is an individual experience, dosing is based on the patient's needs.

IV: intravenous; IM: intramuscular; SC: subcutaneous; CRI: continuous rate infusion; OTM: oral transmucosal.

Source: Adapted from [26]. Reproduced with permission of Elsevier.

A. Opioids

1. Mu-Receptor Agonists

The blood–brain barrier is more permeable to some opioids in the neonate/infant than adults. Lower doses of fentanyl or morphine are required for analgesia in the neonate when compared to the 5-week-old puppy. Very young puppies are also more sensitive to the sedative and respiratory depressant effects of morphine, and it is recommended that fentanyl may be a more suitable opioid in the very young, especially the neonate. This would likely apply to kittens. Lower doses of fentanyl or morphine are required for analgesia in the neonate (0–2 weeks) when compared to the 5-week-old puppy [10] or kitten. Fentanyl may be a more suitable opioid in the young pediatric and neonatal puppy or kitten due to less adverse effects; however, as it is short-acting, continuous intravenous (IV) access and titration are required [10, 11].

Morphine, hydromorphone, methadone and fentanyl all provide potent pain relief. All can cause excessive sedation at higher dosages; morphine and hydromorphone are highly likely to cause vomiting, whereas this is not a problem with methadone. In addition to the opioid (mu-receptor) effect, methadone is also an NMDA receptor antagonist and serotonin reuptake inhibitor, a "mini multi-modal drug". Another advantage to methadone is that it can be administered orally in the cat/kitten. Analgesia from fentanyl only lasts 20 min, but fentanyl is the most potent of these opioids, and the chance of vomiting is minimal. All of these opioids can cause a dose-dependent respiratory depression that is generally mild but may require oxygen supplementation. In addition to vomiting, morphine may cause excessive sedation and hypotension due to histamine release when given IV. In veterinary medicine, recommendations are to administer half the usual adult dose of these agents to puppies and kittens when used as a pre-medication prior to anesthesia. For use as an analgesic, this may not be appropriate. Based on human pediatric studies, dosing depends on the degree of pain and the phase of maturation. Neonates will require less; however, animals a few weeks old may require an adult dosing regimen. Starting at lower dosages and titrating to effect is recommended based on the changing sensitivity of peripheral receptors. Reversal of any adverse effects may be titrated using naloxone (Table 25.1). For the < 4-week-old patient, more than one dose subcutaneously may be required if IV access is not obtained. No veterinary studies are available in this young group of patients assessing the transdermal routes of fentanyl. The dosing recommendations below are ranges published for dogs and cats.

2. Agonist-Antagonist

Where pain is known to be mild and will not increase in severity (e.g. blood collection), aural exam with cleaning, butorphanol or nalbuphine will facilitate the procedure while not affecting cardiovascular and respiratory status, and has anti-emetic and antitussive effects. It is also effective for gastrointestinal (GI) pain with minimal effect on motility. The effect ranges from 30–180 min.

3. Partial Mu-Receptor Agonist

Buprenorphine has a longer duration of action than pure mu-agonists. The problem is, this cannot be titrated to effect due to long duration taken to effect and is only effective for mild to moderate pain. If the degree of pain is known to be mild to moderate without progression to severe, buprenorphine is a good choice as it has only minimal sedative, GI, cardiovascular and respiratory effects. Should the pain be severe, managing this with a mu-agonist will be difficult due to the mu-antagonism of buprenorphine. An advantage of buprenorphine is that it can be administered sublingually or buccally to kittens/cats; however; new data shows that the bioavailability by this route is not as good as once thought, which may mean that an increased dose is warranted.

Sedative/opioid combinations should be avoided in this young age group as the sedation with an opioid alone is extremely profound, especially in younger animals; therefore, where a procedure requires sedation, an opioid is recommended as even blood collection can be painful. Opioids are also readily reversed should this be required.

B. Non-Steroidal Anti-Inflammatory Analgesics

The non-steroidal anti-inflammatory analgesics (NSAIAs) are excellent analgesics; however, are not recommended for animals of less than 6 weeks of age based on the developing hepato-renal systems (refer to Chapter 11). Therefore, these agents should not be administered to animals less than 6–8 weeks of age, or older depending on the NSAIA. Cyclooxygenase-2 (COX-2) is important in renal maturation, sodium and water balance at the level of the kidney and it is important to ensure that this system is fully developed prior to administration of NSAIAs. Prior to administration of an NSAIA, consult the package insert for minimum age as there are differences amongst products with some at 7 months. Dosing for meloxicam should be based on studies in Canada and Europe, where 0.05–0.1 mg/kg has an analgesic effect and can be used for 3–5 days. The recommendation of 0.3 mg/kg once only, in the United States, is not recommended and may potentially cause adverse effects in a compromised situation. The recommended dosages elsewhere in the world provide good analgesia. To avoid overdose, NSAIAs must be based on ideal body weight in the obese patient and actual weight in normal and underweight patients.

C. Ketamine [12–14]

Ketamine may be required in severe pain states (refer to Chapter 13). Although the NMDA system is reported to be underdeveloped in the neonate, ketamine may still be effective. Ketamine also inhibits GABA, and serotonin, norepinephrine and dopamine reuptake in the CNS, enhancing the descending inhibitory pathway. Pre-operative analgesia with ketamine decreases the central sensitization to painful stimuli, reducing morphine requirements in the first 24h in humans. Ketamine is a widely used anesthetic in neonates and children due to its rapid onset and short duration of action, effective anesthetic and analgesic properties and relatively safe respiratory and hemodynamic profile as it does not attenuate the concomitant heart rate or blood pressure (refer to Chapter 12). However, there are no veterinary studies reporting ketamine for analgesia in puppies and kittens. In human pediatric patients an analgesic dose is 0.05–0.25 mg/kg. This may also be an appropriate dose for puppies and kittens; however, this author always titrates ketamine IV to affect analgesia. This is recommended for pediatric patients and is used as an adjunct to opioids, where pain is severe. As a guide to dosing a puppy or kitten, a **quarter to a half of the adult dose** may be used. The suggested **adult dosing is**: titrate loading dose; 0.5–1.0 mg/kg IV followed by continuous rate infusion (CRI) at 0.12–0.6 mg/kg/h; severe pain states will require dosages at the higher end of the range. As dosing is based on careful titration to effect, the initial titration dose will give an assessment of level of pain and drug requirement to manage this on an hourly basis (dose to effect = hourly CRI dose). As liver and kidney maturation is incomplete until at least 4 and 6 weeks of age, respectively, duration of drug action will be longer; therefore, the CRI dosing will have to be reduced. As head trauma is not uncommon in pediatric patients, it is important to note that ketamine is safe, and potentially neuroprotective due to the NMDA antagonistic effect, to use as an adjunct analgesic in this setting. Neuroprotective effects of ketamine have been reported in neonatal rodent models in postnatal day 1 to 4. A long-standing theory is that ketamine raises intracranial pressure (ICP); however, human clinical evidence does not support this and previous claims were due to high CO_2 levels. However, it is essential that hypoventilation resulting in increased CO_2 be avoided. Hallucinations, increased ICP and neuronal death in an immature brain have been reported in rodents after the administration of **repeated extremely high (40 mg/kg), not clinically relevant, doses**. In addition, ketamine also has anti-pro-inflammatory effects (refer to Chapter 13), which have been associated with increased survival in human septic patients. Current clinical evidence favours ketamine's use in human pediatric patients. In addition, it also has weak opioid effects contributing a little analgesia through this mechanism. Dosages of ketamine required for anesthesia and effects of this are discussed in Section VIII.B. Ketamine may produce salivation in cats. With careful titration to a "comfortable analgesic plane", the dissociative adverse effects can be avoided. It is recommended that ketamine be administered/titrated following opioid administration where further analgesia is required for severe pain, where a lower dosage is usually required and to prevent the potential augmented dissociative effect from opioids. Ketamine 0.25 mg/kg PO q4h/PRN is also administered to human babies, mixed with Tylenol® elixir, because ketamine is bitter. Oral administration may be considered for puppies and kittens; however, it should be mixed with something palatable.

D. Alpha$_2$ Adrenoceptor Agonists

No studies investigating this group of analgesics in the younger veterinary pediatric patient have been reported. It is advised not to use this class of analgesics in neonates, infants and weanlings due to the bradycardia produced and associated reduction in cardiac output. Also, the hepato-renal system is not fully developed in the younger animals predisposing to prolonged effect. These may be appropriate, but rarely required, for the juvenile patient and reversal is possible should this be required.

E. Gabapentin

There are no veterinary studies examining gabapentin in pediatric patients; however, it is administered to children at dosages from 9–34 mg/kg/day for seizure control. Also, as an adjunctive analgesic, gabapentin 5 mg/kg q8h decreased pain scores when administered prior to and following spinal fusion surgery in children of 9–18 years of age [15]. Gabapentin appears to be a safe analgesic to use in our pediatric patients where a neuropathic pain component exists in the acute setting (trauma, surgery, etc.) or when a chronic component exists as this results in maladaptive pain with a neuropathic component that may respond to gabapentin. The dose can be titrated up or down from 5 mg/kg q8h with sedation being the limiting factor. Refer to Chapter 3 and Chapter 12 for details.

V. Sedatives

It is not recommended to use sedatives in addition to opioids, or alone where pain is present or anticipated, in young animals, especially when younger than 12 weeks of age [16]. However, sedatives may be included in the pre-operative protocol (see Section VIII.B). The phenothiazine tranquilizers (e.g. acetylpromazine) undergo little hepatic biotransformation and may cause prolonged CNS depression. These agents are not analgesic, and in fact they may mask an increase in the level of pain if analgesics are not co-administered. Acepromazine induce peripheral vasodilation, and hypotension and hypothermia may result. As butorphanol provides moderate sedation this may be effective as a sedative in neonatal/infant, and perhaps weanling, patients. Because the duration of butorphanol-mediated analgesia is short, the drug should be considered more for its sedative rather than its analgesic effects, and analgesia should be provided by other drugs. However, due to the mu-opioid antagonist effects, butorphanol should not be selected in the painful patient unless mild pain only is assessed. Very low-dose benzodiaz-epines (e.g. diazepam, midazolam), which cause minimal to no respiratory and cardiovascular changes at low dosages, and whose effects are reversible, may be indicated alone and can be added to the opioids if more sedation is needed and can be used alone in neonates/infants. Ensure that flumazenil (0.005 mg/kg, repeat if required) is on hand when administered to patients of less than 5 weeks of age just in case there is delay in metabolizing the drug due to hepatic immaturity. However, the benzodiazepines at the higher dosages may result in bradycar-dia and hypotension following IV administration due to sympathetic suppression. Significant CNS depression has been reported in very young animals. On the other hand, excitation, mania, anxiety and potential aggression may occur in the healthy juvenile due to release of inhibition (suppressed behaviour). This also occurs in the healthy young adult animal (personal experience).

VI.   Local Anesthetics for All Age Groups: General Considerations

Local anesthetics are recommended wherever possible, but careful dosing based on accurate body weight is imperative. A maximum dose of local anesthetic is half the adult dose [17, 18] for both kittens and puppies up to 10 days of age. The lower dose is required because of the immatu-rity of peripheral nerves, not because the younger animals are at any greater risk of toxic side effects. This dose should be diluted in sterile water for accurate dosing, ease of administration and distribution over the site; however, this dilutes the local anesthetic and reduces effectiveness. For lidocaine and bupivacaine, concentrations of < 0.125% and < 0.25%, respectively, are not rec-ommended. Infiltration of lidocaine is extremely painful even with 27- to 30-gauge needles, espe-cially in the neonate or pediatric patient [11]. To reduce pain, buffering, warming (37°–42 °C) and slow administration are recommended. As most veterinary practices have a 2% solution, this can be diluted 1:1 with sterile water (1% = 10 mg/mL) and warmed to ~37–42 °C. Should this still be painful, mix with sodium bicarbonate to a further 10:1 ratio (1 mL 1% lidocaine with 0.1 mEq (0.1 mL of 1 mEq/mL) sodium bicarbonate). Lidocaine may be administered as a 4–6 mg/kg total dose in the pediatric puppy and 2–4 mg/kg in the pediatric kitten. Younger puppies should receive 2–4 mg/kg and younger kittens 1–3 mg/kg total dose. Mepivacaine does not induce pain on injec-tion, **a maximum dose is half the adult dose** for both kittens and puppies up to 10 days of age. Bupivacaine may also be used with a 2 mg/kg maximum dose in the older puppy and 1.5 mg/kg in the older kitten, with half of this dose advised for the neonate and weanling. Buffering of a 0.5% bupivacaine solution (5 mg/mL) requires a 20:1 mixture with 1 mEq/mL sodium bicarbonate (~0.5 mL bupivacaine and 0.025 mL sodium bicarbonate) and warmed as described for lidocaine. Lidocaine transdermal patches may be of value when applied over incisions to provide extended pain relief, up to 24 h. Systemic absorption is variable but is reported to below.

A.   Topical Local Anesthetic Creams

EMLA® (Eutectic Mixture of Local Anesthetic) cream is a prescription-only mixture of lido-caine 2.5% and prilocaine 2.5% combined with thickening agents to form an emulsion (EMLA cream, AstraZeneca LP, Wilmington, DE, USA). This product is not sterile and should be used only on intact skin to provide anesthesia for IV catheter placement, blood collection, lumbar puncture and other minor superficial procedures. The prilocaine component may cause methemoglobinemia in cats should this be placed on open or inflammatory areas. EMLA cream should be covered with an occlusive dressing for at least 30 min and preferably longer. In children, the effect is at 2 h; however, our experience in animals is that 30 min facilitates such procedures as jugular catheter placement using the Seldinger technique; however, a longer dwell time may be necessary in the more active animal. Sterile prep is performed just prior to the procedure. In one veterinary study, there was no systemic uptake of the components of EMLA cream and its use appeared effective in preventing signs of discomfort during jugular catheter placement [19]. However, the skin must be intact/normal.

ELA-Max®, LMX™ (Ferndale Laboratories, Ferndale, MI, USA) is an over-the-counter liposome-encapsulated formulation of 4% lidocaine. Transdermal absorption did occur after application of 15 mg/kg of this product, but plasma concentrations remained significantly below toxic values [20]. The area must be covered to prevent licking with subsequent absorption through the oral mucous membrane and concerns for lidocaine toxicity [21]. As prilocaine is not in this product, it is less of a concern when used in the kitten.

Maxiline® 4 (Ferndale Laboratories, Ferndale, MI, USA) is a product containing 4% lidocaine and may be preferred to EMLA cream as the local anesthetic effect occurs faster. This product is only used on intact skin [22].

Lidocaine 2% is also available as a sterile gel and as a cartridge and is useful for sterile local desensitization (e.g. desensitization of the vaginal vault prior to urinary catheter placement in female cats and dogs and may also be applied to the penis prior to urinary catheter placement).

In conclusion, the opioids appear to be the safest class of analgesic in this population of veterinary patients. Morphine is the least desirable of the opioids due to greater potential for associated adverse effects and is not recommended as a bolus in cats. While the NSAIAs may appear safe in the juvenile patient, their use in younger veterinary patients should be withheld due to safety concerns. Please refer to this section when dealing with a specific scenario presented in this book as drugs may, and dosages will, differ depending on the age of the puppy and kitten. In addition, the normal physiological parameters in the pediatric patient differ from the adult and must be maintained to optimize outcome.

VII. Non-Pharmacological Interventions [23, 24]

Nursing care to ensure warmth and comfort prevents discomfort contributing to worsening pain. This includes reducing the noise and lights (Figure 25.1). Gentle massage may also be beneficial, contributing to the "gate effect". Suckling is analgesic in rat and human infants.

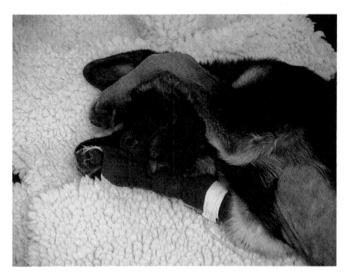

Figure 25.1 A 4-month-old German shepherd puppy requesting that the noise and light be reduced.

Where any painful procedure is required in young animals, contact with the mother as soon as possible is recommended [25]. Bottle feeding/sucking or other feeding procedures can provide distraction-related analgesia and comfort. These procedures should be considered as adjuncts to the analgesics recommended above, not as stand-alone for painful procedures.

VIII. Anesthesia

Because of the previously mentioned physiologic limitations (e.g. higher oxygen demand, lower maximum stroke volume) and the fact that very young patients may have an exaggerated response to anesthetic/analgesic drugs because of the permeable blood–brain barrier, immature hepatic metabolism and decreased albumin for drug protein binding, anesthetic drugs for patients in the neonatal and infant age groups should be chosen carefully and dosed very conservatively. Recommended dosages are based on clinical experience and extrapolation from human neonatal/pediatric pharmacokinetics [27]. Patients in the weanling group can tolerate slightly higher dosages and are closer to adults physiologically. Patients in the juvenile age group are generally considered adults, although drug dosages may still be slightly reduced when compared to dosages used for young and middle-aged adults. In healthy patients of all age groups, most of the currently used anesthetic drugs are appropriate, but in compromised patients drug selection may be more critical and drug **dosage** can be extremely critical. Dosages of anesthetic drugs are generally approximately 50% of adult dosages in neonates/infants and weanlings. Juvenile patients generally require 75–80% of adult dosages. As previously discussed, the dosages of many analgesic drugs are not decreased.

Of special interest is the fact that anesthesia in very young animals has been implicated in neuronal death in rodents, leading to concern that anesthesia in this age group may impair neuronal development [28]. However, this has not been shown in other species, including humans, and the importance of the findings is unclear. The current recommendation from human medicine is to support the patient physiologically, keep anesthesia duration short, utilize low dosages of anesthetic drugs and provide appropriate analgesia using multi-modal techniques that include both systemic and local analgesic drugs [29]. Most veterinary anesthesiologists currently support this approach.

A. Patient Preparation

A thorough physical examination is important for all patients, regardless of age. A complete blood count and serum chemistry evaluation should be considered and an ECG and urinalysis (UA) may be beneficial, especially in patients who may have concurrent disease. Other tests should be performed based on the patient's overall health status.

Hydration status should be critically evaluated (see Section II). Because these patients adapt poorly to hypovolemia, pre-operative fluid therapy may be necessary. However, because normal protein levels are low, resulting in a lower than normal oncotic pressure, and renal clearance may be immature, over-hydration (tissue and pulmonary edema) can occur if fluid needs are not carefully calculated. Weanling and juvenile patients should generally have a short fasting period (4–6h) before surgery but neonates are highly susceptible to hypoglycemia and should not be fasted. Blood glucose concentrations must be evaluated in neonates, and in any patient with prolonged recovery. Because of low oxygen reserve, these patients may need to be pre-oxygenated for 2–5min before induction and receive oxygen for as long as possible after the surgical procedure.

B. Pre-Medication

As previously stated, opioids are a fairly safe class of drugs in veterinary patients and their effects are reversible, adding to their safety. The appropriate opioid from Table 25.1 should be administered to the patient. Opioids alone are often suitable for pre-operative analgesia and tranquilization, especially in dogs. In cats, sedation is generally inadequate with opioids used alone; however, neonatal and infant patients of both species may be sedated with opioids alone. Full mu-agonists like morphine, hydromorphone, methadone and fentanyl should be considered, especially for healthy patients scheduled for painful procedures. Opioid dosages may need to be decreased, and ventilation supported, in the neonatal/infant patients. Partial-agonist opioids like buprenorphine may not provide adequate sedation when used alone but cardiovascular and respiratory effects are almost non-existent, making them safe choices for analgesia for mild to moderate pain. Butorphanol provides moderate sedation and may be effective when used alone for sedation in neonatal/infant patients and perhaps even weanling patients but will require combination with other sedatives in juvenile patients. Because the duration of butorphanol-mediated analgesia is short, and analgesic properties weak, the drug should be considered more for its sedative effects rather than analgesic effects and analgesia should be provided by other drugs or repeat dosages of butorphanol should be administered. Benzodiazepines (e.g. diazepam, midazolam), which cause minimal to no respiratory and cardiovascular changes and whose effects are reversible, can be added to the opioids if more sedation is needed and can be used alone in neonates/infants but may cause paradoxical excitement if used alone in older patients. Because hepatic metabolism is required for termination of drug effect, reversal of benzodiazepines with flumazenil may be necessary in neonatal/infant patients. Acepromazine may be used in some cases but the duration of action can be extremely prolonged and acepromazine-mediated vasodilation is likely to result in hypotension in patients with minimal vascular and baroreceptor control. Also, acepromazine is not reversible and requires hepatic clearance for termination of drug effects. Thus, acepromazine is generally not used in very young patients but is acceptable in juveniles. The alpha$_2$ receptor agonists (e.g. medetomidine, dexmedetomidine) are generally suitable for healthy juvenile patients that need moderate to profound sedation but the alpha$_2$-induced cardiovascular changes make their use in neonates and infants controversial. Fortunately, opioids and benzodiazepines generally provide adequate sedation in this age group so the alpha$_2$ receptor agonists are rarely needed. The effects of the alpha$_2$ receptor agonists are reversible. For all drugs listed, IM administration is usually easiest and requires the least restraint, while IV provides a more rapid and profound effect. The SC route of injection results in uptake that is generally too slow for adequate sedation. Once sedation (or calming; the effect may not be overt sedation) has occurred, an IV catheter should be placed. An intraosseous (IO) catheter is an option where IV access cannot be obtained (see Box 25.1). As previously stated, local anesthetic cream can be applied at the catheter site to decrease the pain of catheterization.

C. Induction Drugs

When used at reduced dosages, any of the currently available injectable induction drugs are appropriate in healthy patients. Because of the multiple routes of elimination, propofol is often the best choice since immature metabolic and clearance mechanisms won't affect elimination of the drug. Both propofol and alfaxalone (not yet available in all countries) can be easily titrated to effect allowing the patient to receive the most appropriate patient-specific dose. Alfaxalone can also be administered IM for sedation and this route provides minimal physiologic impact and moderate sedation of about 10–20 min. Appropriate ventilatory and circulatory support may be needed to compensate for respiratory and cardiovascular depression caused by propofol and alfaxalone when used at induction dosages. Ketamine is cleared, in part, unchanged by the kidney and, therefore, in patients with immature renal clearance may continue to circulate, resulting in prolonged anesthesia. Thus, ketamine is generally reserved for juvenile patients but may be acceptable in very low dosages in patients of other age groups. Mask or chamber induction **is not recommended** because of the high dose of inhalant anesthetic drugs needed to induce anesthesia and because of the potential for struggling/excitement during induction. However, if IV access is not possible, **carefully** titrated mask induction, in patients that have received pre-medication, may be the only option. Concurrent administration of analgesic drugs and/or sedatives is imperative as the use of inhalant anesthetics alone is a risk factor for anesthesia-related mortality [30]. As soon as the patient is induced, or as soon as a mask is applied if inhalant induction is utilized, ophthalmic lubricant should be applied to the eyes.

D. Maintenance Drugs

Isoflurane, sevoflurane and desflurane are appropriate choices for maintenance of anesthesia. As with other patients, inhalant anesthetic concentrations during maintenance of anesthesia should be kept to a minimum since inhalant anesthetics are major contributors to hypotension, hypoventilation and hypothermia. Adequate analgesia can allow a significant decrease in the dose of inhalant anesthetic drugs necessary for anesthesia. **Analgesia is imperative and absolutely should not be withheld from these patients because of misconceptions about pain perception in the very young, or fear of the side effects of analgesic drugs.** Pain itself can cause tachycardia, hypertension, decreased renal blood flow and myriad other effects that may not be well tolerated in very young patients with minimal physiologic reserve. And, as previously stated, pain during nervous system development can lead to lasting pain syndromes. Local anesthetic drugs and opioids can be used in any age group; however, dosage must be calculated carefully and, in neonates and other extremely small patients (at dosages listed in Table 25.1), the drug may need to be diluted with sterile water or sterile saline in order to provide a volume large enough for injection while still maintaining an effective concentration. CRIs of opioids, ketamine, lidocaine or combinations of these drugs are also appropriate in some patients.

E. Monitoring and Support

The limited physiological reserves in neonatal and infant patients increase the possibility of anesthetic complications, and these must be prevented if at all possible, or recognized early if they do occur. A staff member should be dedicated to careful monitoring of the patient throughout the entire procedure. Monitoring should include basics like heart rate, respiratory rate, pulse strength, mucous membrane colour and capillary refill time, and electronic-based monitoring like oxygen-hemoglobin saturation (SpO_2), blood pressure, $ETCO_2$ and ECG analysis. Body temperature should be monitored and normothermia should be vigorously supported as hypothermia causes myriad adverse effects [31]. Neonatal, infant and even weanling patients have a large body surface area compared with body mass, which equates to rapid heat loss. Neonates and infants have an immature thermoregulatory centre which may not respond to hypothermia, and these patients may not be able to shiver and warm themselves. In those patients that can shiver, shivering greatly increases oxygen consumption (up to 200%) and can contribute to hypoxemia. Thus, every attempt should be made to avoid hypothermia.

Table 25.2 Sedation and anesthetic dosages for neonatal: Pediatric patients. (Dosages are suggestions only. Titrate to effect where possible.) Healthy patients of all age groups may require dosages closer to those listed for the next older age group. As previously discussed, the dosages of many analgesic drugs are not decreased.

Dosage (mg/kg)	Neonates, infants and weanlings Dose mg/kg	Juveniles Dose mg/kg	Pediatrics and adults Dose mg/kg	Comments
Pre-operative sedatives: Dosages may be higher when used for sedation without anesthesia				
Acepromazine	Not recommended		0.01–0.03 IM dogs; 0.03–0.05 IM cats	Requires hepatic metabolism for termination of effects and can cause exaggerated, prolonged effect in very young patients
Butorphanol	0.05–0.2 mg/kg IV or IM dogs and cats	0.1–0.3 mg/ kg IV or IM dogs and cats	0.2–0.4 mg/ kg IV or IM dogs and cats	Duration of analgesia short but can be a very effective sedative in younger patients. Effects are reversible
Dexmedetomidine	Not recommended	0.003–0.007 IM dogs; 0.007–0.01 IM cats	0.005–0.01 IM dogs; 0.010–0.015 IM cats	Unlike in adult patients, young patients may need an anticholinergic since heart rate is critical for adequate cardiac output. Effects are reversible
Diazepam	0.05–0.1 IV dogs and cats	0.1 IV dog and cats	0.2 IV dogs and cats	Effects are reversible
Medetomidine	Not recommended	0.005–0.015 IM dogs; 0.01–0.02 IM cats	0.01–0.02 IM dogs; 0.02–0.03 IM cats	Unlike in adult patients, young patients may need an anticholinergic since heart rate is critical for adequate cardiac output. Effects are reversible
Midazolam	0.05–0.1 IV; 0.1–0.2 IM dogs and cats	0.1 IV; 0.1–0.2 IM dogs and cats	0.2 IV; 0.2–0.4 IM dogs and cats	Advantage in very small patients because can be administered IM. Effects are reversible. It is **essential** to have flumazenil on hand when using in neonates, infants and weanlings
Induction drugs: Use the lowest effective dose – **pre-medication should be used to lower the dose**				
Propofol	1–3 IV dogs and cats	1–4 IV dogs and cats	2–6 IV dogs and cats	Titrate carefully to effect
Alfaxalone	0.5–1.5 IV dogs; 1–2.5 IV or 0.5–1.0 IM cats	1–2 IV dogs; 2–3 IV or 1–2 IM cats	2–3 IV in dogs, up to 5 in cats; IM sedation in cats 1–3	Advantage in very small patients because can be administered IM

Table 25.2 (Continued)

Dosage (mg/kg)	Neonates, infants and weanlings Dose mg/kg	Juveniles Dose mg/kg	Pediatrics and adults Dose mg/kg	Comments
Ketamine	Use ½ low end adult dose with caution	1–3 IV; 5–7 IM dogs and cats	1–5 IV; 5–10 IM dogs and cats	Advantage in very small patients because can be administered IM, but does require both hepatic and renal elimination, so use cautiously
Maintenance drugs: **Use lowest effective dose! Pre-medication should be used to lower the dose.** May not be able to administer dosages as low as recommended here without pre-medication				
Isoflurane	1%	1–2%	1–3%	Dose **carefully** to effect
Sevoflurane	1–2%	2–3%	2–4%	Dose **carefully** to effect

Source: Adapted from [32]. With permission.

Box 25.1 Intraosseous (IO) catheter placement

EZ-IO® Technique

- IO catheterization is a very fast and effective technique when performed correctly.
- Ideally, it is used as a short-term alternative until vascular access is available.
- Complication rates in patients with IO catheters is extremely low. However, IO catheters are contraindicated in:
  - recently or previously fractured bones
  - bones where previous catheterization has already been performed
  - bones with an infection at the insertion site.

Indications
- During emergency resuscitation to gain circulatory access.
- When venous or central venous access is not possible due to marked hypotension.

Materials
- Clipper with clean blades
- Antiseptic surgical prep solution
- 2% lidocaine solution
- 3 mL syringe
- 22-gauge hypodermic needle
- #11 scalpel blade
- EZ-IO drill
- EZ-IO stainless steel catheter
- EZ-IO infusion system

Technique
- Place the patient in lateral recumbency.
- Choose access site. Most commonly used sites include the medial surface of the tibial tuberosity, the greater tubercle of the humerus and the trochanteric fossa of the femur.
- Identify landmarks on patient.

(Continued)

Box 25.1 (Continued)

- Shave and aseptically prepare the insertion site.
- Infiltrate the skin with 0.25 mL to 0.5 mL of 2% lidocaine and make a small stab incision.
- Load the appropriate sized IO catheter onto the EZ-IO drill. Two sizes are available for veterinary patients: pediatric: 15-gauge, 15 mm and adult: 15-gauge, 25 mm.
- Position the drill at the insertion site with the needle at a 90° angle to the bone surface. Push the tip of the needle through the skin and gently power the needle until it touches the bone.
- Apply forward pressure to ensure the needle does not slip.
- Depress the power button of the drill to drive the catheter into the bone with steady pressure.
- Once the catheter is placed, apply twisting pressure to the catheter to firmly implant the hub (movement of the hub should also move the patient's leg).
- Remove the stylet and confirm placement by aspiration of bone marrow through the catheter.
- A syringe or fluid administration set can be attached to the catheter hub for administration of emergency drugs or crystalloid/colloid solutions.

Special Notes
- It is important to verify the placement of the catheter prior to the administration of fluid therapy. Aspiration (gentle) of bone marrow into the syringe should be seen. Also, bolus of heparinized saline should pass easily and there should never be accumulation of SC fluid in the surrounding tissue.
- Drug dosages for IO administration are the same as IV dosages.
- Solutions can also be administered at similar IV rates. However, pain may be associated with high rate fluid infusion. An infusion of lidocaine through the catheter (1–2 mg/kg, 2% solution) can reduce the pain.

To Remove IO Catheter
- Gently twist clockwise while applying traction to the catheter.
- Apply a bandage to the insertion site and monitor site for bleeding or signs of infection.

Box 25.2 Intraosseous (IO) catheter placement in neonates (puppy or kitten)

Materials
- Clipper with clean blades
- Antiseptic surgical prep solution
- 2% lidocaine solution
- #11 scalpel blade
- 20- to 22-gauge spinal needle or a 18- to 25-gauge hypodermic needle
- 3 mL syringe with heparinized saline flush
- Sterile gloves

Technique
- Place the patient in lateral recumbency.
- In neonates, the access site most commonly chosen is the trochanteric fossa of the femur.
- Identify landmarks on the patient.
- Shave and aseptically prepare the insertion site.

- Infiltrate the skin with 0.25–0.5 mL of 2% lidocaine and make a very small stab incision in (18-gauge needle is adequate for very small animals) the skin over the trochanteric fossa of the femur.
- Select the appropriate sized needle based on patient and bone size. Use a 20- to 22-gauge spinal needle when available. However, an 18- to 25-gauge hypodermic needle will also work.
- Wearing sterile gloves, position the needle through the skin incision and into the trochanteric fossa.
- Carefully drive the needle through the cortex into the medullary cavity using downward pressure and rotation.
- Once the needle is in place, proper positioning should be checked by manipulation of the femur. The femur and needle should move as a unit. The needle should also be flushed with heparinized saline. If properly positioned, the saline should infuse easily into the medulla of the bone.
- A syringe or burette fluid administration set can be attached to the needle hub for administration of emergency drugs or crystalloid/colloid solutions.
- Cover with a protective bandage.
  IO catheters can remain in place for up to 72 h. However, once the patient is stabilized, IV access should be gained through a peripheral or central venous catheter and the IO catheter removed.

Source: Adapted from [33]. With permission.

F. Recovery

Unfortunately, most anesthetic deaths occur in recovery [30], and many of these deaths are preventable with appropriate monitoring and support. Oxygen and fluid therapy should continue into recovery, and the duration of support depends on the age/health status of the individual patient. Active warming is generally necessary. Blood glucose concentrations should be rechecked, especially in neonatal and infant patients and in any patient that is having a prolonged recovery. In the event of prolonged recovery, the effects of reversible drugs can be antagonized but, if reversing opioids, ensure that pain is controlled by other means.

In conclusion, please refer to this section when dealing with a specific scenario presented in this book as the anesthetic protocol may, and dosages will, differ depending on the age of the puppy and kitten. In addition, the normal physiological parameters in the pediatric patient differ from the adult and must be maintained to optimize outcome.

References

1 Boothe, D. M. and Bucheler, J. (2001) Drug and blood component therapy and neonatal isoerythrolysis. In: Hospkins, J. (ed.), *Veterinary Pediatrics: Dogs and cats from birth to six months*. WB Saunders, Philadelphia: 35–56.

2 For citations on pediatric physiology with respect to analgesia, see: Aarnes, T. K., Muir, III W. W. (2011) Pain assessment and management. In: Peterson, M. E. and Kutzler, M. A. (eds), *Small Animal Pediatrics: The first 12 months of life*. Elsevier, St Louis, MO: 220–232.

3 Lee, B. H. (2002) Managing pain in human neonates: Application for animals. *J Am Vet Med Assoc*, 221: 233–237.

4 Lee, S. J., Ralston, H. J., Drey, E. A., *et al.* (2005) Fetal pain: A systematic multidisciplinary review of the evidence. *JAMA*, 294: 947–954.

5 Fitzgerald, M. and Beggs, S. (2001) The neurobiology of pain: Developmental aspects. *Neuroscientist*, 7: 246–257.

6 Taddio, A., Katz, J., Ilersich, A. L. and Koren, G. (1997) Effect of neonatal circumcision on pain response during subsequent routine vaccination. *Lancet*, 349: 599–603.

7 Berde, C. B. and Sethna, N. F. (2002) Analgesics for the treatment of pain in children. *N Engl J Med*, 347(109): 4–1103.

8 Blanco, J. G., Harrison, P. L., Evans, W. E., *et al.* (2000) Human cytochrome P-450 maximal activities in pediatric vs adult liver. *Drug Metab Dispos*, 28: 379–382.

9 Pascoe, P. J. and Moon, P. F. (2001) Periparturient and neonatal anesthesia. *Vet Clin North Am Small Anim Pract*, 31(2): 315–340.

10 Luks, A. M., Zwass, M. S. and Brown, R. C. (1998) Opioid-induced analgesia in neonatal dogs: Pharmacodynamic differences between morphine and fentanyl. *J Pharmacol Exp Ther*, 284: 136–141.

11 Bragg, P., Zwass, M. S. and Lau, M. (1995) Opioid pharmacodynamics in neonatal dogs: Differences between morphine and fentanyl. *J Appl Physiology*, 79: 1519–1524.

12 Bhutta, A. T. (2007) Ketamine: A controversial drug for neonates. *Semin Perinatol*, 31: 303–308.

13 Himmelseher, S. and Durieux, M. E. (2005) Revising a dogma: Ketamine for patients with neurological injury? *Anesth Analg*, 101: 524–534.

14 Lotx, S., De Kock, M. and Henin, P. (2011) The anti-inflammatory effects of ketamine: State of the art. *Acta Anaesth Belg*, 62: 17–58.

15 Lynn, M., Rusy, L. M., Hainsworth, K. R., *et al.* (2010) Gabapentin use in pediatric spinal fusion patients: A randomized, double-blind, controlled trial. *Anesth Analg*, 110: 1393–1398.

16 Hosgood, G. (1992) Surgical and anesthetic management of puppies and kittens. *Comp Contin Edu*, 14: 345–357.

17 Ball, A. J. and Ferguson, S. (1996) Analgesia and analgesic drugs in paediatrics. *Br J Hosp Med*, 55(9): 586–590.

18 Mathews, K. A., Kronen, P., Lascelles, D., *et al.* (2014) Guidelines for recognition, assessment and treatment of pain. *J Small Anim Pract*, 55(6): E10–E68.

19 Gibbon, K. J., Cyborski, J. M., Guzinski, M. V., *et al.* (2003) Evaluation of adverse effects of EMLA (lidocaine/prilocaine) cream for the placement of jugular catheters in healthy cats. *J Vet Pharmacol Ther*, 26: 439–441.

20 Taddio, A., Soin, H. K., Schuh, S., *et al.* (2005) Liposomal lidocaine to improve procedural success rates and reduce procedural pain among children. *J Can Med Assoc*, 172(13): 1691–1695.

21 Fransson, B. A., Peck, K. E., Smith, J. K., *et al.* (2002) Transdermal absorption of a liposome encapsulated formulation of lidocaine following topical administration in cats. *Am J Vet Res*, 63: 1309–1312.

22 Rodriguez, E. and Jordan, R. (2002) Contemporary trends in pediatric sedation and analgesia: Pediatric emergency medicine: Current concepts and controversies. *Emerg Med Clin North Am*, 1: 199–222.

23 Pillai Riddell, R., Racine, N., Turcotte, K., *et al.* (2011) Non-pharmacological management of procedural pain in infants and young children: An abridged. *Pain Res Manag*, 16: 321–330.

24 Golianu, B., Krane, E., Seybold, J., *et al.* (2007) Nonpharmacological techniques for pain management in neonates. *Semin Perinatol*, 31: 318–322.

25 Gray, L., Miller, L. W., Barbara, B. A., *et al.* (2002) Breastfeeding is analgesic in healthy newborns. *Pediatrics*, 109: 590–593.

26 Mathews, K. A. (2008) Pain management for the pregnant, lactating and neonatal to pediatric cat and dog. *Vet Clin North Am Small Anim Pract*, 38: 191–1308.

27 Hansen, T. G. (2015) Developmental paediatric anaesthetic pharmacology. *Anaesthesia and Intensive Care Med*, 16(8): 417–422.

28 Loftis, G. K., Collins, S. and McDowell, M. (2012) Anesthesia-induced neuronal apoptosis during synaptogenesis: A review of the literature. *AANA J*, 80(4): 291–298.

29 Sinner, B., Becke, K. and Engelhard, K. (2014) General anaesthetics and the developing brain: An overview. *Anaesthesia*, 69(9): 1009–1022.

30 Brodbelty, D. (2009) Perioperative mortality in small animal anaesthesia. *The Veterinary Journal*, 182: 152–161.

31 Clark-Price, S. (2015) Inadvertent perianesthetic hypothermia in small animal patients. *Vet Clin North Am Small Anim Pract*, 45: 983–994.

32 Mathews, K. A. (2008) Analgesia for the pregnant, lactating, and neonatal to pediatric cat and dog. *Vet Clin Small Anim*, 38: 1299–1308.

33 Steele, A., Mathews, K. and Allan, L. (2017) Vascular access techniques, Veterinary. In: Mathews, K. A. (ed.), *Veterinary Emergency & Critical Care Manual*, 3rd edn. LifeLearn, Guelph, Ontario, Canada.

26

Analgesia and Anesthesia for the Geriatric Patient

Karol Mathews, Melissa Sinclair, Andrea Steele and Tamara Grubb

I. General Considerations [1]

Age on its own is not a "disease", but with advanced age it is more typical for cardiovascular or endocrine diseases to develop in an animal. It is the development of these secondary diseases that may complicate the anesthetic or analgesic administration and overall responses in geriatrics and increase the mortality rate in dogs and cats over the age of 12 years. In veterinary medicine, animals living at, or beyond, 75% of their life expectancy, are considered geriatric, but these geriatric patients will typically experience pain as any "average aged" patient would. It is estimated that at least 30% of pet dogs and cats that are seen by veterinarians can be classified as "senior" and many may have chronic pain, which is often mistaken for "getting old". Careful specific questioning of the owner is required to establish whether chronic pain behaviours exist as the changes in behaviour that accompany chronic pain may be insidious in onset and subtle [2]. Chronic pain, with subsequent wind-up components, will potentially increase the acute pain experienced during illness or injury; therefore, veterinarians treating geriatric animals should consider the potential for accompanying chronic pain, even in the absence of immediately obvious signs. This will make pain management very important for the overall success of treatment in this subset of aged patients.

As with any other animal, it is essential to confirm the overall health status and investigate physical findings prior to administering or prescribing certain classes of analgesics or anesthetics. Analgesics should not be withheld, but tailored to the individual needs and findings of the geriatric animal. The selection and dose will likely be the same as those for younger patients unless organ dysfunction is noted. As with other ill or injured animals, a thorough history and physical examination is essential to assess the general health and to identify the problem(s) prompting veterinary care. While physical changes associated with ageing, described below, may be common in the geriatric patient, some older animals may not exhibit these changes. A potential anatomical change that may occur in the very frail patient is a marked decrease in muscle mass. In these patients, avoid intramuscular (IM) administration of analgesics if possible as their body composition limits effective analgesic absorption and distribution [3].

Analgesia and Anesthesia for the Ill or Injured Dog and Cat, First Edition. Karol A. Mathews, Melissa Sinclair, Andrea M. Steele and Tamara Grubb.
© 2018 John Wiley & Sons, Inc. Published 2018 by John Wiley & Sons, Inc.

II.   Physiologic Features of the Geriatric Patient Affecting Dosages, Drug Metabolism and Excretion

A.   Effect of Trauma [1]

Opioids are the first-line analgesic drugs due to their efficacy, ability to carefully titrate to effect and ability to reverse. Immediately following trauma, the presence of a stress and shock response may confer some analgesia for a short period of time. Pain may be difficult to assess during this time as the physiological parameters and mentation changes in response to opioid titration may not be reliable. Depending on the duration from incident to presentation, potentially a lower dose of opioid than one would expect for the degree of injury may be required. As the stress response diminishes over the following hour or two (or less) and the patient becomes more aware, increasing dosages of opioid are required. On the contrary, some geriatric patients may have a decreased receptor response to stress, potentially requiring a higher dose of opioid initially than that anticipated for a similar injury in a younger animal. Regardless of this sympathetic change, geriatric animals typically have other functional and anatomical changes within the central nervous system that may reduce their requirement for all analgesic drug classes. Therefore, required dosing of analgesics, including opioids, should be based on careful titration and close monitoring for response to treatment. Other influencing effects to consider are discussed below. Should the patient be aggressive, and manual restraint is not possible, chemical restraint, for example fentanyl 3–5 µg/kg, IM accompanied by "strategic" manual restraint (refer to Chapter 22), may be administered to facilitate intravenous (IV) catheter placement and further evaluation.

B.   Initial Evaluation

An IV catheter with commencement of fluids at a rate required for the situation should be established immediately prior to analgesic administration. The initial titrated opioid dose should give a sufficient duration of effect for a baseline physical examination, blood sampling for baseline laboratory evaluation and other necessary diagnostics (radiographic/ultrasonographic examination).

C.   Fluids Administration Considerations in Geriatric Trauma Cases [3]

Hydration status may be difficult to assess using the "skin tent" method due to loss of elastin in the geriatric animal; even in hydrated animals, a skin tent may be present. More attention should be paid to moistness and colour of mucous membranes and capillary refill time, pulse, blood pressures and laboratory values. The ageing cardiovascular changes should not be assumed in all geriatric patients as some are extremely fit and maintain an appropriate cardiac index for the reduced muscle mass and metabolic rate. Exercise tolerance is an important positive predictor of a successful anesthetic outcome. However, when the cardiovascular status is questionable, aggressive fluid therapy should not be instituted, and may be potentially dangerous in this population of patients. A careful fluid plan in the peri-anesthetic period is essential and additional inotropic support may be warranted. In the dehydrated patient, IV fluids with a balanced electrolyte solution should be initiated at a conservative rate (3–5 mL/kg/h) until additional laboratory assessment of organ function can be determined. The kidney changes that occur in the geriatric patient frequently result in an increased urine output, potentially requiring measurement to assess replacement.

D. Laboratory Evaluation and Considerations for Analgesic and Anesthetic Administration [1]

Obtaining basic laboratory data is essential to establish the baseline values of any patient, but especially the geriatric patient. Laboratory tests are based on those required for the underlying problem(s) at hand. However, basic tests should include PCV, TS, serum urea, creatinine, alkaline phosphatase (ALP), alanine aminotransferase (ALT), albumin, calcium, glucose, bilirubin, phosphorous, electrolytes and urinalysis [3] or urine stick analysis with urine-specific gravity. Protein assessment is also important. Abnormalities in ALP, ALT, urine-specific gravity/ protein are often detected in the pre-anesthetic assessment of geriatric dogs [4]. Several other laboratory tests may be required based on presenting signs, physical examination and differential diagnoses.

E. Renal and Hepatic Function Considerations for Analgesic and Anesthetic Administration [1]

As renal and hepatic function, as well as albumin levels, influence drug metabolism, overall drug clearance and availability, this information will guide ongoing analgesic and anesthetic decisions. As with the very young animal, the geriatric may have reduced albumin concentration which will affect serum levels of the more protein-bound drugs. This may produce a more profound effect initially and an increased elimination rate.

1. Renal Function [1]

Renal function is affected with ageing due to a loss of cortical mass and functional nephron units. This, together with a reduction in renal plasma flow, results in a decreased glomerular filtration rate (GFR) and drug clearance. Other normal kidney functions – such as antidiuretic hormone function, conservation of sodium and urine concentration – are also decreased, which requires careful assessment of fluid requirements. It is essential to understand that a creatinine value within the high normal range does not mean the patient's kidney is completely "normal" but that it is functioning with little to no reserve. In addition, due to the reduced muscle mass and activity of some geriatric patients, the creatinine value obtained is frequently due to lower production rather than filtration (refer to Chapter 20).

2. Liver Mass

Liver mass and, therefore, blood flow and hepatic function may also decrease over time and this will influence drug metabolism and clearance [1]. Enzyme activity is maintained. However, the reduction in liver mass results in a relative reduction in normal microsomal and non-microsomal enzyme function. This combined with a potentially reduced GFR increases the half-life and duration of effect of many drugs (refer to Chapter 21).

F. Cardiovascular Considerations Impacting Analgesic and Anesthetic Administration [1]

The cardiovascular system in the geriatric patient may appear normal on physical examination; however, occult changes are likely to be present due to normal ageing such as myocardial atrophy and fibrosis, valvular fibro-calcification, ventricular wall thickening and lack of elasticity/ distensibility. These changes reduce pump function and cardiac output and may also affect pacemaker cells, potentially resulting in an abnormal rhythm. Abnormalities in heart rate can occur in geriatric patients [4]. With these changes, diastolic ventricular filling becomes more dependent on the atrial kick and normal sinus rhythm. That is, tachycardia, bradycardia and their associated arrhythmias are not well tolerated in the geriatric animal. Heart rates should be kept to a normal range for the breed and species for awake and anesthetized patients. As analgesics can alter heart rate (reduced from opioids and increased with ketamine), monitoring of heart rate and arterial blood pressure becomes important during analgesic administration in the geriatric. In addition, peripheral arterial stiffness and overall lack of distensibility can result in an increased left ventricular workload and potential hypertrophy. Based on the physiologic changes that may have occurred in the individual geriatric patient, cardiac output may be more dependent on preload and, therefore, the geriatric is less tolerant to volume depletion (see Section II.C and Chapter 19).

G. Pulmonary Considerations Impacting Analgesic and Anesthetic Administration [1]

The lungs are also affected in the ageing process. A reduction in lung elastin, intercostal and diaphragmatic muscle mass and a more rigid thorax results in a reduced pulmonary compliance, ventilatory volume and efficient gas exchange. These changes ultimately result in a decreased PaO_2 when compared to younger animals. With analgesic administration, sedation may also result in compromising effective and overall strength of ventilation. With the reduction in minute ventilation with analgesic administration, monitoring with SPO_2, and where available periodic arterial blood gas analysis, is essential to identify the need and level of flow-by oxygen required. Under general anesthesia, geriatric animals tire more easily during spontaneous ventilation making attention to an appropriate anesthetic depth and strength of ventilation important. Geriatric animals may require manual or mechanical assistance for adequate ventilation. However, over-ventilation will increase anesthetic depth and negatively impact cardiovascular function as with any age. In general, tidal volumes of 10–12 mL/kg with respiratory rates of 6–12 breaths per minute and maximal peak inspiratory pressures of 10–12 cmH_2O will be sufficient.

III. Analgesia and Pain Assessment Considerations [1]

Pain assessment is made based on behaviours exhibited for the various degree of pain experienced (refer to Chapter 8). However, pre-existing arthritic changes may predispose to lameness and/or "abnormal" positioning, which may interfere with pain assessment of the problem at hand. Chronic pain must also be managed. Integrative techniques are highly recommended for this age group (refer to Chapter 15).

- **Opioids** are first-line analgesics in this group of patients. Fentanyl is an excellent analgesic and allows for careful IV titration. The dose required to establish comfort can then be used as an hourly continuous rate infusion (CRI). The initial effective opioid analgesic dose given on presentation can be used to establish an initial CRI with observation for potential increased requirements over time due to additional handling and diagnostic procedures. With ageing, muscle mass tends to decrease and adipose tissue increase. As with other animals with increased adipose tissue, lipid soluble drugs will re-distribute to adipose tissue and this "depot" of drug will result in slower elimination. This is compounded by a reduction in liver mass in the geriatric with reduced hepatic arterial blood flow. A CRI of a lipid soluble drug will require frequent assessment to avoid the potential for overdose over time. Should morphine, methadone or hydromorphone be selected, careful titration is also required. Slow IV injection with morphine is essential, with concurrent monitoring of blood pressure and heart rate for 5–10 min in sick patients as rapid IV administration can result in hypotension for approximately 5 min even in a healthy animal due to histamine release. The dose required to attain comfort can then be used as a 4 h infusion or use one-quarter of this/hour (refer to Chapter 10). Arterial blood pressure should be monitored during analgesic administration and stabilization as the sympathetic response associated with the initial pain will be relieved and a "real" hypotensive condition may be revealed.

- **Alpha$_2$ agonists** in high doses, or as the sole analgesic, should not be used until significant systemic disease, cardiopulmonary disease, with or without arrhythmias or conduction disturbances, pre-existing hypo/hypertension, diabetes mellitus and liver/renal failure have been ruled out. Caution should always be exercised when considering the use of an alpha$_2$ agonist in patients with trauma. A low CRI dose of an alpha$_2$ agonist (i.e. after a 15 min loading dose (IV) of 0.5–1 µg/kg dexmedetomidine, followed by 0.5–1 µg/kg/h) is recommended for a multi-modal analgesic regimen in severe pain, in patients that need light sedation in addition to analgesia and/or in a situation requiring opioid sparing once the patient's cardiovascular and fluid status has been fully assessed, and is normal (refer to Chapter 9).
- **Local anesthetic** infiltration, where appropriate, should be included in the analgesic regimen (refer to Chapter 14).
- **Ketamine** in dogs with normal hepatic function and in cats with normal or minimally affected renal function can be added to the opioid in managing severe pain or to lower the opioid dose to avoid adverse effects (nausea, vomiting, dysphoria and panting, signalling the analgesic effect has maximized). Other adjunct analgesics, case dependent, may also be considered (refer to Chapter 12).
- **Non-steroidal anti-inflammatory analgesics (NSAIAs)** should be avoided until health status is evaluated. Some geriatric patients have chronic pain due to osteoarthritis, or other conditions, and may be receiving an NSAIA. This may have to be discontinued based on the overall health status of the patient; therefore, the pain experienced will increase (refer to Chapter 11) and additional analgesic therapy will be required.
- **Complementary/integrative techniques** should be included where appropriate (refer to Chapter 15).

IV. Anesthetic Considerations [1]

In geriatric animals, the anesthetic drug should be tailored to the status and condition of the patient, and the procedure to be performed and its duration should be considered. It is important to remember that anesthetic requirements are reduced with age, including dose reduction requirements for all induction agents and inhalant MAC reductions of up to 30%. Hence, the key is appropriate dose titration of injectable and inhalant anesthetics and close monitoring of anesthetic depth. Concurrent diseases, and not the age of the animal, may affect the anesthetic choice, for example most forms of cardiac disease will make the use of ketamine or an alpha$_2$ agonist controversial or even contraindicated (refer to Chapter 13).

- **Pre-medication** is always recommended to provide analgesia, reduce the animal's stress and anxiety and also reduce the induction and inhalant dose of anesthetic required.
  - ○ **Opioids** are excellent pre-medicants in older patients as they have mild sedative properties with minimal cardiodepressive effects, and provide analgesia. Fentanyl (1–3 µg/kg, IV), hydromorphone (0.03–0.1 mg/kg, IV or IM), morphine (0.3–0.5 mg/kg, IM), methadone (0.3–0.5 mg/kg, IM), meperidine (3–5 mg/kg, IM only), butorphanol (0.2–0.4 mg/kg, IV or IM) or buprenorphine (0.005–0.02 mg/kg, IV or IM) are acceptable choices depending on the procedure and required level of analgesia.

- o **Sedatives**
  - ▪ **Midazolam** (0.1–0.4 mg/kg, IM or IV) may also be added with the opioids to enhance sedation if required. Sedation with the benzodiazepines is more pronounced in the older animal.
  - ▪ **Acepromazine** can be administered to provide sedation and reduce stress; however, lowered doses may be warranted in the geriatric patient (0.01–0.02 mg/kg, IV or IM), and should be omitted when significant cardiovascular disease or fluid deficits exist.
  - ▪ **Alpha₂ agonists** should not be avoided due to age but a thorough physical exam should be performed to ensure that there are no age-related diseases that might preclude the use of alpha₂ agonists. In general, aged patients require lower dosages than middle-aged and young patients. These drugs may be required in aggressive/vicious animals and can be reversed once restraint and/or general anesthesia has been achieved.
- o **Anticholinergics** (atropine or glycopyrrolate) should not be administered routinely to geriatric animals. Administration should be based on need to treat bradyarrhythmias.
- **General anesthesia**

  Recommended anesthetic induction techniques are:

  - o Propofol (2–6 mg/kg, IV) or alfaxalone (1–3 mg/kg, IV) to effect, **or**
  - o Ketamine with diazepam or midazolam (0.1–0.2 mL/kg, IV). Drugs can be mixed together in the same syringe in a 1:1 ratio.
  - o Etomidate (1–3 mg/kg) causes minimal to no cardiovascular effects and is a good choice for geriatric patients with concurrent cardiovascular disease. Pre-medication with an opioid and a bolus of midazolam or diazepam (0.2 mg/kg, IV of either) should be utilized as etomidate without pre-medications commonly causes muscle rigidity, muscle twitching, paddling and vocalization. Etomidate also causes adrenocortical suppression, and its use in septic patients is controversial.

V. Optimal Nursing Care during Hospital Stay and Influence on Pain Management

- **Comfort:** The recumbent geriatric animal requires attention to detail. As these patients have reduced muscle mass, soft padding and beds are essential to prevent decubitus ulcers. When handling/positioning, be cognizant of potential arthritic joints, even under anesthesia, as the pain caused by "heavy handling" will be felt upon recovery. Frequent side changes, often every 1–2 h whilst awake, are necessary to avoid or reduce positional discomfort; however, do not disturb when sleeping. Place towels or other cushioning between the limbs of the animal in lateral, and prop the head at a natural angle to avoid neck discomfort. When positioning the patient in sternal, maintain the hind limbs in lateral to avoid exacerbation of any arthritic hip pain. Cats that are comfortable like to curl up. For the cats, providing a round padded bed is ideal; however, rolling a large bath towel along its long axis and arranging it in a circle will also suffice.
- **Temperature** support is also important in geriatric animals. The reduced resting metabolic rate results in an overall lower production of body heat and resultant temperature. As with the very young, aged patients become hypothermic more readily and re-warming occurs at a slower rate. Exposure to a cold environment must be avoided as shivering increases oxygen demand by approximately 200–300% which may not be attained in the ill, injured or (especially) perioperative patient. Providing supplemental heat – such as a

microwaveable disk, oat bag or a warm-water-circulating blanket in a portion of the cage that the animal can choose to use – will likely be appreciated. Geriatric cats especially enjoy supplemental heat.

- Many geriatric patients may have issues with senility, blindness or deafness, which can be frustrating for them during hospitalization. The veterinary technician/nurse must always keep in mind that anxiety, cage soiling, digging/chewing at cage bars and vocalizing are common in these patients. Anxiolytics may provide some comfort, and can be considered. Often the geriatric patient can benefit from being removed from the cage and restrained by a harness in a central area where there are lots of people. During less busy times, extra TLC, such as a warm lap or a cuddle, may provide comfort to the distressed patient. Providing bedding or clothing from the owner may also be of comfort. Approach the cage cautiously, calling the patient's name to get their attention, before entering the cage, as a startled patient may bite if they are unable to see or hear you. Cage signs reminding all staff that the patient is blind or deaf, or likely to bite, is important for staff safety.

- **Procedures** such as blood collections and IV catheter placement can be particularly stressful for geriatric patients. Avoid placing the patient on a cold steel table or wash table grate, but instead place on a fleece or blanket. Prior to sampling, surgically prep the site and apply EMLA® cream or Maxilene® local anesthetic cream to reduce the discomfort of the procedure. The restraint technique will need to be tailored to the patient; some will do very well with minimal restraint and a soothing voice; others will resent all restraint and are likely to bite or lash out. Consider sedation for these patients to reduce the stress experienced. Pay particular attention to the position of limbs or neck during blood collection, as some positions may be uncomfortable; for example, allowing the patient to lie in lateral recumbency will optimize access to the saphenous and jugular veins and will also negate the need for dorsiflexion of the neck, which is required when in sternal. Placing a rolled towel under the neck in the lateral position may help to elevate the jugular vein, as the reduced muscle mass of the geriatric causes the jugular to sink deeper into the neck. Drawing blood with the needle directed caudally may also be easier for jugular venipuncture, reducing the need for repetitive attempts, which adds to the patient's discomfort.

- **Feeding:** In general, the geriatric patient requires extra nursing consideration, for example coaxing to eat, by providing ample, palatable food choices for the patient to select from. The patient may benefit from small, frequent feedings, rather than once or twice a day feedings. Questioning the owner about favourite meals, asking them to bring food from home or having the owner spend time coaxing their animal to eat may be necessary. Dental disease is common in geriatric cats and dogs, and dry food may be painful to eat. Water should be freely available, but if the patient is blind or particularly anxious, offering water frequently and leaving the bowl outside of the cage will prevent the patient from hitting the bowl and spilling water on them and the cage.

- **Urination and defecation:** Elderly dogs may benefit from being carried or trolleyed outdoors frequently to urinate and defecate. Geriatric cats would do better with a large, shallow litterbox to help avoid "misses". Where urination or defecation occurs in the cage, clean it immediately and ensure that the soiled patient is bathed and dried to prevent urine scalding. Disposable urine pads or absorbent bedding may help to keep the patient dry. For patients that have difficulty walking and frequently urinate, discuss the risks and benefits of urinary catheterization with a closed collection system with the veterinarian as this will help to reduce patient anxiety associated with frequent urination, prevent urine scalding and hypothermia. Diabetes mellitus and numerous other conditions may be contraindications to urinary catheterization.

References

1 Grubb, T. L., Perez Jiminez, T. E. and Pettifer, G. R. (2015) Senior and geriatric patients. In: Grimm, K. A., Lamont, L. A., Tranquilli, W. J, *et al.* (eds), *Veterinary Anesthesia and Analgesia: The fifth edition of Lumb and Jones*, Wiley-Blackwell: 988–992.

2 Wiseman-Orr, M. L., Nolan, A. M., Reid, J. and Scott, E. M. (2004) Development of a questionnaire to measure the effects of chronic pain on health-related quality of life in dogs. *Am J Vet Res*, 65, 1077–1084.

3 Bookers, S., Bartoszczyk, D. A. and Herr, K. A. (2016) Managing pain in frail elders. *Am Nurse Today*, 11(4).

4 Epstein, M., Kuehn, N. F., Landsberg, G., *et al.* (2005) American Animal Hospital Senior Care Guidelines for Cats and Dogs. *J Am Anim Hosp Assoc*, 41: 81–91.

Further Reading

Mathews, K. A., Kronen, P., Lascelles, D., *et al.* (2014) Guidelines for recognition, assessment and treatment of pain. *J Small Anim Pract*, 55(6): E10–E68.

27

Analgesia and Anesthesia for Head and Neck Injuries or Illness

Karol Mathews, Melissa Sinclair, Andrea Steele and Tamara Grubb

Central nervous system (CNS) depression of varying degrees may be present in patients admitted for emergency care, with or without head and/or neck injuries. It is critical to identify whether a potential traumatic brain injury (TBI), and/or a hypovolemic state, or an underlying medical condition exists as a cause for the CNS changes in order to initiate appropriate resuscitative therapy. In a veterinary study of head trauma patients, 25% had serious TBI. In addition, 14% of cats and 9% of dogs also had a spinal cord injury (SCI) [1], so it is essential to manage all trauma patients as though SCI and TBI is a differential until proven otherwise. Both traumatic and atraumatic causes of head and neck pathological changes require careful selection of analgesics, sedatives and anesthetics with key monitoring points during diagnosis and treatment. Initially, after close examination and assessment of the patient, analgesia with opioids is recommended (Box 27.1). In this group of patients, the potential side effects of opioids are especially important for the clinician to understand (refer to Chapter 10). The pure mu-opioid agonists are preferred as they can be titrated to effect, reversed and used to assess the level of pain by the dose required. Fentanyl intravenous (IV) is preferred by the authors as frequent neurologic assessments are more possible with the shorter duration of action of this opioid, and also it imparts a wider therapeutic index and potentially reduced adverse effects (e.g. vomiting) when compared to other long-acting opioids (e.g. hydromorphone, morphine). Remifentanil is not advised (refer to Chapter 10 for adverse effect information). Methadone is superior to other longer-acting opioids as it also possesses N-methyl-D-aspartate (NMDA) receptor antagonist effects and decreased potential for vomiting. The opioid should **always** be slowly titrated to effect while monitoring. **Do not administer a calculated bolus dose of opioid** in these cases as a bolus will result in a temporary heightened plasma level and potentially result in side effects that will increase intracranial pressure (ICP).

I.   Initial Management

A.   General Emergency

General emergency considerations and assessment of patients with head and/or neck pathology should include the following to avoid worsening of pain in an area not yet identified in both traumatic and atraumatic situations:

1. **Obtain a history** from the owner related to the traumatic incident or, if atraumatic, clinical signs prior to presentation. Question the owner about the general health of the animal, co-morbidities, current medications and when the animal was last fed.

Analgesia and Anesthesia for the Ill or Injured Dog and Cat, First Edition. Karol A. Mathews, Melissa Sinclair, Andrea M. Steele and Tamara Grubb.
© 2018 John Wiley & Sons, Inc. Published 2018 by John Wiley & Sons, Inc.

2. **Position the patient appropriately**. Avoid any compression of the neck. For the trauma patient, assume spinal injuries are present until proven otherwise. If available, place the patient on a 15° slant surface (reverse Trendelenburg position), to accommodate the head, neck and thorax as a unit (Figure 27.1). This will reduce potential exacerbation of pain and worsening neurologic injury.

3. **Provide flow-by oxygen** and determine if positive pressure ventilation is required. Do not place a nasal oxygen catheter as potential sneezing may increase ICP.

4. **Obtain IV access** as soon as possible in **all** patients. Minimize restraint, to avoid stress, movement of neck and inadvertent occlusion of the jugular veins, which will increase ICP. Consider a saphenous catheter if more accessible. Avoid jugular venipuncture or catheterization.

5. **Assess the respiratory status of the patient.** Respiratory depression with resultant increases in $PaCO_2$ can result in a rise in ICP. In the non-depressed patient, respiratory compromise is recognized upon admission and is frequently associated with panic, excitement or anxiety. Flow-by oxygen, calming and sedation may be adequate to facilitate therapy in mild situations. If respiratory compromise is severe, progression to respiratory and cardiac arrest occurs rapidly; therefore, the animal's behaviour and hypoxia must be dealt with immediately. General anesthesia may be necessary for immediate management and diagnosis of the severely distressed patients.

6. **Assessment of CNS depression.** Perform a rapid neurologic examination, including orthopedic examination to ensure this isn't the cause of an abnormal neurologic finding, to obtain baseline data and identify lesion location. It is essential to examine pupil size and function prior to opioid use. The miosis that occurs in dogs, and mydriasis in cats, following opioid administration will be a confounder in the neurologic examination.

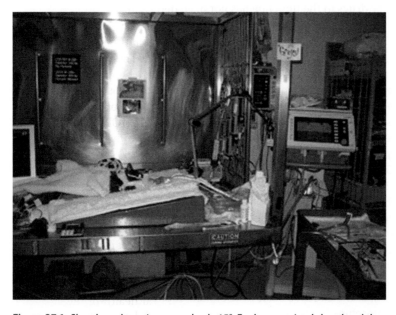

Figure 27.1 Slant board to raise upper body 15°. For larger animals head and thorax are placed on the board where no kinking of the neck will occur. Dimensions to make the slant for 15° [6″ high], 24″ wide, 30″ long. Painted with exterior paint (washable).

7. **Pain assessment** of the animal in relation to their overall condition is important. Analgesia in head-injured patients may be underestimated based on the level of CNS depression caused by TBI; however, pain must be accurately assessed as pain can raise ICP. Where a patient is depressed due to hypovolemia, pain is perceived following resuscitation. Pain associated with intracranial and spinal pathology (e.g. tumour, meningitis) can be significant, requiring caution when handling the patient.

   The clinician should be aware that when administering a standard dose/bolus of an opioid the potential for panting, nausea, vomiting and noise hypersensitivity (may result in increased pain and respiratory compromise) is increased and all these adverse effects increase ICP. However, with careful titration of an opioid this can be avoided, and should not prevent the administration of an opioid when pain exists. At this point another class of analgesic (e.g. ketamine) [2] should be considered if pain is still not controlled.

   Where an upper range, and/or longer duration, of opioid use is required, this may result in urine retention secondary to an increase in external urethral tone. This should not be confused with potential spinal injuries that may have occurred during a traumatic event; however, this must be considered. Monitoring bladder size is essential if a urinary catheter is not in place. Where a full, atonic bladder is present following high-dose opioid administration, naloxone titrated slowly (see Box 27.1) while applying gentle pressure to the bladder will facilitate bladder emptying. When voiding is accomplished, stop the naloxone titration. On the other hand, rarely, urine production may decrease as a result of the enhanced antidiuretic effect of opioids resulting in small volume, high-specific gravity, of urine. If urine volume is not noted, eventually this will be associated with fluid retention and edema, first noticed in the subcutaneous (SC) tissue, particularly in the hock region. SC edema can also be assessed by the "jiggle effect" when moving the skin between the scapulae. Furosemide is indicated in this situation.

8. As **vomiting will increase ICP**, maropitant (Cerenia): dogs: 1–2 mg/kg IV slowly, SC or 2 mg/kg PO q24h; cats: 1 mg/kg IV, SC or PO q24h, for up to five days is recommended to reduce the potential for this to occur. An analgesic effect has also been reported (Chapter 12). Compatibility with other drugs in the fluid line has not been determined.

Box 27.1 Analgesia in general

1. **Opioids**
   Slowly titrate the opioid until the patient appears comfortable. Titration should be halted when early signs of adverse effects appear – nausea, increased respiratory rate, dysphoria. **# Note opioid reversal below.** Dosages for both cats and dogs are within the dose range given unless otherwise stated. Opioids in order of preference for initial administration:
   - **Fentanyl** 2–5 µg/kg, or
   - **Methadone** 0.1–0.5 mg/kg, or
   - **Oxymorphone** 0.02–0.05 mg/kg, or
   - **Hydromorphone** 0.02–0.05 mg/kg only if none of the above is available due to increased potential for vomiting (refer to Chapter 10, Section II.B), or
   - **Morphine** 0.1–0.5 mg/kg only if none of the above is available due to increased potential for vomiting (refer to Chapter 10, Section II.A).
   - **Establish a continuous rate infusion (CRI)**
     - 1 h infusion of the effective bolus dose of fentanyl, or
     - 4 h infusion (or ¼/h) of the effective bolus dose of methadone, hydromorphone oxymorphone or morphine.

- **Fentanyl** is appropriate for pregnant, lactating, pediatric and geriatric patients. Refer to these sections for ongoing analgesia.
  - Sedative, add to opioid, with dosing based on anxiety level of the patient, to reduce opioid requirement initially and to offer sedation in the anxious patient.

Opioids alone may not be effective in cases where neuropathic pain also exists. The adverse effects of an opioid overdose can still occur in the neuropathic painful patient when the mu-receptors are saturated. Caution is required in interpretation of an increase in what appears to be painful behaviour occurring during opioid administration. The patient may be experiencing opioid-induced hyperalgesia requiring addition of a different class of analgesic (e.g. ketamine), versus a dysphoric response (refer to Chapter 8). Should further analgesia be required based on circumstances, especially where neuropathic pain or opioid-induced hyperalgesia is suspected, add ketamine (see point 2 below).

 # Opioid reversal with naloxone where required.

Where excessive nausea, panting or dysphoria is noted, immediately reverse the opioid with naloxone, particularly if using a long-acting opioid. Slowly titrate until the adverse signs of the opioid subside, then stop naloxone administration. With slow titration, the primary effect of opioid analgesia will not be reversed and frequently facilitates calming. Fentanyl is quickly metabolized and it may not be necessary to reverse. Caution is required as it is easy to "over reverse" and reverse the analgesic properties. To ensure accurate dosing for the individual patient and permit slow delivery of the reversal, the following is recommended:

- Dilute naloxone (0.4 mg/mL) using
  - 0.1 mL added to 5 mL saline (=0.008 mg/mL) for small dogs and cats, titrate at 0.5 mL/min
  - 0.25 mL added to 9.75 mL saline (=0.01 mg/mL), titrate at up to 1 mL/min
  - Titrate until signs of dysphoria or nausea are reversed, usually 2–3 mLs of the dilution. Repeat dosing may be required.

2. **Ketamine [2] where pain cannot be managed with an opioid alone**, common where nerve injury is involved. **Not suitable for pregnant or lactating patients.**
   - **Ketamine** 0.2–1 mg/kg titrated to effect.
   - **Establish a CRI** of effective dose/h.

   Ketamine's additive benefit is bronchodilation and anti-inflammatory. However, ketamine should be used with caution as it stimulates the sympathetic nervous system and may exacerbate some arrhythmias. However, ketamine may be considered in some patients with underlying cardiac disease (refer to Chapter 19 for details), but should be avoided where severe hepatic (dogs) or severe kidney (cats) compromise is present. Lidocaine (see point 3 below) may also be considered.

3. **Lidocaine** is the alternative to, or in combination with, ketamine and an opioid.

   Lidocaine intravenous (IV) bolus 1–2 mg/kg followed by 1–2 mg/kg/h – **dogs** can be added to the above regimen where pain is not being controlled or a reduction in the opioid dose is required. This dose must be calculated into the total dose when bupivacaine or lidocaine are used for local anesthesia to avoid toxicity (refer to Chapter 14). The addition of lidocaine may reduce the opioid requirement; therefore, monitoring for potential opioid adverse effects must be noted on the chart and the opioid dose reduced accordingly. Lidocaine has promotility activity, and other benefits, which may be an advantage in patients presenting with abdominal emergencies should the injury/illness and high-dose opioid predispose to ileus. Nausea may develop 9–24 h infusion. Lidocaine IV should be avoided in patients with significant hepatic pathology. Refer to Chapter 12 for guidance on administration to **cats**.

Box 27.1 (Continued)

4. **Non-steroidal anti-inflammatory analgesic (NSAIA) for the stable patient.** Cyclooxygenase-2 (COX-2) preferential/selective NSAIA (refer to Table 11.1, Chapter 11 for dosing), in addition to the opioid above, may be administered parenterally when all concerns for ongoing hemorrhage and hypovolemia (e.g. occult abdominal hemorrhage, kidney injury) or other contraindications (e.g. renal insufficiency, coagulopathy, major crush injuries resulting in rhabdomyolysis) have been ruled out. Do not use in pregnant, lactating (refer to Chapter 24) animals or puppies and kittens less than 6 weeks of age. Consult the NSAIA package insert prior to administration to verify age as this varies with each product.

5. **Gabapentin 10 mg/kg q8h dogs, 10 mg/kg q12h for cats** for severe injuries and where neuropathic pain [3] is suspected, increase or decrease according to response. Where NSAIAs are contraindicated, gabapentin may be beneficial. Commence as soon as possible.

6. **Amantadine 3–5 mg/kg PO q12–24h in dogs and cats** should be commenced 12 h prior to discontinuing the ketamine if assessed as necessary, especially where a neuropathic component to the injury occurred/exists. This dosing may also be prescribed for cats, but it is necessary to compound in chicken-flavour oil due to the reputed terrible taste of amantadine.

7. The **anti-emetic maropitant [Cerenia®] Dogs: 1 mg/kg IV, SC or 2 mg/kg PO q24h, Cats: 1 mg/kg IV, SC or PO q24h, for up to five days** is indicated where N&V is a potential problem. Maropitant may also have analgesic properties that may facilitate a reduction in the opioid dose.

Where additional sedation is required for cats and dogs consider

8. **Dexmedetomidine** administered as a 15 min loading dose (IV) of 0.5–1 µg/kg followed by 0.5–1 µg/kg/h, confers good analgesia with minimal cardiovascular effects at lower doses and rates in stabilized patients. Dexmedetomidine is particularly useful in anxious patients. However, it should be noted that the MAP may increase by 10–20% and HR may decrease slightly with the CRI. A slight increase in arterial blood pressures may be preferred to hypotension in these cases. Human guidelines for TBI cases indicate that raising arterial pressure to maintain MAP above 80 mmHg is of benefit. Also, in human TBI and neurosurgical patients, dexmedetomidine did not raise ICP, in fact it may offer cerebral protection by attenuation of global or focal ischemia. Other important considerations are it produced "co-operative sedation" allowing neurologic examination and was compatible with neurophysiological monitoring. Sedation does not imply analgesia at low dosages. The α_2-agonist induced hyperglycemia at these CRI doses is none to minimal in dogs and may be similar in cats. Ventilated dogs receiving medetomidine 1–1.5 µg/kg/h for 24 h, demonstrated normal blood glucose values. Human medicine guidelines for TBI propose to maintain blood glucose levels between 7.8 and 10 mmol/l (140–180 mg/dl) in the subgroup of patients vulnerable for brain injury. Regardless of species, monitoring is important to ensure excessive hyperglycemia does not occur with or without α_2-agonist administration. As mentioned above, dexmedetomidine has been associated with vomiting, however in the authors' experience, this has not been a concern with such small doses. The decision to use dexmedetomidine is at the discretion of the clinician. Always use lowest effective dose.

II. Specific Injury Management

Assessment of the ABCs in severely compromised patients should be the initial focus followed by specific injury assessment. Immediate management may require endotracheal intubation prior to emergency care of associated injuries. Refer to Chapter 32 for further information on neck injuries not included here.

A. Head

Traumatic injuries to the head area may involve any part of the skull, eyes/orbit, nasal area and/ or mouth, tongue, pharynx, dentition, pinnae/auditory canal/tympanic membrane/middle and inner ear. One can expect the animal to be experiencing a "serious headache" component to be associated with each of these injuries. Injuries associated with other areas of the body must also be considered to avoid manipulation of these areas, and heightening the pain experience, during diagnostics and management. Managing injuries to the head must also include effective patient restraint, analgesia and even anesthesia in the more severe cases to facilitate diagnostic procedures and overall patient assessment. Anesthesia may be necessary for a complete examination/diagnosis of the oral cavity, and associated structures, to allow for endotracheal intubation in cases with oropharyngeal injuries/obstruction, severe head injury and pain, and to support ventilation in the most severe cases.

1. **Initial stabilization:** fluid resuscitation should be initiated prior to analgesic administration where possible. Fluids should be initiated at a maintenance rate (1–2 mL/kg/h), unless obvious and significant blood or fluid loss requires a bolus regimen of 20–60 mL/kg, IV over 20–30 min.

2. **Unapproachable/aggressive patients:** head and neck restraint is not possible in these patients and obtaining IV access may be difficult without chemical restraint. These patients are at a higher risk without knowledge of the specifics of their injury and pre-existing conditions, compounded by sedation with drugs or dosages that would normally not be recommended.

   a. **Dogs:** if the dog is recumbent, try to use a clipboard or other hard, flat object to block the dog's view of a person approaching from behind. The clipboard can be used to very gently lay across the shoulders and head of the dog, to avoid them turning suddenly. Often an aggressive dog will respond better to this gentle pressure instead of human hands trying to restrain. The key is **gentle pressure**, and this method should be avoided if there are obvious skull fractures, to avoid excessive pressure on the fracture sites. In a large dog with head/neck injuries that is standing and acting aggressively, **avoid restraint with a leash or catch pole** as this will place excessive pressure on the jugular veins and possibly increase ICP, or cause additional injury to the neck. Using a large flat object like a backboard may allow for staff to "squeeze" the dog between the board and a wall, and prevent the dog from turning quickly around and biting. For small dogs, often placing a thick towel over the patient will allow the veterinarian technician or nurse (VT/N) to pick the patient up. Once the feet are off the ground the patient will often quiet slightly and an intramuscular (IM) injection will be possible. Place the dog in a quiet area to enhance the sedative action.

   b. **Cats:** as always an aggressive, striking cat can be dangerous. A squeeze cage is ideal, allowing the cat to be squeezed between two vertical surfaces for IM injection. If not available, a clipboard may be used as a barrier if the cat is in a carrier, squeezing the cat to one side, and allowing an IM injection through one of the holes in the cage. This method may also be possible in a small cage but is a little more risky if the cat is very mobile. Initial restraint in these cats with the oral spray method (see point d below) is usually safest for the veterinary team. Even if just mild sedation is achieved, it is often sufficient to allow restraint and an IM injection with additional sedative if necessary. Potential for vomiting is a concern so use only as a last resort.

   c. **Recommended sedation for dogs and cats** consists of choices that do not cause respiratory depression, are unlikely to cause vomiting and are safe for patients with unknown cardiovascular and volume status. It is important to realize that often an IM injection in these patients is a "one-time shot": the patient is unlikely to allow a second attempt once they understand what is happening.

    i. **Fentanyl 3–10 µg/kg IM** – based on pain level. Following IV access, titrate further opioid to effect, and

    ii. **Midazolam 0.2–0.5 mg/kg IM** – offers good sedation when combined with one of the opioids above. Note in a really hostile patient the higher dose may be necessary, and/or

    iii. **Ketamine 2–4 mg/kg IM** – generally will provide adequate sedation when combined with an opioid and midazolam and given IM. Ketamine will increase heart rate (HR), but is usually negligible at the lower doses. Ketamine is not reversible, so consider a lower dose of ketamine and a higher dose of the opioid.

d. **Where there are no other options**, it may be administered via a **spray into the mouth** for both cats and dogs that are mouth-open aggressive; however, alternative approaches are encouraged depending on the situation at hand:

    i. **Ketamine 2–4 mg/kg** (terrible taste), or

    ii. **Dexmedetomidine 2–5 µg/kg.** Dexmedetomidine has the advantage of reversibility, although swallowing will prevent efficacy. **Caution:** dexmedetomidine has been associated with vomiting and therefore is the least-desirable option. Vomiting is a concern in a patient with potential for high ICP; therefore, the clinician must weigh the risk to versus safety of the staff. Low doses would always be preferred. Atipamezole should be readily available.

    iii. **Midazolam 0.2–0.5 mg/kg** is absorbed by the oral mucosa and may provide additional sedation while reducing the ketamine or dexmedetomidine requirements.

3. **Discharge analgesia for head injured patients in general:** where applicable for any patient with a head injury, as the patient improves and is able to take oral medication easily (avoid inciting the gag reflex), and in preparation for discharge home, add:

a. **Gabapentin** 10 mg/kg q8h dogs and cats with titration up or down based on the individual patient. Higher dosages may be required. Consider having these medications compounded into oral liquid form e.g., oil base chicken flavour 200 mg/mL **(caution: human gabapentin formulations often contain xylitol, discuss an alternative vehicle with the compounding pharmacist as xylitol is toxic to cats and dogs)**. AND

b. **Amantadine** 3–5 mg/kg q12–24h for dogs. Pharmacokinetic data for amantadine in cats indicates similar dosing to dogs; however, there is no clinical data on efficacy and adverse effects in this species. Compounding with chicken flavoured oil is suggested to hide the terrible taste! Refer to Chapter 12 for further information. Administration is patient dependent based on veterinarian's assessment. Of interest, a human study reported amantadine accelerated the pace of functional recovery during active treatment in patients with post-traumatic disorders of consciousness; however, the rate of improvement decreased when treatment was discontinued at 4 weeks.

c. **COX-2 preferential/selective NSAIA (Table 1 NSAIA Chapter 11)**, where there are no contraindications, can also be administered in preparation for, and assessment of, a discharge analgesic regimen.

d. At this stage, slowly wean down the injectable analgesics over 48 h, depending on severity of assessed pain. Lidocaine is the first to discontinue, followed by ketamine, while lowering the opioid.

e. **Where an opioid is deemed necessary**

    i. **Fentanyl transdermal patch**, where continuing opioid treatment is required in addition to the NSAIA or where the NSAIA is contraindicated OR where pain is moderate to severe. The patch is unpredictable in duration of onset and effect due to poor epidermal penetration. Continue or commence fentanyl CRI and wean down as the patch becomes effective. Size guidelines below can assist with patch selection.

- Cats 12.5–25 µg/h patch
- Small dogs (<10 kg) 25 µg/h patch
- Medium dogs (10–20 kg) 50 µg/h patch
- Large dogs (20–30 kg) 75 µg/h patch
- Giant dogs (>30 kg) 100 µg/h patch

ii. **Buprenorphine** 0.02–0.04 mg/kg OTM, cats and small dogs (refer to Chapter 10) for mild-to-moderate pain where continuing opioid treatment is required in addition to the NSAIA or where NSAIA is contraindicated, **or**

iii. **Buprenorphine** 24 h duration product (1.8 mg/mL) (Simbadol® Zoetis) approved for SC injection in cats only for three days. The approved dose is 0.24 mg/kg but the dose can be reduced by 25–50% in compromised patients.

B. Oral Cavity and Upper Airway Injury/Obstruction

Porcupine quill injury (refer to Chapter 34).

1. **Traumatic upper airway obstruction:** as any airway obstruction must be relieved immediately, anesthetic induction is required. For these cases, rapid intervention is necessary. Moderate to severe pain will also exist in these cases, but it should be dealt with once an airway is achieved. If airway and ventilatory support is not possible with flow by/mask then anesthetic induction and endotracheal intubation, or tracheostomy, is necessary, as in Figure 27.2c. Patients with upper airway trauma caused by bite wounds (Figures 27.2a, 27.2b) or other trauma will have difficulty breathing and are likely to have concurrent TBI or SCI, and must be handled cautiously. It is advisable to avoid moving the patient excessively for intubation, but rather intubate in the position they are in, with minimal movement of the head and neck.

   a. **Analgesia**

      i. See Box 27.1 and Section II.A where applicable.

   b. **Anesthesia**

      i. **Propofol (2–6 mg/kg, IV) or alfaxalone (1–3 mg/kg, IV)** to effect is ideal as they allow for a rapid sequence anesthetic induction, and endotracheal intubation (15–30 s). This is important for patients with difficulty ventilating and impending hypoxemia. Flow-by oxygen can be administered throughout the induction process; however, gaining the airway should not be delayed for a full minute of pre-oxygenation as is typically recommended.

Figure 27.2a Neck wounds acquired from a dog attack. Oxygen is delivered via a tube passed beyond the injury. *Source:* Courtesy of Dr K. Lamey.

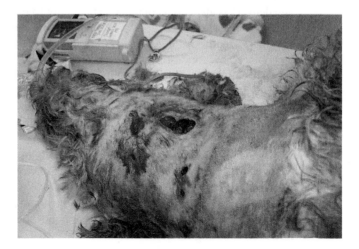

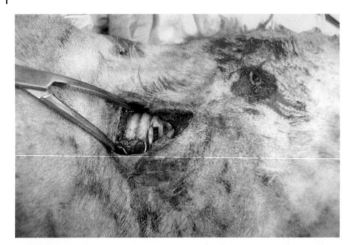

Figure 27.2b Importance of rapid examination of the bite wounds. A tracheal tear is present requiring tracheostomy distal to the tear (Figure 27.2c) to facilitate anesthesia during tracheal repair and healing. *Source:* Courtesy of Dr K. Lamey.

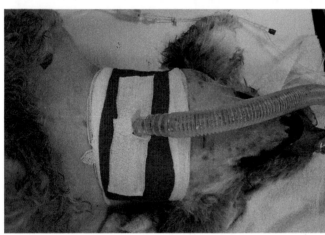

Figure 27.2c Patient in 27.2a upon completion of tracheostomy and tracheal tear repair. *Source:* Courtesy of Dr K. Lamey.

   ii. **Ketamine with diazepam or midazolam** will not be as rapid sequence for endotracheal intubation (45 s to 1 min) so is less ideal than propofol or alfaxalone (refer to Chapter 13 for details).

   iii. If a **tracheostomy** is required, anesthesia using the drugs listed above is appropriate. If possible, orotracheal intubation using a small-diameter endotracheal tube for oxygen delivery is ideal but care must be taken not to move the foreign body (FB) further down the airway. A local block at the incision site should be utilized to allow minimal anesthetic depth. In some patients, a tracheostomy can be done with sedation and a local block at the incision site but this should immediately proceed to general anesthesia (point b.i above) if the patient is struggling. Supplemental oxygen should always be provided regardless of technique.

  c. **Post-surgical analgesia**

    i. **Butorphanol (0.1–0.4 mg/kg)**, if not already administered as an antitussive, may be given as needed to assist recovery extubation where only mild pain/discomfort exists and a pure mu-opioid has/is not given. Mixing opioids will reduce their analgesic efficacy. All opioids confer some antitussive activity, **or**

    ii. **Buprenorphine 0.005–0.02 mg/kg**, IV or IM q(4)6–8h for mild pain. Confers better analgesia than butorphanol with longer duration of action. The peak time to analgesic effect of buprenorphine is longer than a mu-opioid even with IV administration; however, vomiting is not a concern.

   iii. **For local analgesia prior to extubation**, coat the area of the oral lesion with a mixture of 1:1 lidocaine viscous to aluminium hydroxide (64 mg/mL). Mix 50 mL of each for a total volume of 100 mL (aka "**Pink Lady**"), administer at a maximum dose of 0.4 mL/kg q8h; a lower volume is preferred.

  d. **Corticosteroid (0.25 mg/kg dexamethasone)** administration is advised to reduce edema. However, non-steroidal anti- = inflammatory analgesics (NSAIAs) cannot be administered for analgesia.

2. **Foreign body (FB) mouth/pharynx/trachea/esophagus**

   Any degree of pain, with associated anxiousness, is experienced with a FB of the mouth, pharynx, trachea or esophagus. Initial management, as outlined in Section II.A, is required to facilitate assessment of the anatomical involvement of the FB, and any other associated co-morbidities, and to calm the patient while preparing the management plan. Handling the animal may result in increased stress and anxiety that can worsen the situation. Calm the animal while attempting oxygen delivery by mask (with diaphragm removed) or flow-by. **Esophageal FBs**, unless very proximal, may not be immediately life threatening; however, delay in removal will injure the esophageal mucosa and predispose to perforation, esophagitis or esophageal stricture formation. Esophageal injuries can be moderately to excruciatingly painful and analgesia must be provided. See Box 27.1 and refer to Chapter 28, Section V.G for further details.

     a. **Sedation and/or general anesthesia** (see Section II.B.1.a and b) may be necessary to examine and remove FBs. Impaled FBs (i.e. sticks, fish hooks, porcupine quills) require surgical removal. It is mandatory that these patients do not vomit; therefore, very slow titration of the pure mu-agonist opioid is essential. If an IV catheter is established:

       i. **Fentanyl 1–2 μg/kg IV** provides good sedation, confers analgesia, also has antitussive effects and does not pose the risk of inducing vomiting, and is a good adjunct to a balanced anesthetic approach prior to, and during, general anesthesia. Based on the status of the patient.

       ii. **Acepromazine (0.01–0.05 mg/kg, IV or IM) or midazolam (0.2 mg/kg, IV or IM)** may also be added to calm and further sedate these patients during the assessment and stabilization period of the peri-anesthetic phase.

     b. **For situations requiring sedation only**, **with a mild degree of pain**, the sedative, and analgesic agents listed below are recommended for the initial assessment and diagnostic workup. It is important to ensure the patient does not vomit as the FB may prevent the animal from being able to swallow properly, or result in aspiration. Endotracheal intubation supplies should be readily available after sedation. Sedative and analgesic agents – such as, hydromorphone, morphine, and dexmedetomidine – should be used with caution until an airway is achieved, due to the risk of vomiting with IV or IM administration. Once general anesthesia has been induced and the FB has been removed, these sedatives or analgesics can be administered as necessary. Obstructing FBs of mouth and pharynx may be expelled once sedated/relaxed.

       i. **Acepromazine (0.01–0.05 mg/kg, IV or IM)** with or without opioid, if the situation is not critical, administered 20 min prior to the opioid, will reduce the incidence of vomiting.

       ii. **Buprenorphine (0.005–0.02 mg/kg, IV or IM).** This opioid may be a disadvantage for later use of pure mu-agonists if surgery or heightened levels of pain result; however, it does not have the same high risk for vomiting. There is minimal sedation and a lengthy delay to full effect, **or**

       iii. **Butorphanol (0.1–0.4 mg/kg, IV)** can be beneficial when only mild pain/discomfort is assessed, provides sedation and low risk of vomiting. It is typically cited as having the most antitussive benefits; however, if surgery is required, this opioid may be a disadvantage for later use of pure mu-agonists.

c. **Local analgesia** in the oral cavity and esophagus, prior to extubation, coat the area of the lesion with a mixture of 1:1 lidocaine viscous to aluminium hydroxide (64 mg/mL). Mix 50 mL of each for a total volume of 100 mL (aka "**Pink Lady**"), administer at a maximum dose of 0.4 mL/kg q8h, less is preferred. **Pink Lady ≤ 0.4 mL/kg** can be continued PO q8h for 1–2 days.

    i. A caution for an extremely rare reported potential occurrence is pharyngeal desensitization and aspiration; therefore, directions for application to the wound must be explained to the owner.

C. Oral Wounds, Dental Injuries, Electrical Cord Bite and Venomous Injuries Noted within the Mouth or around the Head

Oral wounds, dental injuries, electrical cord bite and venomous injuries noted within the mouth or around the head are painful. Analgesia is important for these animals, and potentially general anesthesia is required to conduct a thorough examination, when the patient is stable, to assess the extent of injury. Continuing analgesia is frequently required to facilitate eating (see Section II.C.1). However, for major injuries and burns, systemic analgesia alone will not be sufficient to facilitate prehension and mastication without pain. During anesthesia place, an esophagostomy or percutaneous gastrostomy tube where appropriate based on anatomical location of injury. A nasoesophageal feeding tube may be used (Figure 27.3) for short duration feeding.

1. **Analgesia**
   a. **See Box 27.1** for initial pain management.
   b. **Pink Lady** mixture of 1:1 lidocaine viscous to aluminium hydroxide (64 mg/mL). Mix 50 mL of each for a total volume of 100 mL, applied to the lesion at a maximum dose of 0.4 mL/kg q8h, or less, is recommended. A caution for an extremely rare potential occurrence is pharyngeal desensitization and aspiration, or
   c. **Topical lidocaine gels** (i.e. lidocaine 2%, viscous lidocaine hydrochloride oral topical solution or injectable lidocaine mixed with amphogel) may be applied q4h.
   d. **NSAIA** (see Table 11.1) where not contraindicated.

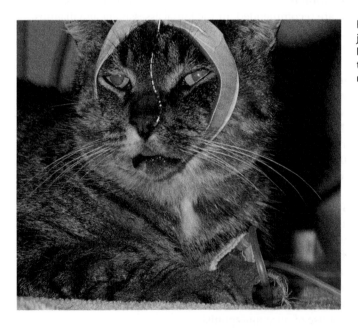

Figure 27.3 Luxated mandibular joint following reduction. Nasoesophageal tube placed due to restriction of prehension and mastication required for ~3 days.

    e. **For venomous lesions** monitor the patient for potential rhabdomyolysis, which is extremely painful and nephrotoxic, NSAIAs are contraindicated should this occur (refer to Chapter 31).

2. **Anesthesia**
    a. As for Section II. point B1b above.
    b. Local anesthetic blocks Chapter 14 where indicated:
        i. maxillary nerve block
        ii. mental nerve block
        iii. mandibular nerve block.

3. **Post-operative analgesia**
    a. An **NSAIA** (see Table 11.1) is recommended where not contraindicated.
    b. Continue with pre-operative opioid (Box 27.1) where appropriate.

4. **Discharge analgesia for all oral and esophageal lesions**
    a. **For local analgesia** in the oral cavity and esophagus, **Pink Lady ≤ 0.4 mL/kg** can be continued PO q8h for 1–2 days. A **caution** for an extremely rare potential occurrence is pharyngeal desensitization and aspiration; therefore, directions for application to the wound must be explained to the owner.
    b. An **NSAIA** (see Table 11.1) should also be prescribed should further analgesia be required and there are no contraindications.
    c. **Buprenorphine 0.02–0.04 mg/kg** oral transmucosal (OTM) cats and small dogs (<10 kg) dosing based on clinical impression and prior to Pink Lady (interferes) or.
    d. A **new transdermal fentanyl patch** if opioid analgesia is required beyond 48 h after discharge. Fentanyl patches should be placed 24 h prior to discharge while weaning down the opioid continuous rate infusion (CRI) to ensure adequate blood levels are present at discharge.

D. Ocular Injuries

1. **Analgesia**
    a. **Box 27.1** and above for II.B.1 initially, and continued post-operatively as described if brain injury is a potential concern. The injury to the eye, and associated pain, can be severe (Figure 27.4) requiring extreme caution in patient handling.

2. **Anesthesia**
    a. As above for I.B.1b.
    b. Local anesthetic blocks (refer to Chapter 14), are encouraged where specific procedures are required. This will reduce the anesthetic requirement and pain upon recovery for several hours.
    c. If injury is localized to the eye, a pure mu-opioid should be administered IV prior to extubation if fentanyl was administered or if the previous dose of long-acting opioid was administered > 3 h ago.

3. **Post-operative analgesia**
    a. An **NSAIA** (see Table 11.1) is recommended where not contraindicated.
    b. Continue with pre-operative opioid (Box 27.1) where appropriate.

4. **Discharge analgesia**
    a. **NSAIA** (see Table 11.1) is preferred, and/or
    b. **Buprenorphine 0·02–0·04 mg/kg OTM** for cats and small dogs(<10 kg due to volume), **or**
    c. **Buprenorphine SC (Simbadol®, Zoetis)** for cats
    d. **Fentanyl transdermal patch. See Section II, point A.3.e.i for patch dosing.** However, response in the dog is variable due to poor epidermal penetration.

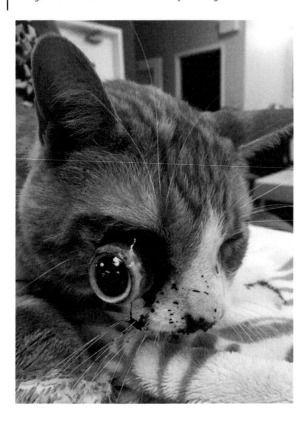

Figure 27.4 Traumatic proptosis immediately prior to enucleation. *Source:* Courtesy of Dr K. Lamey.

E. Auricular Injuries, Hematoma, Acute Severe Otitis

1. **Analgesia**
   a. **Box 27.1** and above for Section II point B.1.b if associated with head trauma. Otherwise, based on patient's general health and no concern for TBI, initial treatment with:
   b. **Dexmedetomidine 0.25–1 µg/kg prior to general anesthesia may be appropriate.**
   c. **The auriculopalpebral block (Figure 27.5a and b)** should be considered for all emergency surgical or medical (e.g. acute severe otitis) procedures of the ear. This reduces anesthetic requirements and post-procedural pain with subsequent reduction in analgesic requirements.

2. **Anesthesia**
   For these cases the anesthetic protocols should be tailored to the individual needs of the patient considering their individual concurrent medical or cardiovascular conditions (refer to Chapter 13, to Chapter 26 if geriatric and Chapters 19, 20 and 21 for associated co-morbidities).
   a. **Appropriate pre-anesthetic sedation** including a pure mu-opioid is preferred to confer optimal analgesia/sedation (Box 27.1) and aid in reduction of the injectable and inhalant anesthetic.
   b. **Induction as for Section II point B.1b** followed by endotracheal intubation and inhalational anesthesia. Mask induction with an inhalant anesthetic is not advised with most patients and is contraindicated in this subset of patients due to the discomfort and pain associated with mask and animal holding.
   c. **Intraoperative:** following general anesthesia, instil 0.25–3.0 mL 0.5% bupivacaine at points 1 & 2 (Figure 27.5a and b) – total dosages of **bupivacaine (0.25–0.75%** concentration) are 2 mg/kg dogs and 1.5 mg/kg cats. Blockade of the auriculotemporal (mandibular) and the

Figure 27.5a Auriculopalpebral block.

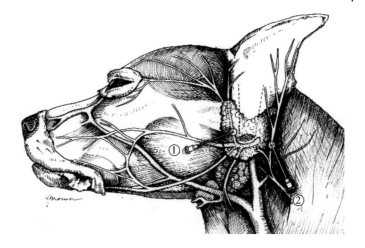

Figure 27.5b Auriculopalpebral block.

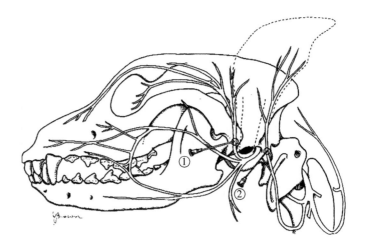

greater auricular nerves will desensitize the inner surface of the auricular cartilage and the external ear canal. For both blocks, a 25-gauge 0.75–1.0 in needle should be inserted SC at the appropriate site. To block the auriculotemporal (mandibular nerve), the needle should be inserted rostral to the vertical ear canal with the tip directed towards the notch, or "V", (1) between the caudal border of the zygomatic arch and the vertical ear canal. The greater auricular nerve can be blocked in the notch or "V" formed by the ventral wing of the atlas and caudal border of the vertical ear canal. (2) The needle should be directed parallel to the vertical ear canal.

3. **Post-operative**
   a. Ensure selected opioid administered pre-op is still effective, if not repeat. Continue where indicated, especially if associated with other injuries incurred during a traumatic event.
   b. Add an **NSAIA, COX-2 preferential/selective** (see Table 11.1) where corticosteroids are **not** prescribed and no other contraindications exist.
4. **Discharge analgesia**
   a. Continue with the **NSAIA**. Contraindicated in otitis externa that is being treated with corticosteroids.

III. Specific Illness Management

A. Non-Traumatic Causes of Airway Obstruction

Non-traumatic causes of airway obstruction are laryngeal paralysis, pharyngeal/laryngeal, tumours, inflammation or edema, brachycephalic syndrome or collapsing trachea. Typically, these conditions are not associated with significant pain, but often benefit from sedation as necessary, most frequently with butorphanol. **Butorphanol** will have the benefit of calming the patient as well as dulling mild pain if present. If necessary, rapid induction and intubation can be achieved using the protocol for upper airway trauma above, with the exception of positioning the patient.

1. **Analgesia and restraint**
   a. **Box 27.1** if butorphanol is inappropriate, with selection based on the patient's general health and co-morbidities.
2. **General anesthesia** is frequently required to facilitate a thorough examination, repair injuries or obtain biopsies. For these cases:
   a. **Anesthetic induction with either propofol (2–6 mg/kg, IV) or alfaxalone (1–3 mg/ kg, IV)** to effect is ideal as they allow for a rapid sequence anesthetic induction, and endotracheal intubation. This is important in cases that have the potential for regurgitation with anesthetic induction and unconsciousness. Both propofol and alfaxalone can be used as total intravenous anesthesia (TIVA), and additional doses do not negatively impact a timely anesthetic recovery.
   b. **Oxygen supplementation and monitoring of cardio-respiratory parameters** are always recommended. In cases where respiratory compromise may still be present after surgery, propofol and alfaxalone are ideal as they have minimal anesthetic hangover and fast recovery times.
3. **Post-operative** analgesia is essential where surgical procedures have been performed.
   a. **Box 27.1**. Continue with pre-operative regimen with adjustment as indicated.
   b. **NSAIA, COX-2 preferential/selective** (see Table 11.1) where no contraindications and corticosteroids have not been administered or recommended.
4. **Discharge analgesia**
   a. **NSAIA, COX-2 preferential/selective** (see Table 11.1) where not contraindicated and corticosteroids are not prescribed, and/or
   b. **Buprenorphine 0.02–0.04 mg/kg (20–40 μg/kg) OTM** for small dogs (<10 kg due to volume) and cats, or
   c. **Fentanyl transdermal. See Section II, point A.3.e.i for patch dosing.** However, response in the dog is variable due to poor epidermal penetration.

B. Neurologic: Meningitis, Neoplasia, Syringomyelia, Other Intracranial Lesions

1. **Meningitis:** various illnesses and syndromes result in inflammation of the meninges. In addition to septic meningitis, several aseptic conditions occur, including the breed associated aseptic meningitis seen in such breeds as the Bernese mountain dog and the Beagle pain syndrome, while being a generalized vasculitis, especially involves the cervical meninges. Other conditions include granulomatous meningoencephalomyelitis (GME).
   a. **Analgesia**
      Meningitis is very painful, and multi-modal analgesia is necessary. Following the neurologic examination
      i. Slowly titrate an opioid **Box 27.1** and follow with the effective dose as a CRI. Frequent neurologic examinations may be required initially; therefore, **fentanyl** is

the best choice due to less chance of vomiting and short duration of action. Timing for neurologic assessment should be made at intervals where the opioid level can be/is reduced, and the examination is conducted expediently, so as to reduce the duration of pain experienced by the patient and the potential difficulty of re-establishing a plane of comfort.

  ii. **Dexmedetomidine 0.25–1 μg/kg** bolus and followed as a CRI is beneficial as an analgesic and sedative. The pain these patients experience makes them very restless, dexmedetomidine is calming and facilitates sleep. The analgesic effects diminish before the sedative effects; therefore, a sedated patient may show signs of pain. Should further analgesia be required, add:

  iii. **Ketamine 0.2–1 mg/kg** titrated until calm appears. Continue with effective dose as an hourly CRI.

  iv. As most of these patients are receiving corticosteroid therapy, NSAIAs **cannot** be administered. After 48 h of corticosteroid therapy, the pain diminishes. If analgesia is still required for discharge home, **See Section II, point A.3.e.i for fentanyl patch dosing**, selecting the regimen appropriate for the individual patient.

b. **Anesthesia is required for cerebrospinal fluid (CSF) collection**
This procedure is typically short in duration and hence anesthetic agents used should be short acting in nature to prevent excessive sedation in the recovery period that may promote respiratory depression. These patients will typically have received an opioid prior to anesthetic induction during their initial examination.

  i. **Pre-medication**
  - **A pure mu-opioid agonist** (fentanyl, methadone, hydromorphone) has the benefit of calming the patient, providing analgesia, is reversible and will also aid in reducing the induction agent, as well as inhalant levels required. An initial bolus of **fentanyl 2–4 μg/kg, IV** can be administered and will not cause vomiting in this subset of patients who would find vomiting painful. After sedation, monitoring can be instituted as patient allows (ECG, Doppler BP, SPO_2).
  - **Butorphanol and buprenorphine** will sedate and calm the patient, but **do not have the same abilities to reduce the injectable or inhalant** agent, hence fentanyl offers advantages. The pre-anesthetic should be based on the patient's condition and veterinarian's comfort with the drug.

  ii. **Induction**
  - **To effect with propofol (2–6 mg/kg, IV) or alfaxalone (1–3 mg/kg, IV).** Attention to depth to prevent coughing and minimize the response to endotracheal intubation, with wire reinforced endotracheal tube if available, is warranted.

  iii. **Maintenance with isoflurane or sevoflurane.**

  iv. **Intraoperative.** Additional monitoring should include end-tidal CO_2 ($ETCO_2$) during the CSF tap to ensure adequate ventilation and observe for airway obstruction when flexion of the head is required for cisternal collections. To prevent tracheal collapse with extreme neck flexion during cisternal CSF collections, a wire-reinforced endotracheal tube can be used for endotracheal intubation. As a cautionary note, the internal diameter of this endotracheal tube is reduced, which will increase resistance to ventilation promoting the need for assisted ventilation during anesthesia. The $ETCO_2$ should be monitored and ventilation assisted as required.

2. **Intracranial Syringomyelia** (see point C Neck Pain).

3. **Brain tumours** also have a high incidence of pain based on careful physical examination. Dogs appear "head-shy", either by avoiding, or being actively resentful of, being touched on the head, sometimes crying out when touched. If these signs are not exhibited, gently press on the temples/forehead and observe if a reaction is elicited indicating a mild to moderate

painful condition. Another feature to examine is that caused by the central pain component. Where intracranial neoplasia is expected, hyperalgesia may occur in other areas of the body. The area of pain experienced is that which is subserved by the location and the pathway involving the neoplastic process.

a. **Analgesia**
   i. **Gabapentin 10 mg/kg** q12h, which should be started prior to surgery/diagnostics.
   ii. Commonly, an **anti-inflammatory dose of corticosteroids (prednisone, 1 mg/kg/ day)** is prescribed by the neurologist to reduce the perilesional vasogenic edema, and will provide some analgesia. Therefore, NSAIAs should **not** be prescribed.
   iii. **An opioid** can be added to the regimen. The opioid selected will depend on whether the patient remains in the hospital as a pre and post-operative patient (**treat as 1. Meningitis**), or refer to discharge home plan (Section II.A.3).

b. **Anesthesia**
   Definitive diagnosis is essential frequently requiring magnetic resonance imaging (MRI) or computed-tomography (CT). The physical examination and mental status of the patient will impact the anesthetic choice of the patient with a suspected brain tumour. In these cases, the potential for an acute increase in ICP from the anesthetic, hypercarbia or inappropriate positioning can be life threatening. Hence, attention to detail and monitoring of arterial blood pressures, HR and $ETCO_2$ are imperative to recognize abrupt changes.

   In severely compromised and depressed patients, minimal to no sedation and anesthesia may be required; however, monitoring is still necessary. For all patients, prior to administration of the opioid, anesthetic and emergency material (e.g. endotracheal intubation and monitoring equipment) should be set and ready in case respiratory depression or apnea occurs. Patients should be pre-oxygenated once relaxed. Flow-by oxygen is acceptable and it is important not to stress the patient with mask application. Sedation and anesthesia will be required to perform an MRI or CT scan.
   i. **Pre-medication: fentanyl** (1–2 µg/kg, IV).
   ii. **Induction: propofol** (2–4 mg/kg, IV to effect).
   iii. **Maintenance with propofol 0.2–0.6 mg/kg/min** during the MRI or CT is preferred in cases where an increase in ICP is present or possible. The patient should have intermittent positive pressure ventilation, and $ETCO_2$ monitored for normocarbia ($ETCO_2$ 30–32 mmHg).

c. **Post-operative**
   i. Continue with selected **opioid** (see **Box 27.1**).
   ii. **Gabapentin** 10 mg/kg (dogs), 6 mg/kg (cats) q8h and increase or decrease based on response/sedation and ketamine.
   iii. Add a **NSAIA (see Table 11.1) if corticosteroids are not prescribed.**
   iv. If an **opioid** is required for home pain management, place the fentanyl patch 24 h prior to discharge to ensure adequate blood levels. However, response in the dog is variable due to poor epidermal penetration. The patch can be in place while receiving systemic opioids. Adjustment to the systemic dose can be made as the transdermal fentanyl slowly reaches adequate blood levels. **See Section II, point A.3.e.i for patch dosing.**

d. **Discharge analgesia**
   i. **Gabapentin** 10 mg/kg q8–12h dogs and cats **titrate up or down** based on response. OR
   ii. **Amantadine** 3–5 mg/kg q12–24h dogs and cats.
   iii. **Buprenorphine** 0.02–0.04 mg/kg (20–40 µg/kg) OTM cats and dogs < 10 kg (due to volume), or
   iv. **Fentanyl transdermal patch** appropriate size for patient. **See Section II, point A.3.e.i for patch dosing.** However, response in the dog is variable due to poor epidermal penetration.

Should/when reduction in analgesia be indicated, wean off all analgesics gradually, especially gabapentin and amantadine even if they may not appear to be effective. Analgesia must not be stopped abruptly.

4. **Miscellaneous intracranial lesions**
   a. **Analgesia**
      i. As for Section II.B.1.
   b. **Anesthesia**
      i. As for Section II.B.1. **However, intraoperative maintenance** with **isoflurane**, as an alternative to propofol, is acceptable in cases that do not have increased ICP or where a brain tumour is not suspected. All other aspects apply.

C. Neck Pain: All Causes

Several medical and traumatic conditions cause neck pain and may be difficult to diagnose [3]. These are excruciatingly painful conditions where the underlying cause must be identified and treated to alleviate the pain. Causes to consider are infectious meningomyelitis, steroid responsive arteritis-meningitis, intracranial tumour, discospondylitis/osteomyelitis, malignant nerve sheath tumour (MNST), bony neoplasia fracture/luxation due to spinal trauma, atlanto-axial luxation, intervertebral disc herniation and a vertebral caudal cervical spondylomyelopathy (CCSM). Caudal occipital malformation syndrome (COMS) is characterized by overcrowding of the caudal fossa, and obstruction of the normal CSF flow, resulting in hydrocephalus. The abnormal CSF flow leads to formation of a fluid filled cavity within the spinal cord known as syringo-hydromyelia (SM). Frequently, herniation of the cerebellar vermis towards the foramen magnum is documented as part of the syndrome. Cavalier King Charles spaniels are the most commonly affected breed.

Breeds with COMS and SM often suffer from other conditions such as atlantoaxial luxation, atlanto-occipital overlapping, meningoencephalomyelitis and arachnoid cysts. Presence of these disorders can complicate a relevant clinical diagnosis for the etiology of neck pain. Other breeds diagnosed with COMS include Griffon Bruxellois, Maltese, Chihuahua, Yorkshire terrier and Boston terrier.

These conditions are excruciatingly painful; **very** careful handling during diagnostic work-up is essential. Signs of pain are low head and neck carriage, neck guarding, stilted and cautious gait and spasms of cervical spinal muscles. A single analgesic cannot manage this degree of pain; multimodal analgesia, and anesthesia in some circumstances, is required. These patients are extremely susceptible to wind-up, and analgesia must be immediate and multimodal. Doses should be titrated as always but are often on the high end or higher than the typically recommended dose.

1. **Analgesia**
   As corticosteroid therapy is prescribed for these conditions, do **not** administer an NSAIA prior to diagnosis and a corticosteroid-dependent diagnosis made. In the rare situation where corticosteroids are not part of the treatment plan, NSAIAs are recommended as part of a multi-modal regimen.
   a. Box 27.1.
   b. Treatment for the specific problem, once established, will also be analgesic.
   c. For cervical vertebral involvement, consider a well-fitting neck brace/splint; however, the owner must be judged as being able to inspect and detect any problems that may arise following discharge.
2. **Anesthesia**
   May be required to manage pain and for specific diagnostic procedures (CSF collection, CT/MRI etc.) (see point B.1 above).

3. **Discharge analgesia**

Commence, as soon as possible:

a. **Gabapentin 6–15 mg/kg q6–8h PO dogs and cats**, (start at 10 mg/kg and increase or decrease dose and/or duration based on response/sedation). Wean off gradually even if not effective. Must not stop abruptly, or

b. **Pregabalin 2–5 mg/kg q8–12h** is an alternative to gabapentin for dogs. Higher doses of 10 mg/kg are reported in the literature but will cause extreme sedation. Do not administer to pregnant animals.

c. **Methocarbamol 22 mg/kg IV q8–12h or 10 mg/kg PO q8–12h** may be of benefit in patients with severe cervical pain when combined with gabapentin and corticosteroids.

References

1 DiFazio, J., Fletcher, D. J. Updates in the management of the small animal patient with neurologic trauma. *Vet Clin Small Anim*, 2013; 43: 915–940.

2 Himmelseher, S. and Durieux, M. E. (2005) Revising a dogma: Ketamine for patients with neurological injury? *Anesth Analg*, 101: 524–534.

3 Sehdev, R. S., Symmons, D. A. D. and Kindl, K. (2006) Ketamine for rapid sequence induction in patients with head injury in the emergency department. *Emergency Medicine Australasia*, 18, 37–44.

Further Reading

Clarke, H., Bonin, R. P., Orser, B. A. *et al.* (2012) The prevention of chronic postsurgical pain using gabapentin and pregabalin: A combined systematic review and meta-analysis. *Anesth Analg*, 115: 428–442.

Duque, C. (2017) Neck pain. In: Mathews, K. A. (ed.), *Veterinary Emergency & Critical Care Manual*, 3rd edn. LifeLearn, Guelph, Ontario, Canada.

Ethier, M., Mathews, K. A., Valverde, A., *et al.* Evaluation of the efficacy and safety of two analgesia and sedation protocols to facilitate assisted ventilation of healthy dogs. *Am J Vet Res.* 2008; 69:1351–1359.

Giacino, J. T., Whyte, J., Bagiella, E., *et al.* Placebo-controlled trial of amantadine for severe traumatic brain injury. *N Engl J Med*, 2012; 366:819–826.

Hossam El Beheiry (2012) Protecting the brain during neurosurgical procedures: Strategies that can work. *Curr Opin Anesthesiol*, 25: 548–555.

Kamtikar, S. and Nair, A. S. (2015) Advantages of dexmedetomidine in traumatic brain injury: A review. *Anaesth Pain & Intensive Care*, 19(1): 87–91.

Maxwell, L. G., Kaufmann, S. C., Bitzer, S., *et al.* (2005) The effects of a small-dose naloxone infusion on opioid-induced side effects and analgesia in children and adolescents treated with intravenous patient-controlled analgesia: A double-blind, prospective, randomized, controlled study. *Anesth Analg*, 100: 953–958.

Otto, K. A., Physiology, pathophysiology and anesthetic management of patients with neurologic disease. In: Grimm, K. A., Lamont, L. L., Tranquilli, W. J., *et al.* (eds), *Veterinary Anesthesia and Analgesia: The fifth edition of Lumb and Jones*. Wiley-Blackwell, Ames, IA: 559–584.

Parr, J. M. and Bersenas, A. M. (2017) Nutritional support plans for the ill or injured cat and dog. In Mathews, K. A. (ed.), *Veterinary Emergency & Critical Care Manual*, 3rd edn. LifeLearn, Guelph, Ontario, Canada.

Schwartz, A., Nossaman, A., Carrolla, D., *et al.* (2013) Dexmedetomidine for neurolosurgical procedures. *Curr Anesthsiol Rep*, 3: 205–209.

Tang, J. F., Chen, P., Tang, E. J., *et al.* (2011) Dexmedetomidine controls agitation and facilitates reliable, serial neurological examinations in a non-intubated patient with traumatic brain injury. *Neurocritical Care*, 15(1): 175–181.

Velayudhan, A., Bellingham, G., Morley-Forster, P. *et al.* (2014) Opioid-induced hyperalgesia. *Cont Educ in Anaesthesia Critical Care & Pain*, 14(3): 125–129.

Wolfe KC, Poma R. (2010) Syringomyelia in the Cavalier King Charles spaniel (CKCS) dog. *CVJ*, 51: 95–102.

28

Torso, Thorax and Thoracic Cavity: Illness and Injury

Karol Mathews, Tamara Grubb and Andrea Steele

Injury or illness involving the thorax frequently interferes with ventilation. The initial management must be directed to ensuring adequate oxygenation by administering oxygen prior to physical examination and considering other procedures. Oxygen flow-by and hood (Figure 28.1) are the least stressful methods of delivery. Secondly, injured patients may be hypovolemic due to blood loss, and ill patients may be hypovolemic due to the primary problem. Intravenous (IV) access and commencement of IV fluids at a rate appropriate for the situation, and halting obvious blood loss, is the second priority. In addition, the extent of trauma is not fully understood until a complete physical examination and diagnostic procedures are complete (Figures 28.3–28.5). Therefore, all patients must be handled carefully to avoid further injury and pain. The third priority is administration of analgesia appropriate for the degree of pain, and to confer sedation to facilitate physical examination and pursue further procedures. Injuries and illness of the thorax, organs and pleura will restrict ventilation and coughing; therefore, appropriate, carefully administered analgesics are essential to facilitate oxygenation and avoid potential compromise to organ function. Excessive work of breathing will increase body temperature, where temperatures may rise to as high as 42 °C (107.6 °F); therefore, including temperature monitoring is essential to avoid the extra heat-induced stress which enhances the pain experience. Where ventilation is compromised (e.g. traumatic injury, neuromuscular

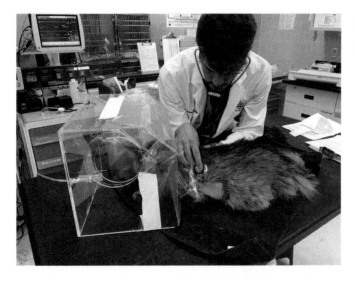

Figure 28.1 A human pediatric oxygen hood allowing oxygenation and physical examination.

Analgesia and Anesthesia for the Ill or Injured Dog and Cat, First Edition. Karol A. Mathews, Melissa Sinclair, Andrea M. Steele and Tamara Grubb.
© 2018 John Wiley & Sons, Inc. Published 2018 by John Wiley & Sons, Inc.

disorders, cervical injury) requiring anesthesia and mechanical ventilation, go directly to Box 28.3 selecting the most appropriate regimen based on patient stability. Boxes 28.1–28.3 are suggestions for the various scenarios given below.

I. Analgesia and Anesthesia

Box 28.1 Analgesia

1. **Opioids**
   Slowly titrate the opioid until the cat or dog appears comfortable, higher dosages may be required. Titration should be halted when early signs of adverse effects appear – nausea, increased respiratory rate (RR), dysphoria or worsening of the signs of pain appear. # Note opioid reversal below. Dosages for both cats and dogs are within the dose range given unless otherwise stated. Opioids in order of preference for initial administration:

   Known moderate to severe pain

   - **Fentanyl** 2–5+ μg/kg, or
   - **Methadone** 0.1–0.5 mg/kg, or
   - **Oxymorphone** or **hydromorphone** 0.02–0.05+ mg/kg (<0.1 mg/kg cats), or
   - **Morphine** 0.1–0.5+ mg/kg, is acceptable should the above not be available but is highly likely to cause vomiting and histamine release (when administered rapidly IV), which can contribute to hypotension.
   - **Where sedation is indicated** to reduce opioid requirement initially, or to offer sedation in the anxious patient, see Box 28.2.
   - **Establish a continuous rate infusion (CRI) where indicated:**
     o 1 h infusion of the effective bolus dose of fentanyl, or
     o 4 h infusion (or ¼/h) of the effective bolus dose of methadone, hydromorphone oxymorphone or morphine.
     Opioids alone may not be effective in cases where neuropathic, or other severe, pain also exists. The adverse effects of an opioid overdose can still occur in these painful patients when the mu-receptors are saturated; the dose received at early signs may be used to calculate the CRI above for continuing care. Caution is required in interpretation of what appears to be painful behaviour occurring during opioid administration. The patient may be experiencing opioid-induced hyperalgesia where the opioid is causing more pain requiring addition of a different class of analgesic, versus a dysphoric response (refer to Chapter 8). Should further analgesia be required based on circumstances, especially where neuropathic pain or opioid-induced hyperalgesia is suspected, add ketamine (see point 2 below).

   Known mild to moderate pain

   - **Butorphanol** 0.1–0.4 mg/kg IV, intramuscular (IM) q2–4h, or to effect, or
   - **Buprenorphine** 5–10 μg/kg IV, IM, 20–50 μg/kg OTM q4–8h. A higher dose may be required.

   # Opioid reversal with naloxone where required
   Where excessive nausea, panting or dysphoria is noted, immediately reverse the opioid with naloxone, particularly if using a long-acting opioid. Slowly titrate until the adverse signs of the opioid subside, then stop naloxone administration. With slow titration, the

(Continued)

Box 28.1 (Continued)

primary effect of opioid analgesia will not be reversed and frequently facilitates calming. Fentanyl is quickly metabolized and it may not be necessary to reverse; caution is required as it is easy to "over reverse" and reverse the analgesic properties. To ensure accurate dosing for the individual patient and permit slow delivery of the reversal, the following is recommended:

- Dilute naloxone (0.4 mg/mL) using
  - 0.1 mL added to 5 mL saline (=0.006 mg/mL) for small dogs and cats, titrate at 0.5 mL/min
  - 0.25 mL added to 9.75 mL saline (=0.01 mg/mL), titrate at up to 1 mL/min
- titrate until signs of dysphoria or nausea are reversed, usually 2–3 mLs.

2. **Ketamine** 0.1–1 mg/kg IV until the patient becomes calm. This dose may also be used to calculate the hourly CRI. Ketamine's additive benefit is bronchodilation. However, ketamine should be used with caution as ketamine stimulates the sympathetic nervous system and may exacerbate some arrhythmias. Ketamine may be considered in patients with underlying cardiac disease (refer to Chapter 19 for details), but should be avoided where severe hepatic (dogs) or severe kidney (cats) compromise is present. Lidocaine (see point 3 below) may also be considered.

3. **Lidocaine** IV bolus 1–2 mg/kg followed by 1–2 mg/kg/h – **dogs** only can be added to the above regimen where pain is difficult to manage or an opioid dose reduction is required. This dose must be calculated into the total dose when bupivacaine or lidocaine is used for local anesthesia to avoid toxicity (refer to Chapter 14). The addition of lidocaine may reduce the opioid requirement; therefore, monitoring for potential opioid adverse effects must be noted on the chart and the opioid dose reduced accordingly. Nausea may develop with 9–24 h infusion. Refer to Chapter 12 for guidelines for use in **cats**.

4. **Non-steroidal anti-inflammatory analgesics (NSAIAs) for the stable patient:** in addition to the opioid above, a cyclooxygenase-2 (COX-2) preferential or selective NSAIA (Chapter 11) may be administered parenterally when all concerns for ongoing hemorrhage and hypovolemia (e.g. occult abdominal hemorrhage, kidney injury) or other contraindications (e.g. renal insufficiency, coagulopathy, major crush injuries resulting in rhabdomyolysis) have been ruled out. Do not use in pregnant animals. Carprofen may be administered to lactating animals, maximum of six days (Chapter 24). Do not administer to puppies and kittens less than 6 weeks of age. Consult the NSAIA package insert prior to administration to verify age as this varies with each product.

5. **Gabapentin 10 mg/kg q8h dogs, 10 mg/kg q12h for cats** for severe injuries and where neuropathic pain is suspected. The dosage can be increased or decreased based on degree of sedation. Where NSAIAs are contraindicated, gabapentin may be beneficial. Commence as soon as possible. May cause mild sedation (generally clinically irrelevant) at higher dosages and/or when combined with other sedating drugs.

Box 28.2 Sedatives

- **Diazepam** 0.2 mg/kg IV or **midazolam** 0.2 mg/kg IV or IM, or
- **Acepromazine** 0.005–0.02 mg/kg, IM, IV. Use with caution in hypovolemic or hypotensive patients, ace-mediated vasodilation may contribute to hypotension.
- **Medetomidine** 0.1–4 μg/kg IM, IV may be considered where no co-morbidities exist.
- **Dexmedetomidine** 0.5–2 μg/kg IM, IV, CRI may be considered where no co-morbidities exist.

Box 28.3 Anesthesia

1. **Anesthesia for hemodynamically stable patients**
   - **Pre-medication** with an opioid plus a sedative for most patients. Dosages for drugs administered for pre-medication are typically higher than those administered for calming/analgesia in the ICU (Boxes 28.1 and 28.2) as more sedation and more analgesia are generally necessary prior to surgery. Use the low end of the dose range for IV administration and/or in mildly compromised patients (see dosages for unstable patients in point 2).
     - ○ **Anesthesia pre-medication dosages of opioids:**
       - ▪ **Methadone** 0.3–0.5 mg/kg (dogs and cats), or
       - ▪ **Oxymorphone** 0.1–0.2 mg/kg (dogs), 0.05–0.1 mg/kg (cats), or
       - ▪ **Hydromorphone** 0.1–0.2 mg/kg (dogs), 0.1 mg/kg (cats), or
       - ▪ **Morphine** IM only 0.3–0.5 mg/kg (dogs), 0.1–0.3 mg/kg (cats)
     - ○ **Anesthesia pre-medication dosages of sedatives:**
       - ▪ **Diazepam** 0.2 mg/kg IV or **midazolam** 0.2 mg/kg IV or IM, or
       - ▪ **Acepromazine** 0.01–0.03 mg/kg, IM, IV, or
       - ▪ **Medetomidine** 2–6 μg/kg IV or 10–20 μg/kg IM (dogs), 4–10 μg/kg IV or 15–30 μg/kg IM (cats), or
       - ▪ **Dexmedetomidine** 1–3 μg/kg IV or 5–10 μg/kg IM (dogs), 2–5 μg/kg IV or 8–15 μg/kg IM (cats)
   - **Induction**
     - ▪ **Propofol** 2–6 mg/kg, IV to effect, or
     - ▪ **Alfaxalone** 1–3 mg/kg, IV to effect, or
     - ▪ **Ketamine with midazolam or diazepam** (1:1): 0.1–0.2 mL/kg, IV to effect (in this case, do not use a benzodiazepine as a pre-medicant)
     - ▪ **Etomidate** (1–3 mg/kg).
   - **Intraoperative maintenance** with inhalant anesthesia (isoflurane or sevoflurane) for procedure > 20 min is recommended. TIVA with propofol or alfaxalone (Chapter 13) may be used for short-term wound lavage or bandage changes; however, ET intubation and oxygen supplementation is recommended.
   - **Local and epidural analgesic/anesthetic procedures** (see Section II) should be considered wherever appropriate.
2. **Anesthesia for patients with mild to moderate hemodynamic compromise**
   - **Pre-medication** with an opioid plus a sedative for most patients. Drug dosages are lower than those used for healthy patients and are in the range of the dosages presented in Boxes 28.1 and 28.2.
   - The opioid may provide adequate sedation; if not, add a sedative from Box 28.2.
   - **Induction:** same drugs as in 1 above but carefully titrate the dose to effect, expect to use the low end of the dose range.
   - **Intraoperative maintenance** same as in 1 above with goal to use the lowest drug dosages possible. Carefully titrate the dose to effect, expect to use the low end of the dose range.
   - **Local and epidural analgesic/anesthetic procedures** (see Section II) should be considered wherever appropriate.
3. **Anesthesia for hemodynamically unstable patients**
   For these patients, all drug dosages are low. Uptake of the drug is slow so administer the dose and give it time to reach the brain – this can take 2–3 times longer than in healthy patients. Patients should be stabilized to the greatest extent possible prior to anesthesia.
   - **Pre-medication**
     - ○ Choose an opioid from Box 28.1
       - ▪ **Fentanyl and methadone** are preferred if vomiting must be avoided. In these instances, also consider administration of maropitant.

(Continued)

Box 28.3 (Continued)

- All drugs should be administered IV through a pre-placed catheter and the patient should be continuously monitored as adverse responses to the drugs may occur.
- If more sedation/calming is needed, add a benzodiazepine from Box 28.2. Occasionally other sedatives may be appropriate and those are discussed with specific scenarios throughout the chapter.
- **Induction**
  - The drugs described for pre-medication often provide adequate sedation to allow intubation in unstable patients. If these drugs alone are used for intubation, **topical lidocaine spray on the larynx** is recommended with this induction technique.
  - If more drug is needed, any of the injectable drugs listed in 1 and 2 above are acceptable but should be **slowly** titrated **to effect**.
  - **Etomidate** (1–3 mg/kg) causes minimal to no cardiovascular effects and may be a good choice for unstable patients. Pre-medication with an opioid and a bolus of midazolam or diazepam (0.2 mg/kg IV of either) should be utilized as etomidate without pre-medications commonly causes muscle rigidity, muscle twitching, paddling and vocalization. Etomidate also causes adrenocortical suppression and its use in septic patients is controversial.
  - Should hypotension develop during anesthesia refer to Chapter 19, Section II.B.3.
4. **Maintenance for mechanical ventilation: based on individual patient requirements**
   - **Fentanyl** up to 10 μg/kg/h plus diazepam up to 1 mg/kg/h plus ketamine 0.1–2 mg/kg/h.
   - **Dexmedetomidine** 0.05–1 μg/kg added to the ketamine propofol if needed, or
   - **Propofol** 2–6 mg/kg/h can be substituted for ketamine, or
   - For very depressed patients fentanyl, dexmedetomidine and diazepam may be adequate.

General anesthesia is required for some ill or injured patients to facilitate diagnostic and surgical procedures. The health status of these patients often ranges from healthy but extremely painful to near death. General recommendations are given in Box 28.3; however, where applicable in the ill or injured scenarios, selection of drugs and dosages will be given.

II. Local and Epidural Analgesic/Anesthetic Techniques

Refer to Chapter 14 to consider when anesthetized for musculoskeletal pain or injury of the thorax. Contraindications for local and epidural blocks are a significant wound or evidence of infection, over the anatomical area where the local block is to be performed with needle insertion.

1. Incisional line blocks.
2. Subcutaneous (SC) infiltration.
3. Intercostal nerve blocks.
4. Epidural injection with morphine into the lumbosacral space is warranted when the patient is anesthetized as analgesia frequently extends to the thoracic cavity, especially when the morphine is diluted with a large volume (>0.02 mL/kg) saline.

   Caution: large volumes of local anesthetic drugs are to be avoided as cranial migration of these drugs may cause phrenic nerve paralysis and further respiratory compromise. In larger dogs, epidural catheters may be considered. Refer to Chapter 14 for details.

5. Epidural/local blocks/infusion catheters/interpleural (chest tube). Local and regional techniques should be administered when possible to supplement systemic analgesics. In small animals, placement of the majority of nerve blocks, infusion catheters or epidurals will require heavy sedation or general anesthesia. Refer to Chapter 14 for details.

6. **Wound diffusion catheters** may be used and have the benefit of repeated administration of local anesthetic into painful incisions. These catheters are placed into the operative site at the end of surgery with the fenestrations on the distal end of the catheter placed into the deepest layer of the incision. Advantages of these catheters include ability to:

   a. desensitize large wounds or incisions;
   b. provide analgesia of the highly-innervated skin and muscle layers long term (days);
   c. reduce dose of systemically administered drugs that may be less than ideal in a particular patient. Refer to Chapter 14 for details.

   The **specifics of local anesthetic agents**, adjuvant analgesics, aseptic and individual technique, equipment required and anatomy are outlined in Chapter 14.

III. Post-Procedural Analgesia

Continue with the pre-operative regimen Box 28.1, with the addition of:

1. **NSAIA, COX 2 preferential/selective** (see Table 11.1) where no contraindications exist.
2. **Ketamine** should be added/continued if needed, and
3. **Gabapentin** continued, or added, if neural tissue is involved in the traumatic incident or during surgical management.
4. The **opioid and ketamine** should be weaned off slowly in preparation for discharge home. Revert to previous dose should the patient appear painful after reduction.
5. **Amantadine**: commence as ketamine is weaned down, 3–5 mg/kg PO q12–24h for dogs to replace ketamine where this is required for continuing analgesia. May also be beneficial at this dose in cats. Refer to Chapter 12 for details on administration.

IV. Nursing Considerations

A. **Sedation:** patients with respiratory compromise secondary to trauma or illness are particularly susceptible to stress, and benefit from a generous sedative regimen prior to handling. Box 28.1 provides analgesia suggestions that will also provide sedation. If the patient has no to mild pain but sedation is necessary due to dyspnea, consider butorphanol 0.2–0.4 mg/kg. For all painful patients, consider the suggestions in Box 28.1. The veterinarian technician/nurse (VT/N) should **always** have intubation supplies ready for rapid sequence intubation in the thoracic trauma/respiratory distress patient, as sedation does not always have the desired effect.

B. **Oxygen therapy:** if nasal catheter or cannulas cannot be placed, consider an oxygen hood, mask or cage – or even "flow-by" oxygen (i.e. hold/tape oxygen hoses from the anesthesia machine or other source near patient's nostrils) – while the patient is being sedated, especially if the drug is given IM or SC. This will reduce stress of handling on the patient, while allowing them to be in an oxygen-rich environment.

C. **Position:** patients with chest wall injury or unilateral lung disease or injury are generally able to ventilate better when positioned with affected side down. This will not be the case for every patient, however, and the VT/N must try various positions to see what works for the individual patient; find a compromise between positions that relieve pain vs positions that allow the best ventilation.

D. **When aspirating chest tubes**, it is imperative that excess negative pressure not be used, as this increases the pain that the patient will feel. Fluid or air flows freely, and in general, no more than 5 "mL" of negative pressure, measured on the syringe, should be used. If it does not flow freely with that pressure, it will not suddenly flow when aspirated with excessive force.

V. Thoracic Cavity Injury

A. **Physical examination:** injury involving structures of the torso frequently include injury to the viscera of the thorax, abdomen and pelvis. Therefore, in addition to musculoskeletal pain, visceral pain is frequently present. Handling and restraining torso-injured patients must be performed very carefully as localized areas of pain will be present. Painful areas to consider are the shoulders, vertebral column, all areas of the thorax, abdomen, pelvis and perineum. Intrathoracic lesions to consider are pericardial, mediastinal and pulmonary hemorrhage, pneumothorax, inflammation and associated lung parenchymal swelling or hemorrhage, all of which result in severe pain.

Pain of various degrees occurs in medical conditions associated with ischemia (thrombus), inflammation ± enlargement of organs resulting in stretching of the capsule (myocarditis, pericarditis, pleuritis, pneumonitis, heptatitis, acute kidney injury), tumours and mediastinal pathology. Common examples occurring in both cats and dogs are neoplasia and esophageal foreign bodies. A careful, focused examination is required to localize the area responsible for causing pain. It is essential to maintain the patient in the least painful position and one that does not compromise ventilation. Careful observation of the patient will assist with position. Frequently sternal is the most comfortable, but right or left lateral may be better with specific and penetrating injuries. Visceral pain tends to be diffuse in nature and is usually perceived as being deep in the body of the thorax; however, pain can also be localized to an area within the cavity when pressure is applied externally (e.g. pleuritis). Thoracic visceral pain may also be exhibited as referred pain at a distant cutaneous site. This site may also exhibit secondary hyperalgesia or an exaggerated pain sensation on palpation of that area. As an example, the pain experienced by inflammation of the lungs and/or pleura may be elicited on abdominal palpation. This response can be confused with acute abdominal pain and potential consideration of treatment for this. Where abdominal pain is elicited, inclusion of caudal lung fields on all abdominal radiographs is essential to rule out potential lung pathology as the cause of pain. When compared to cutaneous pain, visceral pain has a greater motor and autonomic involvement, resulting in an increase in muscle tone, heart and respiratory rate and blood pressure.

B. **Initial management** is also based on inclusion/exclusion of pre-existing problems and co-morbidities, and when the patient was last fed. An additional factor is the aggressive nature of the patient. Frequently, patients require diagnostic imaging and some may require surgical management. Specific analgesic/anesthetic protocols will be required for each circumstance. Preparation for intubation and assisted ventilation is essential. As cardiac arrhythmias may occur within 12–24 h (if not already present) following thoracic trauma, continuous ECG monitoring must be included in the ongoing patient assessment.

C. **Rib fractures/flail chest**

1. Analgesia
    a. opioids, Box 28.1;
    b. intercostal nerve blocks, Chapter 14; and/or
    c. loose, soft bandage wrap (Figure 28.2) to prevent excessive movement. Place patient in lateral recumbency to reduce chest wall movement and associated pain. Patient will often find more comfort lying on the affected side or sternal;
    d. chest tube placement (see D.2 below) for ongoing analgesic delivery where indicated;
    e. placement of nasal catheter. Generous instillation of an **ophthalmic local anesthetic** into the nasal meatus prior to placement and lidocaine gel on the nasal catheter.

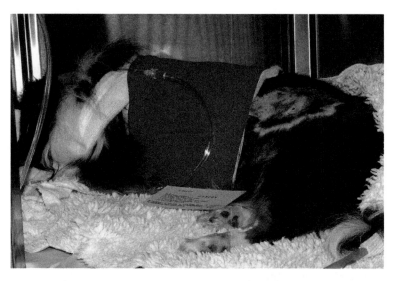

Fig 28.2 A female Shetland sheepdog was referred for management of three fractured ribs and fractured pelvis. In addition, a healing second-degree burn was noted, alerting us to an abusive owner and contact with the Humane Society.

D. **Pneumothorax, hemothorax**
   1. **Thoracocentesis**
      a. **Tension pneumothorax**
         i. **Immediate thoracocentesis** at 7th intercostal space at the junction of upper and middle thirds if in sternal recumbency, or 7th intercostal, highest (mid) point if in lateral recumbency. Placement of local anesthesia may not be an option prior to inserting a 14–16 gauge over-the-needle catheter directly into pleural space to relieve tension as this is a life-saving procedure.
         ii. **If time permits**, quickly pull skin cranially, clip and prep with alcohol, inject **lidocaine 2 mg/kg** into skin, SC, muscle and pleura, wait 5 min, while maintaining the "pulled skin", prior to over-the-needle catheter insertion. If this is not possible, make direct lidocaine injection.
         iii. During this time obtain **IV access, begin appropriate fluid** administration
         iv. Titrate an opioid (**Box 28.1**),
         v. **Ketamine** 0.5–2 mg/kg to effect (potential anesthesia) should further chemical restraint be required to facilitate placement of temporary large-bore IV catheter into the pleural space while preparing for chest tube placement (see point b below).
      b. **Non-tension pneumothorax and hemothorax**
         i. Prep skin.
         ii. Infiltrate warm lidocaine 2 mg/kg through prepped skin, SC, muscle and pleura at the dorsal 7th intercostal space for pneumothorax, or ventral for hemothorax. Avoid the neurovascular bundle at the caudal margin of the ribs as pain and hemorrhage may occur if the injection is made directly into the vessel and nerve, aspirate prior to injection. Where time permits wait 5 min before introducing a needle or catheter.
   2. **Chest tube placement [1]**
      In addition to evacuation of pleural air or fluid, chest tube placement for interpleural instillation of bupivacaine may be considered for pain management of any thoracic, low cervical and diaphragm injury, and inflammation

a. **Analgesia** as in Box 28.1 followed by:
b. **Local anesthesia** should be provided prior to chest tube placement even when the patient is anesthetized.
  i. **Infiltration of lidocaine** as in point 1.b.ii above prior to making a small stab incision through the skin with a scalpel blade for catheter placement.
  ii. **Bupivacaine** in non-emergent situations where there are a few minutes to spare for effect to occur is preferred as it has longer duration of action, **or**
  iii. **Lidocaine** for emergent situations, e.g. tension pneumothorax.
  iv. **Mila™ over-the-guide-wire chest drain placement** [1] is recommended for cats and dogs for pneumothorax and most fluids (transudates, hemorrhage, exudates), for simplicity, minimal discomfort of placement, in-place comfort and not requiring on-going analgesia, unless used for analgesic purposes. However, rarely, where large-volume thick purulent material is present, a large-bore chest tube may be required (see point c below). Patients can be restrained in sternal or lateral recumbency. Sedation combined with a local block is all that is required in almost all cases. Should anesthesia be required for a concurrent procedure, take this opportunity to place the catheter.
c. **Short-term anesthesia**, especially for cats due to the compliant chest wall, is required for a traditional trocar type **(large-bore)** chest tube. This rarely may be indicated with large volume, thick fluid (e.g. purulent) or air where the Mila catheter **was** inadequate.
  i. **Propofol or alfaxalone (1–2 mg/kg increments of either) titrated for induction**, Box 28.3, is preferred for this short procedure due to the rapid recovery. However, if the procedure is predicted to last > 20 min or if more than three dosages of injectable drugs have been administered and the procedure is not complete, consider switching to low-dose isoflurane or sevoflurane for maintenance. The inhalants require minimal metabolism for elimination. Propofol and alfaxalone are potent respiratory depressants so supplemental oxygen is imperative, or
  ii. **Ketamine at 0.5–2 mg/kg** IV incremental doses to effect. If **ketamine** is included in the previous analgesic regimen, but not used alone, continue with incremental doses of 2 mg/kg to effect. A 2.0 mg/kg bolus IV is at the medium-high range. Some patients might need a lower dose or
  iii. **Diazepam/ketamine** slow titration with **1:1 [5 mg/mL diazepam: 100 mg/mL ketamine = 2 mL]** (2.5 mg/50.0 mg per ml of mixture at 0.02 mL/kg of this solution. This is a safe approach in cats with severe respiratory compromise and unknown cardiovascular status. The sympathetic drive and lesser respiratory depression may have a slight advantage over propofol and alfaxalone but supplemental oxygen is still required
  iv. **Interpleural placement of local anesthetics (LA).** Upon completion of chest tube placement, and prior to extubation, instil the local anesthetic through the chest tube. This is a useful adjunct to, or in place of, opioid analgesics for continuous management of traumatic pain, presence of a large drain, thoracic incisional pain or pleuritis. This is not necessary for "tube" analgesia where the small Mila fenestrated chest drains are in place when managing pneumothorax or pleural fluid/blood as these appear to be well tolerated. However, this may be patient dependent.
  v. **Dosing is based on ideal body weight in** the overweight or obese patient. Overdose based on actual weight in these patients may result in toxicity. Refer to Chapter 14.
    • Dilute 0.5% (5 mg/mL) bupivacaine cats: 0.15 mL/kg (= 0.75 mg/kg), dogs: 0.2 ml/kg (=1 mg/kg) with 6–12 mL sterile water for larger dogs (relative to size of dog), 3 mL for tiny dogs and cats. Fill the catheter prior to placement. Aseptic technique is essential, and fresh, single-dose vials should be used. Following

placement, inject the required dose of LA which will displace the required volume from the catheter. After interpleural administration, the animal should be placed with the injured or incision side down for 5 min to enhance the effect at the desired site. The patient can also be rolled onto its back to allow the local anesthetic to flow into the paravertebral gutters to block nerves before entering the spinal cord. Upon recovery, if the patient still appears uncomfortable, adjust their position to facilitate re-distribution of the local anesthetic. Repeat bupivacaine q4–6h dogs, 6h cats. Should the duration of instillation be increased, pain will likely occur upon administration; therefore, it is essential to maintain this timing. Should pain appear at the 6h point, stop delivery for 15 min, then complete delivery. Ensure that the next delivery is at 4h (dogs) to avoid pain upon instillation. As the LA is maintained within the tube, it is maintained at body temperature and pre-warming of the new dose is not required. **After 24h**, reduce to half dose thereafter. The total dose of bupivacaine should not exceed 1.5 mg/kg q6h for dogs; 0.75 mg/kg q6h for cats.

- **For initial placement in the awake patient** prepare a mixture of 0.5% (5 mg/mL) bupivacaine (dogs: 0.2 mL/kg = 1 mg/kg, cats: 0.15 mL/kg = 0.75 mg/kg) based on ideal body weight, and sodium bicarbonate (1 mEq/mL) Buffering of a 0.5% bupivacaine solution (5 mg/mL) requires a 20:0.1 mixture with sodium bicarbonate 1 mEq/mL (~0.2 mL bupivacaine and 0.001 mL sodium bicarbonate) and warmed to ~30 °C, max 35 °C. It is recommended that sterile water be used to dilute bupivacaine.
- Do not add more sodium bicarbonate as this will precipitate out. The sodium bicarbonate reduces the pain associated with local anesthetics at this site by increasing the pH of the solution. Slowly deliver the calculated dose of LA, plus volume of the chest tube initially, via the chest tube. The dose/kg is then used for the following dosages. While the addition of sodium bicarbonate reduces the pain experienced, the positioning required and the local anesthetic itself can cause some pain and certain positions (especially dorsal recumbency) can add to respiratory difficulties in some patients, so be prepared for this. Repeat bupivacaine without bicarbonate as above. Where volume is required for repeat instillation, add sterile water to the bupivacaine dose as described in 2 iv.
- For details on buffering local anesthetics, refer to: https://www.nps.org.au/australian-prescriber/articles/alkalinisation-of-local-anesthetic-solutions

  d. **NSAIA, COX-2 preferential/selective** (Chapter 11) as soon as all contraindications have been ruled out.

3. **Thoracotomy** (intercostal or sternotomy)

Traumatic injuries and dog bite wounds to the thorax frequently require exploratory thoracotomy or a surgical correction. Human patients report a high level of pain following thoracotomy. Based on experience with veterinary patients requiring multi-modal analgesia to effect comfort, this degree of pain can be assumed in cats and dogs. Pain is generated from the underlying problem; therefore, hyperalgesia may also be established depending on cause and duration. The surgical procedure generates massive nociceptive input associated with skin and muscle incision; rib retraction or excision both involve intercostal nerve injury, surgical exploration and manipulation of parietal and visceral pleura, ± resection of lung or neoplasia (vagus nerve). Pain is also established in procedures involving the mediastinum, pericardium and diaphragm (phrenic nerve). Surgical technique also influences nociceptive input. Wire placed around ribs compresses the nerve on the caudal aspect. Sternotomy technique resulting in the potential for segment instability is painful. Entry local anesthetic intercostal nerve blocks (Chapter 14) will reduce the nociceptive input of the thoracotomy procedure; however, pain established by potential nociceptive input via the vagus and phrenic nerves requires ongoing management with interpleural bupivacaine (see point 2.c.iv above) or epidural morphine (Chapter 14).

General anesthesia is required to assess and manage deep bite wounds (Figure 28.3–28.5), and large wounds and removal of penetrating injury/foreign body (Figure 28.6). Wound debridement of gross contaminants is essential to prevent infection and subsequent bacteremia. To safely anesthetize these patients, fluid deficits, including use of blood products where appropriate, should be corrected prior to induction to minimize the negative cardiovascular effects of the injectable and inhalant anesthetics.

E. **Penetrating injury/foreign body/bite wounds**
1. **Analgesia**
   a. **Opioids as Box 28.1.**
   b. **Plan surgical removal of penetrating object** while stabilizing the patient. Diagnostic imaging is not necessary and may result in further injury.
2. **Anesthesia: see Box 28.3 for general anesthesia protocols**

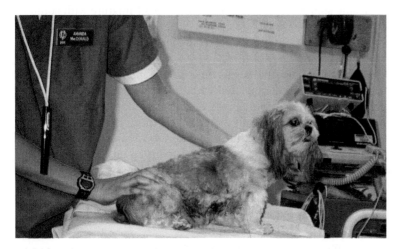

Figure 28.3 A male Shih tzu presented following a dog attack with bite wounds and flail chest.

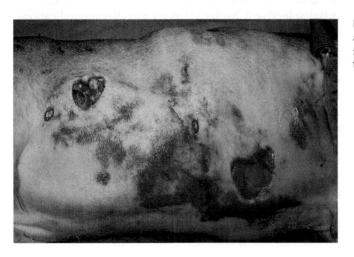

Figure 28.4 The dog above after anesthesia and preparation for surgical exploration and repair of flail chest.

Figure 28.5 The above dog at exploratory thoracotomy

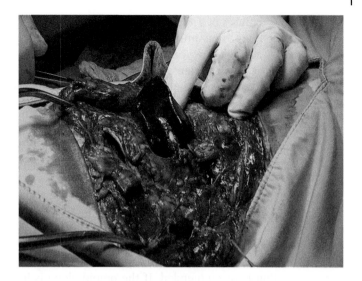

Figure 28.6 A German shorthaired pointer impaled on a tree branch which entered between the forelimbs, skimmed along the sternum and entered the abdomen and pelvis exiting the left lateral to the vulva. Diagnostic imaging was not performed to prevent movement and potential further injury. Minimal movement from the ER to prep room. Exploratory surgery determined extent of injury and appropriate, successful management.

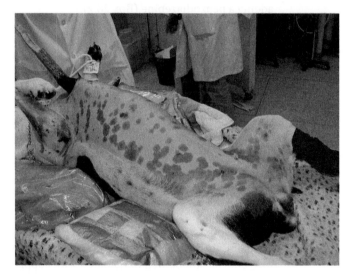

a. Additional comments for anesthesia for patients with unstable hemodynamics:
   i. **Patients should be stabilized** as much as possible; however, some patients may require surgery to control hemorrhage despite being hypovolemic. In these cases, acepromazine and alpha₂ agonists should **not** be administered.
   ii. **Pre-medication**: see Box 28.3 for unstable patients.
   iii. **Induction**
      • **See Box 28.3 for unstable patients.**
      • **Etomidate** (1–3 mg/kg) may be preferred in patients that have been hemorrhaging and are profoundly unstable.
      • **Mask induction with isoflurane or sevoflurane** is contraindicated because deep anesthesia may occur quickly and due to the reduced cardiac output in these patients profound hypotension is likely to occur.
   iv. **Maintenance**
      • During maintenance with an inhalational anesthetic, additional administration of an **opioid** will decrease the amount of inhalant required. IV **lidocaine**

boluses of 2 mg/kg or infusions (50–120 µg/kg/min) may also be beneficial in dogs to minimize inhalant levels and or treat ventricular arrhythmias associated with myocardial contusions (see below).

b. **Anesthesia for patients with lung contusions** requiring immediate surgery. With a traumatic injury, intra-alveolar, interstitial and inter-alveolar hemorrhage occurs resulting in lung contusions. Secondary inflammatory edema also occurs, which collapses pulmonary capillaries further. Lung contusions will usually worsen within the first 24–36 h and may be missed on initial examination and radiographs. Radiographs may not demonstrate the presence of contusions until 4–6 h after the injury. Resolution of pulmonary contusions begins within 3–7 days depending on the patient's lung injury.

   i. **Medical management** of contusions includes oxygen and analgesics to reduce the pain of normal ventilation. Diuretics may be indicated when pulmonary edema is present. Ideally, surgery should be delayed until the degree of lung contusions can be assessed and treated, and have begun to resolve. However, this is not possible with penetrating injuries and large deep (especially bite) wounds.

   ii. **Pre-medication** with an opioid. Box 28.1, and pre-oxygenation prior to induction is recommended. If the opioid alone is insufficient for sedation, consider adding a benzodiazepine (Box 28.2)

   iii. **Induction** with any of the injectable anesthetic drugs (propofol, alfaxalone, ketamine, etomidate; Box 28.3) at the previously recommended dosages. Inhalant induction is not recommended since the time to intubation and initiation of positive pressure ventilation is delayed.

   iv. **Under anesthesia** attention to ventilation, to avoid excessive airway pressures, is essential during assisted or mechanical ventilation. Peak inspiratory pressures should remain < 10 cmH$_2$0, hence lower tidal volumes and higher frequency rates are preferred to prevent further alveolar injury. Manual sighing of the patient during anesthesia is not recommended. Appropriate minute volume (RR × tidal volume) can be determined by measuring end-tidal carbon dioxide (ETCO$_2$), which should be maintained <55 cmH$_2$O (normal is 35–45 cmH$_2$O but some respiratory depression is tolerable) to prevent respiratory acidosis. Pulse oximetry (SpO$_2$) is also recommended but it should be remembered that, in patients receiving supplemental oxygen, pulse oximeters are monitors of oxygenation not ventilation (meaning that the patient may not be ventilating adequately to maintain normal CO$_2$ but can still be well oxygenated with supplemental oxygen).

c. **Anesthesia for patients with myocardial contusions**

   i. **Ventricular dysrhythmias** Premature ventricular contractions and ventricular tachycardia frequently occur within 12–24 h post-trauma in patients with myocardial contusions, which are refractory to all drug treatment in many patients. Therefore, delaying surgery for 1–3 days, if possible, is ideal. Do not expect to always eradicate ventricular tachycardia. The aim is to reduce the high rate to a lower rate (accelerated idioventricular rhythm (<150 in dogs, < 200 in cats) or infrequent premature ventricular contractions, thereby enabling adequate filling of the ventricles and improved cardiac output. If emergent general anesthesia is required prior to arrhythmias resolving, arrhythmic agents such as alpha$_2$ agonists, and thiobarbiturates **must be avoided**. Ketamine should be used with caution as ketamine stimulates the sympathetic nervous system and may exacerbate some arrhythmias.

   ii. **Pre-medication with a neuroleptoanalgesic** combination (i.e. an opioid from **Box 28.1 plus a sedative from Box 28.2**) followed by pre-induction oxygenation. The decision to administer acepromazine in these patients should be made on a case-by-case basis related to their personality and pre-operative status. The advantage of acepromazine is that it has some mild anti-arrhythmic effects. The disadvantage is that it can contribute to hypotension via vasodilatory effects.

  iii. **Anesthetic induction:** ECG and blood pressure monitoring are highly recommended during the induction period since major physiologic changes occur at induction in all patients. ECG and blood pressure monitoring are required during maintenance of anesthesia for all patients.
- **For unstable patients** with **ventricular dysrhythmias, lidocaine boluses** of 2 mg/kg dogs over 30 s, 0.2–1 mg/kg cats **over 5 min** – no more than four boluses within a 10–15 min period, commence an infusion if lidocaine responsive, 30–50 μg/kg/min dogs, 10–20 μg/kg/min cats. This will be required for the emergent patient where delay, to allow myocardial healing and resolution of arrhythmias prior to anesthesia, is not possible. The anti-arrhythmic regimen successfully controlling the arrhythmia should be continued throughout induction and maintenance, and is often necessary into the recovery period.
- **Induction options** listed in **Box 28.3** and dosages for all induction drugs should be kept as low as possible as most of the drugs can have some negative cardiac impact (propofol and alfaxalone – hypotension; ketamine – **maybe** contribution to arrhythmias). Etomidate is preferred because it causes minimal, to no, adverse cardiac effects. Inhalant induction is not recommended as the inhalant drugs are highly likely to cause hypotension when used at induction dosages.
- For the **stable trauma patients**, the anesthetic regimen should be tailored to the patient's co-morbidities, and options are listed in **Box 28.3**.
- **Monitoring** of heart rate (HR), ECG rhythm, RR, SpO$_2$, indirect arterial blood pressure (oscillometric or Doppler) and body temperature should be performed as a minimum standard during all, even short, anesthetics of trauma cases. ETCO$_2$ is also highly useful.

  iv. **Daily wound management** frequently requires heavy sedation/anesthesia, in addition to the ongoing analgesic regimen established:
- **Propofol** 2–6 mg/kg, IV or **alfaxalone** 1–3 mg/kg, IV titrated to effect, or
- **Ketamine** 0.2–1 mg/kg IV.
   If ketamine is part of the multi-modal analgesic therapy, increase the dose to effect.

F. **Tracheobronchial injury/obstruction**
Adults and pediatric patients, primarily dogs, may present with tracheobronchial injury or obstruction. This most commonly occurs following aggressive play with various objects. ET intubation supplies, including sterile catheter for possible bronchial catheterization, should be readily available after sedation.
Endoscopy is required for diagnosis and removal of FBs (foreign bodies).
Where thoracotomy is required see point D.3 above.

1. **Analgesia/sedation: refer to Box 28.1**
2. **Anesthesia for endoscopy**
   a. **Adults**
      i. **Pre-medication** should include pre-oxygenation as well as drug administration.
- **Maropitant** (dogs and cats: 1 mg/kg SC or slowly IV) should be administered for the reason listed above and also because manipulation of the pharyngeal area can induce vomiting.
- **The opioids above (fentanyl or methadone)** are preferred and should be administered through a pre-placed venous catheter so that induction and intubation (if possible) can occur rapidly.

- **Sedatives (Box 28.2)** are not commonly required but a benzodiazepine or a very low-dose acepromazine (0.01 mg/kg) can be utilized. The onset of acepromazine is 10–20 min and so generally too slow in emergency situations, but it is a good addition in some instances because of the acepromazine-mediated long-duration calming effect. Midazolam can be administered IV as part of induction for emergent procedures.
  ii. **Induction + maintenance**
  - **Induction** with midazolam IV (Box 28.3) administered immediately prior to, or concurrently with, a low-dose of **alfaxalone or propofol** titrated to effect, is the most commonly used induction technique.
  - **Maintenance** is then provided by an infusion or repeat boluses of the induction drug. Alternatively, **ketamine plus a benzodiazepine (Box 28.3)** can be titrated to effect and, because of the long duration of action, may provide anesthesia of sufficient duration for the procedure. If not, small boluses of the mixture can be repeated. Placement of an ET tube is recommended if the tube will not interfere with visualization of the injury and if the tube is large enough for the endoscope to pass through.
  iii. **Intraoperative** administration of oxygen is imperative and may be delivered through special ET tube adapters for larger ET tube or can be administered intermittently by stopping the procedure for oxygen delivery if the SpO_2 drops below 90%. SpO2 monitoring is mandatory for this procedure. HR, RR, arterial blood pressure, mucous membrane colour and capillary refill time (CRT) should also be continuously monitored. No specific local blocks are available for this procedure but "blocking what hurts" (i.e. blocking areas of injury with topical lidocaine) will aid in keeping the patient anesthetized with minimal dosages of anesthetic drugs.
  iv. **Recovery and post-operative** pain, excitement and dysphoria must be avoided as they cause the patient to breathe deeply, increasing intra-airway negative pressure, which can then exacerbate areas of airway collapse that may be present.
  - **Opioids (Box 28.1)** are recommended for analgesia; however, if opioid-mediated sedation could be a problem, consider buprenorphine 0.02 mg/kg as it causes only mild to no sedation at this dose.
  - **An NSAIA, COX 2 preferential/selective** should also be administered if not contraindicated, and corticosteroids have not been administered, or planned to be administered, to control airway swelling.
  - **Acepromazine** (0.01 mg/kg dogs; 0.02 mg/kg cats) is safe and effective for calming.
  b. **Pediatric** patients commonly present with tracheobronchial injuries/obstructions following play with a variety of objects. The adult recommendations above can be utilized for the pediatric patient; however, drug dosages are lower. Refer to Chapter 25 for specific information on dosing and duration of the various analgesics, sedatives and anesthetics.
  c. Where thoracotomy is required, see point D.3 above.
- G. **Esophageal lesions/obstruction**
  Adults and pediatric patients, primarily dogs, present with esophageal injuries/obstruction due to the many objects they play with or eat. Clinical presentation is frequently associated with dyspnea; however, some may acquire the "praying position" as this appears to relieve some discomfort/pain (Figure 28.7). Esophageal lesions may occur after eating anything sharp or following general anesthetic where gastric acid refluxed into the esophagus. It is important to ensure the patient does not vomit as the foreign body may prevent the animal from being able to swallow properly, or rapidly result in aspiration.

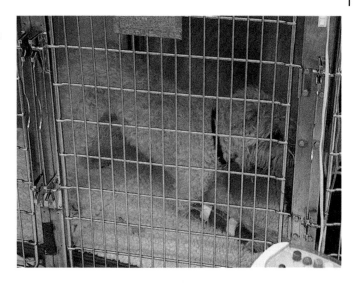

Figure 28.7 The "praying position" due to pain resulting from a foreign body present in the distal esophagus. A similar posture may be noted with abdominal pain.

1. **Maropitant** should be administered to all patients. ET intubation supplies should be readily available after sedation.
2. **Methadone, buprenorphine and fentanyl** are the agents recommended for "analgesic sedation". Due to the risk of vomiting with IV or IM administration, hydromorphone, morphine and dexmedetomidine should be avoided until a protected airway is achieved.
3. **Endoscopy** is required for diagnosis and removal of the foreign body.
4. **Once general anesthesia** (see point D.3 above or endoscopy V.F.2 above) has been induced and the foreign body has been removed, any analgesic in Box 28.1 or sedative in Box 28.2 can be administered as needed for the individual patient.
5. **Where thoracotomy** is required refer to **Box 28.3** above. Assess the severity of the esophageal lesion, and where pain will potentially interfere with eating, place a gastrostomy tube.

H. **Diaphragmatic hernia**

May occur due to trauma but a congenital diaphragmatic defect, in both cats and dogs, may also predispose to intestinal herniation/incarceration into the pleural space. This usually occurs in the pediatric patient but manifestation may not occur until an adult. Where pleural fluid is identified, remove as soon as possible to reduce ventilatory and oxygenation impairment. Associated cardiovascular compromise is also possible in any of these patients and judicial replacement of fluid deficits should begin as soon as IV access is obtained. Analgesic restraint is required for radiography and thoracocentesis. Further respiratory compromise and vomiting must be avoided

1. **Analgesia**
   a. **Opioid (Box 28.1) plus diazepam or midazolam sedation** is the safest approach when significant respiratory compromise is present.
2. **Anesthesia**
   a. **Adults**
      i. **Pre-medication:** to minimize the duration of any pre-medication-mediated respiratory depression, all drugs should be administered IV through a pre-placed venous catheter.
         • **Maropitant** (1 mg/kg IV slowly or SC)
         • **Opioid from Box 28.1**, methadone, buprenorphine and fentanyl are the agents recommended for "analgesic sedation", as the least likely to cause vomiting. Add a **benzodiazepine from Box 28.2**.

- **Monitoring** should start as soon as possible as arrhythmias and hypoventilation are common in these patients and may be exacerbated by anesthetic drugs.
  ii. **Induction + maintenance:** rapid induction with any of the drugs listed in Box 28.3. Inhalant induction is not appropriate as this method is slow and delays the time to securing a protected airway and initiating assisted ventilation. Maintain with either isoflurane or sevoflurane.
  iii. **Intraoperative:** immediately after induction perform intercostal nerve blocks with bupivacaine (refer to Chapter 14).
    - Opioids CRIs, **Box 28.1** above, plus lidocaine (point 3) and/or ketamine (point 2) are highly recommended.
    - **Epidural** administration of morphine may also be beneficial (more information in point D.3 above).
    - **Multi-modal analgesia** intraoperatively will improve anesthetic safety by allowing a lower dosage of inhalant anesthetic drug. It will also improve recovery as the patient will be more comfortable, and therefore decrease the post-operative opioid analgesic requirement and associated sedation which may cause mild respiratory depression).
    - **Monitoring** is critical and should include RR, HR, ECG, arterial blood pressure, SpO_2 and $ETCO_2$. Positive pressure ventilation (as described above in point D.3 above) will be required as long as the thorax is open. If the diaphragmatic hernia is chronic, re-expansion pulmonary edema is a major concern and Intermittent positive pressure ventilation (IPPV) should be delivered using very small tidal volumes (5 mL/kg) with increased RR to maintain the $ETCO_2 < 55$ mmHg.
  iv. **Recovery and post-op:** an interpleural catheter should be placed intraoperatively for the administration of local anesthetics (refer to Chapter 14). Any analgesic infusions initiated intraoperatively should be continued post-operatively for at least several hours if not overnight. An NSAIA, COX 2 preferential/selective, is recommended if there are no contraindications (refer to Chapter 11).
  b. **Pediatrics: traumatic and congenital diaphragmatic herniation** do occur in pediatric patients. The adult recommendations above can be utilized for the pediatric patient; however, drug dosages are lower. Refer to Chapter 25 for specific information on dosing and duration of the various analgesics, sedatives and anesthetics.

VI. Discharge Analgesia Plan for All Injuries

It is anticipated that pain will resolve as the underlying condition improves; therefore, owners must be aware of the requirement for dose reduction of analgesic drugs. The following is suggested based on injury, degree of pain and requirement while in hospital.

A. **NSAIA, COX 2 preferential/selective** (see Table 11.1) where there are no contraindications. The selected drug should be continued at home for a period of time based on the individual injury, and reduced gradually to avoid recurrence of pain. Where pain recurs, return to the dose immediately prior to dose reduction. Refer to Chapter 11.
B. **Fentanyl transdermal patch**, where continuing opioid treatment is required in addition to the NSAIA or where NSAIA is contraindicated or where pain is moderate to severe. The absorption of fentanyl from the patch is unpredictable with onset of action at 12+ h and duration of action up to three days. If a patch is prescribed, the size guideline below can assist selecting the patch size.
  1. Cats 12.5–25 μg/h patch.
  2. Small dogs (<10 kg) 25 μg/h patch.

3. Medium dogs (10–20 kg) 50 μg/h patch.
4. Large dogs (20–30 kg) 75 μg/h patch.
5. Giant dogs (>30 kg) 100 μg/h patch.
C. **Transdermal fentanyl solution** recently approved is now discontinued at time of writing. It is not known whether this will be available in the future.
D. **Buprenorphine** 0.02–0.05 mg/kg **OTM** cats and dogs < 10 kg (refer to Chapter 10) for mild to moderate pain where continuing opioid treatment is required in addition to the NSAIA or where NSAIA is contraindicated, or
E. **Buprenorphine** 24 h duration product (1.8 mg/mL) approved for SC injection in cats only may be used for three days. The approved dose is 0.24 mg/kg but the dose can be reduced by 25–50% in compromised patients.
F. **Gabapentin** 10 mg/kg q8h dogs, 6–10 mg/kg q12h for cats as determined by hospital stay. Dosages may be increased or decreased based on patient response.
G. **Amantadine** 3–5 mg/kg PO q12–24h, dogs and cats, as determined by hospital stay. Refer to Chapter 12 for details on prescribing in cats.
H. **Do not stop analgesia abruptly** unless adverse effects noted with NSAIAs (Chapter 11). The following is a suggested **weaning programme**.
   1. **Buprenorphine** – miss the following scheduled dose and reduce ongoing dose by half. Should pain recur at any time, return to previous dose.
   2. **Gabapentin** – wean gradually by eliminating the q8h schedule and resume with q12h. After one week, reduce dose by one-half or to manageable pill size if not liquid. Continue with weaning based on patient's response. Should pain recur at any point, return to previous effective dose/schedule.
   3. **Amantadine** – as for gabapentin.
   4. **Fentanyl transdermal patch** – instruct owner to return for assessment and patch removal/reduction/replacement as required.

VII. Thoracic Cavity: Illness

A. **Pneumonia/pleuritis**
Smoke inhalation: refer to Chapter 33.
For humane reasons and to assist the patient with ventilation, analgesia is essential. To avoid a peracute increase in pain during inspiration, patients avoid normal chest excursions during inspiration resulting in an ineffective respiratory pattern.
   1. **Analgesia**
      a. Based on severity Box 28.1 above, and/or
      b. NSAIA where no contraindications
      c. CRIs of opioids, lidocaine (refer to Chapter 12 for information on cats) and/or ketamine (Box 28.1, point 2)
      d. Interpleural local anesthesia may be considered in patients with unrelenting dyspnea due to the pain of pleuritis.
B. **Pulmonary edema**
Morphine is no longer recommended as a specific treatment for human patients with pulmonary edema associated with heart failure. This may also apply to non-cardiogenic pulmonary edema; however, the underlying cause for this must be recognized and assume pain exists.
   1. **Analgesia (Box 28.1)** for suggestions.
C. **Cardiovascular**
Approximately 50% of dogs with **pulmonary thromboemboli** (PTE) have multiple underlying disease processes.

1. **Analgesia** for PTE and other thromboses associated with pain:
    a. **Opioids (Box 28.1)**
       If only mild to moderate pain is accurately identified, a lower dose of the opioid is recommended, or
    b. **Butorphanol** 0.4–0.8 mg/kg q2–4h, or to effect, or
    c. **Buprenorphine** 5–10 μg/kg IV, IM, a higher dose may be required, or
    d. **Buprenorphine** 0.02–0.05 mg/kg OTM cats and dogs < 10 kg (refer to Box 28.1) q4–8h for mild to moderate pain where continuing opioid treatment is required in addition to the NSAIA or where NSAIA is contraindicated, or
    e. **Buprenorphine 24 h duration product** (1.8 mg/ml) (Simbadol®, Zoetis) approved for SC injection in cats only, may be used for three days. The approved dose is 0.24 mg/kg but the dose can be reduced by 25–50% in compromised patients.
2. **Anesthesia** for patients with thoracic cavity illness:
    a. **Stabilize** as much as possible prior to anesthesia. Try to delay anesthesia until the SpO_2 can be maintained at > 90%.
    b. **Protocols** the same as those for anesthesia for patients with "lung contusion".

Reference

1 Mila International chest tube placement. YouTube video, https://www.youtube.com/watch?v=jv4kV7fc6dM.

Further Reading

Brandis, K. (2011) Alkalinisation of local anaesthetic solutions. *Austr Prescr*, 34: 173–175, https://www.nps.org.au/australian-prescriber/articles/alkalinisation-of-local-anaesthetic-solutions.

Grubb, T. L. (2016) Respiratory compromise. In: Duke-Novakovski, T., de Vries, M. and Seymour, C. (eds), *BSAVA Manual of Canine and Feline Anaesthesia and Analgesia*, BSAVA, Gloucester: 329–342.

Pascoe, P. J. (2016) Intrathoracic surgery and interventions. In: Duke-Novakovski, T., de Vries, M. and Seymour, C. (eds), *BSAVA Manual of Canine and Feline Anaesthesia and Analgesia*, BSAVA, Gloucester: 343–355.

29

Torso and Abdomen: Illness and Injuries

Karol Mathews, Tamara Grubb and Andrea Steele

Injury involving structures of the torso frequently includes injury to the viscera of the thorax, abdomen and pelvis. Therefore, in addition to musculoskeletal pain, visceral pain is frequently present. Handling and restraining torso-injured patients must be performed very carefully as localized areas of pain will be present. This is especially important where penetrating injuries are present, as excessive movement not only causes pain but also may precipitate further injury. Painful areas to consider are the shoulders, vertebral column, all areas of the thorax, abdomen, pelvis and perineum. Many primary medical, surgical and traumatic problems associated with the abdomen, as well as injuries developing secondarily (e.g. peritonitis), are extremely painful. Blunt or penetrating injury of the abdominal wall frequently results in intra-abdominal injury and subsequent inflammation, resulting in both muscular and visceral pain. Detected muscular pain may be isolated to the abdominal or pelvic wall but may be a reflection of visceral pain; therefore, careful assessment is required for diagnosis. Careful monitoring of the patient with respect to increasing abdominal, pelvic or perineal pain is essential as this may be associated with urological, reproductive or gastrointestinal (GI) injury. Urethral injury results in urine leakage into the perineum and/or hind limbs resulting in severe pain from inflammation and a "compartmental-like syndrome". Assess the penis for pain, and patency, associated with a fractured os penis.

Visceral pain associated with illness is present in conditions associated with distension of hollow, muscular-walled organs (stomach, small intestine, colon, urinary and gall bladder, uterus), ischemia (commonly the bowel) and inflammation of any organ (hepatitis, cholecystitis, pancreatitis, splenitis and pyelonephritis) associated with acute enlargement of solid organs resulting in stretching of the capsule. Subcapsular hematomas following injury confer similar degrees of pain. Other painful conditions are neoplasia, acute kidney injury, inflammatory bowel disease, viral enteritis and GI foreign bodies. Bowel distension and hyper-segmentation has the potential for intussusception. Acute intussusception is painful but with chronicity may not be painful. Small areas of infarcted bowel may not be painful but severe vascular occlusion (volvulus or torsion) is painful. Septic, chemical or bile peritonitis causes severe pain.

On physical examination, visceral pain, especially associated with the bowel, tends to be diffuse in nature and perceived as being deep in the body of the thorax or abdomen. However, pain may be localized to an area when external pressure is applied, especially with a tense, inflamed organ such as the gallbladder or pancreas. Careful application of pressure, while observing the patient's response, is advised to avoid excessive pain and a potential bite reaction by the patient. Visceral pain may also be exhibited as referred pain at a distant cutaneous site from the area of pathology. This site may also exhibit secondary hyperalgesia or an exaggerated pain sensation

Analgesia and Anesthesia for the Ill or Injured Dog and Cat, First Edition. Karol A. Mathews, Melissa Sinclair, Andrea M. Steele and Tamara Grubb.
© 2018 John Wiley & Sons, Inc. Published 2018 by John Wiley & Sons, Inc.

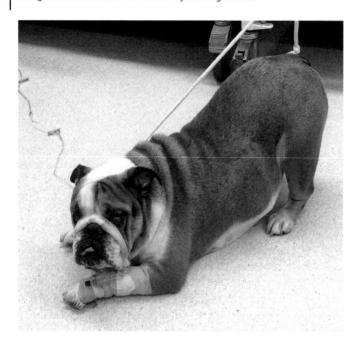

Figure 29.1 Stretched out "praying posture" indicating abdominal or lower esophageal pain.

on palpation of that area. As an example, inflammation of the lungs and/or pleura is very painful and can be elicited on abdominal palpation. This response can be confused with acute abdominal pain and potential consideration of treatment for this. Caudal lung fields must be included on all abdominal radiographs to assist in diagnosing potential lung pathology followed by thoracic radiographs if lung pathology is suspected, or if no abnormal findings are detected on abdominal diagnostic imaging. Back pain and abdominal pain are often confused and may be difficult to differentiate. Patients with abdominal pain may exhibit a stretched out "praying posture" (Figure 29.1). Visceral pain induces a greater motor and autonomic response than that associated with cutaneous pain, resulting in increased muscle tone and changes in heart, respiratory rate and blood pressure, which, in addition to behavioural responses, is letting you know they hurt. However, intense vagal involvement will prevent an increase in heart rate; therefore, heart rate, unless elevated, cannot be used as a marker of pain. The physiological response of pain, especially visceral pain, is extremely detrimental to the patient. Pain activates the sympathetic nervous system causing vasoconstriction and therefore poor splanchnic (especially pancreatic and renal) perfusion. This can cause, or worsen, pancreatitis and reduce glomerular filtration rate. Therefore, good pain control is not only humane but also very important in protecting/improving organ function, reducing nausea and vomiting (N&V) and overall facilitating a more rapid resolution of associated primary illness or co-morbidities.

Abdominal pain associated with illness or injury may prevent deep breathing and coughing due to the pain this may generate; therefore, ensure the patient's pain is controlled as soon as possible.

Initial management is based on the illness or injury at hand and inclusion/exclusion of pre-existing problems/co-morbidities, and when the patient was last fed. Section I outlines details of analgesia, sedation and anesthesia recommended for the various scenarios given in Section IV and V below. The aggressive patient, the pregnant or lactating patient and age also require special consideration. Refer to the individual chapters for sedative (Chapter 9), opioid analgesic (Chapter 10), non-steroidal anti-inflammatory analgesic (Chapter 11), adjunct analgesic (Chapter 12) and anesthetic (Chapter 13) pharmacologic details.

I. Analgesia, Sedation and Anesthesia (General and Local)

A. For All Situations

Box 29.1 Analgesics

---

1. Opioids. For all situations.

Slowly titrate the opioid until the patient appears comfortable; higher dosages may be required. Titration should be halted when early signs of adverse effects appear – nausea, increased respiratory rate, dysphoria. Refer to **# opioid reversal** below. Dosages for both cats and dogs are within the dose range given unless otherwise stated. Opioids in order of preference for initial administration:

- **Fentanyl** 2–5 µg/kg, or
- **Methadone** 0.1–0.5 mg/kg
- **Fentanyl or methadone is preferred as both are less likely to cause N&V**, or
- **Oxymorphone** 0.02–0.05 + mg/kg, or
- **Hydromorphone** 0.02–0.1 mg/kg only if none of the above is available due to increased potential for vomiting (refer to Chapter 10, Section II.B), or
- **Morphine** 0.1–0.5 mg/kg only if none of the above is available due to increased potential for vomiting (refer to Chapter 10, Section II.A)
- **Diazepam intravenously (IV) or midazolam IV, intramuscularly (IM)** 0.2–0.5 mg/kg IV (dose based on anxiety level of the patient) to reduce opioid requirement initially and to offer sedation in the anxious patient.
- **Establish a continuous rate infusion (CRI)**
  - o 1 h infusion of the effective bolus dose of fentanyl, or
  - o 4 h infusion (or ¼ dose/h) of the effective bolus dose of methadone, hydromorphone, oxymorphone or morphine.

Fentanyl is appropriate for pregnant, lactating, pediatric and geriatric patients. Refer to these sections for ongoing analgesia.

Opioids alone may not be effective in cases where neuropathic pain also exists. The adverse effects of an opioid overdose can still occur in the neuropathic painful patient when the mu-receptors are saturated. Caution is required in interpretation of an increase in what appears to be painful behaviour occurring during opioid administration. The patient may be experiencing opioid-induced hyperalgesia requiring addition of a different class of analgesic (e.g. ketamine), versus a dysphoric response (refer to Chapter 8).

 # Opioid reversal with naloxone where required

Where excessive nausea, panting or dysphoria is noted, immediately reverse the opioid with naloxone, particularly if using a long-acting opioid. Slowly titrate until the adverse signs of the opioid subside, then stop naloxone administration. With slow titration, the primary effect of opioid analgesia will not be reversed and frequently facilitates calming. Fentanyl is quickly metabolized and it may not be necessary to reverse; caution is required as it is easy to "over reverse" and reverse the analgesic properties. To ensure accurate dosing for the individual patient and permit slow delivery of the reversal, the following is recommended:

- Dilute naloxone (0.4 mg/mL) using
  - o 0.1 mL added to 5 mL saline (=0.006 mg/mL) for small dogs and cats, titrate at 0.5 mL/min
  - o 0.25 mL added to 9.75 mL saline (=0.01 mg/mL), titrate at up to 1 mL/min
- titrate until signs of dysphoria or nausea are reversed, usually 2–3 mLs.

(Continued)

Box 29.1 (Continued)

---

2. Ketamine

Where pain cannot be managed with an opioid alone. **Not suitable for pregnant or lactating patients.**

- **Ketamine** 0.2–1 mg/kg titrated to effect.
- **Establish a CRI.**
- 1 h infusion of the effective bolus dose.
- Should the patient appear overdosed at any period of time, stop the CRI for 30 min, or less if signs subside, and reinstitute at one-half the previous dose.

3. Lidocaine

Lidocaine in dogs is an alternative to, or in combination with, the above and has shown benefit in humans and horses following abdominal procedures. Lidocaine IV bolus 1–2 mg/kg followed by 1–2 mg/kg/h – **dogs**, can be added to the above regimen where pain is not adequately managed or further reduction in opioid dosing is required. This dose must be calculated into the total dose when bupivacaine or lidocaine is used for local anesthesia (LA) to avoid toxicity (Chapter 14). Refer to Chapter 12 for guidance for use in **cats**. The addition of lidocaine may reduce the opioid requirement; therefore, monitoring for potential opioid adverse effects must be noted on the chart and the opioid dose reduced accordingly. **Lidocaine has promotility** activity which may be an advantage in patients presenting with abdominal emergencies should the injury/illness and high-dose opioid predispose to ileus. Nausea may develop with a 9–24 h infusion. Lidocaine IV should be avoided in patients with significant hepatic pathology.

4. Maropitant

Maropitant should be considered where N&V may be a concern. Dogs and cats: 1 mg/kg SC or 1 mg/kg very slowly IV, every 24 h. Administer into an IV catheter/line where no other drugs are present due to lack of compatibility studies. Maropitant contributes to analgesia, especially in patients with GI pain, through neurokinin (NK)-1 receptor antagonism.

B. Sedatives

Box 29.2

- **Diazepam** 0.2–0.5 mg/kg IV **or midazolam** 0.2–0.5 mg/kg IV or IM, or
- **Acepromazine** 0.005–0.02 mg/kg, IM, IV. Use with caution in hypovolemic or hypotensive patients, ace-mediated vasodilation may contribute to hypotension.
- **Medetomidine** 0.1–4 μg/kg IM, IV may be considered where no cardiac co-morbidities exist.
- **Dexmedetomidine** 0.05–2 μg/kg IM, IV may be considered where no cardiac co-morbidities exist.

C. Anesthesia

Box 29.3

---

1. Adults

a. Pre-medication: any of the opioids in Box 29.1 are appropriate. Low end of the dosages should be used for unstable patients. In very ill patients, an opioid alone may suffice.

In patients that are ill but require more calming, add a benzodiazepine from Box 29.2.

- **Maropitant should be administered to all patients** Dogs and cats: 1 mg/kg SC or slowly IV, **Box 29.1 section 4**.
- **Alpha$_2$ agonist** for patients that are fairly healthy/stable at dosages given below, which are higher than those in Box 29.2, or acepromazine, in addition to an opioid.
  - **Dexmedetomidine** 5–10 µg/kg dogs; 10–15 µg/kg cats IM (use ½ dose for IV), or
  - **Medetomidine** 10–20 µg/kg dogs; 20–30 µg/kg cats IM (use ½ dose for IV), or
  - **Acepromazine** 0.01–0.02 mg/kg dogs; 0.02–0.03 mg/kg cats IM (use ½ dose for IV).
b. **Induction:** any of the injectable anesthetic drugs are acceptable.
  - **Unstable/critical patients**
    - **Propofol and alfaxalone** at the low end of the dose for the stable patient below are preferred as they can be titrated "to effect", or
    - **Etomidate** (1–3 mg/kg IV) causes minimal to no cardiovascular effects and may be a good choice for unstable patients. Etomidate causes adrenocortical suppression, and its use in septic patients is controversial. Etomidate should never be used without adequate pre-anesthetic sedation as it commonly causes muscle rigidity, muscle twitching and vocalization in unsedated patients.
  - **Stable patients**
    - **Propofol** (2–6 mg/kg IV) or **alfaxalone** (1–3 mg/kg IV), or
    - **Ketamine combined with midazolam or diazepam** (1:1 ratio by volume): 0.1–0.2 mL/kg, IV to effect, or
    - **Telazol or Zoletil** (depending on what country you are in) 6–10 mg/kg IM or IV. Use premedicant sedatives to decrease the Telazol dose and to promote smooth recoveries.
  Inhalant induction should never be used whether the patient is stable or not as vomiting is highly likely in patients described in this chapter and a rapid induction with rapid intubation is necessary to assure a protected airway.
c. **Intraoperative maintenance and local blocks:**
  - Anesthesia should be maintained with low dose **inhalant** (sevoflurane or isoflurane) combined with local/regional anesthetics and/or CRIs (Box 29.1).
  - **An epidural** with morphine ± bupivacaine is ideal (refer to Chapter 14). LA in the epidural space is ideal for analgesia but can contribute to hypotension because of vasodilation. Fluid-load the patient prior to the epidural to alleviate this potential. If using CRIs, or an epidural without LA, include **local blockade at the incision site**.
  - **Appropriate fluid therapy and monitoring** are critical. Abdominal pain can often make breathing difficult so positive pressure ventilation (delivered by a mechanical ventilator or a person squeezing the re-breathing bag) may be necessary.
d. Should hypotension develop during anesthesia refer to Chapter 19, Section II.B.3.

2. **Pediatrics**
a. **Pre-medication:** as for adults are appropriate but the dosages may be reduced. Refer to Chapter 25 for more specific information.
b. Induction: as for adults.
c. **Intraoperative:** as for adults, including local blocks.

3. **Local Anesthetic (LA) Techniques**
   These techniques may be required to prevent severe pain. Careful calculation of LAs administered from all techniques is required to avoid overdose (refer to **Chapter** 14).
   a. **Interpleural LA:** nerves from the cranial abdomen enter the spinal cord in the thorax. Where cranial abdominal or diaphragm injury is present, an intrathoracic infusion catheter placed at the 9th intercostal space for interpleural LA administration is suggested (refer to

---

Box 29.3 (Continued)

Chapter 14 and Chapter 28). Or, depending on severity and magnitude of injury, place an epidural catheter.

  b. **Epidural analgesia via epidural catheter** is also an excellent method of controlling severe pain and should be considered for the individual patient's needs where surgical intervention is undertaken. Refer to Chapter 14 for single dose and CRI.

  c. **Entry or exit abdominal LA line blocks** are of value (refer to Chapter 14).

  d. **Interperitoneal LA bupivacaine 2 mg/kg dogs; 1 mg/kg cats** prior to abdominal closure, and for selective medical conditions.

II. Discharge Home Analgesia

Required for injured or ill and post-surgical patients.

A. **Based on the primary problem**, and successful regimen in hospital which may include:
  1. **Buprenorphine** oral transmucosal (OTM) 0.02–0.05 mg/kg cats or dogs < 10 kg (volume limited), or
  2. Cats **buprenorphine** (1.8 mg/ml) 24 h duration product (Simbadol®, Zoetis) approved for SC injection in cats only. The approved dose is 0.24 mg/kg but the dose can be reduced by 25–50% in compromised patients.
  3. **Amantadine** where ketamine was required up to discharge. Amantadine should be started at the time of weaning ketamine, and/or
  4. **Gabapentin 10–20 mg/kg q8h** where additional analgesia is required.
  5. **Non-steroidal anti-inflammatory analgesics (NSAIA)**, cyclooxygenase-2 (COX-2) preferential/selective where there are **no contraindications** including GI injury or illness. Refer to Chapter 11.

III. General Nursing Considerations for the Patient with Abdominal, Pelvic or Perineal Injury or Illness

Patients with abdominal pain are also frequently nauseated (as evidenced by lip smacking, drooling, exaggerated swallowing and inappetence), and may require anti-emetics. The veterinary technician/nurse (VT/N) should report this to the veterinarian to assess for potential problems and begin appropriate anti-emetic therapy. Reducing nausea will help with patient comfort.

Pain may be episodic when abdominal cramping is involved, and this can make pain management difficult, as the patient may be severely painful during cramps and quite comfortable between cramps. Assist the patient with frequent walking when cramping, as this may help move trapped gas along faster, and increase comfort. Also, report this to the veterinarian as an antispasmodic may be warranted.

Patients that are frequently regurgitating are at risk of aspiration, esophageal injury and pain. Regurgitation may be secondary to ileus, and a large dilated, fluid-filled stomach. The VT/N can be invaluable in identifying and notifying the veterinarian of frequent regurgitation, and placement of a nasogastric tube will allow for both removal of gastric residual fluid and small-volume, liquid diet feedings.

The VT/N should always be alert to sudden increased pain in a patient with an abdominal injury or illness. This may indicate a secondary condition such as pancreatitis, a perforation or peritonitis. Any increase in pain should be brought to the veterinarian's attention immediately as it may be indicative of a serious problem.

IV. Injured Patient

IV access and commencement of fluid therapy at an appropriate rate for the patient's condition.

A. Penetrating abdominal foreign body (FB) or puncture bite wound.

The information gained and benefit of diagnostic imaging where a visual penetrating FB is present do not outweigh the risk for increased pain and injury that will occur with these procedures. The authors' experience has been that immediate surgical exploratory offers more definitive assessment and treatment.

These injuries require immediate treatment to prevent further organ injury and reduce potential for extensive infection and ongoing pain. Opioids (fentanyl or methadone) are the authors' choice.

1. **Analgesia: Box 29.1**. It is essential that these analgesics be carefully titrated to avoid excessive dosing resulting in adverse effects. Panting and vomiting must be avoided.
2. **Anesthesia: Box 29.3**. Use protocols listed in Box 29.3 for ill patients. Depending on the location and degree of the injury, these patients may be severely painful and/or severely compromised (see more comments in Section IV.B below).
3. **Post-operative analgesia.**
   a. Continue with **Box 29.1**, titrating to effect. Omit lidocaine IV where intercostal catheters are placed.
   b. **LA** – see **Box 29.3 section 3**.
   c. **NSAIA, COX-2 selective/preferential added** where there are no contraindications, including GI injury (refer to Chapter 11). This will optimize analgesia and reduce opioid and/or the elimination of adjunct analgesics administered.

Refer to Chapter 26 (geriatric), Chapter 23 (pregnant) and Chapter 24 (nursing) cats and dogs for guidance in these patients.

B. **Bowel perforation/rupture** may occur following FB ingestion. In addition to the pain associated with rupture, peritonitis produces severe pain. Immediate surgical exploratory is essential.

1. **Analgesia**
   a. Box 29.1.
2. **Anesthesia**
   a. **Box 29.3**. These patients may be endotoxemic, making appropriate fluid therapy more critical. In addition, by-products of endotoxemia can cause a decrease in cardiac contractility, potentially requiring support with positive inotropes (e.g. dopamine or dobutamine).
   b. **LA** – see **Box 29.3 section 3**.
3. **Post-operative analgesia**
   a. Continue with Box 29.1 with modification based on the LA techniques applied.
   b. **Do not administer an NSAIA.**

C. **Blunt traumatic injury**

Pain may be restricted to torso injury/bruising or may include the vertebral column (refer to Chapter 32), skeletal or visceral injury and the severity of pain will depend on degree and anatomical location of injury.

1. **Analgesia**
   a. **Initially, Box 29.1** while assessing the patient.
   b. **Abdominocentesis** where indicated. In this setting there is time to infiltrate warm lidocaine into the skin, SC tissue and muscle prior to needle/catheter insertion.

2. **Short-acting anesthesia** may be required where diagnostic imaging is indicated
   a. An **opioid (Box 29.1) and a benzodiazepine (Box 29.1**) may be all that is required for very ill patients. This can be followed by careful titration of **propofol or alfaxalone** (Box 29.3) for 10–15 min of anesthesia. Both drugs are respiratory depressants and the patient should receive supplemental oxygen.
   b. The patient should be handled gently while under general anesthesia as aggressive handling results in establishment of pain, which will impact the patient when it regains consciousness.
3. **Anesthesia**
   Where **laparotomy** is required:
   a. Box 29.3 and an opioid Box 29.1, and a sedative Box 29.2, depending on the degree of compromise to the patient.
4. **Intraoperative LA – see Box 29.3 section 3.**
5. **Post-operative analgesia**
   a. Continue with **Box 29.1**, titrating to effect. Omit lidocaine IV where intercostal or epidural catheters are placed.
   b. **LA – see Box 29.3 section 3.**
   c. **NSAIA, COX-2 selective/preferential** where there are **no contraindications** (refer to Chapter 11). This will optimize analgesia and reduce opioid and/or the elimination of adjunct analgesics that may be required for moderate to severe pain. Do not administer following GI surgery.

V. The Ill Patient/Foreign Body Ingestion

Where a cause for abdominal pain is not obvious based on history, physical examination and diagnostic procedures, consider the potential for referred pain from the vertebral column or hips that could be confused with abdominal pain. Hypoadrenocorticism (Addison disease) can also be associated with cranial abdominal pain requiring analgesic (opioid) therapy.

Most patients with **moderate to severe pain** are hospitalized to manage their medical problem. An initial "loading' dose of an opioid, by titration IV over a few minutes is recommended to identify an appropriate dose and avoid potential N&V associated with excessive dosages of opioid. To reduce N&V, **fentanyl or methadone** are recommended. The effective loading dose of the opioid can then be extrapolated to establishing a continuous infusion over the dosing interval for the individual analgesic. The overall analgesic and anesthetic plan is based on the medical problem at hand, age and co-morbidities. The initial treatment, as in **Box 29.1**, is safe for all scenarios. Benzodiazepines should not be administered to patients with significant clinical and laboratory hepatic abnormalities. The addition of **ketamine**, as assessed by severity of pain, should be considered where opioids are inadequate to manage severe pain but avoided where severe compromise of hepatic function in dogs, and renal function in cats, exists, and pregnant animals. Where ileus is present, lidocaine for dogs may be of more benefit than ketamine, although both may be used for severe pain to reduce the opioid dose. Refer to Chapter 12 for guidance for the use of lidocaine in cats.

A. Surgical Management

Several medical conditions involving organs of the abdomen and pelvis require surgical management. LA blocks can be utilized (refer to Chapter 14) and will reduce post-operative pain significantly.

1. **Peritonitis, in general,** increases the level of pain associated with injury or illness requiring multi-modal analgesia, a single analgesic at the initial stage will be inadequate to control this pain and increasing an opioid dose in an attempt to manage this will predispose to N&V.

   a. The **anti-emetic maropitant (Cerenia®) – dogs and cats: 1 mg/kg SC or IV** very slowly, **Box 29.1 section 4 q24h, for up to five days** is indicated where N&V are a feature of visceral pathology/pain. Maropitant may also have analgesic properties that may facilitate a reduction in the opioid dose.

2. **Gastric dilation ± volvulus (GDV)**

   a. **Obtain IV access** immediately, commence with an appropriate loading dose of fluids, titrate opioid to effect (Box 29.1) while fluids are being administered. If the patient is anxious or aggressive, administer an opioid IM and obtain IV access as soon as possible. In the hypotensive, depressed patient, titrate the opioid as the patient responds to fluid resuscitation. Further opioid may be required to facilitate passage of an orogastric tube for gastric decompression, and where gastrocentesis is indicated. Surgery is always indicated.

   b. **Analgesia**

   N&V **must** be avoided. Administer 1 mg/kg maropitant slowly IV.

   i. **For the aggressive,** "walking" dog where IV access cannot be obtained:
   See **Chapter 22**. Remember these are large dogs and safety is important.
   - Follow with an IV opioid titrated to effect **Box 29.1 as soon as possible.**

   ii. For all others, obtain IV access immediately.
   - **Fentanyl*** 2–5 µg/kg IV, or
   - **Hydromorphone 0.05-0.1 mg/kg IV**, or
   - **Methadone 0.1–0.5 mg/kg IV** are the opioids of choice as there is minimal risk for vomiting. **Box 29.1** for guidance on administration. Fentanyl CRI can follow any of the above opioids given IM.
   - **Diazepam** 0.2-0.5 mg/kg IV, or
   - **Midazolam** 0.2-0.5 mg/kg IV to facilitate orogastric intubation.

   c. **Anesthesia**

   i. **Pre-medication:** supplemental oxygen should be delivered to the compromised patient during pre-medication and induction. Pre-medication often consists of a bolus of **fentanyl or methadone (Box 29.1)** IV followed within 30 s to 2 min with:

   ii. **Induction:**
   - **Critical patient:** a bolus of a **benzodiazepine Box 29.2**, just prior to, or with, the **propofol or alfaxalone, Box 29.3**, slowly titrated to effect will reduce the induction drug dose.
   - **For more stable and/or decompressed patients**, pre-medication and induction can occur as in Box 29.3.
   - **Intubation and inflation of the ET tube cuff** must be rapid for all patients with GDV.

   iii. **Intraoperative:** appropriate management is as critical as appropriate choice of anesthetic drugs. Check electrolytes and lactate prior to surgery and intermittently throughout the procedure. Analgesia and aesthesia protocols from Box 29.1 and Box 29.3 are appropriate. Ventilation must be supported, especially until the stomach is decompressed, but over-zealous ventilation will impede cardiac output (and thereby blood pressure) by causing collapse of the intrathoracic vena cava with subsequent decrease in preload. A higher-than-normal respiratory rate with a lower-than-normal peak inspiratory pressure (PIP) is required. A starting point could be 15–20 breaths/min with a 10, potentially down to 5, cmH_2O PIP (this is the pressure indicated on the manometer on the anesthesia machine). Expect large fluid shifts and rapid changes in cardiovascular status with derotation of the the stomach. Lidocaine and dopamine CRIs are commonly needed for treatment of arrhythmias and decreased myocardial contractility, respectively.

    d. Post-operative

    Continue with opioid of choice Box 29.1 as a CRI, reducing the dose based on patient's response. Continue support with antiarrhythmic and inotropic drugs, if necessary.

3. **Gastric FB**

    a. Analgesia

        i. As for GDV.

    b. Anesthesia for endoscopy: depending on the health status of the patient:

        i. Analgesia and anesthesia protocols as described in Box 29.1 and Box 29.3 are appropriate.

    c. Anesthesia for surgery: depending on the health status of the patient:

        i. Analgesia and anesthesia protocols in Box 29.1 and Box 29.3, or

        ii. Those described above for GDV.

    d. Post-operative: continue with an opioid in **Box 29.1** with adjustment as surgical pain subsides.

4. **Splenic torsion/neoplasia/hematoma**

    a. Analgesia

        i. Box 29.1

    b. Anesthesia: depending on the health status of the patient, analgesia and anesthesia protocols in:

        i. Box 29.1 and Box 29.3, or

        ii. Those described above for GDV.

    c. Post-operative analgesia

        i. Continue with Box 29.1 with adjustment as surgical pain subsides.

5. **Portosystemic shunt (PSS)** and hepatic encephalopathy patients.

    a. Analgesia

    Box 29.1, point 1. Hepatic function may be compromised to varying degrees requiring careful assessment of opioid requirement. Initial titration to effect as with other conditions; however, the duration of action may be longer. When establishing a CRI based on initial effective dose, monitor the patient closely to ascertain ongoing requirement, which may be lower due to slower elimination. Do **not** administer benzodiazepines. Do **not** administer ketamine, lidocaine as a CRI (local blocks can still be performed) or NSAIAs. Opioids are recommended; however, dosing intervals may be extended, the duration of which is dependent on degree of functioning liver. Careful monitoring is essential during CRI of an opioid as dosing may decrease due to slower elimination. Refer to Chapter 21 for more in-depth information.

    b. Anesthesia for hepatic disorders: depending on the health status of the patient, analgesia (see point a above) and anesthesia protocols in:

        i. Box 29.3, or

        ii. Those described above for GDV.

        The use of reversible drugs (opioids), drugs that are cleared by multiple routes (propofol) and drugs with minimal need for hepatic metabolism (inhalants) reduce dependency on the liver for recovery from anesthesia. To alleviate the chance of further hepatic compromise during anesthesia, support hepatic oxygen delivery by monitoring and supporting blood pressure and oxygenation.

    c. Post-operative analgesia:

        i. Continue with pre-operative regimen and adjust as pain subsides.

        ii. PSS post-correction frequently results in visceral pain due to redistribution of blood flow, edema, ileus and incisional pain. Due to these factors, careful assessment of dose requirement is essential. Where pain score is increasing, it is essential to assess the abdomen and bowel as ischemia may occur with excessive attenuation of the shunt.

      iii. **Ranitidine** dogs and cats 0.5 mg/kg PO, IV, IM q12h, where ileus is diagnosed, may improve comfort via its promotility function.

6. **Gallbladder distension, rupture and/or cholelithiasis** are extremely painful conditions. Where rupture has occurred, the pain of peritonitis increases the level of pain experienced. Surgical correction is required.

    a. **Analgesia**

      i. Refer to Box 29.1.

    b. **Anesthesia for surgery.** Depending on the health status of the patient:

      i. Analgesia and anesthesia protocols in Box 29.1 and Box 29.3, or

      ii. Those described above for GDV.

      iii. Utilize multi-modal analgesia.

    c. **Anesthesia for laparoscopy.** Depending on the health status of the patient:

      i. Analgesia and anesthesia protocols in Box 29.1 and Box 29.3, or as described for GDV.

      ii. May need to support ventilation since insufflation of the abdomen impairs normal breathing.

    d. **Post-operative analgesia.**

      i. Continue with pre-operative regimen.

    e. **LA** may be required for severe pain. See Box 29.3 section 3.

      i. **Interpleural** bupivacaine via a small thoracostomy tube.

      ii. **Epidural** analgesia via epidural catheter (Chapter 14) is also an excellent method of controlling severe pain and should be considered for the individual patient's needs where surgical intervention is undertaken.

7. **Bowel distension, rupture/perforation/foreign body**

Ascertain cause for **bowel distension**, if this is due to ileus alone a promotility drug is indicated; however, this is contraindicated should any obstruction be present. Refer to Chapter 4 for benefits of adjunct analgesia.

    a. **Mild to moderate pain of distension**

      i. **Analgesia**

        • **Mild pain butorphanol dogs and cats**: 0.2–0.4 mg/kg IM, IV, SC. Duration of action is 1–2 h; therefore, if there is only mild pain continue with effective dose as a 1 h IV CRI, or for mild to moderate pain.

        • **Buprenorphine** 0.02–0.04 mg/kg IV, IM q8h, while treating the underlying cause, or

        • **Buprenorphine** (1.8 mg/ml) 24 h duration product (Simbadol®, Zoetis) approved for SC injection in cats only, for up to three days. The approved dose is 0.24 mg/kg but the dose can be reduced by 25–50% in compromised patients.

    b. **Pain due to bowel rupture/perforation, intussusceptions, foreign body** (Figure 29.2) is severe, requiring immediate surgical correction of the problem.

      i. **Analgesia**

        • **Box 29.1**.

      ii. **Anesthesia**

        • **Box 29.3**, depending on the health status of the patient.

        • Analgesia and anesthesia protocols in Box 29.1 and 29.3, or those described above for GDV.

        • Arrhythmias and hypotension are common with rupture/perforation so the patient should be monitored and the anesthetist should be ready to treat with lidocaine for arrhythmias and/or dopamine for hypotension. **Lidocaine Box 29.1** is also an analgesic and enhances gut motility.

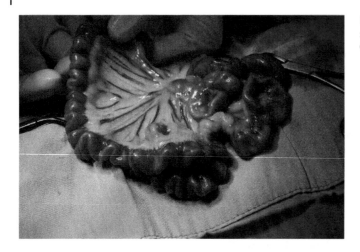

Figure 29.2 Linear FB results in severe abdominal pain. Source: Courtesy Dr Kathy Lamey.

    iii. **Local block ± epidural** ± catheter (refer to Chapter 14).
    iv. **Post-operative.**
        • Box 29.1 with adjustment based on the presence of epidural analgesia.
        • Local anesthesia – see Box 29.3 section 3.

B. Medical Management

Organomegaly frequently occurs with acute pathology and associated inflammation of the **kidney, spleen, liver and pancreas.** The fibrous capsule surrounding these organs is innervated resulting in increasing pain as the swelling occurs. Mild, moderate or severe pain can be expected. Acute kidney injury occurs frequently in veterinary medicine; however, unlike the other organs, pain is frequently overlooked as a problem. Most animals with medical pain will sit very still, cats usually at the back of the kennel, frequently urinating where they lie. When appropriate analgesia is administered, the patient becomes more animated, will move to the front of the cage to meet the caregiver and cats will use their litterboxes. Soon after, an interest in food may develop.

Where inflammation and enlargement are noted on diagnostic imaging, assume the patient is in pain. While treating the underlying condition will reduce the inflammation and pain, this will take time, and in severe situations, this takes several days or more, requiring appropriate analgesia during this period. Opioids are safe to use where kidney and liver pathologies exist. Depending on organ involvement, the duration of analgesic action may be longer; therefore, careful monitoring, to establish an increase in dosing interval or reduction in CRI dose/h may be required.

For analgesic options, refer to Box 29.1 with the exception of NSAIAs with contraindications (Chapter 11).

1. Pancreatitis

Pancreatitis is a relatively common primary problem in both dogs and cats and should be considered in patients with abdominal pain, which is usually moderate to excruciating and may be acute, acute-on-chronic or chronic. Looking at the appearance of acute, severe pancreatitis (Figure 29.3), the pain experienced by the patient can certainly be appreciated. However, overt pain may not always be exhibited, especially in cats (Figure 29.4a), but improvement is noted following analgesia (Figure 29.4b). As neural tissue within the pancreas is involved with the inflammatory process associated with pancreatitis and cancer, a neuropathic component exists resulting in severe pain (refer to Chapter 3 and Chapter 4).

Figure 29.3 Acute, severe pancreatitis at post-mortem examination.

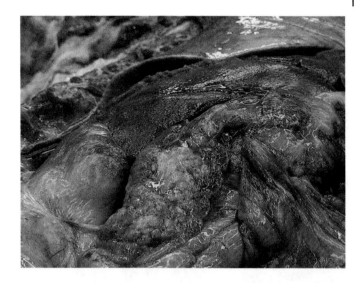

Figure 29.4a Typical position of a cat with abdominal pain. This cat has pancreatitis.

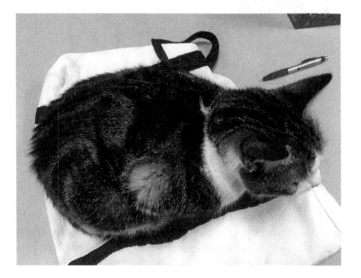

For patients with pancreatitis, the question is often raised regarding the opioid (specifically morphine) effects on sphincter tone and whether the increase in intra-common biliary ductal pressure previously reported in humans can be extrapolated to an increase in pancreatic ductal pressure in dogs. This theory has since been revoked. As the pain associated with pancreatitis results in sphincter contraction, opioid analgesics will relieve this.

a. **Analgesia**

   i. **Mild to moderate pain** may be managed with **buprenorphine (dogs: 0.01–0.02 mg/ kg; cats: 0.02–0.04 mg/kg IV q4–6h)**. Monitoring the patient will dictate whether an increase or decrease is required; however, if the higher dose is ineffective, increasing will not confer greater analgesia. It is important to assess pain accurately as a high dose of a pure mu-agonist will be required to overcome the buprenorphine mu-receptor binding. If there is doubt, treat for moderate to severe pain below.

   ii. **Moderate to severe pain**

     Slowly titrate the opioid until the patient appears comfortable, followed by a CRI. Stop titration should early evidence of nausea, panting and dysphoria appear.

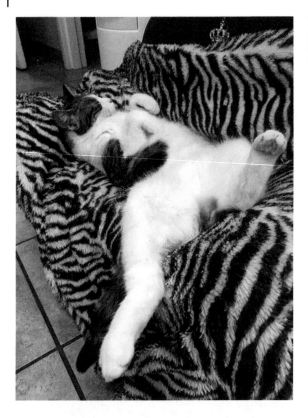

Figure 29.4b The above cat following maropitant and fentanyl analgesia for ~24 h. Fentanyl was replaced with buprenorphine OTM for discharge home.

- **Fentanyl** 2–5 µg/kg preferred due to less potential for N&V. If fentanyl not available:
- **Methadone** 0.1–0.5 mg/kg
  Refer to Box 29.1 for details on establishing a CRI
- **Maropitant** dogs 1–2 mg/kg and cats 1 mg/kg SC or very slowly **IV**, especially where large volumes are required every 24 h. However, it must be administered into an IV catheter/line where no other drugs are present due to lack of compatibility studies.

iii. **Severe pain**
  - **Box 29.1**.
  - **Local anesthesia epidural as for III above**, or
  - **Interperitoneal LA block (bupivacaine 1.5 mg/kg)**, is rarely indicated but is a useful adjunct to opioid analgesics for severe pain associated with pancreatitis.
  - Using aseptic technique prepare a 20:1 mixture of 0.5% (5 mg/mL) bupivacaine with 1 mEq/mL (8.4%) sodium bicarbonate (this would be equivalent to **0.05 mL sodium bicarbonate in 9.95 mL of bupivacaine)**, calculate a **0.3 mL/kg (=1.5 mg/kg bupivacaine) dose for dogs.**
  - **0.15 mL/kg (=0.75 mg/kg) for cats**. Note that a precipitate will form if too much sodium bicarbonate is added or it is allowed to sit for any period. Warm to body temperature and use immediately. Place a bleb of warm **lidocaine prior to catheter placement.** STRICT aseptic technique essential. Slightly elevate abdominal wall and cautiously place a **20-gauge IV catheter into the peritoneal space,** remove the needle, instil the solution via the catheter and gently rock the patient

to distribute this. If the patient still appears uncomfortable, adjust their position to facilitate re-distribution of the LA. While the addition of sodium bicarbonate results in pain reduction, indications of pain may still appear so be prepared for this.

- **Instillation** may be repeated **q6h for up to 24h**. The total dose of bupivacaine should not exceed 1.5 mg/kg q6h for dogs; 0.75 mg/kg q6h for cats.

2. **Hepatitis/hepatomegaly** result in moderate to severe pain depending on illness and duration. Hepatic function may be compromised to varying degrees requiring careful assessment of opioid requirement. Initial titration to effect as with other conditions; however, the duration of action may be longer. When establishing a CRI based on initial effective dose, monitor the patient closely to ascertain ongoing requirement, which may be lower due to slower elimination. Do **not** administer benzodiazepines unless flumazenil is available. Do **not** administer ketamine, lidocaine as a CRI (local blocks can still be performed) or NSAIAs. Opioids are recommended; however, dosing intervals may be extended, the duration of which is dependent on degree of functioning liver. Careful monitoring is essential during CRI of an opioid as dosing may decrease due to slower elimination. Refer to Chapter 21 for more in-depth information.
   a. **Analgesia**
      i. Box 29.1
         - **Fentanyl** is preferred due to duration of action and better control.

3. **Inflammatory bowel disease, colitis**
   a. **Immune-mediated inflammation**
      i. **Analgesia**
         - **Mild to moderate pain**
         - **Buprenorphine** 0.01–0.02 mg/kg IV, IM q4–6h dogs, 0.02–0.04 mg/kg IV, IM, OTM q4–6h cats, or
         - **Buprenorphine** (1.8 mg/mL) 24h duration product (Simbadol®, Zoetis) approved for SC injection in cats only. The approved dose is 0.24 mg/kg but the dose can be reduced by 25–50% in compromised patients, or
         - **Butorphanol** 0.2–0.4 mg/kg q1–2h for both cats and dogs with **mild** pain/discomfort or CRI at 0.2 mg/kg/h after the loading dose.
      ii. **Severe pain:**
         - **Box 29.1**. Anticipate requiring an increased dose of pure mu-opioid if butorphanol or buprenorphine have been administered, due to their antagonistic/partial agonist effect.
         - **Lidocaine dogs** 1–2 mg/kg loading and continued 1–2 mg/kg/h for ~12h, decrease to 1 mg/kg/h. Maximum of 24h. Refer to Chapter 12 for guidance as to use in **cats**. Lidocaine also enhances gut motility, thereby reducing ileus that may be present.
         - **Ketamine** 0.2–1.0 mg/kg. Ketamine has an anti-inflammatory action and is reported to alleviate pain during management of fulminating ulcerative colitis in a young child.
         - **Amitriptyline 1–2 mg/kg orally q12–24h for dogs, and for cats 2.5–12.5 mg/ cat orally q24h** may be beneficial in immune-mediated illness, where corticosteroids are administered but the anti-inflammatory effect cannot manage the acute pain initially. The analgesic effect is not immediate.

4. **Infection-induced inflammation (e.g. parvo enteritis)**
   a. **Analgesia**
      i. As for immune-mediated above.
      ii. No corticosteroids.

VI.   For All Patients

1. Medical massage, and osteopathic techniques of abdominal massage are also recommended where indicated (refer to Chapter 15).
2. Acupuncture utilizes viscero-somatic linkages and reflexes to influence visceral function and pain. Anecdotally, acupuncture may be very useful in GI cases in particular.

VII.   Urogenital System

Refer to Chapter 30, where these injuries and illnesses are presented.

Further Reading

Charles, H. Knowles, A. and Qasim, A. (2009) Basic and clinical aspects of gastrointestinal pain. *Pain*, 141: 191–209.

Hayes, G. M. (2017) Approach to managing the severely traumatized patient- damage control techniques for abdominal injury. In: Mathews, K. A. (ed.), *Veterinary Emergency & Critical Care Manual*, 3rd edn. LifeLearn, Guelph, Ontario, Canada.

Mathews, K. A., Singh, A. M., Boysen, S. (2017) Acute abdomen (abdominal pain). In: Mathews, K. A. (ed.), *Veterinary Emergency & Critical Care Manual*, 3rd edn. LifeLearn, Guelph, Ontario, Canada.

Self, I. (2016) Gastrointestinal, laparoscopic and liver procedures. In: Duke-Novakovski, T., deVries, M. and Seymour, C. (eds), *BSAVA Manual of Canine and Feline Anaesthesia and Analgesia*, BSAVA, Gloucester: 343–355. Refer to Chapter 4 of this book.

30

Pelvic Cavity/Abdomen, Perineum and Torso: Illness and Injuries Urogenital System and Perineum

Karol Mathews, Tamara Grubb and Andrea Steele

Refer to Chapter 29 for general aspects, physical examination and initial management of injury involving structures of the torso including injury to the viscera of the abdomen and pelvis. Many primary medical, surgical and traumatic problems associated with the pelvic cavity, but also those developing secondarily (e.g. peritonitis), are extremely painful. Blunt or penetrating injury of the abdomen, pelvis and perineum frequently results in intra-pelvic and urologic injury and subsequent inflammation resulting in both muscular and visceral pain. Detected muscular pain may be isolated to the abdominal or pelvic wall but may be a reflection of visceral pain; therefore, careful assessment is required for diagnosis. Careful monitoring of the patient with respect to increasing abdominal, pelvic or perineal pain is essential as this may be associated with urological, reproductive or gastrointestinal (GI) injury. Urethral injury results in urine leakage into the perineum and/or hind limbs resulting in severe pain from inflammation and a "compartmental-like syndrome". Assess the penis for pain, and patency, associated with a fractured os penis (Figure 30.1).

Visceral pain associated with illness is present in conditions associated with distension of hollow, muscular-walled organs (colon, urinary bladder, ureter, uterus), ischemia (commonly the bowel) and inflammation of any organ (pyelonephritis) associated with acute enlargement of solid organs resulting in stretching of the capsule. Subcapsular hematomas following injury confer similar degrees of pain. Other painful conditions are neoplasia, acute kidney injury, ureteral, cystic and urethral calculi, inflammatory bowel disease/colitis, viral enteritis, pyometra and intestinal foreign bodies. Bowel distension and hypersegmentation has the potential for intussusception. Acute intussusception is painful but with chronicity may not be as painful. Small areas of infarcted bowel may not be painful but severe vascular occlusion (volvulus or torsion) is painful. Septic or chemical peritonitis causes severe pain.

Initial management is based on the illness or injury at hand and inclusion/exclusion of pre-existing problems/co-morbidities, and when the patient was last fed. The aggressive patient, the pregnant or lactating patient and age also require special consideration; refer to individual chapters for sedative, analgesic and anesthetic details. Section I outlines details for immediate analgesia for the various scenarios given in Sections VII and VIII.

Analgesia and Anesthesia for the Ill or Injured Dog and Cat, First Edition. Karol A. Mathews, Melissa Sinclair, Andrea M. Steele and Tamara Grubb.
© 2018 John Wiley & Sons, Inc. Published 2018 by John Wiley & Sons, Inc.

I. Analgesia, Sedation and Anesthesia (General and Local)

A. Analgesia in General

Box 30.1 Analgesics

1. Opioids. **For all patients.**
   Slowly titrate the opioid IV until the patient appears comfortable, a higher dose than noted below may be required. Titration should be halted when early signs of adverse effects appear – nausea, increased respiratory rate, dysphoria. Refer to # opioid reversal for details. Where indicated, add a sedative (Box 30.2) to reduce opioid requirement and/or to reduce anxiety. Dosages for both cats and dogs are within the dose range given unless otherwise stated. Opioids in order of preference for initial administration:
   - **Fentanyl** 2–5 µg/kg, or
   - **Methadone** 0.1–0.5 mg/kg, or
   - **Oxymorphone** 0.02–0.2 mg/kg, or
   - **Hydromorphone** 0.05–0.2 mg/kg only if none of the above is available due to increased potential for vomiting, or
   - **Morphine** 0.1 – 0.5 mg/kg v. slowly IV only if none of the above is available due to increased potential for vomiting.
   - **Establish a continuous rate infusion (CRI)**
     - 1 h infusion of the effective bolus dose of fentanyl, or
     - 4 h infusion (or ¼ dose/h) of the effective bolus dose of methadone, hydromorphone oxymorphone or morphine.
   - **Fentanyl** is appropriate for pregnant, lactating, pediatric and geriatric patients. Refer to these chapters for ongoing analgesia.
   - **Opioids alone** may not be effective in cases where neuropathic pain also exists. The adverse effects of an opioid overdose can still occur in the neuropathic painful patient when the mu-receptors are saturated. Caution is required in interpretation of an increase in what appears to be painful behaviour occurring during opioid administration. The patient may be experiencing opioid-induced hyperalgesia requiring addition of a different class of analgesic (e.g. ketamine), versus a dysphoric response (refer to Chapter 8).
   # Opioid reversal with naloxone where required.
   Where excessive nausea, panting or dysphoria is noted, immediately reverse the opioid with naloxone, particularly if using a long-acting opioid. Slowly titrate until the adverse signs of the opioid subside, then stop naloxone administration. With slow titration, the primary effect of opioid analgesia will not be reversed and frequently facilitates calming. Fentanyl is quickly metabolized and it may not be necessary to reverse. Caution is required as it is easy to "over reverse" and reverse the analgesic properties. To ensure accurate dosing for the individual patient and permit slow delivery of the reversal, the following is recommended:
   Dilute naloxone (0.4 mg/mL) using:
   - 0.1 mL added to 5 mL saline (=0.008 mg/mL) for small dogs and cats, titrate IV at 0.5 mL/min
   - 0.25 mL added to 9.75 mL saline (=0.01 mg/mL), for medium to large dogs, titrate IV at 1 mL/min
   - Titrate until signs of dysphoria or nausea are reversed, usually 2–3 mLs. Repeat dosing may be required.
2. **Ketamine where pain cannot be managed with an opioid alone**, common where nerve injury, or neuropathic component, is involved. Vagolytic and anti-inflammatory action may also be of benefit. **Not suitable for pregnant or lactating patients.**
   - **Ketamine** 0.2–1 mg/kg titrated IV to effect

- **Ketamine: Establish a CRI**
  - 1 h infusion of the effective bolus dose
  - Should the patient appear overdosed at any time, stop the CRI for 30 min, or less if signs subside, and reinstitute at one-half the previous dose.
3. **Lidocaine** in dogs may be added or as the alternative to ketamine.

    Lidocaine intravenous (IV) bolus 1–2 mg/kg followed by 1–2 mg/kg/h – **dogs**, can be added to the above regimen. This dose must be calculated into the total dose when bupivacaine or lidocaine are used for local anesthesia to avoid toxicity (refer to Chapter 14). Refer to Chapter 12 for guidance for use in **cats**. The addition of lidocaine may reduce the opioid requirement; therefore, monitoring for potential opioid adverse effects must be noted on the chart and the opioid dose reduced accordingly. Lidocaine has promotility activity, and other benefits, which may be an advantage in patients presenting with abdominal emergencies should the injury/illness and high-dose opioid predispose to ileus. Nausea may develop with 9–24 h infusion. Lidocaine IV should be avoided in patients with significant hepatic pathology.
4. **Non-steroidal anti-inflammatory analgesic (NSAIA)** (Table 11.1) following physical examination, stabilization and laboratory information is received and no contraindications are identified. **Do not use in** pregnant, nursing cats or puppies and kittens less than 6 weeks of age, or when corticosteroids are prescribed. Carprofen 2 mg/kg (lean body weight) q12h for up to six days may be considered in lactating dogs (refer to Chapter 24). Consult the NSAIA package insert prior to administration to verify age as this varies with each product. Refer to Chapter 11.
5. **Maropitant may be considered where nausea and vomiting are a concern.** Dogs and cats: 1 mg/kg SC or slowly IV. Maropitant contributes to analgesia, especially in patients with GI pain, through neurokinin (NK)-1 receptor antagonism.

II. Sedatives in General

> **Box 30.2**
>
> - **Diazepam** 0.2 mg/kg IV or **midazolam** 0.2 mg/kg IV or intramuscular (IM), or
> - **Acepromazine** 0.005–0.02 mg/kg, intramuscular (IM), IV Use with caution in hypovolemic or hypotensive patients, ace-mediated vasodilation may contribute to hypotension
> - **Medetomidine** 0.1–4 µg/kg IM, IV may be considered where no co-morbidities exist
> - **Dexmedetomidine** 0.05–2 µg/kg IM, IV may be considered where no co-morbidities exist

III. Local Anesthesia (LA) Techniques

LA techniques may be required/are recommended to prevent severe pain. Careful calculation of local anesthetics administered from all techniques is required to avoid overdose. Refer to Chapter 14.

A. **Epidural analgesia via epidural catheter** is also an excellent method of controlling severe pain and should be considered for the individual patient's needs where surgical intervention is undertaken. Refer to Chapter 14 for epidural technique, for single dose and CRI.
B. Entry or exit abdominal local anesthetic line blocks are of value.
C. **Interperitoneal LA bupivacaine 2 mg/kg, dogs, 1 mg/kg; cats**, prior to abdominal closure, and for selective medical conditions.

IV. Discharge Home Analgesia

Required for injured or ill and post-surgical patients. A single, or combination, analgesic regimen is based on the individual patient's requirement.

A. **Based on the primary problem**, and successful regimen in hospital, including:
1. **Spasmolytics** (see Section VIII.A.2.a.iv).
2. **Amantadine** 3–5 mg/kg q12–24h cats and dogs (refer to Chapter 12 for details) where ketamine was required up to discharge. Amantadine should be started at the time of weaning ketamine.
3. Cyclooxygenase-2 **(COX-2) preferential/selective NSAIA** where there are no contraindications.
4. **Gabapentin** 10–20 mg/kg q8–12h cats and dogs, where a neuropathic component is present, titrate dosage up or down based on patient response/sedation.
5. **Buprenorphine** 0.02–04 mg/kg oral transmucosal (OTM) cats and small dogs (dosing problem with larger dogs), or
6. **Buprenorphine** (1.8 mg/mL) 24h duration product (Simbadol®, Zoetis) approved for SC injection in cats only, for up to three days. The approved dose is 0.24 mg/kg but the dose can be reduced by 25–50% in compromised patients.
7. **NSAIAs where no contraindications.** See Box 30.1 and Chapter 11.

V. Anesthesia in General

Box 30.3

A. Adults

1. **Pre-medication:** any of the opioids in Box 30.1 are appropriate. In very ill patients, an opioid alone may suffice. Where required, opioid dosages can be approximately doubled from those in Box 30.1 in healthy patients.
   In patients that are ill but require more calming, add a benzodiazepine from Box 30.2.
   - **Maropitant should be administered to all patients.** Maropitant, an anti-emetic, contributes to analgesia, especially in patients with GI pain, Box 30.1 section 5.
   - **Alpha$_2$ agonist** for fairly healthy/stable patients at dosages given below, which are higher than those in Box 30.2, or acepromazine, in addition to an opioid.
     - **Dexmedetomidine** 5–10 µg/kg dogs, 10–15 µg/kg cats IM (use ½ dose for IV), or
     - **Medetomidine** 10–20 µg /kg dogs, 20–30 µg /kg cats IM (use ½ dose for IV), or
     - **Acepromazine** 0.01–0.02 mg/kg dogs, 0.02–0.03 mg/kg cats IM (use ½ dose for IV).
     - If **etomidate** is utilized for induction (see point 2 below), pre-medicate with an opioid and a bolus of midazolam or diazepam (0.2 mg/kg IV of either) as etomidate without pre-medications commonly causes muscle rigidity, muscle twitching, paddling and vocalization.
2. **Induction:** any of the injectable anesthetic drugs are acceptable.
   - **Unstable/critical patients**
     - **Propofol** and alfaxalone (to effect, usually 1–3 mg/kg) are preferred as they can be titrated "to effect".
     - **Etomidate** (1–3 mg/kg; low end of dose likely sufficient) causes minimal to no cardiovascular effects and may be a good choice for unstable patients. Etomidate causes adrenocortical suppression and its use in septic patients is controversial.

- **Stable patients**
  - ○ **Propofol** (2–6 mg/kg IV) or alfaxalone (1–3 mg/kg IV), or
  - ○ **Ketamine** combined with midazolam or diazepam (1:1 ratio by volume): 0.1–0.2 ml/kg, IV to effect, or
  - ○ **Telazol** (**or Zoletil**, depending on what country you are in) 6–10 mg/kg IM or IV. Use pre-medicant sedatives to decrease the Telazol dose and to promote smooth recoveries.

  Inhalant induction should never be used whether the patient is stable or not as vomiting is highly likely in patients described in this chapter and a rapid induction with rapid intubation is necessary to assure a protected airway.

3. **Intraoperative maintenance and local blocks:**
   - Anesthesia should be maintained with low-dose inhalant (sevoflurane or isoflurane) combined with local/regional anesthetics and/or CRIs (Box 30.1).
   - An epidural with morphine ± bupivacaine is ideal (refer to Chapter 14). LA in the epidural space is ideal for analgesia but can contribute to hypotension because of vasodilation. Fluid-load the patient prior to the epidural to alleviate this potential.
   - If using CRIs or an epidural without local anesthetic, include local blockade at the incision site (Chapter 14).
   - Appropriate fluid therapy and monitoring are critical. Abdominal pain can often make breathing difficult so positive pressure ventilation (delivered by a mechanical ventilator or a person squeezing the rebreathing bag) may be necessary.
   - Should hypotension develop during anesthesia refer to Chapter 19, Section II.B.3.

B. Pediatrics

1. **Pre-medication**
   - As for adults are appropriate but the dosages may be reduced. See Chapter 25 for more specific information.
2. **Induction**
   - As for adults.
3. **Intraoperative**
   - As for adults, including local blocks.

VI. General Nursing Considerations for the Patient with Pelvic or Perineal Injury or Illness

In addition to the pharmacological management of pain, **nursing care** (Chapter 17) is very important in prevention of hospital-acquired injuries such as urine scalding and decubital ulcers, as well as discomfort associated with constipation or pain upon defecation. A **stool softener** is recommended for all injured patients to facilitate ease, and reduce discomfort, of defecation.

Patients with abdominal and pelvic pain are also frequently nauseated (as evidenced by lip smacking, drooling, exaggerated swallowing and inappetence), and may require anti-emetics. The veterinary technician/nurse (VT/N) should report this to the veterinarian to assess for potential problems and begin appropriate anti-emetic therapy. Reducing nausea will help with patient comfort.

Pelvic pain may be extreme, and can be constant or episodic (associated with moving the patient). Patients will become uncomfortable when immobile in one position for too long, and may express their discomfort by becoming restless, vocalizing, panting or shifting their limbs. Take these cues and move the patient to their other side, or into a different position. Ideally, provide a bolus of opioid prior to moving to prevent a sudden increase in pain upon changing position.

Often when changing position in a pelvic injured patient, the patient will be more comfortable if the hind limbs are left to hang for the position change, rather than trying to bundle up the hind limbs. This seems counterintuitive, but often the bending of the knees and hips will cause more discomfort than allowing them to remain extended. Just ensure when lifting that those limbs are not dragging; the patient must be lifted off the bed sufficiently to ensure this does not happen.

The VT/N should always be alert to sudden increased pain or distress in patients with pelvic injury or disease. The pain could be related to secondary nerve involvement (such as sciatic nerve entrapment), or related to feces in the rectum, which may cause additional anxiety, or pressure-related pain. If the patient needs to urinate, injury or disease in the pelvic area may make this very uncomfortable or difficult, and a urinary catheter is likely warranted. A large distended bladder will put extra pressure on the pelvis, the abdomen and associate nerves as well.

VII. Injuries

A. Pelvic Cavity/Abdomen

For penetrating injuries, refer to Chapter 29, Section IV.A.

1. **Urinary tract**

   Injury of the kidney, ureter, bladder and urethra results in urine leakage. This may not be diagnosed at immediate presentation following injury or there may be a delay in presentation should there be no external injuries and owners aren't aware that the dog or cat may have sustained a blunt injury. Close observation of all abdominal/pelvic injured patients, and assessment for potential urinary tract injury/urine leakage/hemorrhage, is required. Rarely, a ureteral tear associated with a traumatic event will lead to retroperitoneal urine leakage that may dissect to the SC tissue, which is extremely painful (trauma or calculus associated). Where there is a delay in presentation, abdominal fluid may be detected on physical examination. In addition to the pain of injury, urine results in a chemical peritonitis which is very painful. These patients must undergo diagnostic imaging to identify the source of leakage and may require laparoscopy or exploratory laparotomy for repair. Small tears in the bladder may be treated with urinary catheter placement for 7–10 days with analgesia titrated to the requirement of the individual patient where associated injuries will also be painful.

   a. **Analgesia.**
      i. **Box 30.1** initially.
      ii. NSAIA, COX-1 preferential/selective, where there are no contraindications or surgery is planned. Where anesthesia is required proceed to:
   b. **Anesthesia:** check electrolytes prior to induction.
      i. Induction. Choose protocols from **Box 30.3** based on health status.
      ii. Intraoperatively include local anesthetic blocks ± epidural (refer to Chapter 4). Analgesia should include CRIs and/or an epidural as urine is very irritating and these patients are generally very uncomfortable.
   c. **Post-operative**
      i. **Box 30.1**.
      ii. NSAIA, COX-2 preferential/selective where renal function is not compromised. It may be difficult to ascertain kidney injury when based on urea values where uroperitoneum is present as absorption of urea through the peritoneum will alter this. The IDEXX SDMA test is preferred as this assesses glomerular filtration rate. Due to the inflammation that is present, and with administration of appropriate volumes of

Figure 30.1 Degloving motor vehicle injury. An attempt to pass a urinary catheter failed. The os penis was shattered requiring a perineal urethrostomy.

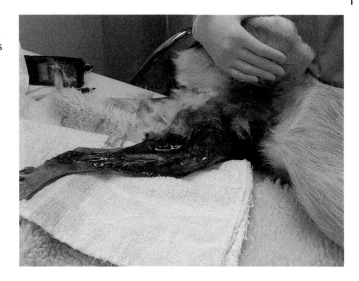

Figure 30.2 Penile hematoma secondary to trauma.

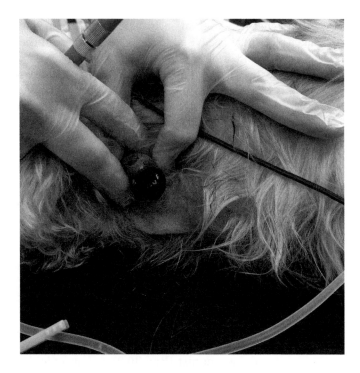

fluid, immediate post-operative NSAIA administration is indicated for 24h, and longer where no contraindications, predominantly GI at this point. The decision to administer an NSAIA is based on overall patient assessment (Chapter 11). Adjustment to opioid dosage may be required.

2. **Penis and prepuce dogs**

   Injuries include wounds caused by automobile accidents, fence jumping, mating, malicious act, dog fights, frostbite (short-legged breeds), fractures of the os penis (Figure 30.1) and paraphimosis due to trauma (Figure 30.2) and post-surgical "trauma" (Figure 30.3), to name a few. Based on the innervation and function of the penis, one can imagine the pain associated

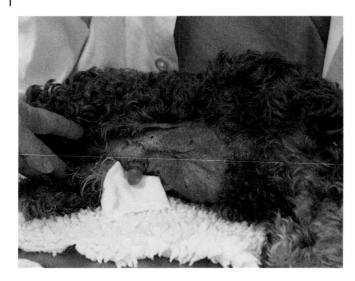

Figure 30.3 "Post-surgical traumatic" paraphimosis. In addition to nursing management, a generous application of granulated sugar applied to the penis will reduce swelling. Rinse well and apply lidocaine gel. Replace penis into prepuce.

with these injuries. Urethral obstruction may be associated with injury; therefore, urinary catheter placement is advised to assess the patency of the urethra, facilitate evacuation of urine and to avoid urine scalding.

a. **Nursing management to reduce pain** upon admission may include cold or warm compresses depending on the injury, sterile lidocaine gel applied to the penis. With paraphimosis, the VT/N must ensure the penis is retracted at all times, and/or covered in sterile lubricant to avoid desiccation. An Elizabethan collar or other deterrent should be used to avoid licking/chewing and self-mutilation.

b. Prior to **urethral catheterization**, cover the catheter tip with **sterile lidocaine gel**. Careful, atraumatic insertion, with an appropriate sized catheter to avoid establishment of urethritis, is essential. Lidocaine is recommended even if catheterization occurs under general anesthesia as the local anesthetic effect will reduce nociceptive input. When suturing of the catheter is required, topical analgesic such as sterile 2% lidocaine gel can be applied to the tip of the prepuce to reduce pain.

c. **Analgesia**

   i. **Box 30.1** initially to facilitate physical examination, assessment and urethral catheterization.

   ii. **NSAIA COX-2 preferential/selective** where no contraindications. See point A.1.c.ii above and Chapter 11.

   iii. **Gabapentin** 10–30 mg/kg q8h dog, 25 mg/kg q12h cat. Increase or decrease to effect.

   iv. **For examination and minimal treatment.** In **healthy** patients, sedation with:
   - An **alpha$_2$ agonist (Box 30.2)** and an **opioid (Box 30.1)**, the sedation can be reversed if the patient isn't going to proceed to anesthesia. If this is insufficient,
   - A dose of **propofol, alfaxalone or ketamine** (Box 30.3), the latter for healthy patients, can be added to the sedation protocol.
   - **Lidocaine 2% gel** for topical analgesia.

   v. **Epidural anesthesia:** survey radiographs should be obtained to ensure lumbosacral spine is intact prior to considering epidural anesthesia (refer to Chapter 14).

d. **General anesthesia** is required to fully assess and manage penile injuries.

   i. **Induction. Box 30.3**. The patients are generally healthy.

   ii. **Intraoperative**
   - **Epidural anesthesia** can be difficult as landmarks may be difficult to identify with lumbosacral injuries. However a sacrococcygeal epidural would work very well for

penile assessment. Skin injuries directly over the epidural injection site preclude the use of epidural analgesia (refer to Chapter 14).

- **CRIs** are an excellent choice for analgesia in these patients, and
- **Local anesthetics** can be used to desensitize the incision site and any lacerations requiring suturing (refer to Chapter 14).

  e. **Post-operative**
    i. **Box 30.1** pre-operative regimen
    ii. **Epidural LA** where indicated (refer to Chapter 14).
    iii. **COX-2** preferential/selective **NSAIA**, where there are no contraindications. See point A.1.c.ii above and Chapter 11.
    iv. **Gabapentin** 10–30 mg/kg q8h, dog; 25 mg/kg q12h, cat.

3. **Uterine injuries**

Uterine and vaginal, depending on location, injuries are rare but where suspected/present, laparotomy is indicated. Should uterine inguinal hernia be present, careful handling of tissue and nerves is essential during surgical repair. Neuropathic pain is reported in humans referable to the ilioinguinal or genitofemoral nerve distribution and is assumed to occur because of injury to the genitofemoral nerves, either at surgery or subsequently by encroachment of scar tissue (refer to Chapter 3).

  a. **Analgesia**
    i. **As for Box 30.1**
  b. **Anesthesia**
    i. **As for Box 30.3**: select the protocol based on the overall health status of the patient.
  c. **LA:** as described in **Section III**.
  d. **Post-operative**
    i. **Box 30.1, pre-operative regimen**
    ii. **NSAIA, COX 2 preferential/selective** where there are no contraindications. See point A.1.c.ii above and Chapter 11.

B. Pelvis

1. **Musculoskeletal** injuries, refer to Chapter 31. Injuries of the vertebral column, sacrum, ischium and acetabulum may involve entrapment/impingement of nerves which would be excruciatingly painful (assessed as 8–10/10) – refer to Chapter 32. The patient will be difficult to examine based on the pain elicited with any movement or handling. It will be necessary to obtain IV access as soon as possible, commence fluids and administer an opioid. Physical examination and diagnostics can be undertaken at this time. Fractures or separation of the **pubis** may be associated with penile injuries and abdominal hernia. As with any fracture, movement of the fractured pubic components results in pain, and careful handling is essential. Urinary tract injuries may be associated with any torso and pelvic trauma. With surgical repair, careful tissue/neural tissue handling is essential to avoid neuropathic pain. Neuropathic pain referable to the ilioinguinal or genitofemoral nerve distribution, potentially due to injury to the genitofemoral nerves, either at surgery or subsequently by encroachment of scar tissue, has been reported in humans (refer to Chapter 3).

  a. **Analgesia**
    i. **Box 30.1**.
    ii. **NSAIA COX-2 preferential/selective** where not contraindicated. See point A.1.c.ii above and Chapter 11.
  b. **Anesthesia**
    i. **Induction Box 30.3**. Protocols should be chosen based on the overall health status of the patient.

    ii. Otherwise, healthy but very painful animals will benefit from sedation with an **alpha₂ agonist Box 30.2, plus an opioid** at the higher dose in **Box 30.1**.

    iii. Analgesia is imperative and must include a **ketamine CRI** (see **Box 30.1, point 2**) if entrapment/impingement of nerves is likely.

    iv. **Intraoperative LA** (see Section III).

  c. **Postoperative Box 30.1**

    i. **LA** (see point A.2.d above).

    ii. **NSAIA, COX-2 preferential/selective NSAIA** where no contraindications. See point A.1.c.ii above and Chapter 11.

C. Perineum

Anatomical structures of the perineum are highly innervated with injuries resulting in severe pain (refer to Chapter 3, Section IV.A.4 and Chapter 4, Section III). Treatment of the specific injury will reduce the pain; however, initial analgesia and possible anesthesia will be required for examination. Specific nursing care procedures are essential to reduce discomfort and pain.

1. **Anus: stool softener**, such as psyllium fibre, is essential to prevent constipation and facilitate normal bowel movements. Diarrhea can cause the perianal area to be very reddened and sore. Gently shaving the area (avoiding further skin irritation), followed by hydrotherapy with warm water and application of zinc-oxide or other barrier cream several times per day. A tail wrap will help to keep the tail clean but must be removed and replaced for hydrotherapy. Ensure the patient has an Elizabethan collar to prevent licking.

2. **Vulva and perivulvar area:** urinary catheter may be required to prevent urine scalding and associated pain. Protective skin care as outlined above should be performed if area is irritated, followed by urinary catheter care to ensure the catheter is kept clean.

3. **Scrotum and testicles, dogs and cats:** a particularly sensitive area, patients will want to lick and chew when irritated, compounding the problem. An Elizabethan collar is a necessity, in addition to protective skin care. Zinc-oxide cream or other barrier cream should cool and soothe, but may need to consider a product that includes topical analgesia such as lidocaine, providing it can be used on broken skin.

4. **Feline penis and prepuce:** cats with urethral obstruction have frequently caused trauma to the penis and prepuce from licking and chewing. Urinary catheterization in these patients will cause further irritation/inflammation. Ensure that the penis fully retracts into the prepuce to avoid damage from drying. Caution with excessive amounts of 2% lidocaine jelly in cats, but small amounts may be used to provide some topical analgesia. An Elizabethan collar is a necessity.

  a. **Analgesia for all.**

    i. **As for Box 30.1.**

    ii. **Sacrococcygeal epidural (Chapter 14)** for the cat or dog where appropriate.

    iii. **NSAIA COX-2 preferential/selective,** when stable, where there are no contraindications. See Section point A.1.c.ii above and Chapter 11.

  b. **Anesthesia**

    As for Box 30.3. Select the appropriate protocol based on overall health of the patient.

  c. **Post-operative**

    i. **Box 30.1 pre-operative regimen**

    ii. **NSAIA COX-2 preferential/selective**, where there are no contraindications. See point A.1.c.ii above and Chapter 11.

VIII. Illness

A. Urologic

1. Kidney

Acute illness (e.g. pyelonephritis) and intoxications (e.g. grape) cause swelling of renal parenchyma and capsular stretch. This, in addition to inflammation, results in moderate to severe pain, the degree of which is patient illness dependent. When looking at the abscessed and swollen kidney (Figure 30.4), one can appreciate the excruciating pain the patient would experience. Grape toxicity results in parenchymal swelling and associated pain (Figure 30.5a). The degree of pain can be assessed using **gentle** palpation of the abdomen and lumbar region during the physical examination. Laboratory and diagnostic imaging findings will rule out lumbosacral pain as a potential etiology for pain. Surgery may be required for some problems (Figure 30.4). Drugs requiring renal excretion (ketamine in cats, Telazol (Zoletil®) cats, potentially dogs) should be avoided if possible or used in very low dosages if there are no other options. An opioid, fentanyl or methadone preferred due to the less chance of nausea, for moderate to severe pain. (Figure 30.5b). It is essential to titrate these opioids and stop when early signs of adverse effects occur (Box 30.1).

a. **Analgesia**
   i. **Mild to moderate pain**
      - **Buprenorphine dogs:** 0.01–0.02 mg/kg IV, IM q4–6 h, **cats:** 0.02–0.04 mg/kg IV, IM, OTM, or
      - **Butorphanol** 0.2–0.4 mg/kg q1–2 h for mild pain in **both cats and dogs** or CRI at 0.2 mg/kg/h after the loading dose.
   ii. **Moderate to severe pain**
      - **Box 30.1**. Anticipate requiring an increased dose of pure mu-opioid if butorphanol or buprenorphine have been administered, due to their antagonistic/partial agonist effect.

2. Ureter cats and dogs

Pain of ureteric origin, due to distension in calculosis, produces a generalized increase in excitability in spinal neurons. Modulation of **mild** to moderate visceral pain has been produced by administration of kappa-opioid receptor agonists such as butorphanol, which appear to dose-dependently attenuate the responses of vagal nerve afferent fibres to noxious visceral distension. This effect was not noted with mu-agonists. Both ketamine at analgesic dosages and lidocaine are also effective (see **Boxes 30.1–30.3**). Mu-agonists (**Box 30.1**) can act at central spinal or supraspinal sites to modulate visceral nociception. Definitive treatment is indicated. In the meantime, analgesia (below) is essential.

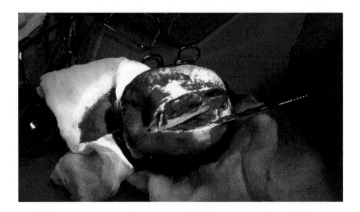

Figure 30.4 Nephrectomized kidney revealing peri-renal abscesses in a 17-month-old male neutered Border collie. *Source:* Courtesy Dr Kathy Lamey.

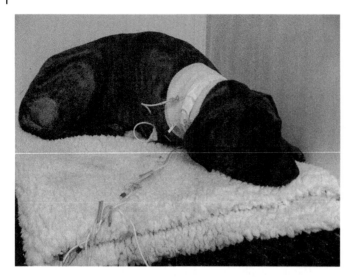

Figure 30.5a Grape toxicity resulted in kidney swelling and pain.

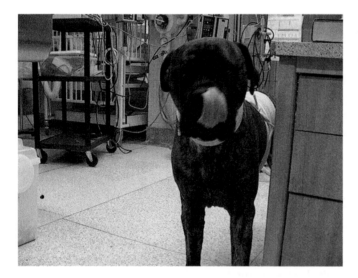

Figure 30.5b Following 24 h fentanyl administration. A gradual improvement in behaviour and appetite was noted during the 24 h period.

a. **Analgesia**
  i. **Severe pain**
      - **Box 30.1**.
      - **Ketamine** (see Box 30.1, point 2).
      - **NSAIA COX-2 preferential/selective once**, in the hydrated patient, and where no contraindications exist. See Section VII.A.1.c.ii and Chapter 11.
  ii. **Moderate to severe pain**
      - **NSAIA COX-2 preferential/selective once**, where pain is not managed with an opioid in the hydrated patient, and where no contraindications exist. An NSAIA was more effective than morphine in humans with ureteral calculosis. See Section VII.A.1.c.ii and Chapter 11.

   iii. **Mild to moderate pain:**
- **Butorphanol**, **dogs** and **cats**: 0.2–0.4 mg/kg q 1–2 h IV or CRI, or
- **Buprenorphine**, **dogs**: 0.01–0.02 mg/kg IV q4–8 h; **cats**: 0.02–0.04 mg/kg IV q4–8 h, or
- **Buprenorphine** (1.8 mg/mL) 24 h duration product (Simbadol®, Zoetis) approved for SC injection in cats only. The approved dose is 0.24 mg/kg but the dose can be reduced by 25–50% in compromised patients.
- **NSAIA COX-2 preferential/selective once**, in the hydrated patient, and where no contraindications exist. See Section VII.A.1.c.ii and Chapter 11.

   iv. **Spasmolytic drugs**: while not classified as an analgesic, the relaxation of smooth muscle reduces pain and facilitates passage of calculus. Only administer to stable patients and monitor blood pressure.
- **Dogs:**
  - **Prazosin**: 0.5–2 mg/animal (1 mg/15 kg) PO q8–12 h, or
  - **Phenoxybenzamine**: 0.25 mg/kg PO q8–12 h or 0.5 mg/kg q24h, or
  - **Tamsulosin**: 0.01 mg/kg/day
- **Cats:**
  - **Phenoxybenzamine**: 2.5 mg/cat orally q12h, or
  - **Prazosin**: 0.5 mg/cat PO q12h, or
  - **Tamsulosin**: 0.004–0.006 mg/kg PO q24h or q12h
- **Amitriptyline**: **Dogs**: 1–2 mg/kg orally q12–24h; **Cats**: 2.5 – 12.5 mg/cat orally q24h also inhibits smooth muscle contraction; however, this may take time to effect.

  b. **Anesthesia**
- i. **Box 30.3**. Choose protocols for pre-medication, induction and maintenance based on health status.
- ii. Intraoperative analgesia should include epidural morphine ± local anesthetic (see Section III).

3. **Bladder**

Cats with interstitial cystitis (FIC) suffer from bladder pain and urinary urgency. This is a very complex syndrome, involving both pathophysiologic and environmental factors, with no definitive effective treatment. These cats have reduced protection of bladder uroepithelium by lowered glycosaminoglycan (GAG) levels resulting in increased contact of urine with the primary afferent nerve terminals innervating the bladder. This subsequently results in increased bladder permeability and neurogenic inflammation (refer to Chapter 4 for further details).

  a. **Analgesia**
- i. **Box 30.1 initially** and until laboratory data is received, or if
- ii. **Mild to moderate pain**, a combination of **buprenorphine** OTM and **acepromazine** PO for 5 to 7 days, this combination of an analgesic and a tranquilizer, also decreases urethral tone and, potentially, the tranquilizer will reduce the activity of the autonomic nervous system which is useful in the initial treatment of FIC.
- iii. **Gabapentin** 10+ mg/kg q8–12h may be effective based on the neurogenic component of pain. Dose adjustment based on the individual response.
- iv. **NSAIA, COX-2 selective/preferential** in the acute stage where there are no contraindications is very effective. Bladder inflammation frequently occurs in patients with normal kidney function. Refer to package insert for contraindications.
  - **Meloxicam** (Metacam®, Boehringer-Ingelheim) 0.1 mg/kg once, q24h later, 0.05 mg/kg, then 24 h later 0.025 mg/kg for both cats and dogs.
  - **Robenicoxib** (Onsior®, Novartis) 6 mg tablet/cat q24h for up to 3 days has been effective for the very painful cat with hemorrhagic interstitial cystitis. See Section VII.A.1.c.ii and Chapter 11.

    v. **Amitriptyline** 2.5–12.5 mg/cat orally q24h has been recommended for the long-term treatment in addition to specific environmental modifications; however, the analgesic effect is not immediate; therefore, a selection from point i–iv above is used initially. If the patient is receiving amitriptyline, this should not be discontinued abruptly as this will result in the abrupt withdrawal syndrome. Amitriptyline, or other in this class, should not be prescribed for an initial episode of FIC or a flare-up of signs that occur infrequently.

4. **Bacterial cystitis** in both cats and dogs is painful, as it is in humans.
   a. **Analgesia**
      i. **NSAIA, COX-2 selective/preferential** in the acute setting may be administered for 24–48 H, where not contraindicated and IV fluids are administered, the patient must be well hydrated. This will reduce the pain of inflammation until antibiotic treatment takes effect. See Section VII.A.1.c.ii and Chapter 11.

5. **Cystic calculi** in both cats and dogs is painful
   a. **Analgesia**
     Surgical removal is recommended, refer to anesthesia below.
   b. **Anesthesia**
      i. **Box 30.3**, choose protocols for **pre-medication, induction and maintenance based on health status**.
      ii. **Intraoperative analgesia should include epidural morphine ± local anesthetic** (see Section III).
   c. **Post-operative**
      i. **Box 30.1** immediately post-operative.
      ii. **NSAIA, COX-2 selective/preferential** where not contraindicated and the patient is normally hydrated. See Section VII.A.1.c.ii and Chapter 11.

B. Reproductive System

1. **Uterine torsion**
   Ovariohysterectomy is required
   a. **Analgesia**
      i. **Obtain IV access immediately then**
      ii. **Box 30.1** during work-up.
        • **Fentanyl** 2–5 µg/kg IV, or
        • **Methadone** 0.1–0.5 mg/kg
      These are the opioids of choice as there is minimal risk for vomiting.
   b. **Anesthesia**
      i. **Box 30.3**: select the protocol based on the health status of the patient.
      ii. **Pre-medication**: supplemental oxygen should be delivered to the compromised patient during pre-medication and induction.
        • **Fentanyl** 2–5 µg/kg IV, or
        • **Methadone** 0.1–0.5 mg/kg
      These are the opioids of choice as there is minimal risk for vomiting. **Box 30.1** for guidance on administration, followed within 30 s to 2 min.
      iii. **Induction**
        • **Propofol** or **alfaxalone** slowly titrated to effect.
        • **Benzodiazepine** bolus just prior to, or with, the propofol or alfaxalone will reduce the induction drug dose.
      iv. **Intraoperative**
        • **Anesthesia and analgesia protocols** from Box 30.3. Include morphine epidural (refer to Chapter 14).

    c. **Post-operative**
       i. **Box 30.1**
      ii. **NSAIA, COX-2 preferential/selective** where no contraindications. See Section VII.A.1.c.ii and Chapter 11.

2. **Pyometra/endometritis**

Medical management, including IV fluids, is commonly used to manage patients with endometritis; however, ovariohysterectomy may be requested. Surgical management is the most common treatment for pyometra

    a. **Analgesia** for both scenarios
       i. **Box 30.1 initially.**
    b. **Anesthesia** – Depending on the health status of the patient, anesthesia and analgesia protocols in **Box 30.3** or those described above for uterine torsion.
    c. **Post-operative analgesia**
       i. Continue with **Box 30.1**.
      ii. **NSAIA COX-2 preferential/selective** when hydrated and no contraindications exist. See Section VII.A.1.c.ii and Chapter 11.

3. **Dogs: Paraphimosis, balanoposthitis, ischemic priapism, urethral obstruction**

All these conditions are very painful. Some require general anesthesia to examine and treat. Some dogs may be difficult to restrain for IV catheter placement requiring intramuscular administration of an analgesic.

    a. **Analgesia**
       i. **For the un-cooperative dog**, to allow placement of an IV catheter and initial examination:
          • **Hydromorphone** 0.05–0.1 mg/kg SC or IM, or
          • **Methadone** 0.1–0.5 mg/kg IM, and if needed select from
          • **Box 30.2**
      ii. **For co-operative patients**
          • **Box 30.1 initially**
          • **NSAIA, COX-2 preferential/selective** when hydrated and no contraindications. See Section VII.A.1.c.ii and Chapter 11.
      iii. **Spasmolytic agents**, in addition to the above, for dogs with urethral obstruction will reduce urethral spasm and associated pain and will also facilitate passage of calculi:
          • **Prazocin**: 0.5–2 mg/animal (1 mg/15 kg) PO q8–12 h, or
          • **Phenoxybenzamine**: 0.25 mg/kg PO q8–12 hr or 0.5 mg/kg q24h, or
          • **Tamsulosin**: 0.01 mg/kg/day
      iv. See Section VII and points A.2.a and b above.
    b. **Anesthesia**

    For the selected patient, and those with major injury requiring emergent surgery (Figure 30.1):
       i. **Box 30.3**. Choose protocols for pre-medication, induction and maintenance based on health status.
      ii. **Intraoperative analgesia** should include epidural morphine ± local anesthetic. Refer to Chapter 14.

C. Perineum

1. **Prolapsed rectum and perineal hernia**
    a. **Analgesia**
       i. **Box 30.1 initially** with immediate nursing care.
    b. **Nursing care for prolapsed rectum** prior to surgery (refer to Chapter 17). It is imperative that the tissues do not become dry, and frequent application of

water-based lubricant. Sterile 2% lidocaine jelly may also be used to reduce pain. Clean bedding or diaper pads should be used to keep patient clean. Gentle hydrotherapy can help to minimize irritation to mucosa and surrounding tissues. Ideally, repair should be performed as soon as possible (emergent) and carefully to avoid neural tissue injury.

  c. **Anesthesia**

    i. **Induction**
- **Box 30.3**: select protocol based on the health status of the patient.

    ii. **Intraoperative**
- An epidural injection of morphine and bupivacaine is highly recommended. Refer to Chapter 14.

    iii. **Post-operative**
- **Box 30.1**
- **NSAIA, COX-2 preferential/selective** where no contraindications. See Section VII.A.1.c.ii and Chapter 11.
- **Local anesthetic gel** where appropriate.
- **Stool softener** (psyllium fibre) to reduce straining.

2. **Perianal fistulae, anal gland abscess**

  a. **Analgesia**

    i. **Opioid Box 30.1 initially**

    ii. **Alpha$_2$ agonist** (dose in Box 30.2) for deep sedation in healthy dogs plus an **opioid** may be adequate for sedation in healthy animals requiring a thorough exam and/or minimally invasive treatment, or

  b. **General anesthesia** is frequently indicated to perform a thorough examination, and for surgical management.

    i. **Box 30.3** select an anesthesia and analgesia protocol depending on the health status of the patient. Consider epidural lumbosacral or sacrococcygeal analgesia/anesthesia where indicated (refer to Chapter 14.)

  c. **Post-operative**

    i. **Box 30.1.**

    ii. **COX-2 preferential/selective NSAIA** where there are no contraindications. See Section VII.A.1.c.ii and Chapter 11.

    iii. **Topical lidocaine** or where appropriate **lidocaine prilocaine analgesic** cream (do not use on broken skin or mucous membranes unless otherwise stated in the package insert).

3. **Testicular torsion**

Surgery is required.

  a. **Analgesia**

    i. **Box 30.1 initially.** Refer to Chapter 22 if the aggressive dog cannot be managed using Box 30.1.

  b. **Anesthesia**

    i. **Box 30.3**. Select anesthesia and analgesia protocols based on the health status of the patient. Include a morphine epidural.

  c. **Post-operative**

    i. **Box 30.1.**

    ii. **NSAIA, COX-2 preferential/selective NSAIA** where there are no contraindications. See Section VII.A.1.c.ii and Chapter 11.

4. **Feline urethral obstruction**

  a. **Analgesia**

    i. **Box 30.1.**

b. **General anesthesia:** electrolytes (particularly potassium) and hydration status should be assessed and corrected prior to anesthesia. Hyperkalemia contributes to patient mortality. Anesthesia techniques are highly variable depending on status of the cat at presentation, which can range from fairly healthy but extremely painful to completely obtunded and near death. Regardless of which category the cat is in, analgesia is crucial. Obstructions are easier to relieve if pain from the muscle spasm at the site of the obstruction is alleviated. Analgesia is commonly provided using systemically administered opioids, epidurally administered local anesthetics (sacrococcygeal, Chapter 14) and by intra-urethrally administered lidocaine gel (which is placed on the urinary catheter).

   i. **For obtunded patients:**
- An opioid in Box 30.1 alone, (fentanyl is preferred) or with a muscle relaxant or spasmolytic below, may be all that is needed to facilitate removal of calculus
- **Lidocaine gel** on the urinary catheter ±
- **Sacrococcygeal epidural** (Chapter 14).
- The patient can then be allowed to **recover and stabilize** prior to general anesthesia for removal of cystic calculi should they be present.
- Administer **supplemental oxygen** and keep the patient warm during the procedure.

   ii. **For more stable patients**
- select a protocol in Box 30.3.

c. **Sacrococcygeal epidural (Chapter 14)** recommended for all, where no contraindications.

d. **Post-procedure if not yet administered**

   i. **Box 30.1**.

   ii. **Spasmolytic**
- **Phenoxybenzamine** 2.5 mg/cat orally q12h or
- **Prazocin** 0.5 mg/cat PO q12h or
- **Tamsulosin** 0.004–0.006 mg/kg PO q24h or q12h.

   iii. **Amitriptyline dogs:** 1–2 mg/kg orally q12–24h; **cats** 2.5–12.5 mg/cat orally q24h inhibits smooth muscle contraction; however, this may take time to effect.

   iv. **COX-2 preferential/selective NSAIA**, where no contraindications, for difficult to manage pain. See Section VII.A.1.c.ii and Chapter 11.

5. **Uterine and vaginal prolapse/uterine inguinal hernia**

a. **Nursing recommendations to reduce injury and pain upon admission.** It is imperative that the tissues do not become dry, and frequent application of water-based lubricant. Sterile 2% lidocaine jelly may also be used to reduce pain. Clean bedding or diaper pads should be used to keep patient clean. Gentle hydrotherapy can help to minimize irritation to mucosa and surrounding tissues. Ideally, repair should be performed as soon as possible.

b. **Ovariohysterectomy** is required for uterine prolapse and uterine inguinal hernia. Injury to pudendal and ilioinguinal nerves during surgical correction will potentially result in chronic neuropathic pain; therefore, caution is required to avoid any handling or suture injury.

c. **Analgesia**

   i. **Box 30.1**.

d. **General anesthesia**

   i. **Box 30.3**: select anesthesia and analgesia protocols based on the health status of the patient.

   ii. **Epidural anesthesia:** epidural injection of morphine + bupivacaine in the lumbosacral space is highly recommended (Chapter 14).

   iii. **Sacrococcygeal epidural (Chapter 14) recommended** where appropriate, e.g. vulvar problems.

Further Reading

Chapter 4 of this book.

Brisson, B. and Gartley, C. (2017) Chapter 96. In: Mathews, K. A. (ed.), *Veterinary Emergency & Critical Care Manual*, 3rd edn. LifeLearn, Guelph, Ontario, Canada.

Gartley, C. and Brisson, B. (2017) Chapter 97. In: Mathews, K. A. (ed.), *Veterinary Emergency & Critical Care Manual*, 3rd edn. LifeLearn, Guelph, Ontario, Canada.

Gartley, C., Defarges, A. and Bichot, S. (2017) Chapter 98. In: Mathews, K. A. (ed.), *Veterinary Emergency & Critical Care Manual*, 3rd edn. LifeLearn, Guelph, Ontario, Canada.

31

Musculoskeletal Injuries and Illness

Karol Mathews, Melissa Sinclair, Andrea Steele and Tamara Grubb

Musculoskeletal pain in dogs and cats may be of traumatic origin or associated with a medical illness. Careful questioning of the owner regarding details of the current painful condition when not traumatic will aid with diagnosis. Following a traumatic event, obtain a detailed history regarding details of the incident as, in addition to the obvious, it may be associated with occult injuries to other areas of the body. A pathological fracture often occurs with minimal trauma, and occasionally there may be no precipitating event. These fractures are extremely painful due to ongoing inflammation and hypersensitivity induced by the neoplastic process, requiring a multi-modal analgesic regimen immediately. It is important to ascertain whether the patient has any co-morbidities or is receiving any medications. This is especially important when selecting analgesics or preparing for general anesthesia. Suggested analgesia and sedation, for all patients, is presented in Section I for scenarios discussed in Section V and VII; however, based on the individual case presentations, there may be additional information given to that in Section I.

I. Analgesia and Sedation

A. Analgesia

Box 31.1 Analgesia in general

1. **Opioids**
   Slowly titrate the opioid IV until the cat or dog appears comfortable. Higher dosages may be required. Titration should be halted when early signs of adverse effects appear (nausea, increased respiratory rate, dysphoria). Refer to # opioid reversal where required. Opioid dosages for both cats and dogs are within the dose range given below unless otherwise stated. Opioids in order of preference for initial administration:
   - **Fentanyl** 2–5 µg/kg, or
   - **Methadone** 0.1–0.5 mg/kg, or
   - **Oxymorphone** or **hydromorphone** 0.02–0.1 mg/kg, or
   - **Morphine** 0.1–0.5 mg/kg only if none of the above is available. If the patient is cardiovascularly unstable, blood pressure monitoring recommended during titration over a minimum of 5 min titration (refer to morphine Chapter 10).

(Continued)

Analgesia and Anesthesia for the Ill or Injured Dog and Cat, First Edition. Karol A. Mathews, Melissa Sinclair, Andrea M. Steele and Tamara Grubb.
© 2018 John Wiley & Sons, Inc. Published 2018 by John Wiley & Sons, Inc.

Box 31.1 (Continued)

- **Establish a continuous rate infusion (CRI):**
  - 1 h infusion of the effective bolus dose of fentanyl, or
  - 4 h infusion (or ¼/h) of the effective bolus dose of methadone, hydromorphone oxymorphone or morphine.
- **Where sedation is indicated** to reduce opioid requirement initially or to offer sedation in the anxious patient. See Box 31.2.
- **Opioids alone** may not be effective in cases where neuropathic pain also exists. The adverse effects of an opioid overdose can still occur in the neuropathic painful patient when the mu-receptors are saturated. Caution is required in interpretation of an increase in what appears to be painful behaviour occurring during opioid administration. The patient may be experiencing opioid-induced hyperalgesia requiring addition of a different class of analgesic (e.g. ketamine), versus a dysphoric response (refer to Chapter 8).

  # Opioid reversal with naloxone where required.
  Where excessive nausea, panting or dysphoria is noted, immediately reverse the opioid with naloxone, particularly if using a long-acting opioid. Slowly titrate until the adverse signs of the opioid subside then stop naloxone administration. With slow titration, the primary effect of opioid analgesia will not be reversed and frequently facilitates calming. Fentanyl is quickly metabolized and it may not be necessary to reverse; caution is required as it is easy to "over reverse" and reverse the analgesic properties. To ensure accurate dosing for the individual patient and permit slow delivery of the reversal, the following is recommended:
  Dilute naloxone (0.4 mg/mL) using
- 0.1 mL added to 5 mL saline (=0.008 mg/mL) for small **dogs** and **cats**, titrate IV at 0.5 mL/min
- 0.25 mL added to 9.75 mL saline (=0.01 mg/mL), titrate at up to 1 mL/min
- Titrate until signs of dysphoria or nausea are reversed, usually 2–3 mLs. Repeat dosing may be required.

2. **Ketamine where pain cannot be managed with an opioid alone**, common with nerve entrapment, bacterial myositis/fasciitis or severe crush injury:
   - **Ketamine** 0.2–1 mg/kg titrated to effect
   - **Establish a CRI:**
     - 1 h infusion of the effective bolus dose.

3. **Lidocaine. Dogs:** IV bolus 1–2 mg/kg followed by 1–2 mg/kg/h (refer to Chapter 12 for information in **cats**) can be added to the above regimen where pain is difficult to manage or a reduction in opioid dosing is required. This dose must be calculated into the total dose when bupivacaine or lidocaine is used for local anesthesia to avoid toxicity (refer to Chapter 14). The addition of lidocaine may reduce the opioid or ketamine requirement; therefore, potential opioid adverse effects and level of sedation must be noted on the chart and the opioid or ketamine dose reduced accordingly. Nausea may develop with > 18–24 h infusion.

4. **Non-steroidal anti-inflammatory analgesics (NSAIAs) for the stable patient.** Cyclooxygenase-2 (COX-2) preferential/selective NSAIA (dosing Table 11.1), in addition to the opioid above, may be administered parenterally when all concerns for ongoing hemorrhage and hypovolemia (e.g. occult abdominal hemorrhage, kidney injury) or other contraindications (e.g. renal insufficiency, coagulopathy, major crush injuries resulting in rhabdomyolysis) have been ruled out. Do not use in pregnant, lactating (refer to Chapter 24) animals or puppies and kittens less than six weeks of age. Consult the NSAIA package insert prior to administration to verify age as this varies with each product.

5. **Gabapentin 10 mg/kg q8h dogs, 10 mg/kg q2h for cats** for severe injuries and where neuropathic pain is suspected, increase or decrease according to response. Where NSAIAs are contraindicated, gabapentin may be beneficial. Commence as soon as possible.
6. **Amantadine 3–5 mg/kg PO q12–24 h in dogs and cats** should be commenced 12 h prior to discontinuing the ketamine if assessed as necessary, especially where a neuropathic component to the injury occurred/exists. This dosing may also be prescribed for cats but it is necessary to compound in chicken flavour oil due to the reputed terrible taste of amantadine.

B. Sedatives

Box 31.2 Sedatives

- **Diazepam** 0.2 mg/kg IV or **midazolam** 0.2 mg/kg IV or IM, or
- **Acepromazine** 0.005–0.02 mg/kg, intramuscularly (IM), IV. Use with caution in hypovolemic or hypotensive patients, acepromazine-mediated vasodilation may contribute to hypotension.
- **Medetomidine** 0.1–4 µg/kg IM, IV may be considered where no cardiac co-morbidities exist. Refer to Chapter 9.
- **Dexmedetomidine** 0.05–2 µg/kg IM, IV may be considered where no cardiac co-morbidities exist.

II. Injury

A. Analgesia for the Injured Patient

1. For the aggressive patient refer to Chapter 22.
2. **Initially**, a mu-agonist opioid (Box 31.1) should be administered and titrated to effect, whilst determining the patient's cardiovascular and volume status.
3. **Pediatric patients** may only require approximately half the adult dose to start with (refer to Chapter 25).
4. **Essential, obtain intravenous (IV) access** and commence fluid therapy, the rate dependent on blood loss, or use at a maintenance rate, prior to opioid titration.

B. Anesthesia for the Injured Patient

Following initial stabilization and opioid administration, general anesthesia is required to assess and manage deep and large wounds and wounds associated with open fractures. While definitive fracture repair should not occur at this time, wound debridement of gross contaminants is essential to prevent infection and subsequent bacteremia. To safely anesthetize these patients, they must be stabilized in advance so that the negative cardiovascular effects of the injectable and inhalant anesthetics are minimized. A minimum of half the fluid deficit should be corrected prior to anesthetic induction in emergency situations. Patients should be stabilized as much as possible with fluid therapy and blood products, where appropriate, prior to anesthesia. However, some patients may require surgery to control hemorrhage despite being hypovolemic. In these cases, acepromazine and alpha$_2$ agonists should **not** be administered. Sedated and or depressed patients may allow placement of monitoring equipment (indirect blood pressure, pulse-oximetry on the toe or ear and ECG pads/clips), which will be beneficial during the induction phase and transfer to inhalant anesthesia.

1. **Stable and Unstable Patients**

Box 31.3 Anesthetic Regimens

a. **Pre-medication with an opioid**
    - **Fentanyl** 2–5 μg/kg, or
    - **Methadone** 0.1–0.5 mg/kg, or
    - **Oxymorphone** or **hydromorphone** 0.02–0.1 mg/kg, or
    - **Morphine** 0.1–0.5 mg/kg (refer to Chapter 10) with or without:
        - **Midazolam:** 0.1–0.5 mg/kg, IM or IV, or
        - **Acepromazine:** 0.01–0.03 mg/kg, IM or IV.
b. **Induction for stable patients**
    - **Propofol** 2–6 mg/kg, IV to effect, or
    - **Alfaxalone** 1–3 mg/kg, IV to effect, or
    - **Ketamine with midazolam or diazepam** (1:1): 0.1–0.2 mL/kg, IV to effect.
    - **Etomidate** (1–3 mg/kg): pre-medication with an opioid and a bolus of midazolam or diazepam (0.2 mg/kg IV of either) should be utilized as etomidate without pre-medications, which commonly causes muscle rigidity, muscle twitching, paddling and vocalization. Etomidate also causes adrenocortical suppression of endogenous cortisol release and its use in septic patients is controversial.
c. **Induction for unstable patients**
    - **Pre-oxygenate** prior to induction.
    - **Induction** utilizing injectable anesthesia is preferred. Mask induction with isoflurane or sevoflurane is not recommended due to the excitement phase during induction, which is deleterious in sick patients. In addition, sick animals may get too deep very quickly with inhalational induction due to a reduced cardiac output in compromised patients. Preferred induction techniques are:
    - **Opioid/benzodiazepine combinations (diazepam or midazolam)** (see Box 31.1 and Box 31.2) should be considered in the extremely **compromised patient** where fluid resuscitation and ideal stabilization are not possible.
    - Topical lidocaine spray should be used 30 s prior to endotracheal intubation attempts with this protocol in both cats and dogs.
    - If the opioid/benzodiazepine is not sufficient for intubation, induction can be accomplished with very careful titration to effect of **alfaxalone** or **propofol** (as in point b above). High-end doses of these drugs must be avoided in unstable patients. If benzodiazepines were not used as pre-medicants, addition of midazolam (0.1–0.5 mg/kg, IV) or diazepam (0.1–0.4 mg/kg, IV) may be beneficial and should be administered after the initial dose of alfaxalone or propofol, or
    - **Ketamine/diazepam or midazolam** (as in point b above), or
    - **Etomidate** (as in point b above).
d. **Maintenance**
    - Anesthesia is generally maintained using an inhalant anesthetic, but if inhalant maintenance is not an option, a CRI of propofol at 0.1–0.4 mg/kg/min can be utilized.
    - Both the inhalant and the propofol dose should be maintained as low as possible to decrease the negative dose-dependent impact on the cardiovascular and respiratory systems. Additional administration of an **opioid** as a bolus or infusion will decrease the amount of maintenance drug required. IV **lidocaine** boluses of 2 mg/kg every 60–90 min or infusions (50–120 μg/kg/min) may also be beneficial in **dogs** to minimize maintenance drug dosages and/or treat ventricular arrhythmias associated with myocardial contusions

> (see below). Doses higher than 50 µg/kg/min may be used under general anesthesia with titration down towards the recovery phase. **For cats** refer to Chapter 12, Section II.A for further information and use.
> - Should hypotension develop under anesthesia refer to Chapter 19, Section II.B.3.

2. Anesthesia for Patients with Lung Contusions

With a traumatic injury, intra-alveolar, interstitial and inter-alveolar hemorrhage occurs, resulting in lung contusions. Secondary inflammatory edema occurs which collapses pulmonary capillaries further. Lung contusions will usually worsen within the first 24–36 h and may be missed on initial physical and radiographic examination. Radiographs may not demonstrate the presence of contusions until 4–6 h after the injury. Resolution of pulmonary contusions typically begins within 3–7 days depending on the case.

a. **Medical management of contusions** includes oxygen and analgesics to reduce the pain of normal ventilation. Diuretics may be indicated when pulmonary edema is present. Ideally, surgery should be delayed until the degree of lung contusions can be assessed and treated, and have begun to resolve.

b. **Pre-medication** with an opioid and pre-oxygenation prior to induction is recommended (refer to Box 31.3).

c. **Induction** (Box 31.3).

d. **Under anesthesia, attention to ventilation**, to avoid excessive airway pressures, is essential during assisted or mechanical ventilation. Peak inspiratory pressures (PIP) should remain at < 10 cmH$_2$0, hence lower tidal volumes and higher frequency rates are preferred to prevent further alveolar injury. Manual sighing (PIP ≥ 20 cmH$_2$O) of the patient during anesthesia is not recommended.

3. Anesthesia for Patients with Myocardial Contusions

a. **Ventricular dysrhythmias** (premature ventricular contractions and ventricular tachycardia) frequently occur within 12–24 h post-trauma in patients with myocardial contusions, which are refractory to all drug treatment in many patients. Ideally, anesthesia would be delayed for 1–3 days to allow healing; however, this, and eradication of ventricular tachycardia, is rarely possible. The aim is to reduce the number of ineffective premature ventricular contractions and to lower the overall heart rate to approximately < 150 in small dogs; 120 in larger dogs, > 30 kg; < 220 in cats. This will enable adequate filling of the ventricles and improved cardiac output to allow the animal to further handle the cardiovascular depressive effects of the general anesthetic. It also lowers the excitability of ventricular myocytes, which is important as all anesthetics have a certain level of arrhythmogenicity. To treat the ventricular dysrhythmias administer **lidocaine boluses** for the **cat** 0.25–1 mg/kg (over 5 min); for the **dog** 2 mg/kg (over 30 s) initially. This can be repeated if no effect is seen within 2 min. A maximum of four doses total may be given within a 10–15 min period. **In cats**, if lidocaine responsive, establish a CRI of 10–20 µg/kg/min, **for dogs** infusions at 30–50 (rarely 60–120 µg/kg/min). Although less commonly available in practice, thiobarbiturates and halothane **must be avoided**.

b. **Pre-medication with a neuroleptoanalgesic (opioid + sedative)** combination **(Box 31.3)** followed by pre-induction oxygenation. The decision to administer acepromazine in these patients should be made on a case-by-case basis related to their personality and pre-operative status.

c. **Anesthetic induction:** ECG and blood pressure monitoring is recommended during the induction period and maintenance of anesthesia for all patients.
  i. **For the unstable emergent patient** where delay to allow myocardial healing and resolution of arrhythmias prior to anesthesia is not possible, commence **lidocaine treatment** (see point a above). The anti-arrhythmic regimen successfully controlling the arrhythmia should be continued in patients where further delay for total resolution is not possible. Induction options listed in **Box 31.3**.
  ii. For the **stable trauma patients**, the anesthetic regimen should be tailored to the patient's co-morbidities, and options are listed in **Box 31.3**.
  iii. **Monitoring** of HR, ECG rhythm, RR, SPO_2, indirect arterial blood pressure (oscillometric or Doppler) and temperature should be performed as a minimum standard during even short anesthetics of trauma cases.
d. **Intraoperative** maintenance with inhalant anesthesia (isoflurane or sevoflurane) for procedure of > 20 min is recommended. **TIVA (total intravenous anesthesia) with propofol (refer to Box 31.3)** may be used for short-term wound lavage or bandage changes, however, endotracheal intubation and oxygen supplementation is recommended [1]. Should hypotension develop during anesthesia refer to Chapter 19, Section II.B.3.

4. Epidural/Local and Regional Anesthesia Details in Chapter 14

Local and regional techniques should be administered when possible to supplement systemic analgesics. In small animals, placement of the majority of nerve blocks, infusion catheters or epidurals will require heavy sedation or general anesthesia.

a. **Contraindications** for local blocks: avoid areas if there is a significant wound or evidence of infection over the anatomical area where the local block would need to be performed.
b. **Wound diffusion catheters** may be used and have the benefit of repeated bolus administration of the local anesthetic into painful wounds. These catheters are placed into the operative site at the end of debridement or surgery with the fenestrations on the distal end of the catheter placed into the wound (Refer to Chapter 14).
c. The **specifics of local anesthetic agents**, aseptic and individual technique, equipment required, and anatomy are outlined in Chapter 14.
  i. **Local techniques** to consider for musculoskeletal pain or fractures of the **thoracic limb** are:
    - Cervical paravertebral nerve block (humerus and below)
    - Brachial plexus nerve block (elbow, antebrachium, distal limb)
    - IV regional anesthesia (distal limb structures below tourniquet).
  ii. **Local techniques** to consider for musculoskeletal pain or fractures of the **pelvic limb** are:
    - Lumbosacral epidural
    - Sacrococcygeal epidural (tail, anus, peri-anal areas)
    - Femoral nerve block (mid-distal femur, medial aspect of the femorotibial joint capsule and skin of the dorsomedial tarsus and first digit)
    - Sciatic nerve block (tarsus and hock)
    - Femoral and sciatic nerve blocked together to achieve anesthesia of the pelvic limb
    - IV regional anesthesia of the distal limb (wounds, toe amputation lacerations).

5. Post-Procedural Analgesia

Continue with the pre-operative regimen (Box 31.1), with the addition of:

a. **NSAIA, COX-2 preferential/selective** (Box 31.1 and Chapter 11 where no contraindications exist).

b. **Ketamine** should be added/continued if needed (Box 31.1), and

c. **Gabapentin** continued, or added if neural tissue is involved in the traumatic incident or during surgical management.

d. The opioid and ketamine should be weaned off slowly in preparation for discharge home. Revert to previous dose should the patient appear painful after reduction. Where ketamine is required for continuing analgesia, replace with:

e. **Amantadine** 3–5 mg/kg PO q24h for dogs, may be beneficial in cats (refer to Chapter 12), commenced as ketamine is weaned down.

f. **Integrative/rehabilitation techniques** (Chapter 15) should be considered where appropriate.

6. **Analgesia and Anesthesia for Daily Wound Management**

a. **Ongoing analgesic regimen established.**

b. **Supplemental sedation** with low doses of propofol 0.5–1 mg/kg, IV or ketamine 0.2–1 mg/kg, IV (this is also suggested where ketamine is part of the multi-modal therapy) may be sufficient for minor control when the patient's pain is adequately managed.

c. **Supplemental oxygen** should be available with pulse-oximetry as a minimum.

d. **When general anesthesia is required** for wound management, endotracheal intubation, oxygen supplementation and further monitoring are necessary:

   i. **Propofol 2–6 mg/kg, IV or alfaxalone 1–3 mg/kg, IV** titrated to effect. Patients may be maintained with repeated IV boluses of **propofol** (0.5–1 mg/kg) or **alfaxalone** (0.3–0.5 mg/kg) as indicated with depth assessment for short procedures, or a CRI can be used (refer to Maintenance in Box 31.1), or

   ii. **Ketamine:** benzodiazepine, see Box 31.3.

7. **Analgesia and Anesthesia for Definitive Fracture Repair**

As the patient's health status is stable at this point and an appropriate regimen and level of analgesia has been reached, the anesthetic protocol should be tailored to the individual needs of the animal. Once the patient is alert and stabilized, the opioid/benzodiazepine regimen is unlikely to work alone.

a. **Anesthesia**
   i. See Box 31.3.

b. **Post-operative analgesia** as required in Box 31.1.

8. **Discharge Analgesia Plan for All Injuries**

Box 31.4 Discharge Analgesia Plan for All Injuries

It is anticipated that pain will resolve as the underlying condition improves; therefore, owners must be aware of the requirement for dose reduction. The following is suggested based on injury, degree of pain and requirement whilst in hospital.

- **Integrative/rehabilitation techniques (Chapter 15)** should be considered where appropriate.
- **NSAIA** (Table 11.1) where not contraindicated. The selected drug should be continued at home for a period of time based on the individual injury, and reduced gradually to avoid recurrence of pain. Where pain recurs, return to the dose immediately prior to dose reduction. Refer to Chapter 11.

(Continued)

Box 31.4 (Continued)

- **Fentanyl transdermal patch**, where continuing opioid treatment is required in addition to the NSAIA or where NSAIA is contraindicated or where pain is moderate to severe. The duration for onset and efficacy is unpredictable due to poor epidermal penetration. Size guidelines below can assist with patch selection.
  - Cats 12.5–25 µg/h patch
  - Small dogs (<10 kg) 25 µg/h patch
  - Medium dogs (10–20 kg) 50 µg/h patch
  - Large dogs (20–30 kg) 75 µg/h patch
  - Giant dogs (>30 kg) 100 µg/h patch
- **Buprenorphine** 0.02–0.05 mg/kg, oral transmucosal (refer to Chapter 10) for mild to moderate pain where continuing opioid treatment is required in addition to the NSAIA or where NSAIA is contraindicated, cats and dogs < 10 kg.
- **Buprenorphine** (1.8 mg/ml) 24 h duration product (Simbadol®, Zoetis) approved for subcutaneous injection in cats only. The approved dose is 0.24 mg/kg, but the dose can be reduced by 25–50% in compromised patients.
- **Gabapentin** 10 mg/kg q8h–12 h dogs and cats, increase or decrease (anecdotal range is 3–40 mg/kg q12h–6 daily)as determined by hospital stay and requirements at home.
- **Amantadine** 3–5 mg/kg PO q24h as determined by hospital stay. Dogs and cats.
- **Do not stop analgesia abruptly** unless adverse effects noted with NSAIAs (refer to Chapter 11). The following is a suggested **weaning programme**:
  - **Buprenorphine:** miss the following scheduled dose and reduce ongoing dose by half. Should pain recur at any time, return to previous dose.
  - **Gabapentin:** wean gradually by eliminating the q8h schedule and resume with q12h. After one week, reduce dose by one-half, or to manageable pill size if not liquid. Continue with weaning based on patient's response. Should pain recur at any point, return to previous effective dose/schedule.
  - **Amantadine:** as for gabapentin.
  - **Fentanyl transdermal patch:** instruct owner to return for assessment and patch removal/reduction/replacement as required.

C. **Injury-Associated Musculoskeletal Pain**

1. Patients with **deep wounds and fractures** will require analgesia, frequently multi-modal; however, initially, the drug and dose chosen will be determined by the overall stability of the patient in addition to the severity and location of the orthopedic and soft tissue injury (especially if accompanied by injuries to genitalia, head and oral cavity, which tend to have a higher degree of pain sensitivity). In addition to potential nerve involvement and movement of fracture segments, skeletal injury also generates a high level of pain due to expansive hemorrhage in a tight periosteal and endosteal environment. **External coaptation of a fractured limb** (see point 5 below) should be applied as soon as possible as this will reduce "movement pain" significantly until definitive repair. Very few, if any, analgesics can stop incident pain produced by movement of fractured bones. Appropriate analgesia is also required to facilitate diagnostic and therapeutic intervention.

2. Traumatic injury also results in muscle pain. Even if lacerations and fractures are not identified, muscular pain can be present. This results from a direct blow to the muscle resulting in contusions, hemorrhage or hematomas, and may compromise neural

structures or result in muscle necrosis, all with varying degrees of pain. This may result in compartmental syndrome, which is excruciatingly painful. Evidence of hemorrhage may be visualized as bruising, but if severe, blood may seep through the skin. Delayed-onset muscular pain is common in people and usually starts several hours following the injury. Muscle contusions are painful and activity should be reduced but not ceased, unless there is a fracture present. Following fracture management, an effective analgesic plan (see Box 31.1) is essential to facilitate movement and physiotherapy to avoid disuse atrophy (refer to Chapter 15). Pain also induces dystrophies (hypotrophy) within hours of injury, not initiated by impaired movement, another important reason to manage the pain as soon as possible. Pain, especially affecting the joints, alters the forces on the limb, and gait, potentially adding to injury. Following surgical procedures, movements that place tension on incisions, flexion and extension of limbs and joints, muscle spasms, all contribute to the painful experience.

3. **To reduce swelling** and further discomfort, local ice pack therapy for the first 24 h; thereafter, heat application, with gentle stretching of injured muscles, may be of benefit for injuries to musculotendinous structures. (refer to Chapter 15 for details).

4. Patients with extreme crush injuries are very painful; however, if on the rare occasion they don't exhibit the expected level of pain initially, this may be due to neuropraxia, the lack of swelling at the time of presentation and massive release of endorphins. This reduced level of pain may mask development of a compartmental syndrome that, within hours or a day, will ultimately cause severe, potentially neuropathic, pain. Ongoing monitoring is essential while anticipating worsening pain. Refer to Chapter 3 for prevention and management of neuropathic pain. Where extensive rhabdomyolysis is noted acute kidney injury may occur; therefore, an NSAIA should not be administered and fluid therapy should be instituted. Acetaminophen is not contraindicated in dogs in these situations; however, when used alone, the analgesia is inadequate.

5. **Limb fractures**
   a. **Analgesia (Box 31.1)** an opioid initially with addition of another analgesic class as required.
   b. **Temporary external coaptation.**
   In addition to **Box 31.1**, external coaptation is considered an essential component of the pain management protocol and should be performed as soon as possible after admission. (Refer to [2] or other appropriate text for guidance as caution and skill are required with the application of coaptation devices to avoid iatrogenic injury and discomfort.) To reduce further injury and pain due to movement, temporary stabilization of closed fractures and luxation distal to the elbow in the forelimb and distal to the stifle in the hind limb is recommended. External coaptation is limited to these areas as the joint proximal and distal to the fracture must be immobilized, and is contraindicated where this is not possible. A reinforced soft padded bandage (modified Robert-Jones) provides good support and facilitates ambulation. Commercial plastic or metal spoon splints, or custom-made splints of fibreglass casting tape, are typically used for bandage reinforcement. This support can be placed on the palmar (thoracic limb), plantar (pelvic limb) or lateral aspect of the limb. Where joint immobilization above and below the fracture or luxation is not possible (e.g. fractures of the humerus, and elbow luxation), a Spica splint that extends over the shoulder and withers region, to achieve stable external coaptation, should be applied. Monitoring should include observations for distal limb swelling, bandage/splint slippage, strike through and ensuring bandage/splint is clean and dry at all times to avoid complications. Should the patient become more painful, assessment of these devices is essential.

III. Medical-Associated Musculoskeletal Pain

Panosteitis, hypertrophic osteodystrophy (HOD), immune-mediated polyarthritis, osteomyelitis and cancer of muscle and bone are very painful. Neoplasia of the central nervous system frequently results in pain distant to the lesion which may manifest as lameness or hyperalgesia and allodynia resulting in vocalization, which is noted by the client. Malignant peripheral nerve sheath tumours (MPNSTs), previously called schwannomas or neurofibromas, are a primary cause of chronic **neurogenic lameness** in dogs and cats. Where a source for limb pain and lameness cannot be identified in either the thoracic or the pelvic limbs, an MPNST should also be considered (refer to Chapter 3 for diagnostic and therapeutic suggestions as these are extensive). Rhabdomyolysis (see **Box 31.1**, point 4). All conditions require a thorough work-up to confirm the diagnosis and direct the owner to specific therapy.

A. Analgesia for Conditions with Definitive Treatment

It is essential to confirm a diagnosis of atraumatic musculoskeletal pathology as the resolution of pain is dependent on eradication of the underlying cause. The following are clinical conditions where a thorough physical examination, and appropriate diagnostic imaging and laboratory testing of aspirates (e.g. cytology C&S and other specific tests), may be performed to confirm a diagnosis.

1. **Osteosarcoma and other tumours of bone and digits**, tumours (sarcoma) of muscles and nerve sheath, require specific therapy with various treatment options. Surgical treatment to remove the tumour offers definitive treatment and elimination of pain. Where limb dysfunction occurs, potentially due to both motor and sensory dysfunction (hyperesthesia or hypoesthesia), and amputation is the suggested treatment, it is essential that the primary lesion also be removed. This may require a hemilaminectomy should the tumour extend into, or beyond, the proximal nerve roots. Leaving the tumour will continue to cause chronic pain, and result in an extremely poor quality of life. Management should be discussed with an oncologist.
   a. **Analgesia**
      i. In the interim if the patient is admitted for evaluation, administer analgesics as recommended for **injury (Box 31.1)**.
      ii. Refer to Chapter 12 for guidelines on lidocaine use in cats. Refer to Chapter 3 for further treatment details.
   b. **Discharge analgesia plan**
      i. As in **Section II.B.8**. Do not stop any analgesic abruptly, weaning over a minimum two-week period or longer. Should pain be noted, return to the previous dose. If there are any adverse effects identified with a particular analgesic, begin weaning that drug first.
      ii. **Bisphosphonate 1–2 mg/kg** IV infusion once/month to palliate bone pain of osteosarcoma if surgery is declined; however, the analgesic efficacy may not be better than placebo.
      iii. **Oxycodone** may be used as a terminal analgesic should surgical treatment be declined. Strict federal regulations must be observed when prescribed.
2. **Immune-mediated polyarthritis** requires corticosteroid therapy, and potentially other immunosuppressive medication, to treat the underlying problem; therefore, NSAIAs should not be administered. Corticosteroids here will be analgesic as a reduction in inflammation occurs.
   a. **Analgesia**
      i. Refer to Box 31.1 above and prescribe as needed.

B. Myositis, Fasciitis

These conditions are excruciatingly painful (Figure 31.1 and 31.2). With early onset, the degree of pain experienced is far greater than the visible lesion would indicate (Figure 31.2); therefore, a high level of suspicion, careful examination and aspirates of the painful area are essential for diagnosis. Plan for immediate surgical management.

1. **Analgesia**
   a. **Box 31.1**. A multi-modal analgesic regimen is required. Initial management with an opioid followed with an NSAIA and ketamine while collecting diagnostic confirmation (based on cytology/Gram stain/submit for C&S) and making arrangements for immediate surgical management. Do not wait for culture results prior to surgical management.
2. **Anesthesia**
   Emergency surgical management, and appropriate empirical antibiotic therapy (based on cytology), is required to prevent the lesion from rapidly progressing, which ultimately will assist in controlling the excruciating pain.
   a. **Box 31.3**.
   b. **Epidural** where indicated (Chapter 14). It is imperative that there are no signs of infection, swelling or gas in the region where the needle is to be placed, and strict attention to technique and asepsis is followed.
   c. **Local anesthetic** blocks where indicated (Chapter 14).
   d. **Intraoperative** maintenance with inhalant anesthesia (isoflurane or sevoflurane) for procedure > 20 min is recommended. TIVA with propofol or alfaxalone (refer to Box 31.3) may be used for short-term wound lavage or bandage changes; however, endotracheal intubation and oxygen supplementation are recommended.

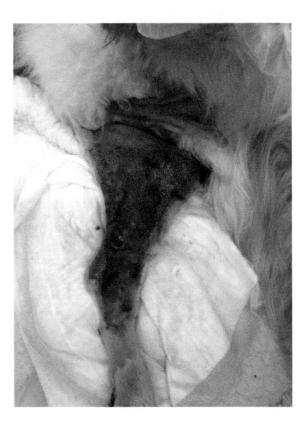

Figure 31.1 *Streptococcal* fasciitis. A 72 h history of lameness with the extent of the integumentary lesion appearing over a 6 h period. *Source:* [3]. Reproduced with permission of John Wiley & Sons

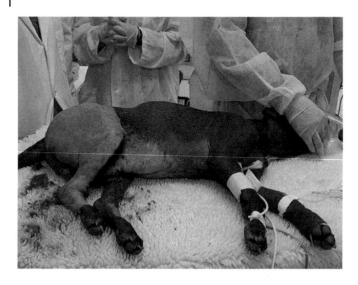

Figure 31.2 A 5-month-old puppy with three-day history of hind limb lameness. Extent of swelling noted here occurred within a one-day period.

3. **Post-operative analgesia**
   a. Due to the extensive inflammation and surgical debridement, severe pain continues for a minimum of 2–3 days requiring continuation of the multi-modal regimen established pre-operatively.
   b. **Box 31.1** select as indicated.
   c. **Weaning off analgesics** should occur slowly, planning to remove ketamine first, followed by the opioid in preparation for discharge home on the NSAIA.
   d. **Wound management:** see Section to II.B.6.

C. Osteomyelitis

As for myositis/fasciitis (see point B above); however, the pain may be moderate to severe but rarely excruciating unless neural tissue is involved.

1. **Analgesic**
   a. Refer to **Box 31.1**.
   b. **NSAIA** where not contraindicated.
   c. Appropriate **antibiotic** to resolve the lesion and associated pain.

D. Thromboembolic (Ischemic Conditions)

These conditions present as acute lameness in either thoracic or pelvic limbs, most commonly in the pelvic limbs of cats. This is excruciatingly painful requiring immediate analgesia to facilitate complete examination and diagnostic imaging.

1. **Analgesia**
   a. Refer to Box 31.1.
   b. If only mild to moderate pain is accurately identified, a lower dose of the **mu-opioid** is recommended, or
      i. **Butorphanol** for mild pain/discomfort 0.2–0.4 mg/kg q2–4 h, or to effect, or
      ii. **Buprenorphine** for mild to moderate pain 0.01–0.02 mg/kg IV, IM, 0.02 mg/kg OTM q4–8 h. A higher dose may be required.
   c. Do not administer an NSAIA in combination with definitive medical therapy.

E. Analgesia for Conditions with No Definitive Therapy

1. **Diabetic neuropathy** may occur in well-controlled diabetics. In addition to motor dysfunction, a sensory neuropathy and radiculopathy may also manifest. Refer to Chapter 3 for diagnosis.
   a. **Analgesia**
      i. **Refer to Box 31.1** select based on requirement.
2. **Polyradiculoneuritis** is most commonly associated with motor and ventral nerve root, and ventral horn motor dysfunction; however, dorsal nerve root and dorsal root ganglial inflammation can result in hyperesthesia with touch and manipulation. As the patient cannot withdraw from the stimulus, pain experience is amplified. **Observing facial expression during examination to identify pain is essential.** Attempts at vocalization may also occur; however, as paralysis of the larynx may be present this will be weak. It is important for the caregiver to be cognizant of this when treating these patients. Treatment is supportive.
   a. **Analgesia**
      i. Prepare an analgesic plan for neuropathic pain as in **Box 31.1**, and refer to Chapter 3 for further details, especially in the first several days of the disease.
      ii. **NSAIA** should be included in the analgesic plan as corticosteroids are of no benefit and so should not be administered.
   b. **Nursing care** (Chapter 17) is the most important aspect of care for these patients.
   c. **Physiotherapy**, a recommended management for these dogs, can be extremely uncomfortable. It is important for the caregiver to be cognizant of this when treating these patients and to consider adding some form of pain management, especially in the first several days of the disease.
3. **Phantom limb** pain clinical signs, other than those occurring in nerve entrapment, may be chewing at the stump, intermittent unprovoked crying or "jumping up or away", indicating lancinating pain due to ectopic firing. Where a neuroma at the amputation site is identified, this should be surgically removed.
   a. **Analgesia** as in Box 31.1 and refer to Chapter 3.
4. **Panosteitis** has no specific therapy and usually resolves over a few weeks. In the interim:
   a. **Analgesic** choice is an NSAIA (Table 11.1, Chapter 11) due to the anti-inflammatory affect; corticosteroids are not recommended.
5. **Hypertrophic osteodystrophy (HOD)** also has no specific therapy.
   a. **Analgesia**
      i. **Most patients respond well to NSAIAs**, the maximum recommended dose should be used initially (Table 11.1, Chapter 11).
      ii. **NSAIA-refractory HOD** tends to occur in Weimaraners, Irish setters and Great Danes but have responded well to high-dose, short-term, corticosteroid therapy. However, infectious disease must be ruled out and radiographic and clinical findings must be consistent with HOD alone.
      iii. **A five-day washout period** after NSAIA use is required prior to a corticosteroid regimen below. A **fentanyl patch** (questionable individual efficacy) or **buprenorphine** is recommended during this period for some relief (Box 31.4).
         • The following regimen has been used successfully:
            o **Prednisone** 0.75 mg/kg, lean body weight PO q12h for 4–5 days, extending to no more than seven days. If signs persist, discontinue. Where prednisone is responsive, gradually wean off over a four- to five-week period, reducing the total daily dose by one-half each week, then administer 5 mg of prednisone every other day for an additional 1–2 weeks.

- In all cases, also administer 3 V Caps (or Derm Caps®) and either Glyco-Flex or Multi-source **Glucosamine**.
- **Supportive care** should be provided as needed.
- **Oral antibiotics**, usually Clavamox, Amoxicillin or Clindamycin for 3–4 weeks are co-administered.
- **Antacids** (famotidine or ranitidine) are also co-administered.
- **Caution:** dogs should not be exposed to possible contagious disease, and owners should be advised not to take their dogs to dog shows, dogs parks, etc.

References

1. Matthews, N. S., Brown, R. M., Barling, K. S., *et al.* (2004) Repetitive propofol administration in dogs and cats. *J Am Anim Hosp Assoc*, 40(4): 255–260.
2. Gibson, T. (2017) Emergency fracture management. In: Mathews, K. A. (ed.), *Veterinary Emergency & Critical Care Manual*, 3rd edn. LifeLearn, Guelph, Ontario, Canada.
3. Aronson, L. R. (2016) *Small Animal Surgical Emergencies*. Wiley-Blackwell, Chichester.

Further Reading

Abeles, V., Harrus, S., Angles J. M., *et al.* (1999) Hypertrophic osteodystrophy in six Weimaraner puppies associated with systemic signs. *Vet Rec*, 145(5): 130–134.

Andress, J. L., Day, T. K. and Day, D. (1995) The effects of consecutive day propofol anesthesia on feline red blood cells. *Vet Surg*, 24(3): 277–282.

Boston, S. (2017) Musculoskeletal neoplasia and limb-sparing surgery. Spencer, A. and Johnston and Tobias, K. M. (eds), *Veterinary Small Animal Surgery*. Saunders-Elsevier, St Louis, MO: 1159–1177.

Jagodzinski, N., Weerasinghe, C. and Porter, K. (2010) Crush injuries and crush syndrome: A review: Part 1: A systemic injury. *Trauma*, 12 (2): 69–88.

Mathews, K. A. (2017) Fasciitis/myositis. In: Mathews, K. A. (ed.), *Veterinary Emergency & Critical Care Manual*, 3rd edn. LifeLearn, Guelph, Ontario, Canada.

Swaim, S. E., Renberg, W. C. and Shike, K. M. (2011) *Small Animal Bandaging, Casting, and Splinting Techniques*. Wiley-Blackwell, Chichester.

32

Vertebral Column (Vertebrae and Spinal Cord)

Karol Mathews, Tamara Grubb and Andrea Steele

The vertebral column, from the first cervical to the last coccygeal vertebrae, may become injured during any traumatic injury and should always be considered in a trauma patient to avoid further injury and exacerbating pain. As an acute intervertebral disc (IVD) herniation/ embolus injures the spinal cord to some degree, and may present as a traumatic incident, approach to diagnosis and management will be presented as an injury. Non-traumatic conditions include IVD disease, disco/osteomyelitis and neoplasia. These conditions always result in moderate to severe pain, and many involve the dorsal horn and peripheral nerves, which can be excruciatingly painful. Myelinated fibres of spinal cord blood vessels in dogs may function in sensory innervation. It may be that innervation of blood vessels shares pathways with nerves supplying other structures in the bony vertebral canal and also play role in pain in this area.

Initial restraint must be well planned and carefully carried out; the specifics of this are presented for each scenario. Refer to Chapter 27 for initial management, placement and nursing care for patients with neck injury. Information contained in Sections I–V is referred to when managing the scenarios in Sections VI and VII.

I. Analgesia

For all injured patients.

Box 32.1 Analgesia in general
1. **Opioids** Initially, a mu-agonist opioid should be administered and titrated to effect, whilst determining the patient's cardiovascular and volume status. Pediatric patients may only require approximately half the adult dose to start with (refer to Chapter 25). Obtain intravenous (IV) access and commence fluid therapy at maintenance rate or as warranted due to blood loss prior to, or during, opioid titration.   **Slowly titrate the opioid IV** until the cat or dog appears comfortable. Higher dosages may be required. Titration should be halted when early signs of adverse effects appear – nausea,

(Continued)

Analgesia and Anesthesia for the Ill or Injured Dog and Cat, First Edition. Karol A. Mathews, Melissa Sinclair, Andrea M. Steele and Tamara Grubb.
© 2018 John Wiley & Sons, Inc. Published 2018 by John Wiley & Sons, Inc.

Box 32.1 (Continued)

increased respiratory rate, dysphoria. **Note # below**. Dosages for both cats and dogs are within the dose range given unless otherwise stated. Opioids in order of preference for initial administration:

- **Fentanyl** 2–5 μg/kg, or
- **Methadone** 0.1–0.5 mg/kg, or
- **Oxymorphone or hydromorphone** 0.05–0.2 mg/kg, or
- **Morphine** 0.1–0.5 mg/kg only if none of the above is available. If the patient is cardiovascularly unstable, blood pressure monitoring is recommended during titration over a minimum of 5 min titration (refer to Chapter 10).
- **Establish a CRI**
  - ○ 1 h infusion of the effective bolus dose of fentanyl, or
  - ○ 4 h infusion (or ¼/h) of the effective bolus dose of methadone, hydromorphone oxymorphone or morphine.

 # Opioid reversal with naloxone where required.

Where excessive nausea, panting or dysphoria is noted, immediately reverse the opioid with naloxone, particularly if using a long-acting opioid. Slowly titrate until the adverse signs of the opioid subside then stop naloxone administration. With slow titration, the primary effect of opioid analgesia will not be reversed and frequently facilitates calming. Fentanyl is quickly metabolized and it may not be necessary to reverse; caution is required as it is easy to "over reverse" and reverse the analgesic properties. To ensure accurate dosing for the individual patient and permit slow delivery of the reversal, the following is recommended:

- **Dilute naloxone** (0.4 mg/mL) using
  - ○ 0.1 mL added to 5 mL saline (=0.008 mg/mL) for small **dogs** and **cats**, titrate IV at 0.5 mL/min
  - ○ 0.25 mL added to 9.75 mL saline (=0.01 mg/mL), titrate at up to 1 mL/min
  - ○ Titrate until signs of dysphoria or nausea are reversed, usually 2–3 mLs. Repeat dosing may be required.
- **Opioids alone** may not be effective in cases where neuropathic, or other severe, pain also exists. The adverse effects of an opioid overdose can still occur in these painful patients when the mu-receptors are saturated. It is essential to titrate the opioid slowly and stop when **very** subtle signs of an increased respiratory rate, nausea, dysphoria or worsening of the signs of pain appear. The dose received at this point may be used to calculate the continuous rate infusion (CRI) for continuing care. Caution is required in interpretation of what appears to be painful behaviour occurring during opioid administration. The patient may be experiencing opioid-induced hyperalgesia where the opioid is causing more pain, requiring the addition of a different class of analgesic, versus a dysphoric response (refer to Chapter 8). Should further analgesia be required based on circumstances, especially where neuropathic pain or opioid-induced hyperalgesia is suspected, add ketamine.

2. **Ketamine where pain cannot be managed with an opioid alone**, common with nerve entrapment, bacterial myositis/fasciitis or severe crush injury:
   a. **Ketamine** 0.2–1 mg/kg titrated to effect.
   b. **Establish a CRI:**
      i. 1 h infusion of the effective bolus dose.
      ii. Ketamine's additive benefit is bronchodilation. However, ketamine should be used with caution as it stimulates the sympathetic nervous system and may exacerbate some arrhythmias.
      iii. Ketamine may be considered in patients with underlying cardiac disease (refer to Chapter 19 for details), but should be avoided where severe hepatic (dogs), severe kidney (cats), compromise is present. Lidocaine may also be considered.

3. **Lidocaine** IV bolus 1–2 mg/kg followed by 1–2 mg/kg/h – **dogs** (refer to Chapter 12 for guidance in **cats**) can be added to the above regimen where pain is difficult to manage or a reduction in the opioid dose is required. This dose must be calculated into the total dose when bupivacaine or lidocaine is used for local anesthesia to avoid toxicity (refer to Chapter 14). The addition of lidocaine may reduce the opioid or ketamine requirement; therefore, monitoring for potential opioid adverse effects and level of sedation must be noted on the chart and the opioid or ketamine dose reduced accordingly. Nausea may develop with 9–24 h infusion.

4. **Non-steroidal anti-inflammatory analgesic** (see Table 11.1, Chapter 11) where indicated following physical examination, stabilization and laboratory information is received and no contraindications are identified. **Do not use** in pregnant or nursing cats or puppies and kittens less than 6 weeks of age (consult package insert as age differs with each non-steroidal anti-inflammatory analgesic (NSAIA)), or when corticosteroids are prescribed. Carprofen 2 mg/kg (lean body weight) q12h for up to six days may be considered in lactating dogs (refer to Chapter 24). Consult the NSAIA package insert prior to administration to verify age as this varies with each product.

II. Sedatives

Box 32.2

Where indicated to assist with restraint or alleviate anxiety

- **Diazepam** 0.2 mg/kg IV or **midazolam** 0.2 mg/kg IV or intramuscularly (IM), or
- **Acepromazine** 0.005– 0.02 mg/kg, IM, IV. Use with caution in hypovolemic or hypotensive patients; acepromazine-mediated vasodilation may contribute to hypotension.
- **Medetomidine** 0.1–4 µg/kg IM, IV may be considered where no co-morbidities exist (refer to Chapter 9).
- **Dexmedetomidine** 0.05–2 µg/kg IM, IV may be considered where no co-morbidities exist (refer to Chapter 9).

III. Post-Assessment and Discharge Analgesia and Management

1. Previous recommendations for high-dose methylprednisolone sodium succinate have proven to be associated with increased morbidity without improvement in the neurologic outcome. Therefore, **the use of corticosteroids is not considered routine**; however, the individual situation may indicate specific corticosteroid therapy.

   a. Where surgery is recommended but is not an option, for the most profoundly neurologic dogs, **dexamethasone at 0.1 mg/kg IV once**, followed by **prednisone starting at 1 mg/kg**, tapering the dose over the following 10–14 days. This treatment is based on an anti-inflammatory effect aiming to reduce vasogenic edema.

2. **Non-steroidal anti-inflammatory analgesics for the stable patient.** In addition to the opioid in Box 32.1, a cyclooxygenase-2 (COX-2) preferential or COX-2 selective NSAIA (see Table 11.1, Chapter 11) may be administered parenterally when all concerns for ongoing hemorrhage and hypovolemia (e.g. occult abdominal hemorrhage, kidney injury) or other contraindications (e.g. renal insufficiency, coagulopathy, major crush injuries resulting in rhabdomyolysis) have been ruled out (refer to Chapter 11). NSAIAs may be the at-home analgesic of choice.

    a. **Do not prescribe** if corticosteroids have/will be administered.

    b. **Do not use in** pregnant or nursing cats or puppies and kittens less than 6 weeks of age, or when corticosteroids are prescribed. **Carprofen** 2 mg/kg (lean body weight) q12h for up to six days may be considered in lactating dogs (refer to Chapter 24). Consult the NSAIA package insert prior to administration to verify age as this varies with each product.

3. **Gabapentin 10 mg/kg q8–12 h dogs and cats** commence as soon as possible. Increase or decrease the dose based on response: decrease with heavy sedation; increase where little to no effect. Gabapentin may be combined with an NSAIA.

4. **Amantadine 3–5 mg/kg PO q12–24 h** should be commenced 12 h prior to discontinuing ketamine if assessed as necessary, especially as a neuropathic component to the injury/illness exists. This dosing may also be prescribed for cats, but it is necessary to compound in chicken-flavour oil due to the terrible taste of amantadine. Can be used in combination with an NSAIA.

5. **Buprenorphine**, selected patients: OTM 0.02–0.04 mg/kg cats or dogs < 10 kg (volume limited) or cats **buprenorphine** (1.8 mg/ml) 24 h duration product (Simbadol®, Zoetis) approved for subcutaneous (SC) injection in cats only. The approved dose is 0.24 mg/kg but this can be reduced by 25–50% in compromised patients.

    a. **Do not stop analgesia abruptly** unless adverse effects noted with NSAIAs (refer to Chapter 11). The following is a suggested **weaning programme**.

        i. **Buprenorphine** – miss the following scheduled dose and reduce ongoing dose by half. Should pain recur at any time, return to previous dose.

        ii. **Gabapentin** – wean gradually by eliminating the q8h schedule and resume with q12h. After one week, reduce dose by one-half or to manageable pill size if not liquid. Continue with weaning based on patient's response. Should pain recur at any point, return to previous effective dose/schedule.

        iii. **Amantadine** – as for gabapentin.

        iv. **Fentanyl transdermal patch** – instruct owner to return for assessment and patch removal/reduction/replacement as required.

6. **Instructions for owners**

    a. **Rest** for four weeks minimum for IVD herniation but up to eight weeks for vertebral column trauma. Outside only on leash ± sling support for urination/defecation.

    b. Bladder care, wound care, changing positions, adequate padding, massage, stretching/range of motion, practice standing/walking (i.e. neurologic rehabilitation; refer to Chapter 15) are all very important for successful recovery of all patients.

IV. Anesthesia

Most anesthetic protocols are acceptable and focus should be on management rather than drugs. Management includes stabilization and **very** careful handling of the injured area. Anesthesia-induced relaxation of the muscles that may be tensed to protect the injured area and inattentive handling of the patient during positioning for intubation, movement on/off gurneys, positioning for imaging/procedures, etc., **can worsen the patient's pain and may even exacerbate the injury**. Management also includes pain management as these patients are generally very painful. Anesthesia can be difficult to maintain at an appropriate plane if pain is not addressed. The goal should be to be very aggressive with pain management so that the patient actually wakes up more comfortable.

Box 32.3

---

1. **Hemodynamically Stable**
   - **Pre-medication** with an opioid plus a sedative for most patients. Dosages for drugs administered for pre-medication are typically higher than those administered for calming/analgesia in the ICU (Box 32.1 and Box 32.2) as more sedation and more analgesia are generally necessary prior to surgery. Use the low end of the dose range for IV administration and/or in mildly compromised patients (see dosages for unstable patients in point 3 below).
   - **Anesthesia pre-medication dosages of opioids:**
     - **Methadone** 0.3–0.5 mg/kg (dogs and cats), or
     - **Oxymorphone** 0.1–0.2 mg/kg (dogs), 0.05–0.1 mg/kg (cats), or
     - **Hydromorphone** 0.1–0.2 mg/kg (dogs), 0.1 mg/kg (cats), or
     - **Morphine** IM **only** 0.3–0.5 mg/kg (dogs), 0.1–0.3 mg/kg (cats)
   - **Anesthesia pre-medication dosages of sedatives:**
     - **Diazepam** 0.2 mg/kg IV or midazolam 0.2 mg/kg IV or IM, or
     - **Acepromazine** 0.01– 0.03 mg/kg, IM, IV, or
     - **Medetomidine** 2–6 µg/kg IV or 10–20 µg/kg IM (dogs), 4–10 µg/kg IV or 15–30 µg/kg IM (cats), or
     - **Dexmedetomidine** 1–3 µg/kg IV or 5–10 µg/kg IM (dogs), 2–5 µg/kg IV or 8–15 µg/kg IM (cats)
   - **Induction**
     - **Propofol** 2–6 mg/kg, IV to effect, or
     - **Alfaxalone** 1–3 mg/kg, IV to effect, or
     - **Ketamine with midazolam or diazepam** (1:1): 0.1–0.2 mL/kg, IV to effect (in this case, do not use a benzodiazepine as a pre-medicant)
     - **Etomidate** (1–3 mg/kg).
   - **Intraoperative maintenance** with inhalant anesthesia (isoflurane or sevoflurane) for procedure > 20 min is recommended. Boluses of propofol or alfaxalone (see Section VII.A.3.b.iii) may be used for short-term wound lavage or bandage changes; however, endotracheal intubation and oxygen supplementation is recommended.
   - Should hypotension develop under anesthesia refer to Chapter 19, Section II.B.3.
2. **Mild to Moderate Hemodynamic Compromise**
   - **Pre-medication** with an opioid plus a sedative for most patients. Drug dosages are lower than those used for healthy patients and are in the range of the dosages presented in Box 32.1 and Box 32.2.
     - Administer an **opioid** from Box 32.1.
     - The opioid may provide adequate sedation. If not, add a **sedative** from Box 32.2.
   - **Induction:** same drugs as in Section IV.1 but **carefully titrate the dose to effect**, expect to use the low end of the dose range.
   - **Intraoperative maintenance:** same drugs as those listed for hemodynamically stable patients with the goal to use the lowest drug dosages possible. **Carefully titrate the dose to effect; expect to use the low end of the dose range.**
3. **Hemodynamically Unstable Patients**
   For these patients, all drug dosages are low. Uptake of the drug is slow so administer the dose and give it time to reach the brain – this can take 2–3 times longer than in healthy patients. **Patients must be stabilized as much as possible prior to anesthesia.**

(Continued)

Box 32.3 (Continued)

- **Pre-medication**
  - **Choose an opioid from Box 32.1**
    - **Fentanyl and methadone** are preferred if vomiting is contraindicated. In these instances, also consider administration of **maropitant**.
    - All drugs should be administered IV through a pre-placed catheter and the patient should be continuously monitored as exaggerated responses to the drugs can occur.
    - If more sedation/calming is needed, add a **benzodiazepine** from Box 32.2. Occasionally, other sedatives may be appropriate and those are discussed with specific scenarios throughout the chapter.
- **Induction**
  - The drugs described for pre-medication often provide adequate sedation to allow intubation in unstable patients. If these drugs alone are used for intubation, **topical lidocaine spray on the larynx** is recommended with this induction technique.
  - If more drug is needed, any of the injectable drugs listed in Section IV.1 are acceptable but they should be **slowly** titrated **to effect**.
  - **Etomidate** (1–3 mg/kg) causes minimal to no cardiovascular effects and may be a good choice for unstable patients. **Pre-medication** with an opioid and a bolus of midazolam or diazepam (0.2 mg/kg IV of either) should be utilized as etomidate without pre-medications commonly causes muscle rigidity, muscle twitching, paddling and vocalization. Etomidate also causes adrenocortical suppression and its use in septic patients is controversial.
- **Intraoperative maintenance** with an infusion of fentanyl (or other potent opioid) and minimal use of inhalant is generally effective and safer than reliance on higher dosages of inhalant in patients with profound cardiovascular dysfunction. The inhalant may drastically contribute to hypotension while the opioid will have minimal to no adverse cardiovascular effects.

V. Nursing Care

Patients with spinal cord and vertebral injury or disease can exhibit myriad pain levels, in addition to frustration and anxiety. Paresis, for example, can be extremely frustrating for many patients, and a patient often becomes stuck in a position that can be very distressing (Figure 32.1). Many patients with hind limb paresis and loss of motor control are unable to urinate, and often suffer from an "overflow bladder" or dribbling as the bladder reaches capacity. This, too, can be distressing for the patient. This anxiety and frustration can compound the pain level and pain scoring of a patient and should be taken into consideration.

Before offering anti-anxiolytic medications, consider the source of the anxiety.

1. **First**, consider pain level and provide appropriate analgesia.
2. **Next**, if a patient is in an uncomfortable position, try to aid them in lying down, and prop limbs or head into a comfortable position. In some cases a small dose of an anti-anxiolytic or sedative may be necessary to facilitate this movement and have the patient relax. Many patients will settle immediately once in a comfortable position.
3. **Palpate the bladder**, and if a urinary catheter is not in place, express the bladder to relieve the dribbling. If the patient is difficult to express, and has a large bladder, ask the veterinarian if a urinary catheter can be placed. This is important as any degree of fullness is uncomfortable but may result in bladder pathology.

Figure 32.1 French bulldog in a typical posture of IVD herniation. Note the dribbling of urine.

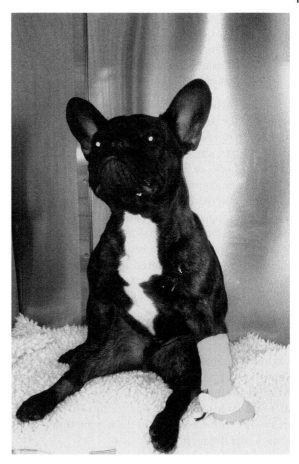

4. **Offer water**, via raised bowl, or by syringe if necessary, as many patients are unable to lower their head to drink from a water bowl.

5. **Feeding** can be carefully offered as well for patients that are not NPO (nothing per os), ensuring that they are in a raised position.

6. **For patients that are completely recumbent**, as often seen in high cervical lesions, **change sides** at set intervals as the patient starts to become restless, but not during sleep.

7. **Ensure that the skin** is monitored closely for urine and/or fecal scalding, irritation over any bony prominences which may be the beginning of ulcer formation or any other issues. Skin irritations must be addressed immediately.

8. **Ensure that respirations** are monitored closely, as respiratory paralysis and/or aspiration can be a concern in these patients. A slant board (refer to Chapter 27) can be used for recumbent patients to help prevent aspiration, and if the patient is swallowing excessively, regurgitating or belching frequently, discuss with the veterinarian as they may prescribe pro-motility medications or a nasogastric tube to reduce stomach size.

9. **For the post-surgical patient**, icing the incision can help to reduce inflammation, and thus pain (Refer to Chapter 15).

10. **Passive range of motion** (PROM) exercises should be performed when the patient can tolerate them, and will help with reducing pain associated with tightening muscles and tendons. Refer to Chapter 15.

11. **Patients with nerve entrapment** may be among the most painful patients a veterinary technician or nurse may care for. **Team discussion and a thorough pain plan** that includes a plan for increased or decreased pain levels is critical. Pain in these patients is often variable and can become excruciating with the slightest movement. As part of a multi-modal treatment plan, acupuncture should be considered.

For all vertebral injuries and post-operative management, it is essential to observe behaviour for potential nerve involvement. As an example, the 7-year-old dog in Figure 32.2a sustained a right-sided ischial/pelvic fracture followed by extensive manipulation during surgical repair. He was extremely painful upon extubation. Meloxicam IV was administered, an additional bolus of fentanyl 6 µg/kg followed as an hourly CRI, and ketamine 1 mg/kg titrated to effect then continued as an hourly CRI. He slept for several hours. At this point ketamine was gradually reduced over ~8 h to 0.3 mg/kg/h. Upon awakening, he was much improved; however, he appeared to be constantly licking his incision. On close observation he was licking the right-sided tail base/anal region. To localize the area of potential pain, a cotton swab was passed over the surgical incision to the tail, and around the anus. A consistent painful yelping (allodynia) reaction was noted at the same anatomical location, the 2 o'clock region of the anus. Pudendal neuritis was suspected.

To prepare for discharge home in 96 h, amantadine 3 mg/kg PO q12h and gabapentin 10 mg/kg q8h PO were given, followed by continuation of fentanyl 6 µg/kg/h, ketamine 1 mg/kg bolus followed by hourly CRI, and meloxicam IV q24h. This was continued for 24 h. A fentanyl patch was applied, followed by a slow reduction of injectable analgesics over a further 24 h. He was much improved. Compare the appearance of the dog in Figure 32.2a to that of Figure 32.2b, where he was pain-free. Ketamine and fentanyl were discontinued. He was monitored on oral meds, including meloxicam, for ~48 h. A new fentanyl patch was applied which was removed after discharge at 96 h. He was continued on amantadine, gabapentin and meloxicam for several weeks with weekly small dose reductions of all analgesics to assess for no return of pain at the lower dosages.

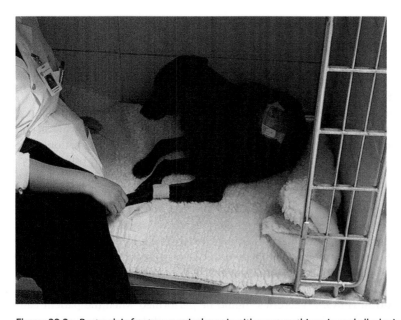

Figure 32.2a Post-pelvic fracture surgical repair with neuropathic pain and allodynia. Compare the appearance of the head down and ears drawn back, to that in Figure 32.2b where the pain has resolved.

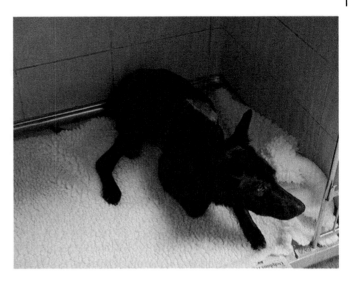

Figure 32.2b The above dog following resolution of the pudendal neuritis. Compare this bright, pain-free appearance to that of 32.2a, when he was in pain.

VI. Injury/Intervertebral Disc Herniation Management

A. Vertebral and Spinal Cord Injury

1. **Traumatic injury** to the vertebral column may or may not result in spinal cord injury. Handle all traumatic patients carefully as vertebral injury may be present. While preparing for IV catheterization, conduct a general primary survey and primary neurologic examination to determine whether underlying neurologic injury is present. Commence fluids at an appropriate rate for the situation at hand, and titrate an opioid carefully to effect. Acute IVD herniation results in a degree of spinal cord injury and is considered in this section.

   a. **Analgesia**

      i. **Box 32.1**, continue at effective dose during work-up and/or referral arrangements.

      ii. **Follow with ketamine and lidocaine (Box 32.1, points 2 and 3)** where indicated for severe pain.

      iii. **Sedative Box 32.2** where indicated following assessment.

      Where possible, survey radiographs of the vertebral column are taken without anesthesia so the animal protects the luxation/fracture site. Severe neck pain is frequently present with vertebral fracture/luxation following spinal trauma, necessitating extreme caution to avoid further pain, injury and dog aggression. See point b. below for the difficult patient or confirmation of a suspect lesion. For transport to the radiographic suite, and during radiography, stabilize the patient on a board with straps to minimize movement. A complete vertebral column (cervical, thoracic, lumbar and sacral) study, with attention to alignment of vertebrae, should be performed. Alignment of vertebrae may appear normal on the lateral views but lateral displacement may still be present on the dorso-ventral (D-V) view. Great care must be taken while positioning the animal for the D-V views as this frequently causes pain. It is preferable to move the radiographic beam instead of moving the patient, if at all possible. Radiographic examination may not always disclose a severe lesion; even if the fracture or luxation are in alignment, complete transection of the cord could still have occurred and should be identified on neurologic examination. If there is collapse vs narrowing of an IVD space, vertebral luxation has likely occurred and instability is present. An MRI (magnetic resonance imaging) scan accurately identifies the severity of vertebral column injury giving the surgeon in-depth pre-operative knowledge of both site and extent of the lesion. Radiographic evaluation of other areas (assessed by physical examination) may be necessary in the trauma patient. **If anesthesia is necessary**, the animal should be moved carefully, as described above when awake, so as not to cause/worsen vertebral displacement.

b. **Anesthesia**

    i. **Radiographic examination for the difficult patient.** Because of the level of pain and/or distress that may be experienced by the patient, general anesthesia may be necessary for imaging for both the patient and the veterinary personnel. Where IV access cannot be obtained:

- Choose an **opioid** at the dosage level suggested for hemodynamically stable patients in Box 32.3. Use the high end of the dose.
- Combine that with a potent **sedative** – preferably an alpha$_2$ agonist – at the high end of the dose (Box 32.2).
- Administer the combination IM and be prepared to wait for sedation, and to administer more drugs, as sedation in excited/agitated/aggressive patients generally takes longer for onset and is less profound than that achieved in the calm patient.
- If this protocol does not achieve adequate sedation:
  - Administer another half dose of each drug IM or IV, or
  - If the patient is manageable and IV access can be achieved, administer any of the injectable induction drugs listed for the hemodynamically stable patients in Box 32.3, or
  - If the patient isn't manageable and/or if the patient isn't likely to be manageable with this protocol from the onset, add:
    - **Ketamine** 2–5 mg/kg ketamine to the opioid and sedative. This dose will create a "dissociated" state but not true anesthesia so IV drugs may be necessary after the patient becomes manageable. Anesthesia can be produced using 5–10 mg/kg **ketamine** IM but this is a very large volume to inject, or
    - **Telazol**° or **Zolatil**° 4–8 mg/kg. This dose will produce general anesthesia. Recoveries from this drug can be prolonged.
- The patient is now deeply sedated or even anesthetized, so use all monitoring and support that would be used for any other patient in this state.
  - Provide supplemental oxygen and intubate if the patient is truly anesthetized.
  - Use all physiologic monitors.
  - Consider IV fluids, depending on the patient's needs.
  - Handle the patient **very carefully** so as not to exacerbate the injury and result in worse pain when awake.

    ii. **For emergent surgical procedures:**

- See Box 32.3. Choose an anesthetic protocol based on the patient's overall health status. The focus should be on provision of adequate analgesia and prevention/treatment of central sensitization.
- **Opioids and ketamine** should be included for all patients unless contraindicated.

2. **IVD herniation, all are painful**, some excruciatingly so. Neurologic dysfunction of varying degrees may also be present. If presenting with recurrence of clinical signs following a previous surgical treatment, rule out: a second disc extrusion, cicatrix formation at the previous surgical site or hyperesthesia resulting from surgical manipulation, residual hemorrhage or disc material. Pain management is extremely important to control continuing acute pain and the establishment of chronic neuropathic pain, although this may be the problem.

   a. **Analgesia**
      i. Box 32.1.
      ii. Continue as for the **injured patient** above.
      iii. An NSAIA COX-2 preferential or selective for the less neurologic and more stable dogs is recommended where corticosteroids **have not** been administered (see Table 11.1, Chapter 11).
      iv. Treatment for the specific problem, once established, will also be analgesic.
         • Where surgery is not an option, for the **most profoundly neurologic dogs, dexamethasone** at 0.1 mg/kg IV then prednisone starting at 1 mg/kg, tapering the dose over 10–14 days. This treatment is based on an anti-inflammatory effect aiming to reduce vasogenic edema. The use of corticosteroids is not considered routine; however, the individual situation may indicate this therapy.
      v. **Acupuncture** is an alternative therapy where surgical correction is declined. Refer to Chapter 15.
   b. **Anesthesia**
      i. As for radiographic examination for the **injured patient**.
      ii. Surgical management: **Box 32.3** and refer to chapters for individual patient concerns:
         • Renal, hepatic, cardiovascular.
         • Intraoperative infusions of **opioids and ketamine ± lidocaine** should be administered to all patients with IVD disease unless otherwise contraindicated.
         • For additional analgesia, topical morphine can be applied to the spinal cord at the surgical site.

3. **Fibrocartilaginous embolic myelopathy (FCEM)**
   FCEM is noted to be painful upon acute disc extrusion as the owners note a yelp followed by the neurologic motor deficits. Pain may also be elicited upon presentation, but pain abruptly subsides in most dogs. Some dogs with FCEM may have sensory as well as motor function involvement and will remain extremely painful for several days (personal observation, KM) requiring constant analgesic administration titrated to effect. As physiotherapy is essential during motor dysfunction, those also exhibiting sensory neurologic involvement will find this very painful. Due to motor deficits they are unable to withdraw; therefore, a multi-modal analgesic regimen is essential for these patients. Also, observe facial expression while conducting physiotherapy to assess whether pain is experienced.
   a. **Analgesia**
      i. **Box 32.1**, continue at effective dose during work-up and/or referral arrangements.
      ii. **Follow with points 1 and 2 above** where indicated for severe pain.
   b. **Anesthesia**
      i. As for radiographic examination as for the **injured patient**.

4. **Coccygeal vertebrae amputation**
   Tail amputation is performed for various traumatic and oncologic conditions but also for unnecessary specific breed cosmetic purposes (e.g. tail-docking; Figure 32.3a). As with any surgical procedure, this must be carefully performed and surgical principles for handling of neural tissue followed to avoid secondary neuroma formation (Figure 32.3b). Effective pre-, intra- and post-operative analgesia are also essential to avoid establishment of chronic (maladaptive) pain, which is especially important in the neonate and young animals where allodynia and hyperalgesia are established following this procedure.

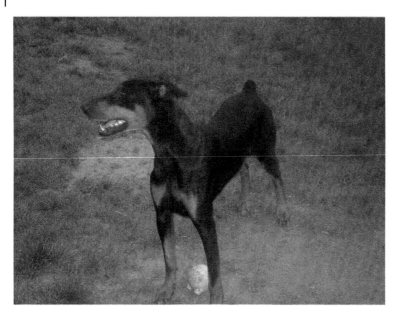

Figure 32.3a A 2-year-old Doberman pinscher with a lifetime history of bizarre behaviour, flank sucking, circling and tail chewing.

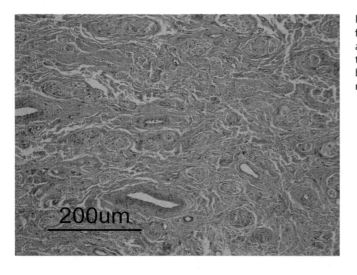

Figure 32.3b Neuroma identified following exploration and amputation of tail docking site of the dog in Figure 32.3a. The dog's behaviour improved following removal of the neuroma.

VII. Illness

A. Vertebral Column/Spinal Cord

Pathology may be due to ischemia, inflammation, infection, hemorrhage, tumours or extra-dural compression (e.g. IVD extrusion) resulting in persistent or intermittent somatic or visceral neuropathic pain.

1. **Neck pain** (also refer to Chapter 27)
   Has many etiologies:
   a. **Trauma, cervical disc protrusion or extrusion** noted in Section VI.
   b. **Inflammatory conditions:**

      i. steroid responsive arteritis-meningitis

      ii. meningomyelitis

      iii. discospondylitis osteomyelitis

  c. **Malformations resulting in:**

      i. caudo-occipital malformation syndrome

      ii. atlantoaxial luxation

      iii. caudal cervical spondylomyelopathy.

  d. **Malignancy:**

      i. malignant nerve sheath tumour

      ii. bony and spinal neoplasia.

Signs of pain for all are low head and neck carriage, neck guarding, stilted and cautious gait, and spasms of cervical spinal muscles. Forelimb lameness may be present due to radicular pain (root signature or referred pain) due to impingement of nerve roots C5 to C8. Pain may also be elicited during the neurologic examination with manipulation of the affected limb. Surgical treatment is recommended as conservative management using corticosteroids, muscle relaxants and cage rest has a high recurrence rate. Refer to Section VI.A.1 cautions above. Based on the pathophysiology of neuropathic pain, and the experience of this severe to excruciating pain, a multi-modal analgesic regimen is necessary for the patient while planning surgical correction, which is essential to prevent further compromise of neurologic function. During work-up for etiology or referral.

2. **Analgesia**

  a. Box 32.1.

  b. Continue as for Section VI.A.1.

  c. Treatment for the specific problem, once established, will also be analgesic.

  d. For cervical vertebral involvement, consider a **well-fitting neck brace/splint**; however, the owner must be judged as being able to inspect and detect any problems that may arise following discharge.

3. **Anesthesia**

  a. **Diagnostic imaging for the difficult patient**

      i. As for radiographic examination for the **injured patient**.

      ii. For longer/more invasive imaging, general anesthesia is recommended and a protocol from Box 32.3 should be chosen based on the patient's health.

  b. **Cerebrospinal fluid collection (CSF tap), biopsy**

      i. In order to prevent injury to the spinal cord, the patient should be completely immobile during these procedures. Thus, general anesthesia is most commonly utilized.

      ii. For long procedures and/or those involving other procedures during anesthesia (e.g. imaging, surgery), a protocol from Box 32.3 should be chosen based on the patient's health status.

      iii. If the tap/biopsy is a stand-alone procedure and will be brief, pre-medication plus small boluses of injectable anesthetic drugs may be appropriate. Incremental boluses of 1–2 mg/kg of either **propofol or alfaxalone** can be used. However, propofol and alfaxalone are potent respiratory depressants so **administration of supplemental oxygen is imperative**.

      iv. If the tap is performed at the atlanto-occipital junction, general anesthesia, intubation and provision of supplemental oxygen is required. For intubation, use of an armoured endotracheal tube (to prevent the tube from kinking) is recommended.

  c. **Surgical procedure**

      i. Choose a protocol from Box 32.3 based on the patient's health.

      ii. Armoured endotracheal tubes are recommended if cervical manipulation is anticipated during the procedure.

      iii. Special consideration: **be very careful with cervical manipulation during intubation**. It is very easy to overextend the neck and exacerbate the patient's injury.

B. Lumbosacral Lesions

There are many causes for lumbosacral lesions (L–S) in addition to injury:

1. Inflammatory conditions
2. Discospondylitis
3. Osteomyelitis
4. Idiopathic stenosis
5. Neoplasia
6. Vascular compromise
7. Congenital abnormalities
8. Degenerative lumbosacral (L–S) stenosis, the most common disease of the cauda equina in large-breed dogs.
   a. A study evaluating severity of cauda equina compression, assessed by diagnostic imaging compared to severity of clinical signs, revealed a lack of correlation. Therefore, in addition to a thorough focused neurologic examination, clinical examination revealing pain on rectal examination, tail elevation and external area compression indicates presence of an L-S lesion. For confirmation, MRI is recommended to accurately identify the underlying disease process and will also give the surgeon pre-operative information on both site and extent of the lesion. In dogs with minimal MRI changes, cauda equina neuritis may be the cause of pain.
9. **For initial pain management**:
   a. **Analgesia**
      i. **Box 32.1**. Where required add.
      ii. **Section VI.A.1**.
   b. **Anesthesia**
      i. Choose an anesthetic protocol based on patient's health from **Box 32.3**.
      ii. Intraoperative infusions of **opioids and ketamine ± lidocaine** should be administered to all patients with inter-vertebral disc disease unless otherwise contraindicated.

C. Discospondylitis and Vertebral Osteomyelitis

Most commonly reported in medium to large-breed dogs, but may occur in any dog, and cat. The most common presenting sign is mild to severe spinal pain that may or may not be associated with neurologic deficits or fever. A definitive diagnosis should be attempted with culture and susceptibility performed on aspirates from the affected area, most important, and blood cultures.

1. **Analgesia**
   a. **Section VI.A.1**.
2. **Anesthesia** for diagnostic imaging and sample collection
   a. As for radiographic examination for the **injured patient or as for CSF collection.**

D. Polyradiculoneuritis

Polyradiculoneuritis is most commonly associated with motor and ventral nerve root, and ventral horn motor dysfunction; however, dorsal nerve root and dorsal root ganglial inflammation can result in hyperesthesia with touch and manipulation. While the origin of these structures is associated with the vertebral column, clinical signs are evident in the musculoskeletal system. Refer to Chapter 31, Section III for pain management and nursing care.

E.   Congenital/Developmental Lesions

Chiari-like malformation with syringomyelia (also known as syringohydromyelia) is a cause for central pain syndrome associated with moderate to severe neuropathic pain in dogs and is a genetic disorder in Cavalier King Charles spaniels. The behaviour exhibited by affected dogs is suggestive of neuropathic pain, since it has the characteristics of allodynia or dysesthesia.

1. **Analgesia**
   a. Box 32.1.

F. Central Pain Syndrome

1. **Neoplasia**
   Tumours involving pathways subserving somatic sensibilities of pain and temperature, such as the dorsal horn, spinothalamic, spinoreticular and spinomesencephalic tracts, and the cerebral cortex, can result in pain. The area of pain experienced is that which is subserved by the location and the pathway involving the neoplastic process. This is referred to as "central pain". In humans, the highest incidence of these tumours is within the spinal cord, lower brainstem and ventro-posterior thalamus. Careful physical examination with comparison to contralateral side, and no radiologic evidence of a problem, warrants further specialty investigation into presence of a central nervous system tumour. Initial pain management
   a. **Analgesia**
      i. Box 32.1.
2. **Meningitis, Arteritis, Vasculitis**
   Vasculitis associated with the meninges and spinal cord can be a cause for central pain. Vasculitis has been identified as a cause of neuropathic pain in Beagle dogs, and has been termed "Beagle pain syndrome". This pain syndrome is associated with a generalized vasculitis, perivasculitis and vascular thrombosis. The small to medium-sized muscular arteries in many organs, including the cervical meninges, are consistently involved. The clinical signs, laboratory abnormalities and vascular lesions suggest that the condition is immune-mediated. There are many other diseases that produce inflammation of the meninges, especially involving the cervical region, resulting in varying severity of cervical pain. These include granulomatous meningoencephalomyelitis aseptic meningitis and breed-associated aseptic meningitis seen in such breeds as the Bernese mountain dog. These lesions result in severe to excruciating pain.
   a. **Analgesia**
      i. **Box 32.1.**
   b. **Anesthesia** should CSF be required. Refer to Section VII.A.3.b.

Further Reading

Aprea, F., Cherubini, G. B., Palus, V., *et al.* (2012) Effect of extradurally administered morphine on postoperative analgesia in dogs undergoing surgery for thoracolumbar intervertebral disk extrusion. *J Am Vet Med Assoc,* 241(6): 754–759.

Brisson, B. A. (2010) Intervertebral disc disease in dogs. *Vet Clin North Am Small Anim Pract,* 40(5): 829–858.

Duque, C. (2017) Neck pain. In: Mathews, K. A. (ed.), *Veterinary Emergency & Critical Care Manual,* 3rd edn. LifeLearn, Guelph, Ontario, Canada.

Harkema, S. J., Hillyer, J., Schmidt-Read, M., et al. (2012) Locomotor training: As a treatment of spinal cord injury and in the progression of neurologic rehabilitation.*Arch Phys Med Rehabil,* 3(9): 1588–1597.

Mathews, K. A. (2008) Neuropathic pain in dogs and cats: Update on management of pain. *Vet Clin North Am Sm Anim Pract*, 38(6): 1366–1414.

Olby, N. (2010) The pathogenesis and treatment of acute spinal cord injuries in dogs. *Vet Clin North Am Small Anim Pract*, 40(5): 791–807.

Posner, L. P., Mariani, C. L., Swanson, C., *et al.* (2014) Perianesthetic morbidity and mortality in dogs undergoing cervical and thoracolumbar spinal surgery. *Vet Anaesth Analg*, 41(2): 137–144.

Singh, A. M., James, F. M. and Mathews, K. A. (2017) Vertebral column: Trauma/ disc herniation/ neoplasia. In: Mathews, K. A. (ed.), *Veterinary Emergency & Critical Care Manual*, 3rd edn. LifeLearn, Guelph, Ontario, Canada.

Wehrenberg, A., Freeman, L., Ko, J., *et al.* (2009) Evaluation of topical epidural morphine for postoperative analgesia following hemilaminectomy in dogs. *Vet Ther*, 10(4): E1–12.

33

Integument Injuries and Illness

Karol Mathews, Tamara Grubb and Andrea Steele

Integumentary lesions may be primary with no secondary involvement, or may be associated with deeper internal injuries. Also, when considering the pain experienced, anatomical location of the lesions require special considerations. Any lesions involving the perineum, scrotum, prepuce, vulva (Figure 33.1), mammary glands, lips and digits will probably hurt more due to the innervation and function. Of importance is to appreciate that **lacerations, shearing, avulsion, penetrating and bite wound** injuries are frequently the tip of the iceberg with respect to potential associated internal injuries. A thorough physical examination and pain assessment of all areas is essential to identify damage to underlying muscle and fascia. Injury involving structures of the torso frequently includes injury to the viscera of the thorax, abdomen and pelvis. Therefore, in addition to musculoskeletal pain, visceral pain is frequently present. Handling and restraining torso-injured patients must be performed very carefully as localized areas of pain will be present. Painful areas to consider are the shoulders, vertebral column, all areas of the thorax, abdomen, pelvis and perineum. Intrathoracic lesions to consider are pericardial, mediastinal and pulmonary hemorrhage, pneumothorax, inflammation and associated lung parenchymal swelling or hemorrhage, all of which result in severe pain. Refer to Chapter 28 for information on managing pain and anesthesia associated with these injuries. Where injuries of the abdominal and pelvic integument may extend into these cavities, refer to Chapters 29 and 30 for information on these injuries. Refer to Chapter 31 where presenting signs of lameness are associated with fasciitis/myositis. Refer to Chapter 32 where vertebral injuries are also involved. Pain of various degrees occurs in medical conditions associated with inflammation of the skin primarily, or secondary to a non-dermatologic lesion, the potential for which should be investigated as this may influence the analgesic regimen (e.g. hepatic).

I. Analgesia, Sedation and Anesthesia

As lavage of wounds and dermatologic lesions is required, to reduce the pain associated with wound lavage, warm solution to ~30 °C, max 35 °C. Room temperature and > 35 °C lavage solution appears to be painful. Initial gentle lavage for non-penetrating, grossly contaminated wounds (i.e. dirt, gravel, etc.), warm tap water (test on palmar surface of wrist where a temperature difference cannot be felt), does not appear to cause, or worsen, pain. However, pain of the injury must be managed with an opioid initially. Refer to Box 33.1.

Analgesia and Anesthesia for the Ill or Injured Dog and Cat, First Edition. Karol A. Mathews, Melissa Sinclair, Andrea M. Steele and Tamara Grubb.
© 2018 John Wiley & Sons, Inc. Published 2018 by John Wiley & Sons, Inc.

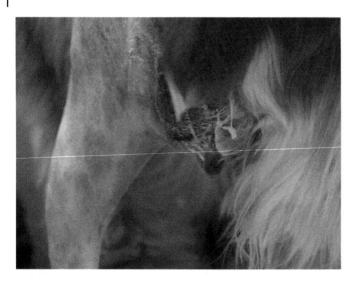

Figure 33.1 Brittany spaniel proximal femoral/iliac fracture with associated perineal/vulva involvement and urinary incontinence. Systemic analgesics could not eliminate the perineal pain. Gentle washing of the area, followed by local application of 4% lidocaine cream (Maxilene 4®), eliminated the pain and prevented urine scald dermatitis.

Box 33.1 Analgesia

1. **Opioids**
   Slowly titrate the opioid IV until the patient appears comfortable. Higher dosages may be required. Titration should be halted when early signs of adverse effects appear – nausea, increased respiratory rate, dysphoria. # **Note opioid reversal below.** Dosages for both cats and dogs are within the dose range given unless otherwise stated. Opioids in order of preference for initial administration:

   Moderate to severe pain

   - **Fentanyl** 2–5 µg/kg, or
   - **Methadone** 0.1–0.5 mg/kg, or
   - **Oxymorphone** 0.02–0.05+ mg/kg, or
   - **Hydromorphone** 0.02–0.1+ mg/kg only if none of the above is available due to increased potential for vomiting (refer to Chapter 10, Section II.B), or
   - **Morphine** 0.1–0.5 mg/kg only if none of the above is available due to increased potential for vomiting (refer to Chapter 10, Section II.A)
   - **Establish a CRI**
     - 1 h infusion of the effective bolus dose of fentanyl, or
     - 4 h infusion (or ¼/h) of the effective bolus dose of methadone, hydromorphone oxymorphone or morphine.
   - **Add a sedative (Box 33.2)** based on the anxiety level of the patient to offer sedation and reduce opioid requirement
   - **Fentanyl** is appropriate for pregnant, lactating, pediatric and geriatric patients. Refer to these chapters for ongoing analgesia.

   Known mild to moderate pain

   - **Butorphanol** 0.2–0.4 mg/kg IV, IM q2–4 h, or to effect, or
   - **Buprenorphine** 5–10 µg/kg IV, IM, 20–50 µg/kg sublingual q4–8 h cats and dogs < 10 kg. A higher dose may be required.

   Opioids alone may not be effective in cases where neuropathic, or other severe, pain also exists. The adverse effects of an opioid overdose can still occur in these painful patients when the mu-receptors are saturated. It is essential to titrate the opioid slowly and stop when **very**

subtle signs of an increased respiratory rate, nausea, dysphoria or worsening of the signs of pain appear. The dose received at this point may be used to calculate the CRI for continuing care. Caution is required in interpretation of what appears to be painful behaviour occurring during opioid administration. The patient may be experiencing opioid-induced hyperalgesia where the opioid is causing more pain requiring addition of a different class of analgesic, versus a dysphoric response (refer to Chapter 8). Should further analgesia be required based on circumstances, especially where neuropathic pain or opioid-induced hyperalgesia is suspected, add ketamine (see point 2 below).

 # Opioid reversal with naloxone where required:
Where excessive nausea, panting or dysphoria is noted, immediately reverse the opioid with naloxone, particularly if using a long-acting opioid. Slowly titrate until the adverse signs of the opioid subside, then stop naloxone administration. With slow titration, the primary effect of opioid analgesia will not be reversed and frequently facilitates calming. Fentanyl is quickly metabolized and it may not be necessary to reverse, caution is required as it is easy to "over reverse" and reverse the analgesic properties. To ensure accurate dosing for the individual patient and permit slow delivery of the reversal, the following is recommended;

- **Dilute naloxone** (0.4 mg/mL) using:
  - 0.1 mL added to 5 mL saline (=0.008 mg/mL) for small dogs and cats, titrate IV at 0.5 mL/min
  - 0.25 mL added to 9.75 mL saline (=0.01 mg/mL), titrate IV at up to 1 mL/min
  - Titrate IV until signs of dysphoria or nausea are reversed, usually 2–3 mLs. Repeat dosing may be required.

2. **Ketamine**
Ketamine, where pain cannot be managed with an opioid alone, common where nerve injury is involved. Ketamine's anti-inflammatory activity and bronchodilation properties will be beneficial, especially where smoke inhalation is associated with thermal burns. Ketamine's additive benefit is bronchodilation and anti-inflammatory. However, ketamine should be used with caution as ketamine stimulates the sympathetic nervous system and may exacerbate some arrhythmias. However, ketamine may be considered in some patients with underlying cardiac disease (refer to Chapter 19 for details), but should be avoided where severe hepatic (dogs), severe kidney (cats) compromise is present. Lidocaine (see point 3 below) may also be considered.
Ketamine should not be administered to pregnant and lactating animals.

- **Ketamine** 0.2–1 mg/kg titrated to effect
- **Establish a CRI**
  - 1 h infusion of the effective titrated dose. Should the patient appear overdosed at any period of time, stop the CRI for 30 min, or less if signs subside, and reinstitute at one-half the previous dose.

3. **Lidocaine**
Lidocaine is the alternative to, or in combination with, ketamine and an opioid.

- Lidocaine 1–2 mg/kg IV titrated followed by 1–2 mg/kg/h – **dogs,** can be added to the above regimen where pain is difficult to manage or a lower opioid dose is required. This dose must be calculated into the total dose when bupivacaine or lidocaine are used for local anesthesia to avoid toxicity (refer to Chapter 14). Refer to Chapter 12 for guidance in cats. The addition of lidocaine may reduce the opioid requirement; therefore, monitoring for potential opioid-adverse effects must be noted on the chart and the opioid dose reduced accordingly. Lidocaine has promotility activity, which may be an advantage in patients with associated abdominal injury/illness or where high-dose opioid predispose to ileus. Nausea may develop with 9–24 h infusion. Lidocaine IV should be avoided in patients with significant hepatic pathology.

4. **NSAIA**
NSAIA (Table 11.1, Chapter 11) following physical examination, stabilization, and laboratory information is received and no contraindications are identified. **Do not use in** pregnant, nursing cats, or puppies and kittens less than six weeks of age, or when corticosteroids are prescribed. Carprofen 2 mg/kg (lean body weight) q12h for up to six days may be considered in lactating dogs (refer to Chapter 24). Consult the NSAIA package insert prior to administration to verify age as this varies with each product.

Box 33.2 Sedatives

- **Diazepam** 0.2 mg/kg IV or **midazolam** 0.2 mg/kg IV or IM, or
- **Acepromazine** 0.005–0.02 mg/kg, IM, IV. Use with caution in hypovolemic or hypotensive patients, acepromazine-mediated vasodilation may contribute to hypotension.
- **Medetomidine** 0.1–4 µg/kg IM, IV may be considered where no co-morbidities exist.
- **Dexmedetomidine** 0.5–2 µg/kg IM, IV, CRI may be considered where no co-morbidities exist.

Box 33.3 Anesthesia

After patient stabilization, anesthesia is required for initial wound management, in addition to the ongoing analgesic regimen established. Supplemental oxygen should be available with pulse-oximetry as a minimum.

1. **Total IV anesthesia (TIVA)** with propofol or alfaxalone may be used for short-term wound lavage or bandage changes.
   - **Propofol 2–6 mg/kg, IV or alfaxalone 1–3 mg/kg, IV** titrated to effect. Patients may be maintained with repeated IV boluses of propofol (0.5–1 mg/kg) or alfaxalone (0.3–0.5 mg/kg) as indicated with depth assessment for short procedures, or a CRI can be used. Repeat dosing of propofol was once thought to cause significant numbers on Heinz bodies but this has since been disproven and propofol CRIs should not be avoided in cats.[1]
   - **Ketamine with midazolam or diazepam** (1:1): 0.1–0.2 mL/kg, IV to effect.
   - **Heavy sedation with dexmedetomidine 2–5 µg/kg IV, with an opioid**, i.e. hydromorphone 0.025–0.05 mg/kg IV, may provide good sedation and analgesia in cardiovascularly stable patients requiring repeat wound care.
2. **When general anesthesia** is required for wound management, endotracheal intubation, oxygen supplementation and further monitoring are necessary.
   - **Isoflurane or sevoflurane** for procedure >20 min is more practical.
   - Should hypotension develop under anesthesia refer to Chapter 19, Section II.B.3.
3. For all patients, analgesia should be a focus for perioperative care.
   - Include infusions as listed **in Box 33.1**, and
   - **Local anesthetic blockade** wherever possible (refer to Chapter 14).
   - **Dexmedetomidine** may also be included in the post-operative analgesic regimen.

II. Injuries

A. Frostbite

Refer to Chapter 34, Section IV.A.

B. Porcupine Quills

Refer to Chapter 34, Section VIII.

C. Burns

These include chemical/caustic and thermal (direct contact with heat including flames, heating pads/blankets, lamps, hot liquids, electrical, radiation). All burn injuries are painful and some can be extensive (Figure 33.2). Refer to emergency text [2] for specific treatment for burns;

Figure 33.2 A young Beagle caught in a barn fire resulting in a third-degree burn from head to tail.

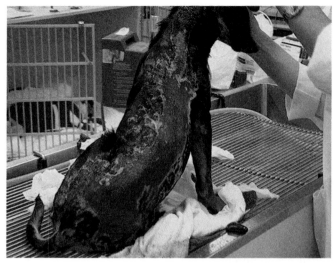

however, the following analgesic regimen applies to all burns. Also consider smoke inhalation and management for that, refer to number 3 in the following list. Do not administer butorphanol where there is smoke exposure, due to the antitussive effects. For oral electrical injuries, refer to Chapter 27, **Section II.C.**

1. **Thermal burns**
   a. **Analgesia**
      i. **Titrated opioid analgesics are absolutely necessary** following intravenous (IV) catheter placement, which should occur immediately upon admission, or intramuscular (IM) if restraint is required to perform catheterization. As pain can be severe, multi-modal analgesia is frequently required.

      Box 33.1 opioids titrated IV to effect if catheter in place: fentanyl, methadone, oxymorphone or hydromorphone; or morphine IM (cat and dog) if no other opiate available, and

      ii. **Ketamine (Box 33.1)** as an adjunct analgesic (cats and dogs) followed by the effective dose as an hourly infusion. Repeat boluses may be needed until a state of relaxation and analgesia is reached, even anesthesia if the situation indicates. Consider with smoke inhalation as it has bronchodilation properties

      iii. **Midazolam or diazepam** (Box 33.2), IV to effect, or

      iv. **Dexmedetomidine 2–5 µg/kg IV**, in conjunction with an opioid, are recommended to decrease anxiety of procedural pain.

      v. **Cool the burned area** with cool, gentle running tap water or light shower spray (12–18 °C (55–64 °F)) as soon as possible after the burn, for at least 20 min. This cooling and stopping of the burning process reduces inflammation and can decrease the need for operative intervention. Cooling is also analgesic. Cooling should take place within 1 h of burn injury but may be beneficial for up to 3 h post burn injury. Assess temperature by degree of discomfort the animal shows (personal experience finds the lower to be less painful!). Cool compresses are not recommended. Do not use ice as this will compromise circulation to the area. Where large areas are involved, monitor the patient's body temperature q5–7 min and avoid hypothermia (<38 °C (100.5 °F)). After cooling, cover wounds with non-adherent dressing to reduce fluid losses and to reduce further painful injury, as a slight bump will hurt. Where eyes are involved, lavage with sterile saline.

      vi. **Consider epidural morphine** if burn injuries are on the hind limbs or perineum and skin at injection site is not injured (refer to Chapter 14).

vii. **Addition of gabapentin** 5–20 mg/kg PO q8h (usually 10 mg/kg to start) is reported to reduce the discomfort and pruritus associated with burn wounds. Also, recommended to manage neuropathic pain associated with injury to neural tissue of the skin.

viii. **Buprenorphine** 0.01–0.02 mg/kg IV or IM q2–4h (cats and dogs) may be effective for **mild first-degree burns**.

ix. **Non-steroidal anti-inflammatory analgesics (NSAIAs):** Box 33.1. Essential to add to the regimen; however, avoid until following initial anesthesia, and the patient is stable with normal renal function.

The effective regimen should be continued throughout hospital stay. Introduce an NSAIA where no contraindications, and gabapentin as soon as possible. Do not stop therapy abruptly, wean off injectable analgesics gradually. Should pain re-appear, return to previous effective dose/regimen. Discharge home with an NSAIA and gabapentin. Following a pain-free period, gradually reduce the NSAIA dose followed by reduction of gabapentin. Return to previous effective dosing should pain re-appear. Refer to Chapter 3 and Chapter 12 for further analgesic guidance if required.

2. **Chemical/caustic burns**
   a. **Analgesia**
   As for thermal burns, caustic burns are excruciatingly painful.
      i. **Box 33.1, select an opioid.**
      ii. **Remove caustic substances.**
         - **Immersion or shower spray** as for thermal burns.
         - **Lavage eyes** with sterile saline.
         - Pursue **removal of specific substances**, as soon as possible. Copious lavage for at least 2h is required for strong acid burns and potentially up to 12h for strong alkali burns. Neutralizing agents can be useful but should be diluted and applied to the wound as a compress [2] (specific antidotes should be pursued).
         - **Removal of hot tar** requires liberal application of an emulsifying agent. Tween-80 (contained in Neosporin ointment, Burroughs-Wellcome) or polysorbate, should be applied during immersion or shower spray. Alternatively, solubilizing with mineral or vegetable oil and then washing with detergent (e.g. Ivory soap) or dishwashing liquid (not dishwasher) has been recommended.
         - Surgical excision may be required if prolonged contact has occurred.
   b. **Anesthesia**
      i. Refer to **Box 33.3** for anesthetic/analgesic protocols.
      ii. Patients with burns may be hypovolemic and/or hypoproteinemic, thus individualized fluid therapy protocols should be developed for each patient. Blood pressure should be monitored and PCV/TS (packed cell volume/total solids) assessed periodically.
      iii. Patients with large areas of debrided skin are very likely to become hypothermic, so active support of body temperature is necessary.
      iv. Debridement of large areas of damaged tissue can lead to hyperkalemia. The ECG should be monitored and serum electrolytes checked as necessary.
      v. Depending on the cause of the burn, smoke inhalation may have occurred with resultant concern for the airway. See specific information under smoke inhalation in point 3 below.
3. **Smoke inhalation**
   a. **Analgesia**
      i. **Box 33.1, select an opioid.**

The pain experienced will vary with severity of injury; therefore, to assess the appropriate analgesic dose, **titrate dosages IV slowly** until the patient is comfortable, and stop at the onset of a slight pant or nausea. The IM route should only be used if IV access cannot be obtained quickly due to patient's behaviour. **Avoid cough suppressants (i.e. butorphanol)** as they prevent expectoration of inhaled smoke particles.

    ii. **Midazolam or diazepam Box 33.2**, in conjunction with an opioid, are recommended to decrease anxiety.

    iii. **Ketamine Box 33.1** for analgesia, bronchodilation and anti-inflammatory properties (Chapter 12).

    iv. **NSAIAs Box 33.1 and Chapter 11. Avoid** until the patient is fully assessed, stable with normal renal function.

b. **Anesthesia** can be very difficult in patients with smoke inhalation, depending on the degree of pathology. Heat damage in the nasal/oral cavity and down to the larynx can result in upper airway edema with the potential for upper airway obstruction. Inhaled toxins, gases and particulate matter can cause pulmonary edema and alveolar atelectasis, with the potential for reduced pulmonary compliance and impaired gas exchange. **Anesthetic techniques and considerations:**

    i. **Anesthesia** can proceed as in Box 33.3 for patients without airway complications.

    ii. **Alternatively**, following an administered opioid above, **propofol** 2–6 mg/kg IV administered to effect to facilitate endotracheal intubation, followed by a continuous rate infusion (CRI) of 0.1–0.4 mg/kg/min and during tracheostomy if indicated (refer to Chapter 27 for details).

c. **For all patients:**

    i. **Analgesia/sedation Box 33.1 and Box 33.2** should be provided to keep the patient calm and comfortable. Excitement and/or pain can cause increased respiratory drive, which can increase the intra-airway negative pressure and exacerbate the altered air flow through narrowed airways (e.g. through an edematous larynx) and exacerbate intra-airway damage.

    ii. **Supplemental oxygen** should be supplied via facemask, nasal cannula, oxygen cage, etc.

    iii. **Patients with upper airway injury** may need a tracheostomy (Chapter 27).

    iv. **Patients with lower airway injury** will need to be ventilated using intermittent positive-pressure ventilation delivered at higher respiratory rates and lower tidal volumes than those traditionally used for patients with unaffected lungs.

    v. **Blood gases** should be used to assess gas exchange and acid-base status. Frequency of blood gas assessment should be based on the health status of the patient.

D. Lacerations, Shearing and Avulsion

1. Of importance is to appreciate that these traumatic injuries are frequently associated with other injuries. A thorough physical examination and pain assessment of all areas is essential to identify damage to underlying muscle and fascia, which may be extensive, and limb fractures, both open and closed. Refer to Chapter 31. Wounds require hemostasis, debridement, lavage and surgical exploration as soon as stable (Figure 33.3). Some may require surgery as a stabilizing procedure due to traumatic lesions [3].

a. **Analgesia**

    i. **Box 33.1 opioids.**

    ii. Where indicated, follow with: **local anesthesia** where appropriate (refer to Chapter 14).

    iii. **NSAIAs, Box 33.1** and Chapter 11, are very effective and may be administered in stable patients where no contraindications exist and anesthesia not planned.

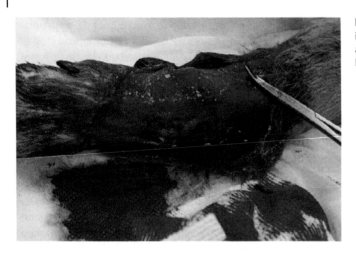

Figure 33.3 Degloving injury incurred during an automobile accident. *Source:* Courtesy of Dr K. Lamey.

   b. **Anesthesia**
      i. **Box 33.3**.
      ii. **For extensive lacerations**, consider epidural morphine if injuries are on the hind limbs or perineum and skin at injection site is not injured (refer to Chapter 14).
   c. **Post-operative**
      i. Continue with **established regimen**, and/or
      ii. **NSAIAs** (Box 33.1 and Chapter 11) recommended where all concerns for ongoing hemorrhage and hypotension, and other contraindications based on history or biochemical profile, have been ruled out.

E. Bite Wounds and Crush Injuries

  1. These wounds can be extensive and deep, all are painful and require debridement, lavage ± closure/reconstruction. These injuries may communicate with the thoracic, abdominal or pelvic cavity. If there is evidence/suspicion of this, refer to the anatomical chapters in this book for guidelines for ongoing analgesic and anesthetic requirements.
     All patients upon admission:
     a. **Analgesia**
        i. **Box 33.1, opioids.**
        ii. Where indicated follow with: **local anesthesia** (Chapter 14 for appropriate technique).
        iii. **NSAIAs** (Box 33.1 and Chapter 11) following debridement etc., where anesthesia is not required and there are no contraindications, the NSAIAs are excellent analgesics for these patients.
     b. **Anesthesia**
        i. **Box 33.3**.
        ii. **For extensive wounds, consider epidural morphine** if injuries are on the hind limbs or perineum and skin at injection site is not injured (refer to Chapter 14).
     c. **Post-op analgesia**
        i. Continue with **established regimen**.
        ii. **NSAIAs** should be avoided until all concerns for ongoing hemorrhage and hypotension, and other contraindications based on history or biochemical profile, have been ruled out. Refer to Box 33.1 and Chapter 11.

F. Penetrating Injuries

1. All require surgical debridement, lavage ± closure. Some may require diagnostic imaging (e.g. bullets) prior to surgical exploration. However, impalement injuries should go straight to surgery for exploration and specific removal technique warranted by the situation observed at surgery (Figure 33.4 went straight to surgery). Movement incurred during imaging will be painful with added risk of further injury.
    a. **Analgesia**
        i. **Box 33.1, opioids.**
        ii. For **deep foreign body injuries** refer to the anatomical chapters for guidelines for ongoing analgesic and anesthetic requirements.
    b. **Anesthesia** for integument involvement only (epidermis/dermis torso) or penetration of limbs.
        i. **Box 33.3**.
        ii. **Local/regional anesthetic blocks** should be utilized wherever possible. Refer to Chapter 14.
    c. **Post-operative analgesia**
        i. Based on the individual patient and injury, continue with established regimen (**Box 33.1 opioids** ± an NSAIA).
        ii. **NSAIAs:** where there are no contraindications the NSAIAs are excellent analgesics for these patients. Refer to Box 33.1 and Chapter 11.

G. Pressure Necrosis

A common complication of bandage applied too tightly (typically on limbs), and of immobilized, recumbent animals (typically on bony prominences). Manage as for wounds above.

H. Urine Scald

1. Nursing care is important for all patients; however, where illness or injury results in recumbency, this has to include urinary care, frequent cage monitoring and a scheduled body rotation where possible. Where these procedures are not followed serious

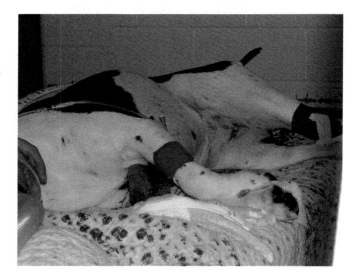

Figure 33.4 A German shorthaired pointer impaled on a tree branch which entered between the forelimbs, skimmed along the sternum and entered the abdomen and pelvis exiting lateral to the vulva. Diagnostic imaging procedures were not performed prior to immediate surgical exploration where the branch was easily visualized and removed without complications.

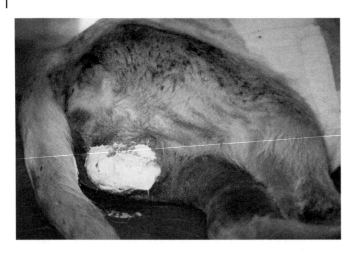

Figure 33.5 Golden retriever three days post right femoral fracture appears to have been left in right lateral recumbency while waiting for referral for fracture repair. The hind limb urine scald was as painful as the contralateral fractured femur. A zinc-based cream is shown on the associated scrotal dermatitis.

dermatologic urine scald occurs and the pain is severe when occurring for > 24 h (Figure 33.5). When present:

a. **Analgesia**
   i. analgesia given **for the primary problem**, refer to Box 33.1. In addition:
   ii. **Gentle wash with shampoo** (such as an oatmeal based calming shampoo), ensure complete rinse and dry.
   iii. **Local application of 4% lidocaine cream** (Maxilene 4®), or a calming barrier type ointment such as zinc-based baby diaper cream. Ensure that the patient cannot lick the area.
   iv. **NSAIA** where no contraindications. Refer to Box 33.1 and Chapter 11.

III. Illness

A. Medical Dermatologic Emergencies

1. **Dermatologic Pain**
   The majority of dermatologic diseases cause inflammation and are, therefore, a source of discomfort and, for some, excruciating pain. The etiology must be determined as specific therapy to treat the underlying problem may alleviate the discomfort. Where moderate to severe pain is suspected, and there are rare cases:

   a. **Analgesia**
      i. **Box 33.1, opioid.**
      ii. Add **ketamine Box 33.1** where the opioid alone is not effective.
      iii. **NSAIA** where pain is severe and not controlled with (i) and (ii) while waiting for culture and susceptibility (C&S) or biopsy results, and no contraindications are present. Refer to Box 33.1 and Chapter 11. Should biopsy indicate immune-mediated process and an NSAIA has been administered, commence omeprazole therapy and wait for 96 h prior to corticosteroid therapy, commence planned corticosteroid therapy at half the intended dose for two days.

B. Myositis and Fasciitis

At presentation, may (Figure 33.6 and Figure 33.7) or may not (Figure 33.8) be associated with an integumentary lesion as this is an advanced presentation. However, severe pain and a degree of swelling are detected on physical examination of the area involved and immediate surgery is required. Refer to **Chapter 31** for analgesia and anesthesia recommendations.

Figure 33.6 *Streptococcal* fasciitis. A 72 h history of lameness with the extent of the integumentary lesion appearing over a 6 h period. *Source:* [4]. Reproduced with permission of John Wiley & Sons.

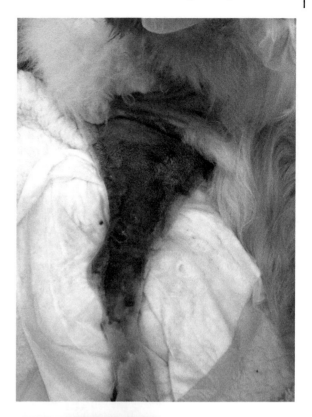

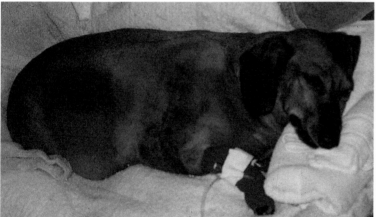

Figure 33.7a *Pseudomonas* fasciitis following subcutaneous fluid administration to treat a vaccine anaphylactic reaction two days prior to referral. *Source:* [4]. Reproduced with permission of John Wiley & Sons.

C. Immune-Mediated Disease

1. Where **immune-mediated disease** is suspected, corticosteroid therapy will be prescribed which will alleviate the inflammation and pain. However, while waiting for biopsy results and pain is moderate to severe when lesions are disseminated, treat as in:
   a. **Analgesia** Box 33.1

   Caution: refer to Box 33.1 and Chapter 11 where an NSAIA may be contemplated prior to diagnosis. See **point A.1** above.

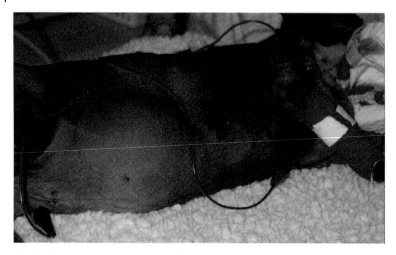

Figure 33.7b Within 2 h following Figure 33.7a, while awaiting surgical management, the lesion rapidly expanded. *Source:* [4]. Reproduced with permission of John Wiley & Sons.

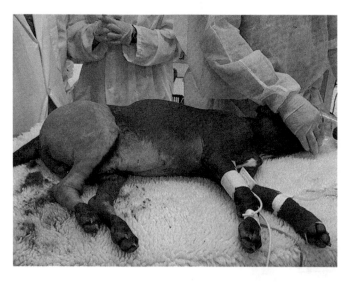

Figure 33.8 *Streptococcal* fasciitis. Five-month-old puppy with three-day history of hind limb lameness. Extent of swelling noted here occurred within a one-day period.

D. Bacterial Dermatitis

Where a **bacterial dermatitis** is highly suspected, appropriate antibiotic therapy, based on C&S, will reduce inflammation and pain. An **NSAIA Box 33.1 and Chapter 11** is beneficial while waiting for results should pain be moderate to severe.

E. Drug Eruption

Where there is a history of a recent event and drug administration, **drug eruption** may be the diagnosis. This is frequently disseminated and very painful. Treat as in **Box 33.1** while waiting for biopsy results. An NSAIA may be required during this period as opioids may not be adequate to manage the pain (KM experience). See point A.1 above. **Caution: refer to Chapter 11**.

F. Mastitis

Mastitis is a painful lesion most commonly associated with bacterial infection (Figure 33.9a).

See **Section I** to avoid further pain when cleaning. Treat as in Box 33.1. **Local anesthetic**, where appropriate after lavage and prior to topical therapy**: bupivacaine 0.5% (5 mg/mL)** at 0.2 mL/kg (=1 mg/kg) based on ideal body weight, and sodium bicarbonate (1 mEq/mL). Buffering of a 0.5% bupivacaine solution (5 mg/mL) requires a 20:0.1 mixture with sodium bicarbonate 1 mEq/mL (~0.2 mL bupivacaine and 0.001 mL sodium bicarbonate) and warmed to ~30 °C, max 35 °C. Based on wound size and to cover the area, it may be necessary to dilute bupivacaine with 6–12 mL sterile water for larger dogs (relative to size of dog); 3 mL for tiny dogs and cats.

Frequently local treatment for approximately 5–7 days sloughs the necrotic tissue (Figure 33.9b). Anesthesia is required to close the wound. Refer to **Box 33.3**.

Figure 33.9a Gangrenous mastitis upon presentation.

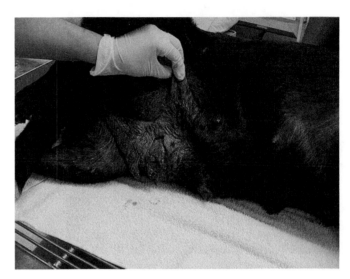

Figure 33.9b Patient above after six days of raw honey treatment prior to closure.

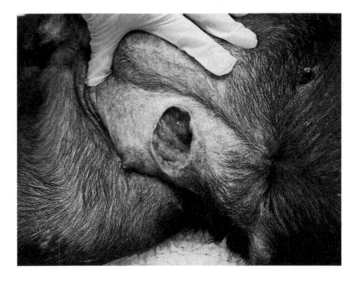

For large surgical wounds (Figure 33.10a and b), there may be an opportunity to place a **wound diffusion catheter**. Refer to Chapter 14 for detailed instructions.

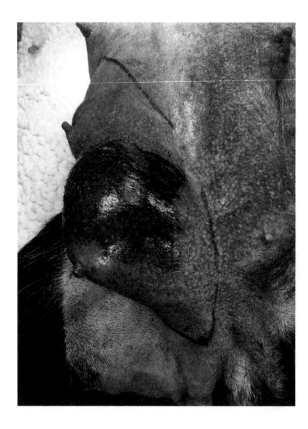

Figure 33.10a Mastitis. *Source:* Courtesy of Dr K. Lamey.

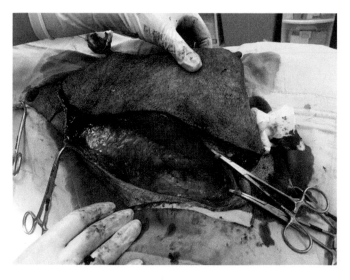

Figure 33.10b Above patient during mastectomy. Placement of a wound diffusion catheter (Chapter 14) is suggested where "mesh incisions" are not required to reduce tension on the suture line. *Source:* Courtesy of Dr K. Lamey.

References

1 Bley, C. R., Roos, M., Price, J. *et al.* (2007) Clinical assessment of repeated propofol-associated anesthesia in cats. *J Am Vet Med Assoc*, 231(9):1347–1353

2 Bersenas, A., Mathews, K. A. (2017) Burn injuries. In: Mathews, K. A. (ed.), Veterinary Emergency & Critical Care Manual, 3rd edn. LifeLearn, Guelph, Ontario, Canada.

3 Wright, T. and Brisson, B. (2017) Wounds. In: Mathews, K. A. (ed.), Veterinary Emergency & Critical Care Manual, 3rd edn. LifeLearn, Guelph, Ontario, Canada.

4 Aronson, L. R. (2016) *Small Animal Surgical Emergencies*. Chichester, Wiley-Blackwell.

Further Reading

Mathews, K. A. and Binnington, A. G. (2002) Wound management using honey. *Compendium Cont Edu for Pract Vet – North America Small Animal/Exotics*, 24(1): 53–60.

Valentine, B. (2017) Dermatologic emergencies. In: Mathews, K. A. (ed.), *Veterinary Emergency & Critical Care Manual*, 3rd edn. LifeLearn, Guelph, Ontario, Canada.

34

Environmental Injuries
Karol Mathews, Tamara Grubb and Andrea Steele

There are many, and an assortment of, environmental injuries that cats and dogs may incur. The ones presented here tend to be the most common; however, for others the analgesic and anesthetic protocols included here, and other scenarios in this book where applicable, may be applied. Sections I, II and III contain guidelines for the management of scenarios presented in Sections IV–IX.

I. Analgesia

Box 34.1   Analgesia in general

1. **Opioids**
   Slowly titrate the opioid until the patient appears comfortable. Titration should be halted when early signs of adverse effects appear – nausea, increased respiratory rate, dysphoria. **# Note opioid reversal below.** Dosages for both cats and dogs are within the dose range given unless otherwise stated. Opioids in order of preference for initial administration:
   - **Fentanyl** 2–5 μg/kg, or
   - **Methadone** 0.1–0.5 mg/kg, or
   - **Oxymorphone** 0.02–0.05 mg/kg, or
   - **Hydromorphone** 0.02–0.05 mg/kg only if none of the above is available due to increased potential for vomiting (refer to Chapter 10, Section II.B), or
   - **Morphine** 0.1–0.5 mg/kg only if none of the above is available due to increased potential for vomiting (refer to Chapter 10, Section II.A).
   - **Establish a continuous rate infusion (CRI)**
     o 1 h infusion of the effective bolus dose of fentanyl, or
     o 4 h infusion (or 0.25/h) of the effective bolus dose of methadone, hydromorphone oxymorphone or morphine.
   - **Fentanyl** is appropriate for pregnant, lactating, pediatric and geriatric patients. Refer to these sections for ongoing analgesia.
     o Sedative Box 34.2 add to opioid, with dosing based on anxiety level of the patient, to reduce opioid requirement initially and to offer sedation in the anxious patient.
   - **Where sedation is indicated** to reduce opioid requirement initially, or to offer sedation in the anxious patient. Box 34.2.

Analgesia and Anesthesia for the Ill or Injured Dog and Cat, First Edition. Karol A. Mathews, Melissa Sinclair, Andrea M. Steele and Tamara Grubb.

Opioids alone may not be effective in cases where neuropathic pain also exists. The adverse effects of an opioid overdose can still occur in the neuropathic painful patient when the mu-receptors are saturated. Caution is required in interpretation of an increase in what appears to be painful behaviour occurring during opioid administration. The patient may be experiencing opioid-induced hyperalgesia requiring addition of a different class of analgesic (e.g. ketamine), versus a dysphoric response (refer to Chapter 8). Should further analgesia be required based on circumstances, especially where neuropathic pain or opioid-induced hyperalgesia is suspected, add ketamine (see point 2 below).

 # Opioid reversal with naloxone where required.

Where excessive nausea, panting or dysphoria is noted, immediately reverse the opioid with naloxone, particularly if using a long-acting opioid. Slowly titrate until the adverse signs of the opioid subside, then stop naloxone administration. With slow titration, the primary effect of opioid analgesia will not be reversed and frequently facilitates calming. Fentanyl is quickly metabolized and it may not be necessary to reverse. Caution is required as it is easy to "over reverse" and reverse the analgesic properties. To ensure accurate dosing for the individual patient and permit slow delivery of the reversal, the following is recommended:

- Dilute naloxone (0.4 mg/mL) using:
  o 0.1 mL added to 5 mL saline (=0.008 mg/mL) for small dogs and cats, titrate IV at 0.5 mL/min
  o 0.25 mL added to 9.75 mL saline (=0.01 mg/mL), titrate IV at up to 1 mL/min
  o Titrate until signs of dysphoria or nausea are reversed, usually 2–3 mLs. Repeat dosing may be required.

2. **Ketamine where pain cannot be managed with an opioid alone**, common where nerve injury is involved. **Not suitable for pregnant or lactating patients.**
   - **Ketamine** 0.2–1 mg/kg titrated to effect.
   - **Establish a CRI** of effective dose/h.

   Ketamine's additive benefit is bronchodilation and anti-inflammatory. However, ketamine should be used with caution as it stimulates the sympathetic nervous system and may exacerbate some arrhythmias. However, ketamine may be considered in some patients with underlying cardiac disease (refer to Chapter 19 for details), but should be avoided where severe hepatic (dogs) or severe kidney (cats) compromise is present. Lidocaine (see point 3 below) may also be considered.

3. **Lidocaine** is the alternative to, or in combination with, ketamine and an opioid.
   Lidocaine intravenous (IV) bolus 1–2 mg/kg followed by 1–2 mg/kg/h – **dogs** can be added to the above regimen where pain is not being controlled or a reduction in the opioid dose is required. This dose must be calculated into the total dose when bupivacaine or lidocaine are used for local anesthesia to avoid toxicity (refer to Chapter 14). The addition of lidocaine may reduce the opioid requirement; therefore, monitoring for potential opioid adverse effects must be noted on the chart and the opioid dose reduced accordingly. Lidocaine has promotility activity, and other benefits, which may be an advantage in patients presenting with abdominal emergencies should the injury/illness and high-dose opioid predispose to ileus. Nausea may develop with > 24 h infusion. Lidocaine IV should be avoided in patients with significant hepatic pathology. Refer to Chapter 12 for guidance on administration to **cats**.

4. **Non-steroidal anti-inflammatory analgesic (NSAIA) for the stable patient.** Cyclooxygenase-2 (COX-2) preferential/selective NSAIA (refer to Table 11.1, Chapter 11 for dosing), in addition to the opioid above, may be administered parenterally when all concerns for ongoing hemorrhage and hypovolemia (e.g. occult abdominal hemorrhage, kidney injury) or other contraindications (e.g. renal insufficiency, coagulopathy, major crush injuries resulting in rhabdomyolysis) have been ruled out. Do not use in pregnant, lactating (refer to Chapter 24) animals or puppies and kittens less than 6 weeks of age. Consult the NSAIA package insert prior to administration to verify age as this varies with each product.

Box 34.1 (Continued)

5. **Gabapentin 10 mg/kg PO q8–12 h initially in dogs and cats** for severe injuries and where neuropathic pain is suspected, increase or decrease according to response. Where NSAIAs are contraindicated, gabapentin may be beneficial. Commence as soon as possible.
6. **Amantadine 3–5 mg/kg PO q12–24 h in dogs and cats** should be commenced 12 h prior to discontinuing the ketamine if assessed as necessary, especially where a neuropathic component to the injury occurred/exists. This dosing may also be prescribed for cats, but it is necessary to compound in chicken-flavour oil due to the reputed terrible taste of amantadine.

II. Sedatives

Box 34.2

- **Diazepam** 0.2 mg/kg IV or **midazolam** 0.2 mg/kg IV or intramuscular (IM), or
- **Acepromazine** 0.005–0.02 mg/kg, IM, IV Use with caution in hypovolemic or hypotensive patients, acepromazine-mediated vasodilation may contribute to hypotension.
- **Medetomidine** 0.1–4 µg/kg IM, IV may be considered where no cardiac co-morbidities exist.
- **Dexmedetomidine** 0.05–2 µg/kg IM, IV may be considered where no cardiac co-morbidities exist.

III. Anesthesia

Box 34.3

A. Anesthesia for Healthy Patients

- **Pre-medication** with an opioid plus a sedative for most patients. Dosages for drugs administered for pre-medication in healthy patients are typically higher than those administered for calming/analgesia in the ICU (Box 34.1) as more sedation and more analgesia are generally necessary prior to surgery. Use the low end of the dose range for IV administration and/or in mildly compromised patients.
  - ○ **Anesthesia pre-medication dosages of opioids:**
    - ▪ **Methadone** 0.3–0.5 mg/kg (dogs and cats), or
    - ▪ **Oxymorphone** 0.1–0.2 mg/kg (dogs), 0.05–0.1 mg/kg (cats), or
    - ▪ **Hydromorphone** 0.1–0.2 mg/kg (dogs), 0.1 mg/kg (cats), or
    - ▪ **Morphine** IM **only** 0.3–0.5 mg/kg (dogs), 0.1–0.3 mg/kg (cats).
  - ○ **Anesthesia pre-medication dosages of sedatives:**
    - ▪ **Diazepam** 0.2 mg/kg IV or midazolam 0.2 mg/kg IV or IM, or
    - ▪ **Acepromazine** 0.01–0.03 mg/kg, IM, IV, or
    - ▪ **Medetomidine** 2–6 µg/kg IV or 10–20 µg/kg IM (dogs), 4–10 µg/kg IV or 15–30 µg/kg IM (cats), or
    - ▪ **Dexmedetomidine** 1–3 µg/kg IV or 5–10 µg/kg IM (dogs), 2–5 µg/kg IV or 8–15 µg/kg IM (cats).
- **Induction**
  - ○ **Propofol** 2–6 mg/kg, IV to effect, or
  - ○ **Alfaxalone** 1–3 mg/kg, IV to effect, or
  - ○ **Ketamine with midazolam or diazepam** (1:1): 0.1–0.2 mL/kg, IV to effect (in this case, do not use a benzodiazepine as a pre-medicant).

- ○ **Telazol** 6–10 mg/kg IM or IV.
- ○ **Etomidate** (1–3 mg/kg).
- **Intraoperative maintenance** with inhalant anesthesia (isoflurane or sevoflurane) for procedure >20 min is recommended. **TIVA** (total intravenous anesthesia) with propofol or alfaxalone (refer to Chapter 13) may be used until the patient can be intubated and placed on inhalants. The ketamine induction dose should provide 20 min of anesthesia and could be repeated twice if necessary. The Telazol induction dose should provide 30–45 min of anesthesia but should not be repeated as rough recoveries can occur.
- Should hypotension develop under anesthesia refer to Chapter 19, Section **II.B.3.**
- **Recovery** is likely to be uncomplicated but analgesia should be addressed. Patients can be sedated with a low dose of alpha$_2$ agonist if dysphoric.

IV. Injury

A. Hypothermia Induced/Associated Injuries

Analgesic requirements must be based on the patient at hand, the level of consciousness, core temperature, associated injuries and pain behaviours exhibited. Opioids are the analgesic of choice and must be titrated to affect to avoid a "relative" overdose. Avoid IM and subcutaneous (SC) administration of analgesics unless the rare situation indicating this route prior to IV access is necessary. Opioids are more slowly metabolized in a hypothermic patient, which in turn prolongs the hypothermic event. When stable and an analgesic state is established, commence secondary survey examination for injuries and treatment of frostbite.

1. **Frostbite**
   a. **Rapid warming** of frostbitten tissues should be carried out as soon as possible while monitoring core temperature. Immerse the affected area in water of no more than 40–42 °C (104–108 °F) for at least 20 min or until thawing is complete. This may confer comfort; however, this is patient dependent. Placing the patient in a "bath" may be required should the torso be affected. If this is not possible due to other injuries and for areas that cannot be immersed such as ears and head, apply moist warmed 40–42 °C (104–108 °F) towels to the lesion. Dry heat should not be used. Never rub or massage the tissues.
   b. **Analgesia**
      i. **Box 34.1.**
      ii. **Ketamine.** Box 34.1, point 2 may be required in addition to the opioid as pain may worsen when sensation returns to the tissues.
      iii. **Aloe vera**, a potent anti-prostaglandin agent is recommended to cover the frostbitten areas q6h. The local anti-inflammatory affect will also reduce progression of pain.
      iv. Application of a **loose, soft, dry bandage** to the injured part is required to protect the area from self-inflicted, or other, trauma. Where digits are affected further pain reduction may be achieved with padding between the digits to avoid lateral digital pressure. A splint may be required (refer to Chapter 31). Padding between the limbs when in lateral recumbency is also required to elevate the upper limb and avoid dependent, re-perfusion edema which is also painful (Figure 34.1).
      v. **Cage rest** is required to reduce injury and pain.
      vi. **NSAIAs:** a COX-2 preferential (e.g. meloxicam, as a minimal amount of COX-1 activity may be beneficial to reduce thrombosis) can be administered when re-warming

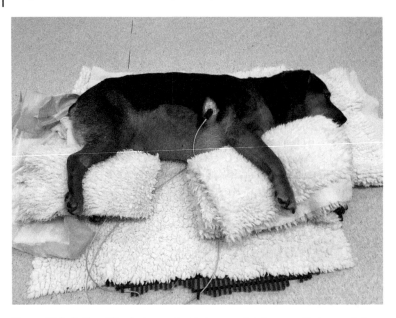

Figure 34.1 Soft padding between the limbs to maintain upper limbs parallel.

is complete, perfusion is established, gastrointestinal and renal abnormalities are ruled out and rhabdomyolysis is not occurring. In addition to analgesia, the systemic anti-prostaglandin activity has been shown to limit the cascade of the inflammatory effects of hypothermic injury in humans.

- **Do not use in** pregnant, nursing cats, or puppies and kittens less than 6 weeks of age, or when corticosteroids are prescribed. **Carprofen** 2 mg/kg (lean body weight) q12h for up to six days may be considered in lactating dogs (refer to Chapter 24). Consult the NSAIA package insert prior to administration to verify age as this varies with each product.

c. **Anesthesia.**

Surgical management should be delayed until spontaneous amputation of necrotic tissue has occurred and is complete. Definitive surgical management is based on the individual injury. Minor procedures can often be performed with opioids and local blocks with no general anesthesia necessary. However, should anesthesia be required for any emergency diagnostic, medical or surgical procedure:

i. **Pre-medication and induction:**
   - **Refer to Box 34.3.**

ii. **Maintenance and intraoperative.**
   - Extreme hypothermia causes a reduction in MAC (minimum alveolar concentration; the "dose" of the inhalant gas) so inhalant concentrations should be kept low.
   - In **extremely hypothermic patients a fentanyl infusion** as described in Box 34.1 may be effective at maintaining anesthesia with no or minimal inhalant necessary. The advantage of this technique is a reduced impact on the body temperature since inhalants contribute significantly to hypothermia.
   - **Active warming** should be continued as inhalant-induced vasodilation and anesthesia-induced impairment of the thermoregulatory system will lead to further decreases in body temperature. Hypothermia can also lead to hypotension, hypoventilation and bradycardia that is **not** responsive to anticholinergic therapy. Thus, support of normotension using positive inotropes and pressors and support of normoventilation using assisted ventilation may be necessary.

- Use appropriate analgesic techniques such as infusion of opioids and local anesthetic blockade.

iii. **Post-operative:**
  - Expect to continue physiologic support well into recovery, which will be prolonged when compared to recovery of a normothermic patient.
  - Re-address analgesia as appropriate for the particular injury.
  - Hypothermia can cause clotting dysfunction and immunosuppression so check clotting times if concerned about bleeding.

B. Nursing Considerations

1. **Monitoring pain:** as mentioned, pain level may increase as the patient warms and becomes more aware. It is important to be prepared to deal with this pain as it occurs. Consider a CRI of an opioid that can be titrated easily as needed during the re-warming phase.

2. **Monitoring concerns:** hypothermic patients in the re-warming phase must be monitored closely.
   a. **Temperature:** as mentioned, most standard thermometers will not read below 32 °C, and a dedicated **precision** thermometer should be used. Some thermometers available on multi-parameter monitors will read lower temperatures. If continuous temperature is not available, temperatures should be taken every 10–15 min while warming. Avoid actively warming the patient beyond 37 °C (104 °F) or when the patient stops shivering, but passive measures can be maintained.
   b. **Shivering** can result in not only tremendous muscle pain but also increased oxygen demands. Providing oxygen supplementation during the shivering phases may be warranted.
   c. **ECG** monitoring will facilitate a rapid response to arrhythmias should they arise. Hypothermic patients may be bradycardic and prone to arrhythmias and cardiovascular collapse during re-warming.

3. **Warming types** are "passive" or "active".
   a. **Passive re-warming** relies on insulation and allowing the patient to generate its own heat. Covering with warm or reflective blankets will help the patient to slowly warm itself; however, this method is only successful with mild hypothermia. If the patient is wet, drying with a hair dryer will provide some supplemental heat (external re-warming) while avoiding further heat loss.
   b. **Active re-warming** involves either external or internal re-warming. External re-warming is easy to perform and involves the use of warming devices such as microwavable rice or oat bags, IV fluid bags or warming systems such as forced air, or blanket systems. **Caution** must be used with external warming devices as burns may occur more easily in hypothermic, recumbent patients. Items warmed in a microwave should be mixed thoroughly to avoid hot spots, and electric type heating pads or conductive warmers should only be placed on the patient, never under the patient.
   c. **Active internal warming** may be accomplished with warmed IV fluids using balanced crystalloid solutions warmed to 40 °C (104 °F). Depending on the fluid rate, this may be accomplished using a bowl of warm water, in which the IV line is coiled close to the patient or a blood warmer. Microwaves should be avoided, but storing some fluids in a warming cabinet would be ideal. If using slow flow rates, fluids will likely cool before reaching the patient. Other methods of active re-warming include peritoneal lavage with warmed, sterile isotonic NaCl or lactated Ringer's solution (do not use PlasmaLyte or Normosol solutions, these are painful) and gastric lavage or enemas with warm water.

V. Hyperthermia

Causes include increased activity, hot environmental conditions and impaired heat dissipating mechanisms (i.e. inability to pant). Hyperthermia, associated with hot environmental situations (worsened by increasing humidity), may be exhibited as:

1. **Heat stress:** thirst, discomfort associated with physical activity, and may progress to:
2. **Heat exhaustion:** intense thirst, weakness, discomfort, anxiety, fainting/collapse, associated with physical activity, or
3. **Heatstroke (classical):** severe illness associated with abnormal brain function and multi-internal organ involvement, not associated with exercise (locked in a car), or
4. **Exertional heatstroke:** similar clinical presentation as classical heatstroke but associated with physical activity.

While pain is not associated with hyperthermia, associated injuries, either traumatic or subsequent to organ involvement, will cause pain.

1. **Analgesia**
   a. **Box** 34.1 where pain is identified with associated illness and injuries.
   b. For **continuing analgesia**, refer to sections related to identified illness and injury.
2. **Anesthesia**
   Depending on the body temperature, these patients may be at extreme risk for anesthesia-related adverse events. Anesthesia should be delayed until the body temperature is stable and either normal or only slightly above normal. Should anesthesia be required due to associated injuries prior to achieving normothermia:
   a. **Pre-medication:** depending on the body temperature, hyperthermic patients may be agitated and require sedation. If possible, the patient should be sedated with an **opioid from Box** 34.1 administered IV. The mu-agonist opioids can cause hyperthermia in cats; therefore, buprenorphine or butorphanol (with dosages repeated as necessary to compensate for the short duration) may be better choices until the temperature is normal. Combine with a sedative.
   b. **Sedation with midazolam or diazepam** 0.2 mg/kg. If more sedation is needed, consider **acepromazine** (0.02 mg/kg IV or IM) as acepromazine is a vasodilator, which can aid in heat dissipation. Sedation with an **alpha₂ agonist (Box** 34.2) may be necessary and is reversible should adverse effects occur.
   c. **Induction:** the patient should be rapidly induced to anesthesia with any of the induction drugs listed in Box 34.3.
   d. **Maintenance and intraoperative:** anesthesia can be maintained with isoflurane or sevoflurane and the vasodilatory properties of the inhalants may help to dissipate heat. However, inhalants impair the response of the thermoregulatory centre so other heat dissipating responses, like panting, will be absent. Monitor body temperature closely so that normothermia is achieved but hypothermia is avoided. Cardiovascular support is critical since hyperthermia causes decreased cardiac output, hypotension and tachyarrhythmia. Cardiac arrest can also occur. Hyperthermia-related acid-base and electrolyte abnormalities can also adversely affect the heart. Ventilation may need to be supported to ensure that anesthesia-induced hypoventilation with subsequent respiratory acidosis does not occur and compound any heat-induced metabolic acidosis. As with other patients, address pain with opioids and local blocks.
   e. **Post-operative:** continue oxygen and fluid support with any anti-arrhythmic or other support instituted during anesthesia. Hyperthermia can cause agitation or even seizures, so be prepared to dose the patient with sedatives, benzodiazepines and/or propofol. These effects are less likely to occur if the patient is normothermic, which is likely by recovery, but they should still be anticipated.

VI. Immersion (Near Drowning)

Pain is not associated with immersion unless very cold (see Section **IV**.A) and/or associated with injury or subsequent illness. However, "near-drowning" will result in a degree of respiratory distress where intubation and oxygenation may be indicated and general anesthesia required.

A. Respiratory Distress

1. **Analgesia**
   a. **Opioids Box 34.1**. If physical findings identify pain, refer to the sections these associated findings indicate for specific ongoing analgesic management.
2. **Anesthesia**
   a. If at all possible, these patients should not be anesthetized until they can maintain a normal SpO_2.
   b. **Pre-medication and induction:** refer to Box 34.3.
3. **Maintenance:** depending on why the patient is anesthetized, **inhalants or a propofol CRI of 0.1–0.4 mg/kg/min** should be administered. Oxygen therapy is critical and positive pressure ventilation may be required. Analgesia should be added as needed for painful conditions/procedures. The patients will likely be hypothermic so low-end dosages of reversible drugs, e.g., opioids, should be considered. If being anesthetized solely for oxygen and ventilator support, analgesia may not be necessary but body temperature support should be provided. The propofol CRI is the preferred method of anesthesia for ventilator support.
4. **Recovery:** this may be the most critical phase of anesthesia for these patients. Keep the patients calm and pain-free to avoid increased respiratory work. Do not remove the endotracheal (ET) tube until the patient can no longer tolerate it. Maintain the patient on oxygen support. The pulse oximeter can be used to determine whether or not the patient is oxygen dependent.

B. Emergent Surgical Procedures

Analgesia and anesthesia as for respiratory distress (see point A above).

VII. Snake Envenomation

Pain associated with envenomation results mostly from local and systemic myolysis. These patients are often recumbent with an impaired gag reflex and significant ventilatory dysfunction. If the patient is showing respiratory compromise, have supplies ready for intubation prior to administering an analgesic and if possible delay analgesic administration until the antivenin has been administered.

A. Analgesia

1. **Opioids Box 34.1.**
   A set dose of an opiate may be excessive for some patients and is potentially dangerous. To ensure safety, slowly titrate methadone or fentanyl. Buprenorphine can also be used; however, titration to effect is difficult due to delay in onset of action. Hydromorphone administered slowly to effect can also be considered but it should be administered cautiously given its known propensity to cause vomiting.
2. **NSAIA:** where rhabdomyolysis is noted, acute kidney injury may occur; therefore, it should not be administered. Acetaminophen is not contraindicated in dogs.

VIII. Porcupine Quill Injury

Usually, these patients are healthy and may only have a few quills. The most frequent locations for quills are head and neck region (Figure 34.2), followed by the oral cavity then limbs and trunk. Frequently, quills land in multiple locations and it is essential to conduct a slow, careful examination/palpation of the entire body to locate potential hidden quills. While the majority of quills may be easily visualized, there is always one or more that is detected by palpation/stroking in a retrograde direction. **Minimize movement** as quills embedded in the chest and legs may migrate further through tissues. To facilitate a thorough examination, analgesia is essential.

A. Analgesia

1. **Opioids Box 34.1**. A set dose of an opiate may be excessive for some patients and is potentially dangerous. To ensure safety, slowly titrate methadone or fentanyl. Hydromorphone administered slowly to effect can also be considered but it should be administered cautiously given its known propensity to cause vomiting. The **ocular and periocular** regions are frequently involved. Do not use force to open a painful blepharospastic eye. Place a single drop of **topical anesthetic (e.g. 1% proparacaine HCl)** into the eye if the dog cannot open their eyes because of pain.
2. **In general** the dog should be anesthetized to allow ease of removal and thorough oral examination. However, this is case dependent based on the number and location of quills, and the co-operation of the dog. If anesthesia is not possible, deep sedation with analgesia should be utilized.
3. **Mouth and pharynx:** anesthesia is required to thoroughly examine. Quills are frequently located in the hard palate, gingiva, buccal mucosa, muzzle and nose (Figure 34.3). A few may make it to the pharyngeal area as well. Careful examination, including the nares, is required as some quills may be damaged/broken due to the dog scratching. These quills must be found and removed as they will migrate and be a constant source of inflammation, abscessation and pain.

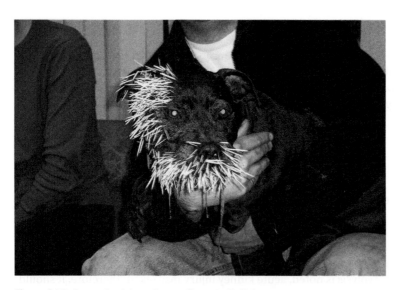

Figure 34.2 Porcupine injury. *Source:* Courtesy Dr K. Lamey.

B. Anesthesia

1. These are often young, healthy patients and anesthetic choices for this patient population are provided in **Box** 34.3.
2. If the **quills extend through the mouth and into the pharynx**, intubation is not recommended until quills that might be pushed into the trachea by the ET tube have been removed. In this case, use an **injectable protocol** and provide "flow by" oxygen by placing the end of the rebreathing hoses near the patient's nose or mouth and flowing oxygen only (no inhalant) through the anesthetic machine. Alternatively, a tube that is small and can be easily passed through the arytenoids can be placed and oxygen delivered by the machine as described for "blow by". If the tube is smaller than what the patient would be intubated with, do not inflate the cuff, as breathing through a very small airway increases the work of breathing. **Intubate with an appropriately sized tube** and inflate the ET tube cuff (to prevent aspiration of blood) as soon as possible.

   These patients **will be painful**. An NSAIA should be included in the therapy since there will be a large amount of inflammation. Opioids are also required, at least intraoperatively.

C. Quill Removal

1. When removing quills, use mosquito forceps and pull the quill slowly, while applying counter-pressure with the non-dominant hand. Quills can break easily. Also, counter-pressure prevents tenting of the skin, which may bury nearby quills, making them almost impossible to remove. **Where quills cannot be removed** due to penetration/swelling/abscess etc., a surgical approach is required. To identify quill location in a large area of swelling, in a joint or intrathoracic or other area, ultrasonographic guidance is recommended/essential.
2. **Surgical exploration** must be performed cautiously so as to not damage the quill, as quill splinters may be difficult to find and will be a continual source of inflammation and pain. Referral to a speciality centre is recommended for the difficult to access areas.

   For the majority of cases, the patient is discharged home after recovery from anesthesia unless there is concern for migration into the thorax. In this case, 24 h observation is recommended.
3. **Discharge analgesia** is dependent on degree of injury. The patient in Figure 34.2 and Figure 34.3 will be moderately painful requiring an NSAIA for a minimum of three days to

Figure 34.3 Severe porcupine quill injury to the level of the pharynx. *Source:* Courtesy Dr K. Lamey.

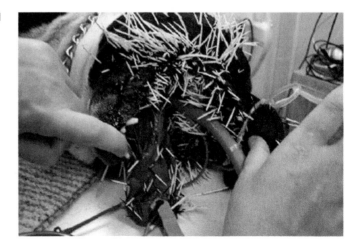

facilitate eating and sleeping and to avoid self-mutilation. **Do not use in** pregnant, nursing cats, or puppies and kittens less than 6 weeks of age, or when corticosteroids are prescribed. Carprofen 2 mg/kg (lean body weight) q12h for up to six days may be considered in lactating dogs (refer to Chapter 24). Consult the NSAIA package insert prior to administration to verify age, as this varies with each product.

4. **Owners should be warned** about the potential of a hidden quill; clinical signs will depend on location. If there is the potential for intrathoracic migration, alert the owner of clinical signs. A recent case report described a 5-year-old Boston terrier following a porcupine attack. More than 100 quills were removed on initial visit from head, limbs, chest and flank; however, many quills were palpated beneath the skin. Five days later, the dog demonstrated extraocular pain and was referred to a speciality centre for further evaluation. Computed tomography (CT) and magnetic resonance imaging (MRI) scans identified pulmonary and abdominal involvement requiring abdominal and thoracic surgery. Six days after discharge, the dog died. At post-mortem quill migration was noted in the right ventricle, pulmonary artery, vertebral canal at C4/C5, foramen magnum an base of the brain, trachea and in the cortex and medulla of the kidney.

IX.   Smoke Inhalation

A.   Analgesia

1. **Opioids (Box 34.1).** The pain experienced will vary with severity of injury (refer to Chapter 33, Section II.C); therefore, to assess the appropriate analgesic dose, **titrate dosages IV slowly** until the patient is comfortable – stop at the onset of a slight pant. Only use the IM route if IV access cannot be obtained due to patient's behaviour. **Avoid cough suppressants (i.e. butorphanol)** as they prevent expectoration of inhaled smoke particles.
2. **Benzodiazepines (Box 34.2)**, in conjunction with an opioid, are recommended to decrease anxiety.
3. **NSAIAs (Box 34.1): avoid** until the patient is stable and with normal renal function. Avoid COX-1 selective due to potential interference with PG bronchodilation.
4. **Ketamine (Box 34.1)** added to the opioid for potential moderate to severe pain associated with injuries is recommended as ketamine has bronchodilation properties.

B.   Anesthesia

1. **Propofol 2–6 mg/kg, IV,** following an opioid above, should be administered to effect to allow ET intubation followed by a **CRI of 0.1–0.4 mg/kg/min**.
2. **If general anesthesia** is needed for surgical procedures, use the protocols listed in Section VI.A. Anesthesia should be postponed if at all possible until the patient can maintain normal SpO_2.

Further Reading

Flesher, K., Lam, N. and Donovan, T. A. (2017) Diagnosis and treatment of massive porcupine quill migration in a dog. *Can Veterinary J*, 58: 28–284.

Mathews, K. A. (ed.) (2017) *Veterinary Emergency & Critical Care Manual*, 3rd edn. LifeLearn, Guelph, Ontario, Canada.

Index

Note: Page numbers in *italic* denote figures/boxes, those in **bold** denote tables.

a

abdomen block, local anesthetics   190–198
abdominal pain
   analgesia   57
   gastrointestinal (GI) and pelvic
      neurophysiology   51–55
   gastrointestinal system   55–56
   inflammatory bowel disease   56
   pancreatitis/pancreatic pain   56–57
   sources of pain   55–59
   spleen   56
   urogenital system   57–59
A-beta Fibre Mediated Inhibition, neuropathic
   pain   21
acepromazine   113–114, 248, 273, **274**
   adverse effects   113
   cardio-respiratory effects   113
   contraindications   114
   environmental injuries   *456*
   geriatric patients   333
   head/neck injuries   345
   integument injuries   *442*
   kidney disease   259
   liver disease   267
   musculoskeletal pain   *411, 412*
   nursing patients   301
   pregnant patients   287
   thorax   358, 359
   torso/abdomen   *378, 379, 393, 394*
   vertebral column   *425*
acetaminophen (paracetamol), nursing
   patients   300
acupuncture   205–207
   neuropathic pain   24, 43

acute kidney injury/failure (AKI/F), anesthetic
   considerations   257–261
acute pain management, neuropathic
   pain   36–43
adjunctive analgesics   **102**, 144–161
   case example   161
   nursing patients   300–301
adjunct medications, kidney disease   260–261
adverse effects
   see also compatibility of drugs
   acepromazine   113
   analgesics   2–5, 146–147, 150–152,
      154–159
   tramadol   131
   venlafaxine   159–160
affective visceral co-morbidities,
   pathophysiology   61–62
aggressive patients   270–277
   cats   271–272
   dogs   270–271
   handling strategies   270–272
   initial presentation   3–4
   protocols   273–277
   risk factor for anesthesia- adverse events   **273**
   sedation/anesthesia   272–277
airway obstruction   343–346, 350
alfaxalone   166–167, 249, 273, **274**, 277
   cesarean section   291
   environmental injuries   *456*
   musculoskeletal pain   *412*
   nursing patients   303
   pregnant patients   288
   thoracic cavity injury   364
   torso/abdomen   *379*

Analgesia and Anesthesia for the Ill or Injured Dog and Cat, First Edition. Karol A. Mathews, Melissa Sinclair,
Andrea M. Steele and Tamara Grubb.
© 2018 John Wiley & Sons, Inc. Published 2018 by John Wiley & Sons, Inc.

alfentanil   128

allodynia   73, 74

  neuropathic pain test   25

alpha₂ adrenergic receptor function   21

alpha₂ adrenoceptor agonists   114–116, 248, **275**, 284, 287, 316

  bradycardia   151–152

  dexmedetomidine   151–152

  geriatric patients   332, 333

  kidney disease   256, 259

  liver disease   267

  neuropathic pain   23–24, 41

  nursing patients   302

  pediatric patients   316

  pregnant patients   284, 287–288

  torso/abdomen   *379, 394*

alveolar block, local anesthetics   179–180

amantadine   153–154

  adverse effects   154

  chronic pain   43

  dosing   154

  environmental injuries   *456*

  head/neck injuries   *339*, 342

  indications   153

  kidney disease   257

  liver disease   264

  mode of action   153

  musculoskeletal pain   *411, 416*

  neuropathic pain   23, 39, 40, 43

  nursing patients   301

  pregnant patients   284

  thorax   361

  torso/abdomen   *380*, 394

amitriptyline   158–159

  kidney disease   257

  liver disease   264

  nursing patients   300

  pregnant patients   285

amputation

  cancer pain   65–66

  coccygeal vertebrae amputation   433, *434*

  neuropathic pain   29–31

analgesia

  abdominal pain   57

  initial presentation   6

analgesia considerations

  kidney disease   256–257

  liver disease   263–264

analgesic orders   217–218

analgesic regimens

cats   **103–109**

dogs   **90–94, 100–102**

analgesics   230–242

  adverse effects   2–5, 146–147, 150–152, 154–160

  bolus dosing   230–231

  burette delivery   233–234

  cardiovascular disease   244–246

  compatibility of drugs   239–242

  continuous rate infusion (CRI)   231–233

  diluting drugs   237–239

  elastomeric pump delivery   236

  fluid bag delivery   232–233

  masking signs of patient deterioration   2

  nursing patients   295–300

  pediatric patients   311–316

  pregnant patients   279–285

  standardized concentration infusions   235–236

  syringe pump delivery   237–239

anal gland abscess   406

anesthesia

  cesarean section   288–292

  pregnant patients   286–292

anesthetic induction, cesarean section   290

anesthetic maintenance, cesarean section   290–291

anesthetic plans   *251–253*

  chronic kidney disease (CKD)   *260–261*

  liver disease   *268*

anesthetic recovery, nursing care plans   227–228

anticholinergics, geriatric patients   333

anti-nociception

  dexmedetomidine   115

  opioids/opiates   120–121

antitussive effects, opioids/opiates   121–122

arteritis, neuropathic pain   35

ascending analgesic pathway, physiologic pain   12

aspirin (salicylates), nursing patients   299

assessing pain *see* pain assessment

auricular injuries   348–349

avulsion   445–446

axillary approach, brachial plexus block   184–185

axillary block, local anesthetics   187

b

bacterial dermatitis   450

balanoposthitis   405

benzodiazepines   117–118, **274, 275**

  cardio-respiratory effects   117

co-induction with injectable anesthetics
117–118, 168–169
  dose recommendations   117, 118
  kidney disease   259
  liver disease   267
  nursing patients   301
  reversal   118
Bier block, local anesthetics   199
bite wounds   366–369, 446
bladder   403
blood pressure, anesthetic considerations   250
bolus dosing, analgesics   230–231
bowel distension   385
bowel rupture/perforation, intussusceptions,
    foreign body   385, *386*
brachial plexus block
  axillary approach   184–185
  local anesthetics   184–185
  paravertebral approach   185–186
bradycardia, alpha$_2$ adrenoceptor
    agonists   151–152
breakthrough pain (BTP)   15, 68–69, 73–74
bupivacaine   172
  nursing patients   302
  prolonged-release bupivacaine   201
  thoracic cavity injury   364
buprenorphine   129–130, **276**
  head/neck injuries   343–345, 347
  integument injuries   *440*
  musculoskeletal pain   *416*
  nursing patients   297–298
  pediatric patients   **312**
  pregnant patients   282
  thorax   357
  torso/abdomen   *380*, 394
burette delivery, analgesics   233–234
burns   442–445
  chemical/caustic burns   444–445
  thermal burns   443–444
butorphanol   130, **276**
  head/neck injuries   344, 345
  integument injuries   *440*
  nursing patients   296–297
  pediatric patients   **312**
  pregnant patients   282
  thorax   357

c

cancer pain   64–67
  gait abnormalities   65
  management   64–67

physiology   64–67
cannabinoids, neuropathic pain   45
cardio-respiratory effects
  acepromazine   113
  benzodiazepines   117
  dexmedetomidine   115–116
  ketamine   167–168
cardio-respiratory systems, pregnant
    patients   286
cardiovascular disease   244–253
  analgesics   244–246
  anesthetic considerations   246–253
  co-morbidity for anesthesia   244–253
cardiovascular effects, opioids/opiates   121
catheters
  intraosseous (IO) catheter placement,
    neonate patients   *324–325*
  intraosseous (IO) catheter placement,
    pediatric patients   *323–325*
  wound diffusion catheters   361
  wound infusion catheter block, local
    anesthetics   200–201
central nervous system
  congenital/developmental lesions   35
  neuropathic pain   19–20, 34–35
  tumours   34–35
central pain syndrome   437
  neuropathic pain   34–35
cesarean section   288–292
  see also pregnant patients
chemical/caustic burns   444–445
Chinese herbs   207
chronic kidney disease (CKD)   255–261
  anesthetic plans   *260–261*
  proton pump inhibitors (PPIs)   140
chronic pain, neuropathic pain   17, 43–44
CKD *see* chronic kidney disease
clonidine   **274**
coccygeal vertebrae amputation   433, *434*
co-induction agents, injectable
    anesthetics   117–118, 168–169
co-induction with injectable anesthetics,
    benzodiazepines   117–118
Colorado State University (CSU), pain
    scale   76
colostrum   294–295
common peroneal block, local
    anesthetics   197–198
compatibility of drugs
  see also adverse effects
  analgesics   239–242

conditions, pain levels associated with **82**
congenital/developmental lesions, neuropathic pain 35
constipation, opioids/opiates 122
continuous rate infusion (CRI)
   analgesics 231–233, 357
   environmental injuries *454*
   integument injuries *440*
   musculoskeletal pain *410*
   thorax 357
   torso/abdomen *377, 392*
   vertebral column *424*
corticosteroids 160
   head/neck injuries 345
corticotropin-releasing hormone (CRH) 61
cosmetic surgery, pediatric patients 309
COX-1,2,3 *see* cyclooxygenase…
CRH (corticotropin-releasing hormone) 61
CRI *see* continuous rate infusion
crush injuries 446
cryotherapy 210–211
cyclooxygenase 1 (COX-1) 134–135, **137**
   nursing patients 299
   selective NSAIA administration 2
cyclooxygenase 2 (COX-2) 135, **137**
   nursing patients 299
   thorax 361
   torso/abdomen 394
cyclooxygenase 3 (COX-3) 135, **137**

d

defecation/urination, patient comfort 224–225
degloving injuries *397, 446*
dermatologic pain 448
descending inhibitory pathway
   neuropathic pain 20–21
   pathologic pain 14
   physiologic pain 11
detomidine, nursing patients 302
dexamethasone 160
dexmedetomidine 115–116, 151–152, 273, **274**
   adverse effects 151–152
   anti-nociception 115
   cardio-respiratory effects 115–116
   dose recommendations 115
   environmental injuries *456*
   head/neck injuries *339, 342*
   indications 151

integument injuries *442*
   mode of action 151
   musculoskeletal pain *411*
   reversal 116, 152
   thorax 358–360
   torso/abdomen *378, 379, 393, 394*
   vertebral column *425*
diabetic neuropathy 421
   neuropathic pain 34
diagnosis, neuropathic pain 24–27
diaphragmatic hernia 371–372
diazepam 117–118, **275**
   environmental injuries *456*
   integument injuries *442*
   musculoskeletal pain *411*
   thoracic cavity injury 364
   thorax 358, 359
   torso/abdomen *377, 378, 393*
   vertebral column *425*
diluting drugs, analgesics 237–239
diphenylhydramine **274**
direct injection block, local anesthetics 200
discharge analgesia and management
   thorax 372–373
   torso/abdomen *380*, 394
   vertebral column 425–426
discospondylitis, neuropathic pain 33
dopamine 260
dose recommendations
   benzodiazepines 117, 118
   dexmedetomidine 115
   thoracic cavity injury 364–365
drug eruption 450
duloxetine 160
   neuropathic pain 45
dysphoria
   opioids/opiates 122
   pain assessment 72

e

ECG monitoring, initial presentation 1
elastomeric pump delivery, analgesics 236
emergence delirium, pain assessment 72
EMLA® (eutectic mixture of local anesthetic) cream 201–202
   pediatric patients 201–202, 317–318
emotional component to pain management 213–214
endogenous analgesic pathways, physiologic pain 11–12

endogenous descending facilitatory systems, neuropathic pain   20
environmental injuries   454–464
   hyperthermia   460
   hypothermia induced/associated injuries   457–459
   immersion (near drowning)   461
   nursing considerations   459
   porcupine quill injury   462–464
   smoke inhalation   464
   snake envenomation   461
EP4 receptor   136
epidural analgesia, cesarean section   291
epidural block   414
   local and regional anesthesia   414
   local anesthetics   190–195
   opioids/opiates   **191**
   repeated drug administration   193–194
   sacrococcygeal epidural block   194–195
   single lumbosacral epidural block   191–193
   thorax   360–361
   torso/abdomen   *379, 380*
esophageal lesions/obstruction   370–371
etomidate   249
   environmental injuries   *457*
   musculoskeletal pain   *412*
   nursing patients   303
   thoracic cavity injury   367
   thorax   359, 360
   torso/abdomen   *379*
eye block, local anesthetics   180–182

f

fasciitis   419–420, 448, *449, 450*
FCEM (fibrocartilaginous embolic myelopathy)   33, 433
femoral block, local anesthetics   195
fenoldopam   261
fentanyl   126–127
   cesarean section   289
   derivatives   128
   environmental injuries   *454*
   head/neck injuries   *338, 339,* 342, 345
   integument injuries   *440*
   musculoskeletal pain   *409, 412*
   neuropathic pain   36–37
   nursing patients   295–296
   pediatric patients   **312, 313**
   pregnant patients   281
   thorax   357

   torso/abdomen   *377, 392*
   transdermal (Recuvyra®, Elanco)   127
   vertebral column   *424*
fentanyl transdermal patches   127
   head/neck injuries   342–343, 347
   musculoskeletal pain   *416*
fibrocartilaginous embolic myelopathy (FCEM)   33, 433
flecainide, neuropathic pain   41
fluid bag delivery, analgesics   232–233
foreign body (FB)   366–369
   mouth/pharynx/trachea/ esophagus   345
   torso/abdomen   384, 385, *386*
fractures   415–417
   pelvic fractures   28
   rib fractures/flail chest   362, *363*
frostbite   457–459
future therapeutic modalities, neuropathic pain   45

g

GABA-mediated inhibition, neuropathic pain   21
gabapentin   154–156, **274**
   adverse effects   155–156
   cardiovascular disease   246
   chronic pain   43–44
   dosing   156
   environmental injuries   *456*
   head/neck injuries   *339,* 342
   indications   154–155
   kidney disease   257
   liver disease   264
   mode of action   155
   musculoskeletal pain   *411, 416*
   neck pain   354
   neuropathic pain   22, 42–44
   nursing patients   300
   opioid adjunct   111
   pediatric patients   316
   pregnant patients   284
   thorax   358
   torso/abdomen   *380,* 394
gait abnormalities, cancer pain   65
gallbladder distension, rupture and/or cholelithiasis   385
gastric dilation   383
gastrointestinal (GI) and pelvic neurophysiology   51–55

gastrointestinal system, abdominal
    pain   55–56
general anesthesia
    geriatric patients   333
    initial presentation   4–5
    nursing patients   303–304
geriatric patients   328–334
    anesthetic considerations   332–333
    cardiovascular considerations   330–331
    comfort   333–334
    feeding   334
    fluids administration   329
    general anesthesia   333
    hepatic function consideration   330
    initial evaluation   329
    laboratory testing prior to anesthesia   330
    nursing care   333–334
    opioids/opiates   329
    pain assessment   331–332
    pain management   333–334
    pre-medication   332–333
    pulmonary considerations   331
    renal function considerations   330
    sedatives   333
    temperature   333–334
    trauma effect   329
    urination/defecation   334
Glasgow Composite Measure Pain Scale
    (CMPS-SF)   76, 87
grape toxicity   401

h
head blocks, local anesthetics   173–182
head/neck injuries   336–354
    airway obstruction   343–346, 350
    auricular injuries   348–349
    cats   341
    dogs   341
    foreign body (FB) mouth/pharynx/trachea/
        esophagus   345
    initial management   336–340
    meningitis   35, 350–353, 437
    neck pain   353–354
    neoplasia   350–353
    ocular injuries   347–348
    oral cavity and upper airway injury/
        obstruction   343–346
    pain assessment   338
    syringomyelia   350–353
heart rate, pain assessment   71

heat stress, heat exhaustion, heatstroke,
    exertional heatstroke   460
hematoma   348–349
hemodynamically unstable patients,
    anesthesia   359–360
hemothorax   363
hepatitis/hepatomegaly   389
    see also liver disease
herbal pain medication   207
    pregnant patients   285
HOD (hypertrophic osteodystrophy)
    421–422
hunger/thirst, patient comfort   225, *226*
hydrocodone   132
hydromorphone   125–126, **276**
    cesarean section   289
    environmental injuries   *454, 456*
    head/neck injuries   *338*
    integument injuries   *440*
    musculoskeletal pain   *409, 412*
    neuropathic pain   36–37
    nursing patients   295
    pediatric patients   **312, 313**
    pregnant patients   282
    torso/abdomen   *377, 392*
    vertebral column   *424*
hyperalgesia   74
    neuropathic pain test   25
hyperthermia   460
    opioids/opiates   123
hypertrophic osteodystrophy (HOD)   421–422
hypothermia induced/associated
    injuries   457–459

i
immersion (near drowning)   461
immune-mediated disease   449–450
immune-mediated polyarthritis   418
immune response mechanisms, neuropathic
    pain   18–19
incisional line blocks, cesarean section   291
induction agents, liver disease   267–268
induction drugs/considerations
    see also co-induction agents
    cardiovascular disease   248–249
    kidney disease   261
    musculoskeletal pain   *412*
    nursing patients   304
    pediatric patients   320–321
    torso/abdomen   *394–395*

induction options, pregnant patients   288
infection-induced inflammation   389
inflammation, initial presentation   5
inflammatory bowel disease   56, 389
inflammatory conditions, non-steroidal anti-
  inflammatory analgesics (NSAIAs)   138
inflammatory pain   74
infraorbital block, local anesthetics   176–178
inguinal hernia repair, neuropathic pain   28
inhalational anesthesia   169–170, 249–250
  environmental injuries   *457*
  kidney disease   261
  liver disease   268–269
  torso/abdomen   *395*
initial presentation
  aggressive patients   3–4
  analgesia   6
  ECG monitoring   1
  general anesthesia   4–5
  inflammation   5
  non-steroidal antiinflammatory analgesics
    (NSAIAs)   2
  nursing patients   5
  pain management   1–6
  pediatric patients   5
  pregnant patients   5
  sedation   5–6
  sleep   6
injectable anesthetics   165–169
  co-induction agents   117–118, 168–169
integrative therapy   204–214
integument injuries   *397*, 439–452
intercostal block, local anesthetics   188
interpleural block, local anesthetics   188–190
intervertebral disc herniation/extrusion
    (IVDH/E), neuropathic pain   32
intra-articular block, local anesthetics   198–199
intraosseous (IO) catheter placement
  neonate patients   *324–325*
  pediatric patients   *323–325*
intravenous regional anesthesia (IVRA), local
    anesthetics   199
ischemic priapism   405
isoflurane, integument injuries   *442*
IVDH/E (intervertebral disc herniation/
    extrusion), neuropathic pain   32

k
kappa- agonist, mu-antagonist   130
ketamine   148–150, 167–168, 249, **276**

adverse effects   150
cardio-respiratory effects   167
cardiovascular disease   245
case example   38–39
with diazepam   167–168
dosing   150, 167
environmental injuries   *455, 456*
geriatric patients   332
head/neck injuries   *339, 342, 344*
indications   148–149
integument injuries   *441, 442*
kidney disease   256–257
with midazolam   167–168
mode of action   149
musculoskeletal pain   *410, 412*
neuropathic pain   22, 38–39
nursing patients   302, 303
patient comfort properties   149–150
pediatric patients   315–316
pregnant patients   283–284
thoracic cavity injury   364, 369
thorax   358, 359, 361
torso/abdomen   *378, 379, 392*
vertebral column   *424*
ketamine benzodiazepine, pregnant
    patients   288
kidney disease   255–261, 401
  adjunct medications   260–261
  analgesia considerations   256–257
  anesthetic considerations   257–261
  co-morbidity for anesthesia   255–261
  laboratory testing prior to anesthesia   258
  pre-operative examination prior to
    anesthesia   258
kidney injury, non-steroidal anti-inflammatory
    analgesics (NSAIAs)   140

l
lacerations   445–446
laser therapy (phototherapy)   212
lidocaine   145–148, 172
  adverse effects   146–147
  cardiovascular disease   245
  cats   147–148
  dogs   147
  environmental injuries   *455*
  head/neck injuries   *339, 346*
  indications   145–146
  integument injuries   *441*
  kidney disease   257

lidocaine (*cont'd*)
  liver disease   264
  mode of action   146
  musculoskeletal pain   *410*
  neuropathic pain   39–40
  nursing patients   301
  patches   148
  pediatric patients   318
  pregnant patients   284–285
  thoracic cavity injury   364
  thorax   358
  torso/abdomen   *378, 393*
  vertebral column   *425*
limb nerve entrapment, neuropathic pain   29
5-lipoxygenase (5-LOX) pathway   136
liver disease   263–269
  analgesia considerations   263–264
  anesthetic considerations   264–266
  anesthetic plans   *268*
  biotransformation   266
  co-morbidity for anesthesia   263–269
  drug elimination   266
  hepatic blood flow with anesthesia and
    surgery   266
  hepatitis/hepatomegaly   389
  laboratory testing prior to
    anesthesia   265–266
  pre-operative examination prior to
    anesthesia   265–266
  sedative and anesthetic
    considerations   267–268
local anesthetics   171–202
  abdomen block   190–198
  axillary block   187
  Bier block   199
  brachial plexus block   184–185
  cesarean section   291
  common peroneal block   197–198
  direct injection block   200
  EMLA® (eutectic mixture of local anesthetic)
    cream   201–202
  epidural block   190–195
  eye block   180–182
  femoral block   195
  geriatric patients   332
  head blocks   173–182
  head/neck injuries   346, 347
  infraorbital block   176–178
  intercostal block   188
  interpleural block   188–190

  intra-articular block   198–199
  intravenous regional anesthesia (IVRA)   199
  mandibular block   178–179
  maxillary block   174–176
  median block   187
  mental block   179–180
  musculocutaneous block   187
  neuropathic pain   23
  nursing patients   301–302
  opioids/opiates   **191**
  pediatric patients   201–202, 317–318
  pelvic limb block   190–198
  perineum block   190–198
  pregnant patients   284–285
  preparation for blocks   172–173
  prolonged-release bupivacaine   201
  radial block   187
  rostral mandibular block   179–180
  rostral maxillary block   176–178
  saphenous block   195–197
  sciatic block   197
  thoracic block   187–190
  thoracic limb block   182–187
  thorax   360–361
  tibial block   197–198
  topical local anesthetic creams   201–202
  torso/abdomen   *379–380*, 393
  toxicity   171–172
  ulnar block   187
  wound infusion catheter block   200–201
  wound management block   200–201
lumbosacral lesions, neuropathic pain   31
lung contusions, anesthesia   413

m
MAC (minimum alveolar concentration)
  requirements, pregnant patients   286
magnesium   160
maladaptive pain   8, 43, 74, 81
malignant peripheral nerve sheath tumours
  (MPNSTs), neuropathic pain   34
mandibular block, local anesthetics   178–179
mannitol   260–261
manual therapy techniques   207–208
MAOIs *see* monoamine oxidase inhibitors
maropitant   152–153
  head/neck injuries   *339*
  pancreatitis/pancreatic pain   388
  torso/abdomen   *378, 379, 393, 394*
mastectomy   148–149, *452*

mastitis   451, *452*
maxillary block, local anesthetics   174–176
MBST® Nuclear Magnetic Resonance
     Therapy   213
medetomidine
  see also dexmedetomidine
  environmental injuries   *456*
  integument injuries   *442*
  musculoskeletal pain   *411*
  thorax   358, 359
  torso/abdomen   *378, 379, 393, 394*
  vertebral column   *425*
median block, local anesthetics   187
medical pain   74
meningitis   350–353, 437
  neuropathic pain   35
mental block, local anesthetics   179–180
meperidine   129
  cesarean section   289
  nursing patients   296
  pediatric patients   **312**
methadone   129, **276**
  environmental injuries   *454, 456*
  head/neck injuries   *338*
  integument injuries   *440*
  musculoskeletal pain   *409, 412*
  neuropathic pain   36–37
  nursing patients   295
  pediatric patients   **312, 313**
  pregnant patients   281
  thorax   357, 359
  torso/abdomen   *377, 392*
  vertebral column   *424*
methocarbamol, neck pain   354
methylprednisolone   160
mexiletine, neuropathic pain   41
midazolam   117–118, 273, **275**, 277
  environmental injuries   *456*
  geriatric patients   333
  head/neck injuries   342
  musculoskeletal pain   *412*
  thorax   358
  torso/abdomen   *393*
minimum alveolar concentration (MAC)
     requirements, pregnant patients   286
modulation
  pathologic pain   13
  physiologic pain   10–11
monoamine oxidase inhibitors (MAOIs)
     157–160

adverse effects   157–158
  mode of action   157
morphine   124–125, **276**
  environmental injuries   *454, 456*
  head/neck injuries   *338*
  integument injuries   *440*
  musculoskeletal pain   *409, 412*
  neuropathic pain   36–37
  nursing patients   296
  pediatric patients   **312, 313**
  pregnant patients   282
  thorax   357, 359
  torso/abdomen   *377, 392*
  vertebral column   *424*
movement-evoked pain   15, 68–69, 73
MPNSTs (malignant peripheral nerve sheath
     tumours), neuropathic pain   34
mu opioid agonists   99–109, 124–130
  pediatric patients   314
musculocutaneous block, local
     anesthetics   187
musculoskeletal injuries   399–400
musculoskeletal pain   409–422
myocardial contusions, anesthesia   413–414
myositis   419–420, 448, *449*

n

nalbuphine, nursing patients   298
naloxone
  environmental injuries   *455*
  integument injuries   *441*
  musculoskeletal pain   *410*
  opioids/opiates   123–124
  thorax   357–358
  torso/abdomen   *377*
  vertebral column   *424*
neck pain   353–354
  see also head/neck injuries
neonatal/pediatric pain   14
neonate patients, intraosseous (IO) catheter
     placement   *324–325*
neoplasia   350–353, 384, 437
neuropathic pain   14, 17–46, 74
  acute pain management   36–43
  amputation   29–31
  assessing   26–27
  associated conditions   27–33
  categories   27
  central nervous system   19–20, 34–35
  central pain syndrome   34–35

neuropathic pain (*cont'd*)
  chronic pain   17, 43–44
  defining   17
  diagnosing   24–27
  features   26
  future therapeutic modalities   45
  immune response mechanisms   18–19
  inguinal hernia repair   28
  limb nerve entrapment   29
  lumbosacral lesions   31
  managing   17–46
  patient's experience   18
  pelvic fractures   28
  peripheral nervous system   19, 33–34
  physiology   18–21
  pudendal nerve entrapment   28–29
  sensitivity, altered   18–19
  serotonin and norepinephrine re-uptake
    inhibitor mixed compound   45
  spinal cord injury   32–33
  tests   25
  trauma   27–28
  tricyclic antidepressants (TCAs)   44
  vanilloid receptor 1 (TRPV1)
    antagonists   45
neurophysiology, gastrointestinal (GI) and
    pelvic neurophysiology   51–55
NMDA receptor antagonists
  neuropathic pain   22–23, 38–39
  nursing patients   302
nociception   70
  anti-nociception   115, 120–121
  vs pain   8–9
nociceptive pain   73
non-obstetrical procedures, pregnant
    patients   287
non-pharmacological interventions, pediatric
    patients   318–319
non-pharmacologic methods, pregnant
    patients   285
non-steroidal anti-inflammatory analgesics
    (NSAIAs)   134–140
  cardiovascular disease   246
  chronic pain   44
  contraindications   139–140
  environmental injuries   *455*
  geriatric patients   332
  head/neck injuries   *339*, 347
  indications   136–138
  inflammatory conditions   138

  initial presentation   2
  integument injuries   *441*
  kidney disease   257
  kidney injury   140
  liver disease   264
  musculoskeletal pain   *410, 415*
  neuropathic pain   24, 42, 44
  nursing patients   298–300
  osteoarthritis   138
  pediatric patients   315
  pharmacology   134–136
  post-operative pain   137
  pregnant patients   282–285
  pyrexia   138
  safety   138–139
  thorax   358, 361
  torso/abdomen   *380, 393*, 394
  trauma   137
  vertebral column   *425*
  veterinary-approved NSAIAs
    136, **137**
NSAIAs *see* non-steroidal anti-inflammatory
    analgesics
numerical rating scales (NRS)   75–76, 87
nursing care
  geriatric patients   333–334
  vertebral column   428–431
nursing care plans   219–228
nursing considerations
  environmental injuries   459
  pelvic injury/illness   395–396
  perineal injury/illness   395–396
  thorax   361
  torso/abdomen   380
nursing patients   294–304
  adjunctive analgesics   300–301
  analgesics   295–300
  anesthetics   302–303
  colostrum   294–295
  general anesthesia   303–304
  induction drugs/considerations   304
  inhalational anesthesia   303
  initial presentation   5
  intraoperative anesthesia   304
  local anesthetics   301–302
  NMDA receptor antagonists   302
  pre-medication   303
  recovery from general anesthesia   304
  relative infant dose (RID)   294
  sedatives   301

o

ocular injuries 347–348
opioid antagonism, pregnant patients 282
opioid immunosuppressive effects 2–3
opioid-induced hyperalgesia, pain
    assessment 72–73
opioid receptor function, neuropathic
    pain 20–21
opioids/opiates 119–132, 273, **276**, 277
    anti-nociception 120–121
    antitussive effects 121–122
    bolus dosing 230–231
    cardiovascular disease 244–245, 248
    cardiovascular effects 121
    cesarean section 292
    constipation 122
    dysphoria 122
    environmental injuries *454–455*
    epidural block **191**
    geriatric patients 329, 331–332
    head/neck injuries 336, *338–339*
    hyperthermia 123
    integument injuries *440–441*
    kappa- agonist, mu-antagonist 130
    kidney disease 256, 259
    liver disease 263–264, 267
    local anesthetics **191**
    mu opioid agonists 99–109,
        124–130
    musculoskeletal pain *409–410, 412*
    naloxone 123–124
    neuropathic pain 21–22, 36–38
    nursing patients 295–298
    oral opioids 131–132
    pediatric patients **312–313**, 314–315
    pharmacologic and clinical
        application 119–132
    pregnant patients 281–282, 287
    respiratory effects 121
    reversal 123
    sedation 119–120
    sphincter tone effects 122
    thorax 357
    torso/abdomen *377, 392*
    urinary retention 123
    vertebral column *423–424*
    vomiting 122
oral cavity and upper airway injury/
        obstruction 343–346

organomegaly 386
osteoarthritis, non-steroidal anti-inflammatory
        analgesics (NSAIAs) 138
osteomyelitis 420
osteosarcoma 418
otitis, acute severe 348–349
oxymorphone 126
    environmental injuries *454, 456*
    head/neck injuries *338*
    integument injuries *440*
    musculoskeletal pain *409, 412*
    nursing patients 296
    thorax 357, 359
    torso/abdomen *377, 392*
    vertebral column *424*

p

pain
    behavioural characteristics **83–84**
    defining 8, 70
    misconceptions 77–78
    vs nociception 8–9
    objective markers 71–73
    pathophysiology 8–15
    physiological parameters 71–73
    physiology 8–15
    types 14–15
    understanding pain 70–78
pain assessment 88–109
    adjunctive analgesics **102**
    analgesic regimens **90–94, 100–109**
    cats 89–95, 111
    clinical utility of methods 87–88
    dogs 88, 109–111
    geriatric patients 331–332
    head/neck injuries 338
    key points 82–87
    pediatric patients 310
    scales 75–78
pain levels associated with conditions **82**
pain management 17–46, 95–109
    acute pain management 36–43
    cancer pain 64–67
    geriatric patients 333–334
    inappropriate management 74
    initial presentation 1–6
    pediatric patients 309–310
    slow weaning 99
pain mechanisms 73–74

pain pathways
  pathologic pain 12–14
  physiologic pain 9–12
pain plan, nursing care plans 226–227
pain prevention, pediatric patients 308–309
pain scoring systems 75–78
pancreatitis/pancreatic pain 56–57, 386–389
panosteitis 421
paracetamol (acetaminophen), nursing
  patients 300
paraphimosis 405
paravertebral approach, brachial plexus
  block 185–186
partial mu-receptor agonist, pediatric
  patients 314–315
parvo enteritis 389
pathophysiology,
  affective visceral co-morbidities 61–62
patient advocates, veterinary technician or
  nurse (VT/N) 218
patient comfort, nursing care plans
  221–226
patient preparation, anesthetic
  considerations 246–247
pediatric patients 308–325
  analgesics 311–316
  anesthesia 319–325
  anesthetic dosages **322–323**
  cosmetic surgery 309
  EMLA® (eutectic mixture of local anesthetic)
    cream 201–202, 317–318
  induction drugs/considerations 320–321
  initial presentation 5
  intraosseous (IO) catheter
    placement *323–325*
  local anesthetics 201–202, 317–318
  maintenance drugs 321
  monitoring and support 321
  non-pharmacological
    interventions 318–319
  opioids/opiates **312–313**
  pain assessment 310
  pain management 309–310
  pain prevention 308–309
  patient preparation 319
  pre-medication 320
  recovery from general anesthesia 322–325
  sedatives 316–317
  topical local anesthetic creams 201–202,
    317–318

pelvic and gastrointestinal (GI)
  neurophysiology 51–55
pelvic cavity/abdomen injuries 396–399
pelvic fractures, neuropathic pain 28
pelvic injury/illness, nursing
  considerations 395–396
pelvic limb block, local anesthetics 190–198
pelvis 59–60
pelvis injuries 399–400
PEMF (Pulsed Electromagnetic Field)
  Therapy 213
penetrating injuries 447
penetrating injury/foreign body/bite
  wounds 366–369
penis and prepuce dogs 397–399
perception
  pathologic pain 14
  physiologic pain 11
perianal fistulae 406
perineal hernia 405–406
perineal injury/illness 400, 405–407
  nursing considerations 395–396
perineum 59–60
perineum block, local anesthetics 190–198
peripheral nervous system, neuropathic
  pain 19, 33–34
peritonitis 383
pethidine *see* meperidine
phantom limb 29–30, 421
phototherapy (laser therapy) 212
physical rehabilitation 208–213
placental blood barrier, pregnant
  patients 287
pneumonia/pleuritis 373
pneumothorax 363–364
polyradiculoneuritis 421
  neuropathic pain 33
porcupine quill injury 462–464
portosystemic shunt (PSS) 384–385
post-operative pain, non-steroidal anti-
  inflammatory analgesics (NSAIAs) 137
post-procedural analgesia, thorax 361
prednisone 160
pregabalin 156
  neck pain 354
  neuropathic pain 44
  pregnant patients 284
pregnant patients
  see also cesarean section
  analgesia 279–285

anesthesia   286–292

initial presentation   5

non-pharmacologic methods   285

non-steroidal anti-inflammatory analgesics
(NSAIAs)   282–285

opioids/opiates   281–282

physiological changes   279–281

pre-medication

cesarean section   289–290

environmental injuries   *456*

geriatric patients   332–333

nursing patients   303

pediatric patients   320

thorax   359

torso/abdomen   *378–379, 394*

pressure necrosis   447

prolapsed rectum   405–406

propofol   166, 249

cesarean section   290

environmental injuries   *456*

integument injuries   *442*

musculoskeletal pain   *412*

nursing patients   302

oral cavity and upper airway injury/
obstruction   343

pregnant patients   288

smoke inhalation   464

thoracic cavity injury   364, 369

torso/abdomen   *379*

proton pump inhibitors (PPIs), chronic kidney
disease (CKD)   140

PSS (portosystemic shunt)   384–385

PTE (pulmonary thromboemboli)   373–374

pudendal nerve entrapment, neuropathic pain
28–29

pulmonary edema   373

pulmonary thromboemboli (PTE)   373–374

Pulsed Electromagnetic Field (PEMF)
Therapy   213

pupillary dilation, pain assessment   72

pyometra/endometritis   405

pyrexia, non-steroidal anti-inflammatory
analgesics (NSAIAs)   138

q

quill injury, porcupine   462–464

r

radial block, local anesthetics   187

recovery from general anesthesia

nursing patients   304

pediatric patients   322–325

regimens, analgesic *see* analgesic regimens

regional analgesia, neuropathic pain   41

relative infant dose (RID)   294

remifentanil   128

renal disease *see* kidney disease

reproductive system   404–405

respiratory distress   461

respiratory effects, opioids/opiates   121

respiratory rate, pain assessment   71–72

reversal

benzodiazepines   118

dexmedetomidine   116

opioids/opiates   123

rib fractures/flail chest   362, *363*

rostral mandibular block, local anesthetics
179–180

rostral maxillary block, local anesthetics
176–178

s

salicylates (aspirin), nursing patients   299

saphenous block, local anesthetics   195–197

scales, pain assessment   75–78

sciatic block, local anesthetics   197

scrotum   59–60

sedation, initial presentation   5–6

sedatives   112–118

nursing patients   301

pediatric patients   316–317

pharmacologic and clinical application
112–118

routes of administration   112–113

thorax   358

selective serotonin reuptake inhibitors
(SSRIs)   157–160

adverse effects   157–158

mode of action   157

nursing patients   300

serotonin and norepinephrine re-uptake
inhibitor mixed compound, neuropathic
pain   45

sevoflurane, integument injuries   *442*

shearing   445–446

simple descriptive scales (SDS)   75–76, 87

sleep

initial presentation   6

nursing care plans   222–223

slow weaning, pain management   99

snake envenomation   461

sodium channel blockers, neuropathic
   pain   39–41

spasmolytics, torso/abdomen   394

sphincter tone effects, opioids/opiates   122

spinal cord injury
   discospondylitis   33
   fibrocartilaginous embolic myelopathy
      (FCEM)   33
   intervertebral disc herniation/extrusion
      (IVDH/E)   32
   neuropathic pain   32–33
   vascular innervation   33
   vertebral osteomyelitis   33
   visceral pain   60

spleen, abdominal pain   56

splenic torsion/neoplasia/hematoma   384

SSRIs *see* selective serotonin reuptake
   inhibitors

standardized concentration infusions,
   analgesics   235–236

stimulus-evoked/movement-evoked pain   15,
   68–69, 73

stress reduction, nursing care plans   221–222

sufentanil   128
   pregnant patients   281–282

surgical pain   74

syringe pump delivery, analgesics   237–239

syringomyelia   350–353

systolic hypertension, pain assessment   72

t

tachycardia   2

TCAs *see* tricyclic antidepressants

TCVM (traditional Chinese veterinary
   medicine)   205–207

telazol, environmental injuries   *457*

Telazol/Zoletil, torso/abdomen   *379*

TENS (Transcutaneous Electrical Nerve
   Stimulation)   212–213

teratogenicity, pregnant patients   287

testicular torsion   406

thermal burns   443–444

thirst/hunger, patient comfort   225, *226*

thoracic block
   epidural block   190
   intercostal block   188
   interpleural block   188–190
   local anesthetics   187–190

thoracic cavity illness   373–374

thoracic cavity injury   362–372
   anesthesia   368–369
   diaphragmatic hernia   371–372
   esophageal lesions/obstruction   370–371
   hemothorax   363
   initial management   362
   penetrating injury/foreign body/bite
      wounds   366–369
   physical examination   362
   pneumothorax   363–364
   rib fractures/flail chest   362, *363*
   thoracocentesis   363
   thoracotomy   365–366
   tracheobronchial injury/
      obstruction   369–370

thoracic limb block, local anesthetics   182–187

thoracocentesis   363

thoracotomy   365–366

thorax   356–374
   analgesia   357–358
   anesthesia   359–360
   discharge analgesia and management
      372–373
   nursing considerations   361
   post-procedural analgesia   361

thromboembolic (ischemic conditions)   420

tibial block, local anesthetics   197–198

tibial plateau levelling osteotomy (TPLO)   3

tiletamine   249

tiletamine-zolazepam   **276**

TIVA (total intravenous anesthesia),
   environmental injuries   *457*

tocainide, neuropathic pain   41

topical local anesthetic creams, pediatric
   patients   201–202, 317–318

torso/abdomen   375–390
   analgesia   377–380
   anesthesia   377–380
   discharge analgesia and management
      380, 394
   foreign body   384, 385, *386*
   ill patient   382–389
   injured patient   381–382
   nursing considerations   380
   sedation   377–380
   visceral pain   14–15, 60, 375–376

touch-evoked pain   73

TPLO (tibial plateau levelling osteotomy)   3

tracheobronchial injury/obstruction 369–370
traditional Chinese veterinary medicine
    (TCVM) 205–207
tramadol 131–132
    adverse effects 131
    neuropathic pain 37–38
    nursing patients 298
Transcutaneous Electrical Nerve Stimulation
    (TENS) 212–213
transduction
    pathologic pain 12–13
    physiologic pain 10
transmission
    pathologic pain 13
    physiologic pain 10
trauma, non-steroidal anti-inflammatory
    analgesics (NSAIAs) 137
trauma effect, geriatric patients 329
trazodone **274**
tricyclic antidepressants (TCAs) 157–160
    adverse effects 157–158
    mode of action 157
    neuropathic pain 22, 44
TRPV1 (vanilloid receptor 1) antagonists,
    neuropathic pain 45
tumours, central nervous system 34–35

u
ulnar block, local anesthetics 187
UNESP-Botucatu, pain scale 76
University of Melbourne Pain Scale 76, 88
ureter cats and dogs 401–403
urethral obstruction 405–407
urinary retention, opioids/opiates 123
urinary tract injuries 396–397
urination/defecation
    geriatric patients 334
    patient comfort 224–225
urine scald 447–448
urogenital system, abdominal pain 57–59
urologic illness 401–404
uterine and vaginal prolapse/uterine inguinal
    hernia 407
uterine injuries 398–399
uterine torsion 404–405

v
vanilloid receptor 1 (TRPV1) antagonists,
    neuropathic pain 45

vascular innervation, neuropathic pain 33
vasculitis, neuropathic pain 35
venlafaxine
    adverse effects 159
    neuropathic pain 45
verbal rating scales (VRS) 75–76
vertebral column 423–437
    analgesia 423–425
    anesthesia 426–428
    arteritis 437
    central pain syndrome 437
    coccygeal vertebrae amputation
        433, *434*
    congenital/developmental lesions 437
    discharge analgesia and
        management 425–426
    disc herniation management 431–434
    discospondylitis 436
    fibrocartilaginous embolic myelopathy
        (FCEM) 433
    hemodynamically stable/unstable
        patients *427–428*
    illness 434–437
    lumbosacral lesions 436
    meningitis 35, 350–353, 437
    neoplasia 437
    nursing care 428–431
    polyradiculoneuritis 436
    sedatives 425
    vasculitis 437
    vertebral osteomyelitis 436
    visceral pain 60
vertebral osteomyelitis, neuropathic
    pain 33
veterinary technician or nurse (VT/N)
    see also nursing…
    nursing care plans 219–228
    role 217–218
visceral nociception, modulatory
    influences 60–62
visceral pain 14–15, 375–376
    illness-associated 389
    pelvis 60
    spinal cord injury 60
    vertebral and spinal cord injury 60
visual analogue scale (VAS) 75–76, 87
vomiting, opioids/opiates 122
VT/N *see* veterinary technician or nurse
vulva 60, 400, *440*

W
warm therapy 211–212
wound diffusion catheters, thorax 361
wound infusion catheter block, local
    anesthetics 200–201, 414
wound management 415
  local anesthetics 200–201

X
xylazine, nursing patients 302

Z
Zoletil/Telazol, torso/abdomen *379*

Printed and bound by CPI Group (UK) Ltd, Croydon, CR0 4YY

16/04/2025

14658464-0004